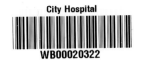

MUSCULOSKELETAL
ASSESSMENT

Joint Motion and Muscle Testing

Third Edition

Hazel M. Clarkson, M.A., B.P.T.

Formerly Assistant Professor, Department of Physical Therapy, Faculty of Rehabilitation Medicine, University of Alberta, Edmonton, Alberta, Canada

Wolters Kluwer | Lippincott Williams & Wilkins
Health

Philadelphia • Baltimore • New York • London
Buenos Aires • Hong Kong • Sydney • Tokyo

Acquisitions Editor: Emily Lupash
Product Manager: Meredith L. Brittain
Interior Design: Terry Mallon
Compositor: Aptara, Inc.
Photography: Jacques Hurabielle, P.P.O.C., Ph.D., Sandra Bruinsma, and Thomas Turner
Illustrations: Heather K. Doy, B.A., B.F.A., Joy D. Marlowe, M.A., C.M.I., and Kimberly Battista, M.A., B.A.

Copyright © 2013, 2000, 1989 by LIPPINCOTT WILLIAMS & WILKINS | a WOLTERS KLUWER business
Two Commerce Square
2001 Market Street
Philadelphia, PA 19103 USA
LWW.com

Printed in China

Not authorized for sale in United States, Canada, Australia and New Zealand.

Library of Congress Cataloging-in-Publication Data
Clarkson, Hazel M.
    Musculoskeletal assessment : joint motion and muscle testing / Hazel M. Clarkson. – 3rd ed.
        p. ; cm.
    Includes bibliographical references and index.
    ISBN 978-1-4511-7571-4 (alk. paper)
    I. Title.
    [DNLM: 1. Musculoskeletal Diseases–diagnosis.   2. Musculoskeletal Physiological Phenomena.   3. Musculoskeletal System–anatomy & histology.   4. Physical Examination–methods. WE 141]
    616.7'2075–dc23
                                            2011040088

To purchase additional copies of this book, call our customer service department at (800) 638-3030 or fax orders to (301) 223-2320. International customers should call (301) 223-2300.

Visit Lippincott Williams & Wilkins on the Internet: at LWW.com. Lippincott Williams & Wilkins customer service representatives are available from 8:30 am to 6:00 pm, EST.

10 9 8 7 6 5 4 3 2

Dedicated to my parents,
Dr. and Mrs. Graham and
June Clarkson,
who have so generously given so
much of themselves for so many in
such a quiet way

Preface

I am delighted to introduce the third edition of *Musculoskeletal Assessment: Joint Motion and Muscle Testing*. This edition continues the quest to convey new information, methodology, experience, and wisdom to students and professionals alike. New approaches that facilitate learning elevate the existing status of this title as an important educational tool and clinical resource. The third edition is updated to include the latest research findings and assessment techniques.

New to This Edition

Some of the more significant additions to the third edition include the following.

Practical testing forms for the assessment and measurement of joint range of motion (ROM), muscle length, and assessment of muscle strength are found on this book's companion website at http://thepoint.lww.com/Clarkson3e. These forms list the criteria for each assessment and measurement technique in a chart/checklist format. Judging from my teaching experience, these forms will be an invaluable tool for students to become proficient in the clinical assessment and measurement techniques, allow for evaluation of student proficiency, and serve as a handy review. **Practice Makes Perfect** icons appear next to clinical assessment and measurement techniques throughout the textbook to cross-reference the corresponding online practical testing forms. (For information on other ancillary materials available with this text, see section on "Additional Resources" in this preface.)

Further noteworthy additions to the third edition include more in-depth reviews of articulations, arthrokinematics, the SFTR method, and illustration of normal and reverse scapulohumeral rhythm resulting from restricted glenohumeral joint ROM. Normal ranges of motion are now emphasized in red font in the text. New techniques are described and illustrated to measure active range of motion (AROM) of the temporomandibular joint (TMJ) using the ruler and calipers, and the spine using the tape measure, standard inclinometers, the Cervical Range-of-Motion Instrument (CROM), and the universal goniometer. For the assessment and measurement of muscle length, muscle origins and insertions are included with each procedure. A more concise description of grading muscle strength is presented. A new chart of patient positioning for the assessment and measurement of joint ROM, muscle length, and muscle strength is added as Appendix C.

Many new photographs and illustrations augment the written text. Of special note are unique illustrations of the measurement of joint passive range of motion (PROM) showing the universal goniometer and therapist's hand positions in relation to the deep anatomy, and those of the noncontractile normal limiting factors (NLF) that limit movement. Illustrations of the deep bony anatomy that accompany the photographs of surface anatomy are also new.

Need for This Textbook

Assessment of joint ROM and muscle strength are important clinical skills in the practice of physical and occupational therapy. These evaluations form two component parts of the physical assessment of a patient with a musculoskeletal disorder. This book has evolved in response to a need for a comprehensive textbook that contains the principles and methodology of joint ROM and manual muscle strength evaluation in one volume. The content is written on the assumption that the student possesses prerequisite knowledge of the anatomy of the musculoskeletal system.

Organizational Philosophy and Use of Visual Material

Section I: Principles and Methods (Chapters 1 and 2)

Chapter 1 of this volume focuses on the principles and methodology of evaluation. The overview of the principles and methods provided here contains knowledge prerequisite for the remaining chapters.

Chapter 2 (Chapter 9 in the previous edition) of this volume illustrates how specific assessment methods are utilized and adapted to serve as treatment methods. Using description and illustration, the principles and methodology of joint ROM, muscle length, and manual muscle strength evaluation are shown to be the same as those used for selected treatment techniques. The content of this chapter relates directly to the principles and methodology presented in Chapter 1. This unique presentation blends the topics of assessment and treatment to facilitate learning and application of these skills as practiced clinically.

Section II: Regional Evaluation Techniques (Chapters 3 through 9)

Chapters 3 through 9 focus on the specific methodology of ROM and muscle strength evaluation of the extremities, head, neck, and trunk. Each of these chapters is devoted to a specific joint complex, and all are organized in an identical format.

Articulations and Movements

Each chapter begins with a review of the articulations, shapes of the articular surfaces, joint movements, and axes of movement pertaining to the specific joint complex. A summary of joint structure, movements, and NLF to joint movements are presented in tabular form. This table provides reference information pertinent to assessment, measurement, and interpretation of findings. Line drawings accompany the table to enable the reader to visualize the noncontractile NLF that normally limit joint motion.

Surface Anatomy

Through illustration and description, the pertinent landmarks for the assessment of joint ROM and muscle strength are identified. Muscles are excluded from this description, as precise points of palpation are presented in the description of each muscle test later in the chapter.

Range of Motion Assessment and Measurement

Following the surface anatomy is the methodology for assessing and measuring each movement at the particular joint complex. In some chapters, AROM scans used to guide the need for subsequent assessment procedures are described and illustrated.

A consistent method of assessing and measuring joint ROM is essential for accurate assessment of a patient's present status, progress, and effectiveness of the treatment program. Learning is promoted through consistency in documentation and illustration of methods.

The assessments of ROM are described under the main headings of joint movements. In *Chapters 3 through 8*, the description of the assessment and measurement of the ROM normally begins with a reminder to assess the AROM and identifies the substitute movements to be avoided, when applicable. For a select few peripheral joint movements, the measurement of the AROM is also described and illustrated.

For the joints of the extremities, description and illustration of the assessment of PROM that includes determination of the end feel is followed by description and illustration of the measurement of PROM using the universal goniometer and in some cases the OB "Myrin" goniometer.

Chapter 9 (Chapter 2 in the previous edition) covers the assessment and measurement of AROM for the TMJ and spine. This chapter is extensively revised to describe and illustrate many new measurement techniques using the ruler and calipers to measure AROM of the TMJ, and the tape measure, standard inclinometers, CROM, and universal goniometer to measure spinal AROM.

Muscle Length Assessment and Measurement

Following the assessment and measurement of joint ROM, assessment and measurement of muscle length is described and illustrated under the main headings of the muscle(s) being assessed.

Muscle Strength Assessment

The next section of the chapter focuses on manual muscle strength assessment. The section begins with a review of the relevant anatomy of the region, including muscle actions, attachments, and nerve supply.

In each chapter, the muscle strength tests are described under the main headings of joint movements. The prime mover(s) and accessory muscle(s) are identified. Through illustration and description, the against gravity tests are presented, followed by the gravity eliminated tests. The sequence is consistent for each movement.

For each muscle strength test, the first against gravity photograph illustrates the start position and stabilization. The next photograph illustrates the patient's position at the end of the ROM and the best point for muscle palpation. The resistance test follows with a photograph of the therapist applying manual resistance. An illustration of the muscle being tested and the location of the therapist's hand relative to deep anatomical structures when applying resistance accompanies the resistance photograph. The illustration also provides a visual review of muscle attachments and direction of muscle fibers to assist the student in visualizing the deep structures.

The first gravity eliminated test photograph illustrates the start position and stabilization. A second photograph illustrates the end position for the gravity eliminated test and the best point for palpation of the muscle(s) being assessed.

Normally, the assessment or measurement procedures for joint ROM and muscle strength first give the optimal start position that could be used to perform the procedures based on the position that offers the best stabilization. In some instances, there may be more than one position that could be used to assess or measure the joint ROM or assess the muscle strength. These positions are termed alternate positions and are documented if they are common in clinical practice or if the preferred start position is impractical or contraindicated for some patients.

Functional Application

The final section of each chapter is devoted to the functional application of assessment. The specific function of the joint complex is described. The functional ROM at the joint is documented. Emphasis is placed on those ranges required for performance of daily activities. The function of the muscles is described according to biomechanical principles and daily activities. Assessments of joint ROM and muscle strength are not performed in isolation of function. Through knowledge of the ROM and muscle function required in daily activities, the therapist can elicit meaningful information from the assessments. The therapist correlates the assessment findings with the patient's ability to perform daily activities and, in conjunction with other physical assessment measures, determines an appropriate treatment plan to restore or maintain function.

Section III: Appendices

Appendices A and B present sample recording forms for ROM Assessment and Measurement, and Manual Muscle Strength Assessment, respectively. A new chart of patient positioning for the assessment and measurement of joint ROM, muscle length, and muscle strength has been added as Appendix C. Appendix D describes joint positions and motions of the lower limb throughout the gait cycle.

Additional Resources

Musculoskeletal Assessment: Joint Motion and Muscle Testing, Third Edition, includes additional resources for both students and instructors that are available on the book's companion website at http://thepoint.lww.com/Clarkson3e.

Students

Students who have purchased *Musculoskeletal Assessment: Joint Motion and Muscle Testing*, Third Edition, have access to the following additional resources:

- **Practical testing forms** (mentioned earlier in this preface) for the assessment and measurement of joint ROM, muscle length, and assessment of muscle strength; these forms list the criteria for each assessment and measurement technique in a chart/checklist format.
- **Video clips** illustrating assessment techniques

Instructors

Approved adopting instructors will be given access to the following additional resources:

- An image bank containing all the images and tables in the book
- A WebCT and Blackboard Ready Cartridge

In addition, purchasers of the text can access the searchable Full Text Online by going to the *Musculoskeletal Assessment: Joint Motion and Muscle Testing*, Third Edition, website at http://thePoint.lww.com/Clarkson3e. See the inside front cover of this text for more details, including the passcode you will need to gain access to the website.

A Final Note

It is my hope this textbook continues to serve as a valuable resource in the classroom, laboratory, and clinical environments to promote a high level of standardization and proficiency in the clinical evaluation of joint ROM and muscle strength.

Hazel M. Clarkson

Acknowledgments

The development and success of each new edition of *Musculoskeletal Assessment: Joint Motion and Muscle Testing* has come about because of the efforts of many people. I want to again thank all who worked with me to produce the first and second editions of this textbook. These editions served as the beginning to the third edition. I am now pleased to be able to thank those who assisted me with the production of the third edition.

I am most grateful for the unconditional support and encouragement I received from my family once again, as "we" took on yet another edition! A great many thanks to my husband Hans Longerich, parents Graham and June Clarkson, and brother Ronald Clarkson, who have given unselfishly of their time and expertise to edit the text, assist to manage photography sessions, serve as models for photographs and illustrations, and for always being there. It was always a great support for me to know you were there to help whenever needed.

I thank my clinical and academic colleagues who provided helpful reviews of my work and so generously shared their experience and expertise. A special thanks to Bob Haennel, Chairman, Department of Physical Therapy, Faculty of Rehabilitation Medicine, University of Alberta, for his support.

A special thanks to my good friend and colleague, Liza Chan, for giving so generously her time and expertise to assist with literature searches and the organization of research materials. Jess Chan, thank you for your assistance with collecting reference materials.

To my photographer for this edition, Thomas Turner, thank you for producing such high quality photographs. It was a pleasure to work with you. Ron Clarkson, my model, thanks for serving in this role again. I thank you for your thoughtfulness as you went above and beyond your modeling role.

To my artist, Kim Battista; it was a pleasure to work with you to create the new line art for this third edition.

Last but not least, I wish to extend my thanks to the entire Lippincott Williams & Wilkins team, and in particular to Meredith Brittain for having been such a dedicated team leader—thanks for your helpful suggestions and patience throughout the process.

Reviewers

Denise Donica, PhD
Assistant Professor
Occupational Therapy
East Carolina University
Greenville, North Carolina

Carol Fawcett, PTA, MEd
PTA Program Director
PTA Department
Fox College
Tinley Park, Illinois

Bradley Michael Kruse, DPT, OCS, SCS, Cert. MDT, ATC, CSCS
Instructor
Physical Therapy
Clarke College
Dubuque, Iowa

Clare Lewis, BSPT, MSPT, MPH, PsyD
Associate Professor
Physical Therapy
California State University, Sacramento
Sacramento, California

Lee N. Marinko, PT, ScD, OCS, FAAOMPT
Clinical Assistant Professor
Department of Physical Therapy and Athletic Training
Boston University
Boston, Massachusetts

Jennifer McDonald, PT, DPT, MS
Associate Professor
PTA
SUNY Canton
Canton, New York

Cindy Meyer, OTA-AAS, OT-BS, MS
COTA retired, OTR, Associate Professor,
    Academic Fieldwork Coordinator
OTA Program
South Arkansas Community College
El Dorado, Arkansas

Shannon Petersen, DScPT, OCS, COMT
Assistant Professor of Physical Therapy
Physical Therapy
Des Moines University
Des Moines, Iowa

Hamdy Radwan, PhD
Professor of Physical Therapy
Physical Therapy
Winston Salem State University
Winston Salem, North Carolina

S. Juanita Robel, MHS
Associate Professor
Doctor of Physical Therapy Program
Des Moines University
Des Moines, Iowa

Susan Rogers, MOT
Assistant Professor
Allied Health/ Occupational Therapy
Tuskegee University
Tuskegee, Alabama

Theresa Schlabach, PhD
Dr. OTR/L Board Certified in Pediatrics
Master of Occupational Therapy
St. Ambrose University
Davenport, Iowa

Susan Shore, PhD
Professor
Physical Therapy
Azusa Pacific University
Azusa, California

Contents

SECTION I
Principles and Methods

Chapter 1:
Principles and Methods

Chapter 2:
Relating Assessment to Treatment

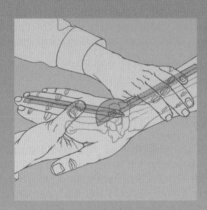

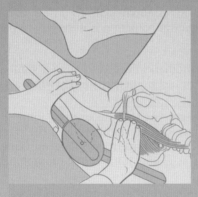

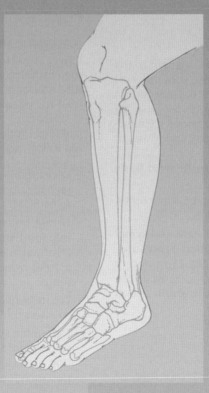

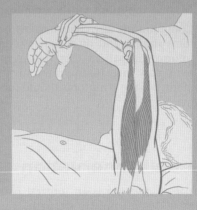

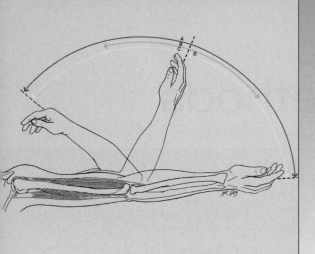

Chapter 1

Principles and Methods

A fundamental requisite to the study of evaluation of joint range of motion (ROM) and muscle strength is the knowledge of evaluation principles and methodology. This chapter discusses the factors pertinent to the evaluation of ROM and strength. A firm foundation in the principles, methods, and associated terminology presented in this chapter is necessary knowledge for the specific techniques presented in subsequent chapters.

Communication

When conducting a physical assessment, explain to the patient the rationale for performing the physical assessment and the component parts of the assessment process as these are carried out. Speak slowly, use lay terms, provide concise and easily understood explanations, and encourage the patient to ask questions at any time.

It is essential the patient understands the need to do the following:

1. Expose specific regions of the body and assume different body positions for the examination.
2. Communicate any change in his/her signs and symptoms during and after the examination procedures. Inform the patient that he/she might experience a temporary increase in symptoms following an assessment, but the symptoms should subside within a short period.

Visual Observation

Visual observation is an integral part of assessment of joint ROM and muscle strength. The body part being assessed should be adequately exposed for visual inspection. Throughout the initial assessment of the patient, the therapist gathers visual information that contributes to formulating an appropriate assessment plan and determining the patient's problems. Information gained from visual observation includes such factors as facial expression, symmetrical or compensatory motion in functional activities, body posture, muscle contours, body proportions, and color, condition, and creases of the skin.

Palpation

Palpation is the examination of the body surface by touch. Palpation is performed to assess bony and soft tissue contours, soft tissue consistency, and skin temperature and texture. Visual observation and palpation are used to "visualize" the deep anatomy.[1]

Palpation is an essential skill to assess and treat patients. Proficiency at palpation is necessary to perform the following:

- Locate bony landmarks needed to align a goniometer, tape measure, or inclinometer correctly when assessing joint ROM.
- Locate bony segments that make up a joint so that one joint surface can be stabilized and the opposing joint surface can be moved to isolate movement at a joint when assessing joint ROM or mobilizing a joint.
- Locate bony landmarks that are used as reference points to assess limb or trunk circumference.
- Determine the presence or absence of muscle contraction when assessing strength or conducting reeducation exercises.
- Identify bony or soft tissue irregularities.
- Localize structures that require direct treatment.

Proficiency at palpation is gained through practice and experience. Practice palpation on as many subjects as possible to become familiar with individual variations in human anatomy.

Palpation Technique

- Ensure the patient is made comfortable and kept warm, and the body or body part is well supported to relax the muscles. This allows palpation of deep or inert (noncontractile) structures such as ligaments and bursae.
- Visually observe the area to be palpated and note any deformity or abnormality.
- Palpate with the pads of the index and middle fingers. Keep fingernails short.
- Place fingers in direct contact with the skin. Palpation should not be attempted through clothing.
- Use a sensitive but firm touch to instill a feeling of security. Prodding is uncomfortable and may elicit tension in the muscles that can make it difficult to palpate deep structures.
- Instruct the patient to contract a muscle isometrically against resistance and then relax the muscle to palpate muscle(s) and tendon(s). Palpate the muscle or tendon during contraction and relaxation.
- Place the tips of the index and middle fingers across the long axis of the tendon and gently roll forward and backward across the tendon to palpate a tendon.

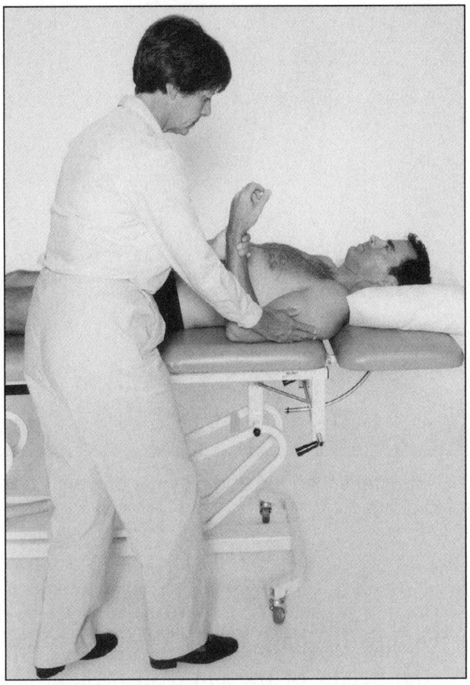

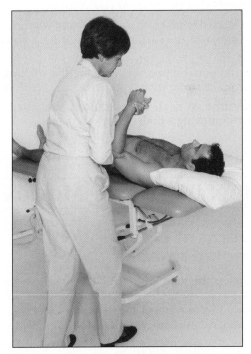

Figure 1-1 Therapist's stance when performing movements parallel to the side of the plinth.

Therapist Posture

Apply biomechanical principles of posture and lifting when performing assessment techniques. Therapist posture and support of the patient's limb are described.

Posture

Stand with your head and trunk upright, feet shoulder width apart, and knees slightly flexed. With one foot ahead of the other, the stance is in the line of the direction of movement. *Maintain a broad base of support* to attain balance and allow effective weight-shifting from one leg to the other. When performing movements that are:

- Parallel to the side of the plinth, stand beside the plinth with the leg furthest from the plinth ahead of the other leg (Fig. 1-1).
- Perpendicular to the side of the plinth, face the plinth with one foot slightly in front of the other (Fig. 1-2).
- Diagonal movements, adopt a stance that is in line with the diagonal movement with one foot slightly ahead of the other.

Protect your lumbar spine by assuming a neutral lordotic posture (the exact posture varying based on comfort and practicality) and avoiding extreme spinal flexion or extension.[2] Gain additional protection by the following:

- Keeping as close to the patient as possible.
- Avoiding spinal rotation by moving the feet to turn.

Figure 1-2 Therapist's stance when performing movements perpendicular to the side of the plinth.

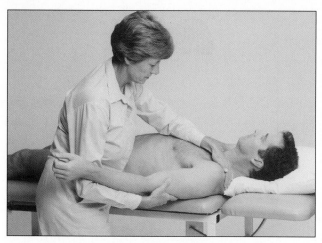

Figure 1-3 The limb supported at the center of gravity using a relaxed hand grasp.

- Using your leg muscles to perform the work by flexing and extending the joints of the lower extremity.

Adjust the height of the plinth to assume a neutral lordotic posture, keep close to the patient, and avoid fatigue.

Supporting the Patient's Limb

To move a limb or limb segment easily, perform the following:

- Support the part at the level of its center of gravity, located approximately at the junction of the upper and middle third of the segment (Fig. 1-3)[3].
- Use a relaxed hand grasp, with the hand conforming to the contour of the part, to support or lift a body part (Fig. 1-3)[3].
- Give additional support by cradling the part with the forearm.
- Ensure that all joints are adequately supported when lifting or moving a limb or limb segment.

JOINT RANGE OF MOTION

Movement Description: Osteokinematics

Kinematics is the term given to the study of movement.[4] *Osteokinematics* is the study of the movement of the bone in space.[4] The movement of the bone is assessed, measured, and recorded to represent the joint ROM. *Joint ROM* is the amount of movement that occurs at a joint to produce movement of a bone in space. To perform *active range of motion (AROM),* the patient contracts muscle to voluntarily move the body part through the ROM without assistance. To perform *passive range of motion (PROM),* the therapist or another external force moves the body part through the ROM.

A sound knowledge of anatomy is required to assess the ROM at a joint. This includes knowledge of joint articulations, motions, and normal limiting factors. These topics are discussed separately.

Joint Articulations and Classification

An *anatomical joint* or *articulation* is formed when two bony articular surfaces, lined by hyaline cartilage, meet[5] and movement is allowed to occur at the junction. The movements that occur at a joint are partly determined by the shape of the articular surfaces. Anatomical articulations are classified as described and illustrated in Table 1-1 (Figs. 1-4 to 1-10).

In addition to classifying a joint according to the anatomical relationship of the articular surfaces, a joint may also be classified as a syndesmosis or a physiological or functional joint. A *syndesmosis* is a joint in which the opposing bone surfaces are relatively far apart and joined together by ligaments (Fig. 1-11).[7] Movement is possible around one axis. A *physiological*[5] or *functional*[8] joint consists of two surfaces, muscle and bone (scapulothoracic joint) or muscle, bursa, and bone (subdeltoid joint), moving one with respect to the other (Fig. 1-12).

Movements: Planes and Axes

Joint movements are more easily described and understood using a coordinate system (Fig. 1-13) that has its central point located just anterior to the second sacral vertebra, with the subject standing in the anatomical position. The *anatomical position* is illustrated in Figures 1-14 through 1-16. The "start" positions for assessing ranges of movement described in this text are understood to be the anatomical position of the joint, unless otherwise indicated.

The coordinate system consists of three imaginary cardinal planes and axes (Fig. 1-13). This same coordinate system can be transposed so that its central point is located at the center of any joint in the body. Movement in, or parallel to, the cardinal planes occurs around the axis that lies perpendicular to the plane of movement. Table 1-2 describes the planes and axes of the body. Many functional movements occur in diagonal planes located between the cardinal planes.

TABLE 1-1 Classification of Anatomical Articulations[6]

Ball-and-socket (spheroidal)

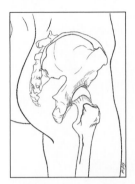

Figure 1-4 Ball-and-socket articulation (hip joint). A ball-shaped surface articulates with a cup-shaped surface; movement is possible around innumerable axes.

Hinge (ginglymus)

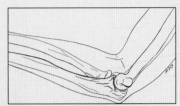

Figure 1-5 Hinge articulation (humeroulnar joint). Two articular surfaces that restrict movement largely to one axis; usually have strong collateral ligaments.

Plane

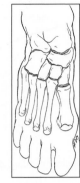

Figure 1-6 Plane articulation (intertarsal joints). This articulation is formed by the apposition of two relatively flat surfaces; gliding movements occur at these joints.

Ellipsoidal

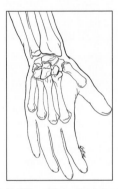

Figure 1-7 Ellipsoidal articulation (radiocarpal joint). This articulation is formed by an oval convex surface in apposition with an elliptical concave surface; movement is possible around two axes.

Saddle (sellar)

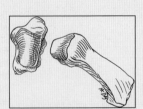

Figure 1-8 Saddle articulation (first carpometacarpal joint). Each joint surface has a convexity at right angles to a concave surface; movement is possible around two axes.

Bicondylar

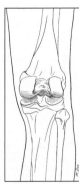

Figure 1-9 Bicondylar articulations (femorotibial joint). Formed by one surface having two convex condyles, the corresponding surface having two concave reciprocal surfaces; most movement occurs around one axis; some degree of rotation is also possible around an axis set at 90° to the first.

Pivot (trochoid)

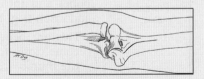

Figure 1-10 Pivot articulation (superior radioulnar joint). Formed by a central bony pivot surrounded by an osteoligamentous ring; movement is restricted to rotation.

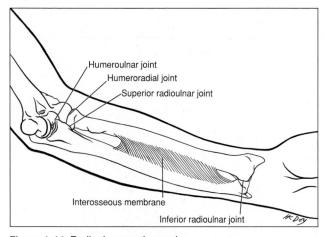

Figure 1-11 Radioulnar syndesmosis.

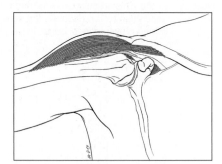

Figure 1-12 Physiological or functional joint (subdeltoid joint).

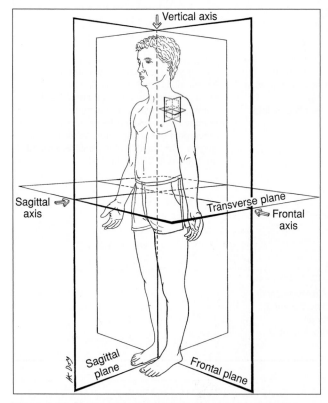

Figure 1-13 Planes and axes illustrated in anatomical position.

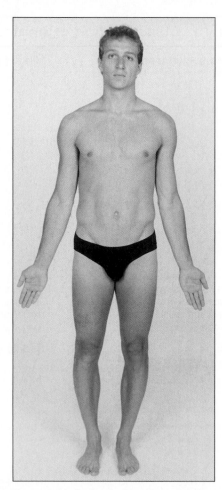

Figure 1-14 Anatomical position—anterior view. The individual is standing erect with the arms by the sides, toes, palms of the hand, and eyes facing forward and fingers extended.

Movement Terminology

Angular Movements

Angular motions refer to movements that produce an increase or a decrease in the angle between the adjacent bones and include flexion, extension, abduction, and adduction (Fig. 1-17).[6]

Flexion: bending of a part so the anterior surfaces come closer together. *Special considerations:* Flexion of the thumb—the thumb moves across the palm of the hand. Knee and toe flexion—the posterior or plantar surfaces of the body parts, respectively, come closer together. Ankle flexion—when the dorsal surface of the foot is brought closer to the anterior aspect of the leg, the movement is termed *dorsiflexion*. Lateral flexion of the neck and trunk—bending movements that occur in a lateral direction either to the right or left side.

Extension: the straightening of a part and movement is in the opposite direction to flexion movements. *Special*

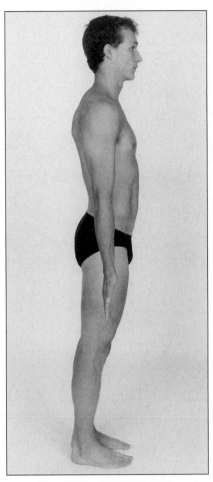

Figure 1-15 Anatomical position—lateral view.

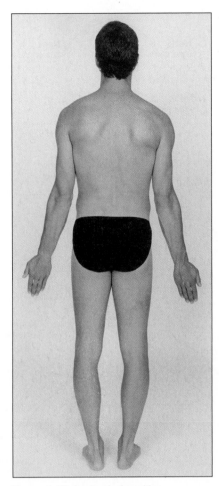

Figure 1-16 Anatomical position— posterior view.

consideration: Ankle extension—when the plantar aspect of the foot is extended toward the posterior aspect of the leg, the movement is termed *plantarflexion.*

Hyperextension: movement that goes beyond the normal anatomical joint position of extension.

Abduction: movement away from the midline of the body or body part. The midline of the hand passes through the third digit, and the midline of the foot passes through the second digit. *Special considerations:* Abduction of the scapula is referred to as *protraction* and is movement of the vertebral border of the scapula away from the vertebral column. Abduction of the thumb—the thumb moves in an anterior direction in a plane perpendicular to the palm of the hand. Abduction

TABLE 1-2	Planes and Axes of the Body			
Plane	**Description of Plane**	**Axis of Rotation**	**Description of Axis**	**Most Common Movement**
Frontal (coronal)	Divides body into anterior and posterior sections	Sagittal	Runs anterior/ posterior	Abduction, adduction
Sagittal	Divides body into right and left sections	Frontal (transverse)	Runs medial/lateral	Flexion, extension
Transverse (horizontal)	Divides body into upper and lower sections	Longitudinal (vertical)	Runs superior/ inferior	Internal rotation, external rotation

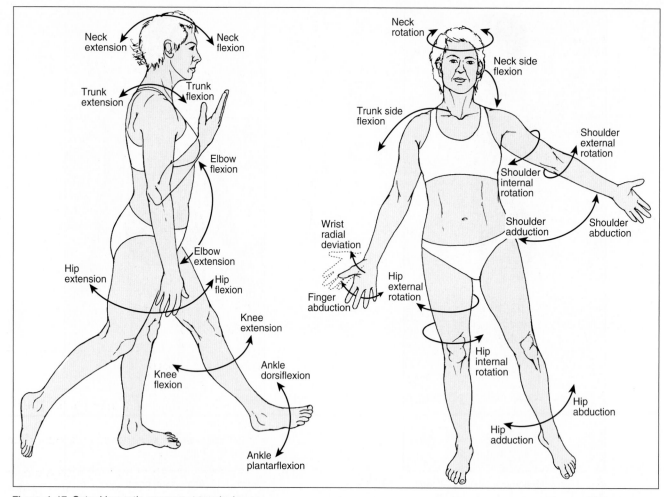

Figure 1-17 Osteokinematic movement terminology.

of the wrist is referred to as *wrist radial deviation.* Eversion of the foot—the sole of the foot is turned outward; it is not a pure abduction movement because it includes abduction and pronation of the forefoot.

Adduction: movement toward the midline of the body or body part. *Special considerations:* Adduction of the scapula, referred to as *retraction,* is movement of the vertebral border of the scapula toward the vertebral column. Adduction of the thumb—the thumb moves back to anatomical position from a position of abduction. Adduction of the wrist is referred to as *wrist ulnar deviation.* Inversion of the foot—the sole of the foot is turned inward; it is not a pure adduction movement because it includes adduction and supination of the forefoot.

Shoulder elevation: movement of the arm above shoulder level (i.e., 90°) to a vertical position alongside the head (i.e., 180°). The vertical position may be arrived at by moving the arm through either the sagittal plane (i.e., shoulder flexion) or the frontal plane (i.e., shoulder abduction), and the movement is referred to as *shoulder elevation through flexion* or *shoulder elevation through abduction,* respectively. In the clinical setting,

these movements may simply be referred to as *shoulder flexion* and *shoulder abduction.*

The plane of the scapula lies 30° to 45° anterior to the frontal plane,[9] and this is the plane of reference for diagonal movements of shoulder elevation. *Scaption*[10] is the term given to this midplane elevation (Fig. 1-18).

Rotation Movements

These movements generally occur around a longitudinal or vertical axis.

Internal (medial, inward) rotation: turning of the anterior surface of a part toward the midline of the body (Fig. 1-17). *Special consideration:* Internal rotation of the forearm is referred to as *pronation.*

External (lateral, outward) rotation: turning of the anterior surface of a part away from the midline of the body (Fig. 1-17).

Special consideration: External rotation of the forearm is referred to as *supination.*

Neck or trunk rotation: turning around a vertical axis to either the right or left side (Fig. 1-17).

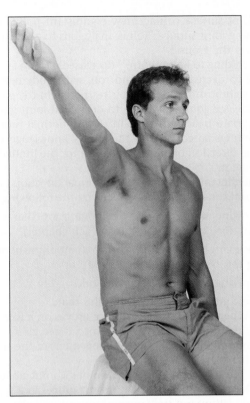

Figure 1-18 Shoulder elevation: plane of the scapula.

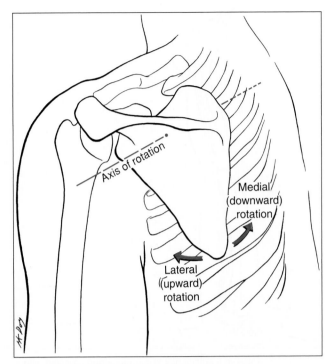

Figure 1-19 Rotation of the scapula.

Scapular rotation: described in terms of the direction of movement of either the inferior angle of the scapula or the glenoid cavity of the scapula (Fig. 1-19).

Medial (downward) rotation of the scapula—movement of the inferior angle of the scapula toward the midline and movement of the glenoid cavity in a caudal or downward direction.

Lateral (upward) rotation of the scapula—movement of the inferior angle of the scapula away from the midline and movement of the glenoid cavity in a cranial or upward direction.

Circumduction: a combination of the movements of flexion, extension, abduction, and adduction.

Opposition of the thumb and little finger: the tips of the thumb and little finger come together.

Reposition of the thumb and little finger: the thumb and little finger return to anatomical position from a position of opposition.

Horizontal abduction (extension): occurs at the shoulder and hip joints. With the shoulder joint in 90° of either abduction or flexion, or the hip joint in 90° flexion, the arm or the thigh, respectively, is moved in a direction either away from the midline of the body or in a posterior direction.

Horizontal adduction (flexion): occurs at the shoulder and hip joints. With the shoulder joint in 90° of either abduction or flexion, or the hip joint in 90° flexion, the arm or the thigh, respectively, is moved in a direction either toward the midline of the body or in an anterior direction.

Tilt: describes movement of either the scapula or the pelvis.

Anterior tilt of the scapula—"the coracoid process moves in an anterior and caudal direction while the inferior angle moves in a posterior and cranial direction,"[11(p. 303)]

Posterior tilt of the scapula—the coracoid process moves in a posterior and cranial direction while the inferior angle of the scapula moves in an anterior and caudal direction.

Anterior pelvic tilt—the anterior superior iliac spines of the pelvis move in an anterior and caudal direction.

Posterior pelvic tilt—the anterior superior iliac spines of the pelvis move in a posterior and cranial direction.

Lateral pelvic tilt—movement of the ipsilateral iliac crest in the frontal plane either in a cranial direction (elevation or hiking of the pelvis) or in a caudal direction (pelvic drop).

Shoulder girdle elevation: movement of the scapula and lateral end of the clavicle in a cranial direction.

Shoulder girdle depression: movement of the scapula and lateral end of the clavicle in a caudal direction.

Hypermobility: an excessive amount of movement; joint ROM that is greater than the normal ROM expected at the joint.

Hypomobility: a reduced amount of movement; joint ROM that is less than the normal ROM expected at the joint.

Passive insufficiency of a muscle occurs when the length of a muscle prevents full ROM at the joint or joints that the muscle crosses over (Fig. 1-20).[12]

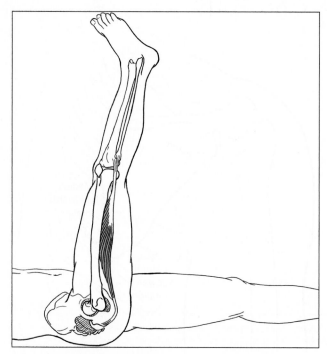

Figure 1-20 Passive insufficiency of the hamstring muscles. Hip flexion range of motion (ROM) is limited by the length of the hamstring muscles when the knee joint is held in extension.

Movement Description: Arthrokinematics

The study of movement occurring within the joints, between the articular surfaces of the bones, is called *arthrokinematics*.[4] Arthrokinematic motion can be indirectly observed and determined when assessing active and passive joint ROM by knowing the shape of the articular surfaces and observing the direction of movement of the bone.

Joints are classified on the basis of the general form of the joint (see Table 1-1). Regardless of the joint classification, the shape of all articular surfaces of synovial joints is, to varying degrees, either concave or convex, even for articulations classified as plane.[4] All joint surfaces are either concave or convex in all directions, as in the hip joint (see Fig. 1-4) (i.e., the acetabulum is concave and the head of the femur is convex), or sellar (i.e., saddle-shaped). The saddle-shaped surface has a convexity at right angles to a concave surface, as in the first carpometacarpal joint (i.e., formed by the distal surface of the trapezium and base of the first metacarpal) (see Fig. 1-8). At all joints, concave articular surfaces mate with corresponding convex surfaces.

When movement occurs at a joint, two types of articular motion—glide (i.e., slide) and roll—are present.[4] Both glide and roll occur together in varying proportions to allow normal joint motion. *Glide* is a translatory motion that occurs when a point on one joint surface contacts new points on the opposing surface. Glide at a joint is analogous to a car tire sliding over an icy surface when the brakes are applied. *Roll* occurs when new points on

one joint surface contact new equidistant points on an opposing joint surface. Roll is analogous to a car tire rolling over the ground.

According to Kaltenborn,[13] decreased motion at a joint is due to decreased glide and roll, with glide being the more significant motion that is restricted. In the presence of decreased joint ROM due to decreased joint glide, an appropriate treatment plan to restore normal motion is determined based on the therapist's knowledge of the normal direction of glide at the joint for the limited joint movement.

The therapist determines the normal direction of glide at a joint for a specific movement by the following:

1. Knowing the shape of the moving articular surface (described at the beginning of each chapter).

2. Observing the direction of movement of the bone during the assessment of the PROM.

3. Applying the concave–convex rule.

   The concave–convex rule[13] states that:
   a. When a convex joint surface moves on a fixed concave surface, the convex joint surface glides in the opposite direction to the movement of the shaft of the bone (Fig. 1-21A).

   Example: During glenohumeral joint abduction ROM, the shaft of the humerus moves in a superior direction and the convex humeral articular surface moves in an inferior direction on the fixed concave surface of the scapular glenoid fossa. Restricted inferior glide of the convex humeral head would result in decreased glenohumeral joint abduction ROM.
   b. When a concave joint surface moves on a fixed convex surface, the concave joint surface glides in the same direction as the movement of the shaft of the bone (Fig. 1-21B).

   Example: During knee extension ROM, the shaft of the tibia moves in an anterior direction and the concave tibial articular surface moves in an anterior direction on the fixed convex femoral articular surface. Restricted anterior glide of the concave tibial articular surface would result in decreased knee extension ROM.

Arthrokinematics, specifically the glide that accompanies the bone movement for normal ROM at the extremity joints, is identified in subsequent chapters. The normal joint glide is introduced to facilitate integration of osteokinematic (i.e., bone movement) findings with arthrokinematics (i.e., the corresponding motion between the joint surfaces) when assessing and measuring ROM of the extremity joints. The techniques used to assess and restore joint glide are beyond the scope of this text.

Spin,[4] the third type of movement that occurs between articular surfaces is a rotary motion that occurs around an axis. During normal joint ROM, spin may occur alone or accompany roll and glide. Spin occurs alone during flexion and extension at the shoulder (Fig. 1-22A) and hip joints, and pronation and supination at the humeroradial joint (Fig. 1-22B). Spin occurs in conjunction with roll and glide during flexion and extension at the knee joint.

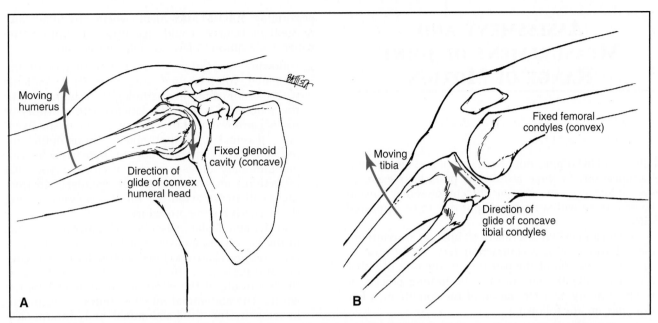

Figure 1-21 Arthrokinematic movement: the concave–convex rule. **A.** A convex joint surface glides on a fixed concave surface in the opposite direction to the movement of the shaft of the bone. **B.** A concave joint surface glides on a fixed convex surface in the same direction as the movement of the shaft of the bone.

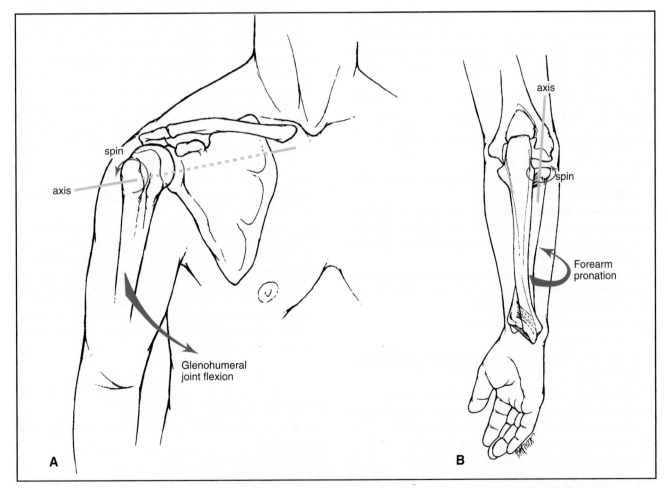

Figure 1-22 Arthrokinematic movement: **A.** Spin at the glenohumeral joint when the shoulder is flexed or extended. **B.** Spin at the humeroradial joint when the forearm is supinated or pronated.

ASSESSMENT AND MEASUREMENT OF JOINT RANGE OF MOTION

Contraindications and Precautions

AROM or PROM must not be assessed or measured if contraindications to these assessment procedures exist. In special instances, the assessment techniques may have to be performed with a modified approach to be employed safely.

AROM and PROM assessment techniques are contraindicated where muscle contraction (i.e., in the case of AROM) or motion of the part (i.e., in the case of either AROM or PROM) could disrupt the healing process or result in injury or deterioration of the condition. A few examples are the following:

1. If motion to the part will cause further damage or interrupt the healing process immediately after injury or surgery.

2. If the therapist suspects a subluxation or dislocation or fracture.

3. If myositis ossificans or ectopic ossification is suspected or present, AROM and PROM should not be undertaken without first ensuring the patient is assessed by a professional who has expertise in the management of these conditions.[14]

After ensuring no contraindications to AROM or PROM exist, the therapist must take extra care when assessing AROM and PROM if movement to the part might aggravate the condition. A few examples are as follow:

1. In painful conditions.

2. In the presence of an inflammatory process in a joint or the region around a joint.

3. In patients taking medication for pain or muscle relaxants, because the patient may not be able to respond appropriately and movement may be performed too vigorously.

4. In the presence of marked osteoporosis or in conditions where bone fragility is a factor, perform PROM with extreme care or not at all.

5. In assessing a hypermobile joint.

6. In patients with hemophilia.

7. In the region of a hematoma, especially at the elbow, hip, or knee.

8. In assessing joints if bony ankylosis is suspected.

9. After an injury where there has been a disruption of soft tissue (i.e., tendon, muscle, ligament).

10. In the region of a recently healed fracture.

11. After prolonged immobilization of a part.

After ensuring no contraindications to AROM or PROM exist, the therapist must take extra care when performing AROM assessment where strenuous and resisted movement could aggravate or worsen the patient's condition. A few examples are as follow:

1. Following neurosurgery[15] or recent surgery of the abdomen, intervertebral disc, or eye[16]; in patients with intervertebral disc pathology,[15] or herniation of the abdominal wall; or in patients with a history or risk of cardiovascular problems (e.g., aneurysm, fixed-rate pacemaker, arrhythmias, thrombophlebitis, recent embolus, marked obesity, hypertension, cardiopulmonary disease, angina pectoris, myocardial infarctions, and cerebrovascular disorders). Instruct these patients to avoid the *Valsalva maneuver* during the strength testing procedure.

   Kisner and Colby[15] describe the sequence of events in the Valsalva maneuver, which consists of an expiratory effort against a closed glottis during a strenuous and prolonged effort. A deep breath is taken at the beginning of the effort and held by closing the glottis. The abdominal muscles contract, causing an increase in the intra-abdominal and intrathoracic pressures, and blood is forced from the heart, causing a temporary and abrupt rise in the arterial blood pressure. The abdominal muscle contraction may also put unsafe stress on the abdominal wall.

   To avoid the Valsalva maneuver, instruct the patient not to hold his or her breath during the assessment of AROM. Should this be difficult, instruct the patient to breathe out[17] or talk during the test.[15]

2. If fatigue may be detrimental to or exacerbate the patient's condition (e.g., extreme debility, malnutrition, malignancy, chronic obstructive pulmonary disease, cardiovascular disease, multiple sclerosis, poliomyelitis, postpoliomyelitis syndrome, myasthenia gravis, lower motor neuron disease, and intermittent claudication), strenuous testing should not be carried out. Signs of fatigue include complaints or observation of tiredness, pain, muscular spasm, a slow response to contraction, tremor, and a decreased ability to perform AROM.

3. In situations where overwork may be detrimental to the patient's condition (e.g., patients with certain neuromuscular diseases or systemic, metabolic, or inflammatory disease), care should be used to avoid fatigue or exhaustion. Overwork[15] is a phenomenon that causes a temporary or permanent loss of strength in already weakened muscle due to excessively vigorous activity or exercise relative to the patient's condition.

Assessment of AROM

Assessment of the AROM can provide the following patient information:

- Willingness to move
- Level of consciousness
- Ability to follow instructions

- Attention span
- Coordination
- Joint ROM
- Movements that cause or increase pain
- Muscle strength
- Ability to perform functional activities

AROM may be decreased due to the following patient factors:

- Unwillingness to move
- Inability to follow instructions
- Restricted joint mobility
- Muscle weakness
- Pain

To perform a scan of the AROM available at the joints of the upper and lower limb, instruct the patient to perform activities that include movement at several joints simultaneously. Scans of the AROM for the upper and lower extremity joints are described and illustrated in this text.

Example: a scan of upper extremity joint AROM is illustrated in Figure 1-23 A and B: instruct the patient to try and touch the fingertips of each hand together behind the back.

- As the hand reaches down the back, observe the AROM of scapular abduction and lateral (upward) rotation, shoulder elevation and external rotation, elbow flexion, forearm supination, wrist radial deviation, and finger extension.
- As the hand reaches up the back, observe the AROM of scapular adduction and medial (downward) rotation, shoulder extension and internal rotation, elbow flexion, forearm pronation, wrist radial deviation, and finger extension.
- Elbow extension is observed as the patient moves from position A to position B. If required, to scan wrist, finger, and thumb AROM – instruct the patient to make a fist, and then open the hand and spread the fingers as far apart as possible.

The results of the scan(s) are used to guide the need for subsequent assessment procedures.

For a more detailed assessment of the AROM, instruct the patient to perform all of the active movements that normally occur at the affected joint(s) and at the joints immediately proximal and distal to the affected joint(s). Observe the patient's ability to perform each active movement, if possible, bilaterally and symmetrically (Fig. 1-24A). Bilateral and symmetrical movement allows comparison of the AROM with the unaffected side, if available. When the patient actively moves through the range, emphasize the exactness of the movement to the patient so that substitute motion at other joints is avoided. The AROM can be measured using a universal goniometer or OB "Myrin" goniometer to provide an objective measure of the patient's ability to perform functional activity.

In the presence of full joint movement (i.e., full PROM) and muscle weakness, the effect of gravity on the

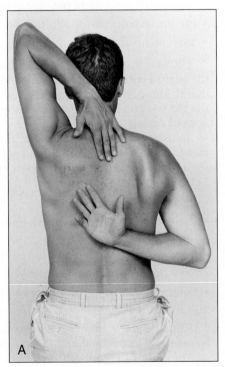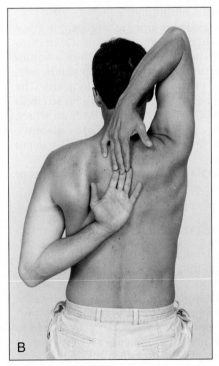

Figure 1-23 A and B. End positions: scan of active range of motion (AROM) of the upper extremities.

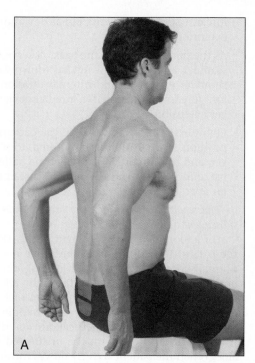
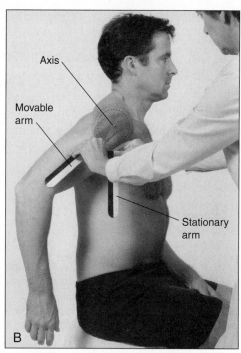

Figure 1-24 Assessment and measurement of active range of motion (AROM) using glenohumeral joint extension as an example. **A.** Observe and evaluate the AROM. **B.** Use an instrument such as a universal goniometer to measure the AROM.

part being moved may affect the AROM. When the part is moved in a vertical plane against the force of gravity rather than in a horizontal plane when gravity is not a factor, the AROM may be less. Consider the patient's position and the effect of gravity on the movement to interpret the AROM assessment findings.

When manually assessing muscle strength, a grade is assigned to indicate the strength of a muscle or muscle group. The grade indicates the strength of a voluntary muscle contraction and the AROM possible relative to the existing PROM available at the joint. The muscle grade assigned to indicate muscle strength provides a general indication of the AROM from which to extrapolate the patient's functional capability. Assessment of muscle strength is discussed in detail later in this chapter.

Assessment of AROM is followed by an assessment of PROM and muscle strength.

Measurement of AROM

The measurement procedures for the universal goniometer (Fig. 1-24B) and the OB "Myrin" goniometer are described in the section "Measurement of ROM," later in this chapter. The measurement of AROM may use the same or different positions to those used for PROM; for example, functional positions or activities may be used to measure AROM. When the patient actively moves through the range, emphasize the exactness of the movement to the patient so that substitute motion at other joints is avoided.

Assessment of PROM

Assessment of the PROM provides information about the following:

- Amount of movement possible at the joint
- Factors responsible for limiting movement
- Movements that cause or increase pain

PROM is usually slightly greater than AROM, owing to the slight elastic stretch of tissues and in some instances due to the decreased bulk of relaxed muscles. However, the PROM can also be greater than the AROM in the presence of muscle weakness.

To assess the PROM at a joint, for each joint movement, stabilize the proximal joint segment(s) and move the distal joint segment(s) through the full PROM (Fig. 1-25) and do the following:

- Visually estimate the PROM
- Determine the quality of the movement throughout the PROM
- Determine the end feel and factors that limit the PROM
- Note the presence of pain
- Determine whether a capsular or noncapsular pattern of movement is present

If the PROM is either less than or greater than normal, measure and record the PROM using a goniometer.

The following concepts and terms are important to understanding joint motion restriction when assessing PROM.

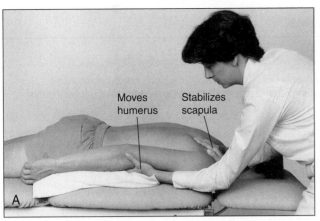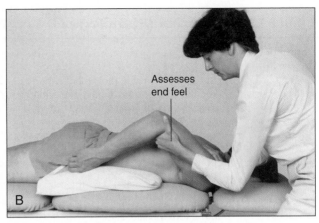

Figure 1-25 Assessment of passive range of motion (PROM) using glenohumeral joint extension as an example. **A.** The patient is comfortable, well supported, and relaxed with the joint in the anatomical position. The therapist manually stabilizes the proximal joint segment (e.g., scapula) and moves the distal joint segment (e.g., humerus). **B.** The distal joint segment is moved to the end of PROM and gentle overpressure is applied to determine the end feel.

Normal Limiting Factors and End Feels

The unique anatomical structure of a joint determines the direction and magnitude of its PROM. The factors that normally limit movement and determine the range of the PROM at a joint include:

- The stretching of soft tissues (i.e., muscles, fascia, and skin)
- The stretching of ligaments or the joint capsule
- The apposition of soft tissues
- Bone contacting bone

When assessing the PROM of a joint, observe whether the range is full, restricted, or excessive, and by feel determine which structure(s) limits the movement. The *end feel* is the sensation transmitted to the therapist's hand at the extreme end of the PROM that indicates the structures that limit the joint movement.[18] The end feel may be normal (physiological) or abnormal (pathological).[19]

A normal end feel exists when there is full PROM at the joint and the normal anatomy of the joint stops movement. An abnormal end feel exists when there is either a decreased or an increased passive joint ROM or when there is a normal PROM, but structures other than the normal anatomy stop joint movement. Normal and abnormal end feels are presented in Tables 1-3 and 1-4. The end feel(s) for joint movements are documented in subsequent chapters based on knowledge of the anatomy of the region, clinical experience, and available references. Although several different end feels may be possible for a particular joint motion, only one end feel will be present. When several different end feels are possible at a joint, this will be indicated using a "/" between each possible end feel. For example, the end feel for elbow flexion may be soft/firm/hard (i.e., soft, firm, or hard).

Method to Assess End Feel

Movement is isolated to the joint being assessed (Fig. 1-25A). With the patient relaxed, stabilize the proximal

TABLE 1-3   Normal (Physiological) End Feels[18-20]

End Feel General Terminology (Specific Terminology)	Description
Hard (Bony)	A painless, abrupt, hard stop to movement when bone contacts bone; for example, passive elbow extension, the olecranon process contacts the olecranon fossa.
Soft (Soft tissue apposition)	When two body surfaces come together a soft compression of tissue is felt; for example, in passive knee flexion, the soft tissue on the posterior aspects of the calf and thigh come together.
Firm (Soft tissue stretch)	A firm or springy sensation that has some give when muscle is stretched; for example, passive ankle dorsiflexion performed with the knee in extension is stopped due to tension in the gastrocnemius muscle.
(Capsular stretch)	A hard arrest to movement with some give when the joint capsule or ligaments are stretched. The feel is similar to stretching a piece of leather; for example, passive shoulder external rotation.

TABLE 1-4	Abnormal (Pathological) End Feels[18-20]
End Feel	**Description**
Hard	An abrupt hard stop to movement, when bone contacts bone, or a bony grating sensation, when rough articular surfaces move past one another, for example, in a joint that contains loose bodies, degenerative joint disease, dislocation, or a fracture.
Soft	A boggy sensation that indicates the presence of synovitis or soft tissue edema.
Firm	A springy sensation or a hard arrest to movement with some give, indicating muscular, capsular, or ligamentous shortening.
Springy block	A rebound is seen or felt and indicates the presence of an internal derangement; for example, the knee with a torn meniscus.
Empty	If considerable pain is present, there is no sensation felt before the extreme of passive ROM as the patient requests the movement be stopped, this indicates pathology such as an extra-articular abscess, a neoplasm, acute bursitis, joint inflammation, or a fracture.
Spasm	A hard sudden stop to passive movement that is often accompanied by pain, is indicative of an acute or subacute arthritis, the presence of a severe active lesion, or fracture. If pain is absent a spasm end feel may indicate a lesion of the central nervous system with resultant increased muscular tonus.

joint segment and move the distal joint segment to the end of its PROM for the test movement (Fig. 1-25B). Apply gentle overpressure at the end of the PROM and note the end feel.

When assessing the PROM at a joint, in addition to determining the end feel, visually estimate the available PROM for each movement at the joint, and establish the presence or absence of pain.

Capsular and Noncapsular Patterns

If there is a decreased PROM, assess the *pattern of joint movement restriction*. The description of capsular and non-capsular patterns is derived from the work of Cyriax.[18]

Capsular Pattern

If a lesion of the joint capsule or a total joint reaction is present, a characteristic pattern of restriction in the PROM will occur: the capsular pattern. Only joints that are controlled by muscles exhibit capsular patterns. When painful stimuli from the region of the joint provoke involuntary muscle spasm, a restriction in motion at the joint in the capsular proportions results. Each joint capsule resists stretching in selective ways; therefore, in time, certain aspects of the capsule become more contracted than others do. The capsular pattern manifests as a proportional limitation of joint motions that are characteristic to each joint; for example, the capsular pattern of the shoulder joint differs from the pattern of restriction at the hip joint. The capsular pattern at each joint is similar between individuals. Joints that rely primarily on ligaments for their stability do not exhibit capsular patterns, and the degree of pain elicited when the joint is strained at the extreme of movement indicates the severity of the total joint reaction or arthritis. The capsular pattern for each joint is provided in each chapter, with

movements listed in order of restriction (most restricted to least restricted). However, be advised that research[21-23] indicates capsular patterns may not be relied upon as much as previously thought.

Noncapsular Pattern

A noncapsular pattern exists when there is limitation of movement at a joint but not in the capsular pattern of restriction. A noncapsular pattern indicates the absence of a total joint reaction. Ligamentous sprains or adhesions, internal derangement, or extra-articular lesions may result in a noncapsular pattern at the joint.

Ligamentous sprains or adhesions affect specific regions of the joint or capsule. Motion is restricted and there is pain when the joint is moved in a direction that stretches the affected ligament. Other movements at the joint are usually full and pain-free.

Internal derangement occurs when loose fragments of cartilage or bone are present within a joint. When the loose fragment impinges between the joint surfaces, the movement is suddenly blocked and there may be localized pain. All other joint movements are full and pain-free. Internal derangements occur in joints such as the knee, jaw, and elbow.

Extra-articular lesions that affect nonarticular structures, such as muscle adhesions, muscle spasm, muscle strains, hematomas, and cysts, may limit joint ROM in one direction while a full and painless PROM is present in all other directions.

Measurement of ROM

Instrumentation

A *goniometer* is an apparatus used to measure joint angles.[7] The goniometer chosen to assess joint ROM

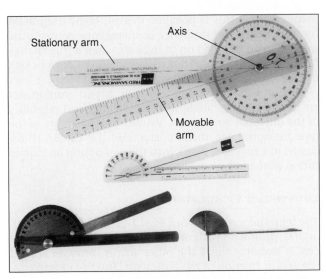

Figure 1-26 Various sizes of 180° and 360° universal goniometers.

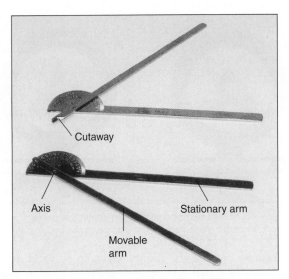

Figure 1-27 Universal goniometer with a 180° protractor. *Top:* range of motion (ROM) cannot be read as the cutaway portion of the movable arm is off the scale. *Bottom:* With the cutaway portion of the movable arm on the scale, the ROM can be read.

depends on the degree of accuracy required in the measurement, the time, and resources available to the clinician, and the patient's comfort and well-being. Radiographs, digital images, photographs, photocopies, and the use of the electrogoniometer, flexometer, or plumb line may give objective, valid, and reliable measures of ROM but are not always practical or available in the clinical setting. When doing clinical research, the therapist should investigate alternative instruments that will offer a more stringent assessment of joint ROM.

In the clinical setting, the universal goniometer (Figs. 1-26 and 1-27) is the goniometer most frequently used to measure ROM for the extremity joints. In this text, the universal goniometer is described and illustrated for the measurement of the ROM for the joints of the extremities and spine. The OB "Myrin" goniometer[24] (OB Rehab, Solna, Sweden) (Fig. 1-28), although less commonly used in the clinic, is a useful tool and is described and illustrated for the measurement of selected ROM at the forearm, hip, knee, and ankle.

The universal goniometer, tape measure (Fig. 1-29), standard inclinometer (Fig. 1-30), and the Cervical Range-of-Motion Instrument (CROM)[25] (Performance Attainment Associates, Roseville, MN) (Fig. 1-31), are the tools used to measure spinal AROM as presented in this text. AROM measurements of the temporomandibular joints (TMJs) are performed using a ruler or calipers. These instruments and the measurement procedures employed when using these instruments to measure spinal and TMJ AROM are described and illustrated in Chapter 9.

Validity and Reliability

Validity

Validity is "the degree to which an instrument measures what it is supposed to measure".[26(p. 171)] Validity indicates the accuracy of a measurement. A goniometer, inclinometer, or tape measure is used to provide measurements of the number of degrees or distance in centimeters, of movement or the position of a joint. Measurements must

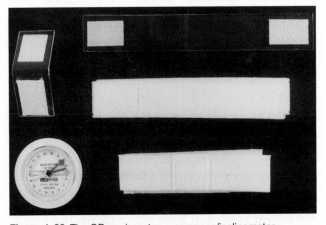

Figure 1-28 The OB goniometer, a compass/inclinometer, includes Velcro straps and plastic extension plates used to attach the goniometer to the body part being measured.

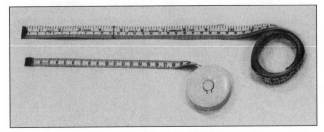

Figure 1-29 Tape measures used to measure joint range of motion (ROM).

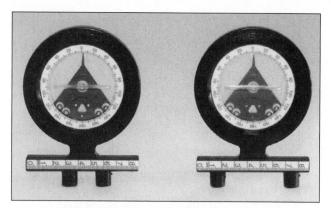

Figure 1-30 Standard inclinometers with adjustable contact points to facilitate placement on the surface of the body.

be accurate because the results, taken to be valid representations of actual joint angles, are used to plan treatment and determine treatment effectiveness, patient progress, and degree of disability.

Criterion-related validity is one means of assessing the accuracy of the instruments for assessing joint angles or positions. To establish this validity, the measures of the instrument being assessed are compared to the measures obtained with an instrument that is an accepted standard (criterion) for the measurement of joint angles; for example, a radiograph. When the supporting evidence from the accepted standard is collected at the same time as the measurement from the test instrument, concurrent validity is assessed. If a close relationship is found between the measures obtained with the instrument and the accepted standard, the instrument measures are valid.

Reliability

Reliability is "the extent to which the instrument yields the same measurement on repeated uses either by the same operator (intraobserver reliability) or by different operators (interobserver reliability)".[27(p. 49)] Reliability indicates the consistency or repeatability of a measurement.

The therapist measures ROM and compares measurements taken over time to evaluate treatment effectiveness and patient progress. It is important for the therapist to know that joint position and ROM can be measured consistently (i.e., with minimal deviation due to measure-

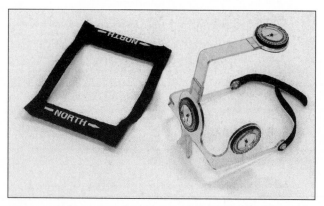

Figure 1-31 The Cervical-Range-of-Motion Instrument (CROM) consists of two gravity inclinometers, a magnetic compass inclinometer, and a magnetic yoke.

ment error). If this is possible, then in comparing ROM measurements, the similarity or divergence between the measures can be relied on to indicate when a true change has occurred that is not due to measurement error or lack of measurement consistency.

The universal goniometer and OB "Myrin" goniometer are described here, along with the validity and reliability of the universal goniometer. Validity and reliability of the tape measure/ruler, inclinometer, and the CROM is discussed in Chapter 9, along with the description and application of these instruments.

Universal Goniometer

The *universal goniometer* (see Figs. 1-26 and 1-27) is a 180° or 360° protractor with one axis that joins two arms. One arm is stationary and the other arm is movable around the axis or fulcrum of the protractor. The size of universal goniometer used is determined by the size of the joint being assessed. Larger goniometers are usually used for measurement of joint range at large joints.

Validity and Reliability—Universal Goniometer

Radiographs, "the most accurate means of assessing joint motion",[28(p. 116)] and photographs are accepted standards used for comparison to determine the accuracy of the universal goniometer. When the supporting evidence from the radiographs or photographs is collected at the same time as the measurement from the universal goniometer, concurrent validity can be assessed.

There has been little study of the criterion-related validity of the universal goniometer. Using x-ray bone angle measurements compared to goniometric measurements of knee joint position,[29,30] high criterion-related validity has been found, along with disparate findings of goniometric accuracy in only a small part of the range, thought to be due to the increased complexity of movement in approaching terminal extension. Using a photographic reference standard to assess elbow joint positions, the "results indicate that relatively inexperienced raters should be able to use goniometers accurately to measure elbow position when given standardized methods to follow".[31(p. 1666)]

Reliability of joint position and ROM using the universal goniometer depends on the joint being assessed but has generally been found to be good to excellent. Reliability study results indicate that:

1. The universal goniometer is more reliable than visual estimation of joint ROM.[32–37] The use of the goniometer becomes even more critical when the examiner is inexperienced.[36,38]

2. The reliability of goniometric measurement varies depending on the joint and motion assessed.[34,39–42]

3. Intratester reliability is better than intertester reliability; therefore, the same therapist should perform all measures when possible.[32,33,39,40,43–45] Different therapists should not be used interchangeably to obtain ROM measurements on the same patient unless the intertester reliability is known.[46]

4. The size of the goniometer selected to assess ROM at a joint does not affect measurement reliability.[47,48]

5. The findings are mixed on whether taking the average of repeated measures improves[33,44,49] or makes no difference to[41,42,47,50] the reliability of goniometric measures.

6. Research[50-56] regarding the reliability of goniometric measurement in the presence of spasticity appears inconclusive.

Joint ROM can be measured reliably using a universal goniometer when preferably the same therapist performs the repeated measures using a "rigid standardized measurement protocol",[43(p. 57)] in the absence of spasticity. Miller[28] provides a method for clinicians to determine the intratester and intertester reliability within their clinical facility. Knowing the measurement error factor allows therapists to better determine patient progress.

Joint ROM Assessment and Measurement Procedure

Expose the Area

Explain to the patient the need to expose the area to be assessed. Adequately expose the area and drape the patient as required.

Explanation and Instruction

Briefly explain the ROM assessment and measurement procedure to the patient. Explain and demonstrate the movement to be performed and/or passively move the patient's uninvolved limb through the ROM.

Assessment of the Normal ROM

Initially assess and record the ROM of the uninvolved limb to determine the patient's normal ROM and normal end feels, and to demonstrate the movement to the patient before performing the movement on the involved side. If there is bilateral limb involvement, use your clinical knowledge and experience to judge the patient's normal PROM, keeping in mind that PROM is usually slightly greater than the AROM.

Use the tables of normal AROM values provided by the American Academy of Orthopaedic Surgeons[57] and the suggested normal AROM values derived from an evaluation of the research literature by Berryman Reese and Bandy,[58] as a guide to normal AROM. These "normal" AROM values are presented in table form at the beginning of each chapter.

"Normal" ranges can be misleading because joint ROM can vary between individuals depending on gender, age, occupation, and health status.[59] Therefore, "normal" ranges should be used only as a guide when assessing and treating patients. More importantly, determine the essential functional ROM required by the patient to perform activities of daily living (ADL) and the patient's ability to meet these requirements.

Assessment and Measurement Procedure

Patient Position. Ensure the patient is:
• Comfortable.
• Well supported.
  Position the patient so that the:
• Joint to be assessed is in the anatomical position.
• Proximal joint segment can be stabilized to allow only the desired motion.
• Movement can occur through the full ROM unrestricted.
• Goniometer can be properly placed to measure the ROM.

If the patient's position varies from the standard assessment position outlined in this text, make a special note on the ROM assessment form.

Substitute Movements. When assessing and measuring AROM and PROM, ensure that only the desired movement occurs at the joint being assessed. Substitute movements may take the form of additional movements at the joint being assessed or at other joints, thus giving the appearance of having a greater joint ROM than is actually present. An example of substitute movements used when performing a functional activity is illustrated in Figure 1-32.

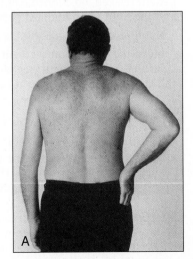 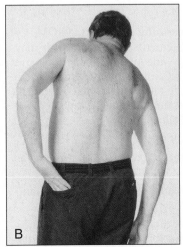

Figure 1-32 **A.** Patient reaches into a back pocket using normal right upper extremity. **B.** Substitute motions at the left shoulder girdle and trunk compensate for restricted left shoulder joint range of motion (ROM) as the patient attempts to reach into a back pocket.

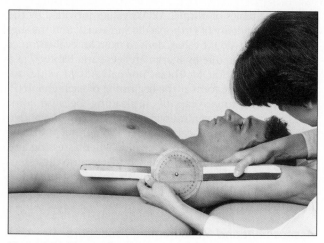

Figure 1-33 The weight of the trunk on the plinth serves to stabilize the scapula as the therapist measures the passive range of motion (PROM) of shoulder elevation through flexion.

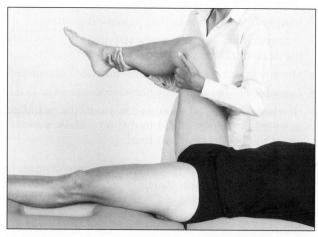

Figure 1-34 The weight of the trunk and position of the pelvis on a firm surface serves to stabilize the pelvis as the therapist assesses hip internal rotation passive range of motion (PROM) and end feel.

When assessing and measuring AROM and PROM, try to eliminate substitute movements. For AROM, this may be accomplished through adequate explanation and instruction to the patient regarding the movement to be performed and the substitute movement(s) to be avoided. In addition, substitute motion(s) may be avoided for AROM and PROM by the following:

- Using proper patient positioning
- Adequately stabilizing the proximal joint segment as required
- Acquiring substantial practice in assessing AROM and PROM

To assess joint ROM accurately, the therapist must know and recognize the possible substitute movements. If the presence of substitute movements results in inaccurate AROM or PROM assessment and measurement, the treatment plan may be inappropriate.

Stabilization. Stabilize the proximal joint segment to limit movement to the joint being assessed or measured and prevent substitute movement for lack of joint range by making use of the following:

1. The patient's body weight.

   Examples:
   - To measure shoulder elevation through flexion PROM, position the patient supine on a firm plinth so that the weight of the trunk stabilizes the shoulder girdle (Fig. 1-33).
   - To assess hip internal rotation PROM, position the patient supine on a firm plinth so that the weight of the body stabilizes the pelvic girdle (see Fig. 1-34).

2. The patient's position.

   Example:
   - To assess hip abduction ROM (Fig. 1-35), position the patient supine on a firm plinth with the contralateral leg over the opposite side of the plinth and the foot resting on a stool. This leg position prevents the tilting or shifting of the pelvis toward the test side, which would give the appearance of a greater hip abduction PROM than actually exists.

3. External forces in the form of external pressure applied directly by the therapist and devices such as belts or sandbags. Ensure that manual contacts or devices avoid tender or painful areas, for example, in some viral diseases (i.e., poliomyelitis) muscle bellies may be tender.

   Examples:
   - Manually stabilize the pelvis to assess hip extension PROM (Fig. 1-36) and employ a belt to stabilize the pelvis when both hands are needed to place the goniometer to measure hip extension PROM (Fig. 1-37).
   - Manually stabilize the tibia and fibula to assess ankle (i.e., talocrural) joint dorsiflexion and plantarflexion PROM (Fig. 1-38).

Assessment of Passive ROM and End Feel. With the patient relaxed, positioned comfortably on a firm surface, and the joint in anatomical position:

- Stabilize the proximal joint segment (see Fig. 1-39A)
- Move the distal joint segment to the end of the PROM for the test movement (see Fig. 1-39B and apply slight (i.e., gentle) overpressure at the end of the PROM
- Visually estimate the PROM
- Note the end feel, presence of pain
- Return the limb to the start position
- Following the assessment of the PROM for all movements at a joint, determine the presence of a capsular or noncapsular pattern of movement.

Measurement. It is not necessary to measure the joint ROM when the involved joint has a full AROM and PROM. Record the full ROM as full, normal (N), or within normal limits (WNL).

The *neutral zero method*[57] is used to assess and measure joint ROM. All joint motions are measured from a defined

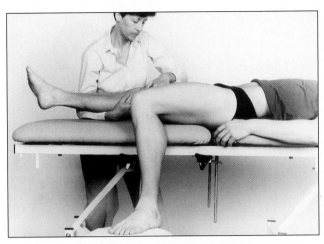

Figure 1-35 The position of the patient's nontest leg stabilizes the pelvis when testing hip abduction passive range of motion (PROM).

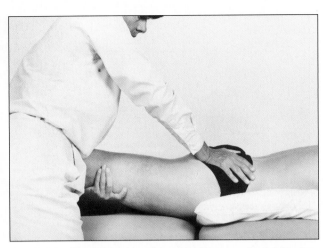

Figure 1-36 The therapist applies external pressure to stabilize the pelvis to assess hip extension passive range of motion (PROM).

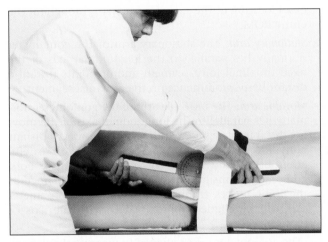

Figure 1-37 A belt may be used to stabilize the pelvis to measure hip joint extension passive range of motion (PROM).

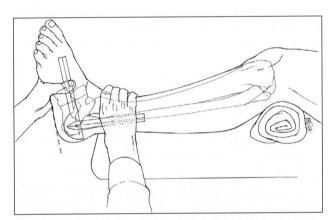

Figure 1-38 The therapist manually stabilizes the tibia and fibula proximal to the ankle joint to measure ankle dorsiflexion and plantarflexion passive range of motion (PROM).

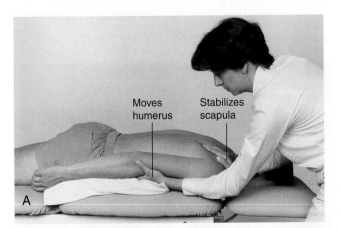

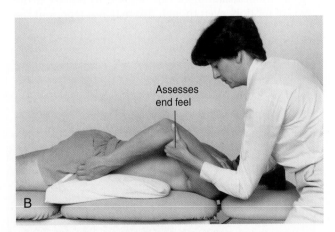

Figure 1-39 Assessment of passive range of motion (PROM) using glenohumeral joint extension as an example. **A.** The patient is comfortable, well supported, and relaxed with the joint in the anatomical position. The therapist manually stabilizes the proximal joint segment (e.g., scapula) and moves the distal joint segment (e.g., humerus). **B.** The distal joint segment is moved to the end of joint PROM and gentle overpressure is applied to determine the end feel.

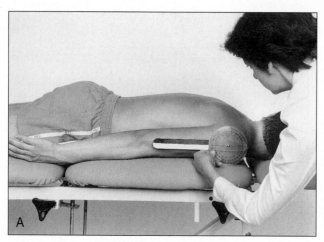
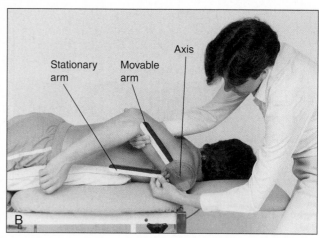

Figure 1-40 Measurement of passive range of motion (PROM) using glenohumeral joint extension as an example. **A.** Start position: the universal goniometer is aligned with the joint in anatomical position (0°). **B.** End position: measurement of shoulder extension PROM (60°).

zero position, either the anatomical position (see Figs. 1-14 to 1-16) or a position specified as zero. Any movement on either side of zero is positive and moves toward 180°.

Measurement Procedure—Universal Goniometer

- *Goniometer placement:* The preferred placement of the goniometer is lateral to the joint, just off the surface of the limb (see Fig. 1-40), but it may also be placed over the joint (see Fig. 1-41) using only light contact between the goniometer and the skin. If joint swelling is present, placing the goniometer over the joint may give erroneous results when assessing joint ROM as the degree of swelling changes.

- *Axis:* The axis of the goniometer is placed over the axis of movement of the joint. A specific bony prominence or anatomical landmark can be used to represent the axis of motion, even though this may not represent the

exact location of the axis of movement throughout the entire ROM.

- *Stationary arm:* The stationary arm of the goniometer normally lies parallel to the longitudinal axis of the fixed proximal joint segment and/or points toward a distant bony prominence on the proximal segment.

- *Movable arm:* The movable arm of the goniometer normally lies parallel to the longitudinal axis of the moving distal joint segment and/or points toward a distant bony prominence on the distal segment. If careful attention is paid to the correct positioning of both goniometer arms and the positions are maintained as the joint moves through the ROM, the goniometer axis will be aligned approximately with the axis of motion.[59]

The goniometer is first aligned to measure the defined zero position for the ROM at a joint (see Figs. 1-40A and 1-41A). If it is not possible to attain the defined zero position, the joint is positioned as close as possible to the zero position, and the distance the movable arm is positioned

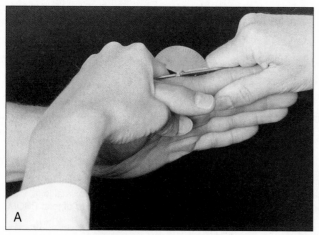
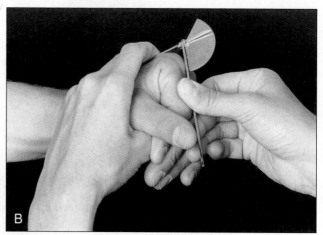

Figure 1-41 **A.** Start position (0°) for metacarpophalangeal (MCP) joint flexion with the universal goniometer placed over the dorsum of the MCP joint. **B.** End position: MCP flexion PROM (90°) with the goniometer aligned over the joint.

away from the 0° start position on the protractor is recorded as the start position.

To Measure AROM. To measure the AROM, have the patient move actively through the full AROM and either move the movable arm of the goniometer along with the limb through the entire range of movement to the end of the AROM, or realign the goniometer at the end of the AROM (see Fig. 1-24B).

To Measure PROM. One of the following two techniques is used to measure the PROM at a joint:

1. Have the patient actively move through the joint ROM, and realign the goniometer at the end of the AROM. Have the patient relax and passively move the goniometer and the limb segment through the final few degrees of the PROM.

2. Passively move the movable arm of the goniometer and the limb segment through the entire range of movement to the end of the PROM.

Using either technique, the distance the movable arm moves away from the 0° start position on the protractor is recorded as the joint ROM. When using a goniometer with a 180° protractor (see Fig. 1-27), ensure the goniometer is positioned such that the cutaway portion of the moving arm remains on the protractor so that the ROM can be read at the end of the assessed joint ROM.

To avoid parallax when reading a goniometer, look directly onto the scale and view the scale with both eyes open or by closing one eye. Be consistent and use the same methodology on subsequent readings.

Proficiency in assessing and measuring joint ROM is gained through practice. It is important to practice the techniques on as many persons as possible to become familiar with the variation between individuals.

OB "Myrin" Goniometer

The OB "Myrin" goniometer (see Fig. 1-28), a compass inclinometer, consists of a fluid-filled rotatable container mounted on a plate.[24] The container has the following:

- A compass needle that reacts to the Earth's magnetic field and measures movements in the horizontal plane.
- An inclination needle that is influenced by the force of gravity and measures movements in the frontal and sagittal planes.
- A scale on the container floor is marked in 2° increments.

Two straps with Velcro fastenings are supplied to attach the goniometer to the body segment, and two plastic extension plates are also supplied to position the goniometer for certain joint measurements.[24] When using the OB goniometer, magnetic fields other than those of the earth will cause the OB goniometer compass needle to deviate, and therefore must be avoided.

The *advantages* of using the OB goniometer for measuring joint ROM are as follow:

- It is not necessary to align the inclinometer with the joint axis.

- Rotational movements using a compass inclinometer are measured with ease.
- Assessment of trunk and neck ROM is measured with ease.
- There is little change in the alignment of the goniometer throughout the ROM.
- PROM is more easily assessed using the OB goniometer, as the therapist does not have to hold the goniometer and can stabilize the proximal joint segment with one hand and passively move the distal segment with the other.

The *disadvantages* of the OB goniometer are as follow:

- It is expensive and bulky compared to the universal goniometer.
- It cannot be used to measure the small joints of the hand and foot.
- Magnetic fields other than those of the earth will cause the compass needle to deviate and must be avoided.

Measurement Procedure—OB "Myrin" Goniometer

- *Velcro strap and/or plastic extension plate:* Apply the Velcro strap to the limb segment proximal or distal to the joint being assessed. Attach the appropriate plastic extension plate to the Velcro strap for some ROM measurements.

- *OB Goniometer:* Attach the goniometer container to the Velcro strap or the plastic extension plate. The goniometer is positioned in relation to bony landmarks and placed in the same location on successive measurements.[60] With the patient in the start position, rotate the fluid-filled container until the 0° arrow lines up directly underneath either the inclination needle, if the movement occurs in a vertical plane (i.e., the frontal or sagittal planes) (Fig. 1-42A), or the compass needle, if the movement occurs in the horizontal plane[24] (Fig. 1-43).

- Ensure the needle is free to swing during the measurement.[24] Do not deviate the goniometer during the measurement by touching the strap or goniometer dial or by applying hand pressure to change the contour of the soft tissue mass near the OB goniometer.

- At the end of the AROM or PROM, the number of degrees the inclination needle (Fig. 1-42B) or the compass needle (Fig. 1-44) moves away from the 0° arrow on the compass dial is recorded as the joint ROM.

- The OB goniometer is especially useful for measuring forearm supination and pronation, tibial rotation, and hamstring and gastrocnemius muscle length. The ROM measurements of these movements are described and illustrated in this text as examples of how to apply the OB goniometer.

Sources of Error in Measuring Joint ROM

Read the goniometer scale carefully to avoid erroneous ROM measurements. Sources of error to be avoided when measuring joint ROM are[61] the following:

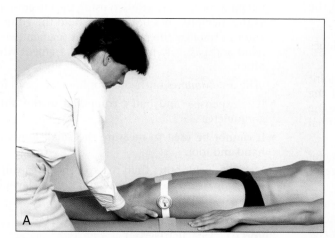

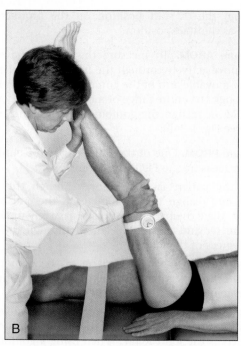

Figure 1-42 A. Start position: length of hamstrings utilizing the OB goniometer. **B.** End position: OB goniometer measurement of hip flexion angle, that indirectly represents the hamstrings length.

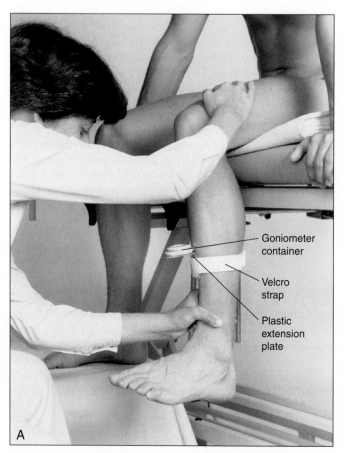

Goniometer container

Velcro strap

Plastic extension plate

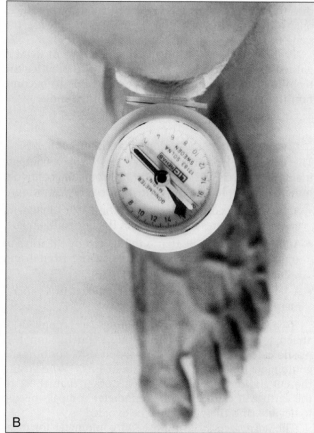

Figure 1-43 A and B. Start position for total tibial rotation: tibial internal rotation.

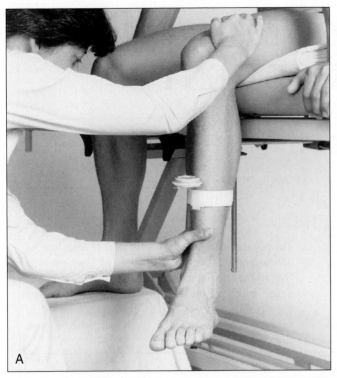

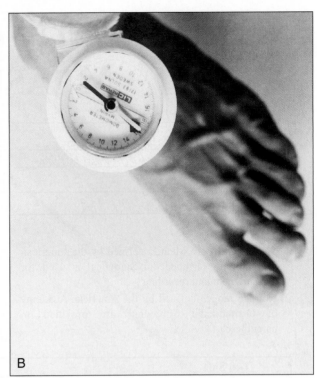

Figure 1-44 **A and B.** End position for total tibial rotation: tibial external rotation.

• Reading the wrong side of the scale on the goniometer (e.g., when the goniometer pointer is positioned midway between 40° and 50°, reading the value of 55° rather than 45°).

• A tendency to read values that end in a particular digit, such as zero (i.e., "_0°").

• Having expectations of what the reading "should be" and allowing this to influence the recorded result. For example, the patient has been attending treatment for 2 weeks and the therapist expects and sees an improvement in the ROM that is not actually present.

• A change in the patient's motivation to perform.

• Taking successive ROM measurements at different times of the day.

• Measurement procedure error: Make sure sources of error do not occur or are minimized so that ROM measurements are reliable and the patient's progress will be accurately monitored.

For reliable ROM measurements the following are essential:

• The same therapist should assess the ROM.

• Assess the ROM at the same time each day.

• Use the same measuring tool.

• Use the same patient position.

• Follow a standard measurement protocol.[59]

• Treatment may affect ROM; therefore, assess the ROM in a consistent manner relative to the application of treatment techniques.

If upper or lower extremity ROM is measured by the same therapist, a 3° or 4° increase in the ROM indicates improvement.[42] If different therapists measure the ROM, an increase of more than 5° for the upper extremity and 6° for the lower extremity would be needed to indicate progress.[42]

Recording of ROM Measurement

Standard information on a ROM recording form include the following:

• Patient name

• Date of birth or age

• Diagnosis

• Date of examination

• Assessing therapist's name, signature, and credentials

• Type of ROM being recorded, that is, AROM or PROM.

Different conventions are used internationally when listing the date numerically (either day/month/year or month/day/year); to ensure clear communication when recording dates, write the month in full or abbreviated form, as shown in Figures 1-45 and 1-46.

Numerical or pictorial charts are used to record ROM. See Figure 1-45 and Appendix A for examples of a numerical recording form; Figure 1-46 gives examples of selected joint motion recordings from a pictorial recording form.

If the AROM and PROM are full, the joint ROM does not have to be measured with a goniometer or tape measure and the ROM may be recorded as full, normal (N), within normal limits (WNL), or numerically.

RANGE OF MOTION MEASUREMENT

Patient's Name   *Jane Donner*   Age   *31*

Diagnosis   *# Ⓡ distal humeral shaft,*   Date of Onset   *July 10/11*
             depressed # Ⓡ tibial plateau

Therapist Name   *Tom Becker*   AROM or PROM   *PROM*

Signature   *T Becker BPT, MA*

Recording:

1. The Neutral Zero Method defined by the American Academy of Orthopaedic Surgeons[1] is used for measurement and recording.

2. Average ranges defined by the American Academy of Orthopaedic Surgeons[1] are provided in parentheses.

3. The columns designated with asterisks (*) are used for indicating limitation of range of motion and referencing for summarization.

4. Space is left at the end of each section to record hypermobile ranges and comments regarding positioning of the patient or body part, edema, pain, and/or end feel.

Left Side				Date of Measurement		Right Side		
*	Oct 8/11	*			*	Oct 8/11	*	
				Shoulder Complex				
	0-180°		Elevation through flexion (0–180°)		*	0-160°		
	N		Elevation through abduction (0–180°)			N		
			Shoulder Glenhumeral Joint					
			Extension (0–60°)					
			Horizontal abduction (0–45°)					
			Horizontal adduction (0–135°)					
			Internal rotation (0–70°)					
	↓		External rotation (0–90°)			↓		
			Hypermobility:					
			Comments: *end feel: Ⓡ Shoulder flexion firm*					
			Elbow and Forearm					
	0-150°		Flexion (0–150°)		*	10-120°		
	N		Supination (0–80°)			N		
	↓		Pronation (0–80°)			↓		
			Hypermobility: Ⓛ *elbow hyperextension 5°*					
			Comments: *end feels: Ⓡ elbow extension firm; flexion firm*					
			Knee					
	0-135°		Flexion (0–135°)		*	0-75°		
	NT		Tibial rotation			NT		
			Hypermobility:					
			Comments: *end feel: Ⓡ knee flexion firm*					

Figure 1-45 Example of recording range of motion (ROM) using a numeric recording form.

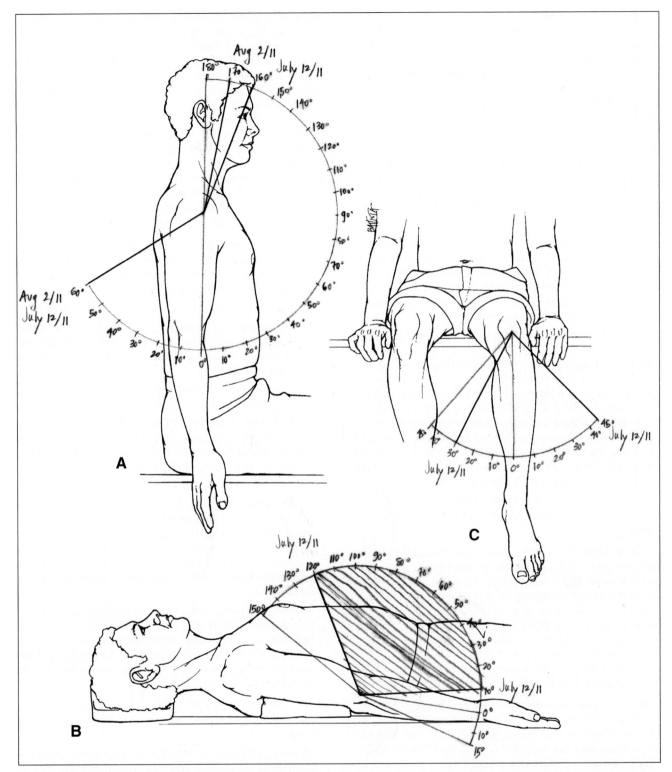

Figure 1-46 Examples of recording range of motion (ROM) using a pictorial recording form: **(A)** right shoulder flexion and extension, **(B)** right elbow flexion and extension/hyperextension, and **(C)** left hip internal and external rotation. The use of shading to show the available elbow flexion ROM is illustrated in **B.**

If the ROM is less than or greater than the normal ROM, the existing ROM is indicated on a pictorial chart, or the number of degrees of motion is recorded on a numerical chart.

Every space on the ROM recording form should include an entry.[8] If the measurement was not performed, not tested (NT) should be entered and a line may be drawn from the first such entry to the end of several adjacent entries so that NT does not have to be recorded in every space.[8]

Any changes from the standard method of assessing joint ROM as presented in this text should be noted on the assessment form.

The ranges of motion are recorded on the *numerical chart* as follow (Fig. 1-45).

- When it is possible to begin the movement at the 0° start position, the ROM is recorded by writing the number of degrees the joint has moved away from 0°—for example, right shoulder elevation through flexion (i.e., shoulder flexion) 160° or 0°–160°, right knee flexion 75° or 0°–75°, right knee extension 0°.

- When it is not possible to begin the movement from the 0° start position, the ROM is recorded by writing the number of degrees the joint is away from the 0° at the beginning of the ROM, followed by the number of degrees the joint is away from 0° at the end of the ROM— for example, the patient cannot achieve 0° right elbow extension due to a contracture (abnormal shortening) of the elbow flexor muscles; the end feel is firm. More specifically, the right elbow cannot be extended beyond 10° of elbow flexion and can be flexed to 120°. The ROM would be recorded as right elbow flexion 10°–120°.

- For a joint that is in a fixed position or ankylosed, this is recorded on the chart along with the position of the joint.

On *pictorial charts* (Fig. 1-46), the therapist extends lines from the joint axis on the diagram to the appropriate number of degrees marked on the arc of movement at the start and end positions for the movement. The area between the two lines may be shaded in to provide a visual image of the ROM (see Fig. 1-46B). The date is recorded at the end of each line drawn to a degree marking on the arc of movement.

Figure 1-46 provides examples of ranges of motion recorded using a pictorial chart for the following:

- Right shoulder elevation through flexion (i.e., shoulder flexion) 160° or 0°–160° and right shoulder extension 60° or 0°–60° as assessed on July 12, 2011. The patient was reassessed on August 2, 2011, and the ROM for right shoulder elevation through flexion increased to 170° or 0°–170°, and there was no change in the ROM for right shoulder extension.

- Right elbow flexion 10°–120° assessed on July 12, 2011.

- The July 12, 2011 assessment of left hip external rotation of 30° or 0°–30° and left hip internal rotation of 45° or 0°–45°.

The *SFTR Method*[62] is a less commonly used method of recording joint ROM. The letters S, F, and T represent the plane of motion (sagittal, frontal, and transverse, respectively; see Fig. 1-13) of the joint ROM assessed; the R represents rotational motions. To record ROM, the letter identifying the plane of motion or rotational motion is noted. The letter is followed by three numbers that represent the start position, 0° with normal movement, and the ROM present on either side of the start position. The start position is recorded as the middle number. The ROM present on either side of the start position is recorded before and after the start position using the conventions indicated below.[62] If a joint is ankylosed, only two numbers are recorded, 0° and the joint position to either the right or left of 0° using the conventions.

Conventions and examples of recording ROM using the SFTR method are as follows:

- Motion occurring in the S (i.e., sagittal plane) is extension and flexion. The number to the left of the start position represents extension ROM, and the number to the right represents flexion ROM.

Example: Shoulder left S:60-0-180° right S:60-0-80°.

Interpretation: Left shoulder ROM is WNL, with 60° extension and 180° shoulder elevation through flexion. Right shoulder extension is 60° and shoulder elevation through flexion 80°.

Example: Elbow left S:0-0-150° right S: 0-10-120°.

Interpretation: The ROM recorded indicates motion in the sagittal plane. Left elbow ROM is WNL with a start position of 0°, 0° extension, and 150° flexion. Right elbow extension and flexion has a start position of 10°, elbow flexion is 10° to 120°, or right elbow flexion is 120°.

Example: Knee right S: 0-15°.

Interpretation: The use of only two numbers indicates the knee joint is ankylosed. The S indicates the ankylosed position is in the sagittal plane; therefore, the joint is in either an extended or flexed position. The number is to the right of the 0 and by convention represents flexion. Thus, the knee is ankylosed in 15° flexion.

- Motion occurring in the F (i.e., frontal plane) is abduction and adduction. The number to the left of the start position represents abduction, eversion, or left spinal lateral flexion ROM and the number to the right of the start position represents adduction, inversion, or right spinal lateral flexion ROM.

Example: Hip right F:45-0-30°.

Interpretation: Right hip abduction is 45° and adduction is 30°.

- Motion occurring in the T (i.e., transverse plane) is horizontal abduction and horizontal adduction, and retraction and protraction. The number to the left of the start position represents horizontal abduction or retraction ROM and the number to the right of the start position represents horizontal adduction or protraction ROM.

Example: Shoulder left T(F90):35-0-90°.

Interpretation: (F90) following the T indicates frontal plane 90°, meaning the motions of horizontal abduction

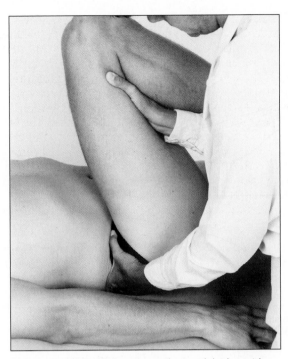

Figure 1-47 Knee flexion places the two-joint hamstring muscles on slack so that hip flexion range of motion (ROM) is not restricted by the length of the hamstrings.

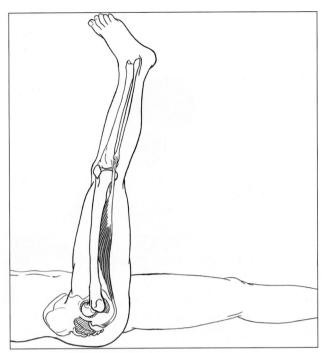

Figure 1-48 Passive insufficiency of the hamstring muscles. Hip flexion range of motion (ROM) is limited by the length of the hamstring muscles when the knee joint is held in extension.

and adduction were performed with the left shoulder in a start position of 90° abduction. Left shoulder horizontal abduction is 35° and horizontal adduction is 90°.

- An R indicates rotational motion. The number left of the start position represents external rotation, forearm supination, or spinal rotation to the left. The number right of the start position represents internal rotation, forearm pronation, or spinal rotation to the right.

Example: Hip right R(S90):45-0-30°.

Interpretation: The (S90) after the R indicates hip rotation was measured with the hip in the sagittal plane 90° (i.e., with the hip flexed 90°). Right hip external rotation ROM is 45° and internal rotation is 30°.

Assessing and Measuring Joint ROM with a Two- or Multi-joint Muscle in the Region

If during the assessment of joint ROM the movement will lengthen or stretch a two- or multi-joint muscle, move the nontest joint crossed by the muscle into position so that the two-joint or multi-joint muscle is placed on slack. This prevents the muscle from becoming passively insufficient and restricting the assessed joint ROM.

Example: When the hip is flexed to assess hip flexion ROM (Fig. 1-47), the knee is positioned in flexion to place the hamstrings on slack and prevent restriction of the hip flexion ROM due to passive insufficiency of the hamstrings (Fig. 1-48).

Passive joint ROM must be assessed before assessing muscle strength. The full available PROM at the joint then becomes the range the muscle(s) can be expected to move the limb through, and is therefore defined as the full available ROM for the purpose of grading muscle strength.

ASSESSMENT AND MEASUREMENT OF MUSCLE LENGTH

To assess and measure the length of a muscle, passively stretch (i.e., lengthen) the muscle across the joint(s) crossed by the muscle. When the muscle is on full stretch, the end feel will be firm, and the patient will report a pulling sensation or pain in the region of the muscle. Use a universal goniometer, inclinometer (e.g., OB goniometer), or tape measure to measure the PROM possible at the last joint moved to place the muscle on full stretch, or note any observed limitation in joint PROM due to muscle tightness. The PROM measurement indirectly represents the length of the shortened muscle. Retesting the joint PROM with the nontest joint crossed by the muscle placed into position so that the two- or multi-joint muscle is on slack, will normally result in an increased PROM at the joint. Procedures used to assess and measure specific muscle length are described and illustrated for each joint complex in Chapters 3–9.

One-Joint Muscle

To assess and measure the length of a muscle that crosses one joint, the joint crossed by the muscle is positioned so

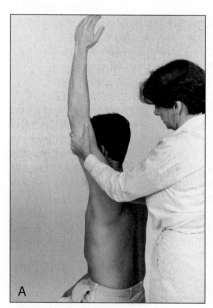
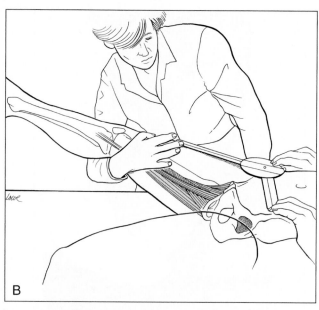

Figure 1-49 A. Hip abduction places the one-joint hip adductor muscles on stretch. **B.** Goniometer measurement: length of the hip adductors as the muscles limit hip abduction passive range of motion (PROM).

that the muscle is lengthened across the joint. The position of the joint is measured and this represents an indirect measure of the muscle length. The end feel will be firm.

Example: To assess and measure the length of the one-joint hip adductor muscles, passively abduct the hip to the limit of range to place the hip adductors on stretch. If the hip adductor muscles limit the motion (Fig. 1-49A), the end feel will be firm. To measure the length of the hip adductor muscles, use a universal goniometer and measure the hip abduction PROM (Fig. 1-49B). This measurement serves an indirect measurement of hip adductor muscle length.

Two-Joint Muscle

To assess and measure the length of a two-joint muscle, position one of the joints crossed by the muscle so as to lengthen the muscle across the joint. Then move the second joint through a PROM until the muscle is placed on full stretch and prevents further joint motion. Assess and measure the final position of the second joint; the joint position represents an indirect measure of the muscle length.

Example: To assess and measure the length of the two-joint triceps muscle, place the shoulder in full elevation to stretch the triceps across the shoulder joint (Fig. 1-50A).

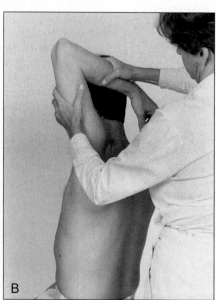
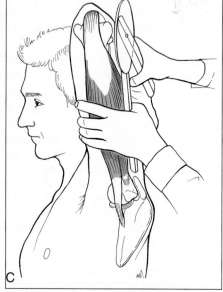
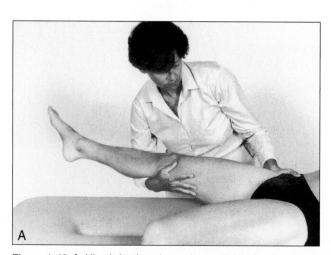

Figure 1-50 A. Start position: length of triceps, the muscle is stretched across the shoulder joint. **B.** The elbow is flexed to place triceps on full stretch. **C.** Goniometer measurement: length of the triceps as the muscle limits elbow flexion range of motion (ROM).

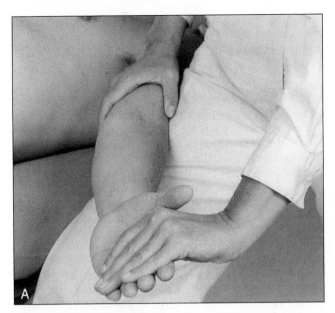

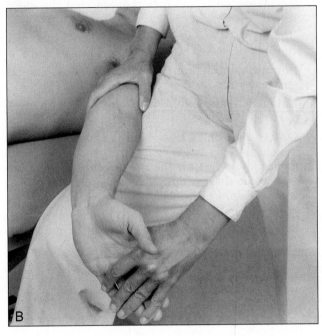

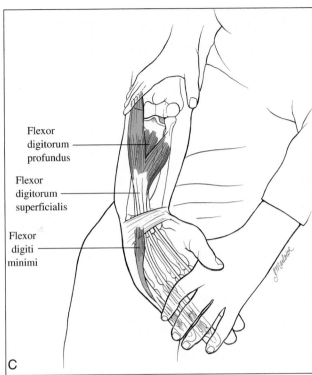

Figure 1-51 A. Start position: length of multi-joint finger flexors (i.e., flexor digitorum superficialis, flexor digitorum profundus, and flexor digit minimi). Elbow and finger joint extension places the muscles on stretch across these joints. **B.** The wrist is extended to place the finger flexors on full stretch. **C.** The therapist observes the passive range of motion (PROM) and assesses a firm end feel at the limit of wrist extension PROM.

Then flex the elbow to place triceps on full stretch (Fig. 1-50B). If the triceps muscle limits the motion, the end feel will be firm. The elbow flexion PROM measured using a universal goniometer (Fig. 1-50C) indirectly represents the triceps muscle length.

Multi-joint Muscle

To assess and measure the length of a multi-joint muscle, position all but one of the joints crossed by the muscle so that the muscle is lengthened across the joints. Then move the one remaining joint crossed by the muscle through a PROM, until the muscle is on full stretch and prevents further motion at the joint. Assess and measure the final position of the joint; the joint position represents an indirect measure of the muscle length.

Example: To assess and measure the length of the multi-joint finger flexor muscles, place the elbow and fingers in full extension to stretch the muscles across these joints (Fig. 1-51A). Extend the wrist to place the flexors on full stretch (Fig. 1-51B and C). The end feel will be firm if the finger flexors limit wrist extension PROM. The position of wrist extension PROM can be measured using a universal goniometer to indirectly represent the muscle length of the finger flexors.

MANUAL ASSESSMENT OF MUSCLE STRENGTH

Definition—Manual Muscle Testing

"Manual muscle testing is a procedure for the evaluation of the function and strength of individual muscles and muscle groups based on effective performance of a movement in relation to the forces of gravity and manual resistance."[63(p. 466)]

Manual muscle testing (MMT) can be used to assess most medical conditions but has limitations in the treatment of neurological disorders where there is an alteration in muscle tone if reflex activity is altered[64] or if there is a loss of cortical control due to lesions of the central nervous system.[65]

To assess muscle strength, a sound knowledge of anatomy (including joint motions, muscle origins and insertions, and muscle function) and surface anatomy (to know where a muscle or its tendon is best palpated) is required. Keen observation and experience in muscle testing is essential to detect muscle wasting, minimal muscle contraction, movement, and substitute movement. It is important to apply a consistent method of manually testing muscle strength to accurately assess a patient's present status, progress, and the effectiveness of the treatment program.

Muscle Testing Terminology

Muscle Strength

Strength is the maximal amount of tension or force that a muscle or muscle group can voluntarily exert in one maximal effort,[66] when type of muscle contraction, limb velocity, and joint angle are specified.[67] Use of the term muscle strength in the clinical setting actually represents torque.[68]

Torque

Torque (Fig. 1-52) is the tendency of a force (i.e., muscle tension, a therapist's pull or push, or gravity) to turn a lever (i.e., a limb or limb segment) around an axis of rotation (i.e., the joint axis of rotation) in either a clockwise (cw) or counterclockwise (ccw) direction. The magnitude of the torque (T) is the product of the force (F) and the perpendicular distance (d) between the axis of rotation and the force: $T = F \times d$. In Figure 1-52, the $T_{cw} = F_1 \times d_1$ and $T_{ccw} = F_2 \times d_2$.

Types of Muscle Contraction

- **Isometric (Static) Contraction.** An isometric contraction occurs when tension is developed in the muscle but no movement occurs, the origin and insertion of the muscle do not change position, and the muscle length does not change.[66]

  In Figure 1-52, when the $T_{ccw} = T_{cw}$ no movement occurs and the biceps muscle contracts isometrically.

- **Isotonic Contraction.** The muscle develops constant tension[69] against a load or resistance.

- **Isokinetic Contraction.** The muscle contracts at a constant rate of movement[70] or velocity.

- **Concentric Contraction.** Tension is developed in the muscle and the origin, and insertion of the muscle move closer together; the muscle shortens. In Figure 1-52, when the $T_{ccw} < T_{cw}$ the biceps contracts concentrically and the elbow flexes.

- **Eccentric Contraction.** Tension is developed in the muscle and the origin and insertion of the muscle move farther apart; the muscle lengthens.

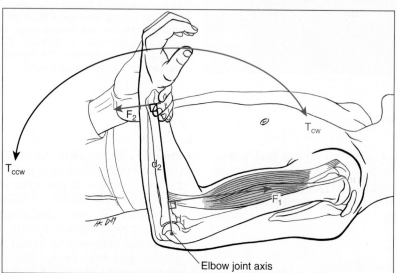

Figure 1-52 Manually assessing biceps muscle strength, the therapist applies a resistance force (F_2) at the distal end of the forearm (lever) that acts to turn the forearm around the elbow joint axis (axis of rotation), in a counterclockwise (T_{ccw}) direction to extend the elbow, and oppose the force of the biceps muscle contraction (F_1) that acts to turn the forearm (lever) in a clockwise (T_{cw}) direction around the elbow joint axis (axis of rotation) to flex the elbow.

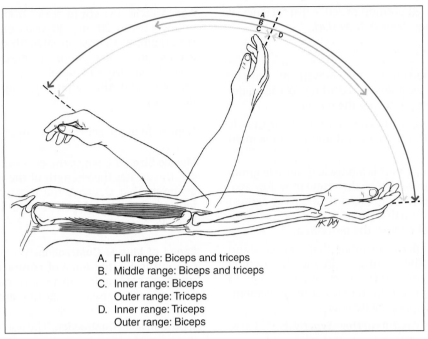

A. Full range: Biceps and triceps
B. Middle range: Biceps and triceps
C. Inner range: Biceps
   Outer range: Triceps
D. Inner range: Triceps
   Outer range: Biceps

Figure 1-53 Ranges of muscle work.

In Figure 1-52, when the $T_{ccw} > T_{cw}$ the biceps contracts eccentrically and the elbow slowly extends.

Muscle Endurance

Endurance is the ability of a muscle or a muscle group to perform repeated contractions, against a resistance, or maintain an isometric contraction for a period of time.[66]

Muscle Fatigue[16]

Fatigue is a diminished response of the muscle to generate force that may be due to a lack of energy stores or oxygen, a buildup of lactic acid, protective inhibitory influences from the central nervous system, or a decrease in conduction impulses at the myoneural junction.

Overwork[15]

Overwork is a phenomenon that causes a temporary or permanent loss of strength in already weakened muscle due to excessively vigorous activity or exercise relative to the patient's condition. Avoid fatigue or exhaustion in patients with certain neuromuscular diseases, or systemic, metabolic, or inflammatory disease that increase susceptibility to muscle fatigue. Patients with certain neuromuscular diseases are more susceptible to this condition because of their lack of the normal sensation of discomfort that accompanies fatigue and puts a natural stop to performance of the activity or exercise before damage occurs.

Ranges of Muscle Work[71]

The **full range** in which a muscle works refers to the muscle changing from a position of full stretch and contracting to a position of maximal shortening. The full range can be more precisely described if it is divided into parts: outer, inner, and middle ranges (Fig. 1-53).

- **Outer range** is from a position where the muscle is on full stretch to a position halfway through the full range.

- **Inner range** is from a position halfway through the full range to a position where the muscle is fully shortened.

- **Middle range** is the portion of the full range between the midpoint of the outer range and the midpoint of the inner range.

Employ this terminology to clearly convey the position(s) used to test muscle strength.

Active Insufficiency

The active insufficiency of a muscle that crosses two or more joints occurs when the muscle produces simultaneous movement at all of the joints it crosses and reaches such a shortened position that it no longer has the ability to develop effective tension (Fig. 1-54).[12] When a muscle

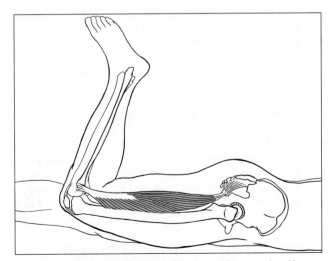

Figure 1-54 Active insufficiency of the hamstring muscles. Knee flexion performed with the hip in extension results in a shortening of the hamstring muscles that in turn decreases the ability of the hamstrings to develop tension.

is placed in a shortened position of active insufficiency, it is described as putting the *muscle on slack*.[72]

Functional Classification of Muscle

Muscles work in groups to produce movement. Muscles may be categorized as follows, according to the major role of the muscles in producing the movement.

- **Prime Mover or Agonist.** This is a muscle or muscle group that makes the major contribution to movement at the joint.

- **Antagonist.** An antagonist is a muscle or muscle group that has an opposite action to the prime mover or agonist. The antagonist either relaxes to allow the agonist to move the part through a ROM, or may contract concurrently to control or slow the movement.[73]

- **Synergist.** A synergist is a muscle that contracts and works along with the agonist to produce the desired movement. Synergists function in different ways to assist the prime mover to produce the movement. Three types of synergists are described.

  Neutralizing or Counteracting Synergists.[12] These are muscles that contract to prevent unwanted movements produced by the prime mover. For example, when the long finger flexors contract to produce finger flexion, the wrist extensors contract to prevent wrist flexion from occurring.

  Conjoint Synergists.[12] Conjoint synergists are two or more muscles that work together to produce the desired movement. The muscles contracting alone would be unable to produce the movement. For example, wrist extension is produced by contraction of extensor carpi radialis longus and brevis and extensor carpi ulnaris. If only the extensor carpi radialis longus and brevis contract, the wrist extends and radially deviates. If only the extensor carpi ulnaris contracts, the wrist extends and ulnar deviates. When the muscles contract as a group, the radial and ulnar deviation actions of the muscles cancel out and the common action of wrist extension results.

  Stabilizing or Fixating Synergists.[12] These muscles prevent movement or control the movement at joints proximal to the moving joint to provide a fixed or stable base from which the distal moving segment can effectively work. For example, if the elbow flexors contract to lift an object off a table anterior to the body, the muscles of the scapula and glenohumeral joint must contract to either allow slow controlled movement or no movement to occur at the scapula and glenohumeral joint, to provide the elbow flexors with a fixed origin from which to pull. If the scapular muscles do not contract, the object cannot be lifted because the elbow flexors would act to pull the shoulder girdle downward toward the table top.

Factors Affecting Strength

It is commonly recognized that a number of factors affect strength.[12,66,68,74,75] These factors must be considered when assessing a patient's strength.

Age. Muscle strength increases from birth to a maximum point between 20 and 30 years of age.[70] Following this maximum, a decrease in strength occurs with increasing age due to a deterioration in muscle mass. Muscle fibers decrease in size and number, connective tissue and fat increase, and the respiratory capacity of the muscle decreases.

Gender. Men are generally stronger than women.[76]

Muscle Size. The larger the cross-sectional area of a muscle, the greater the strength of the muscle. When testing a muscle that is small, the therapist would expect less tension to be developed than if testing a large, thick muscle.

Speed of Muscle Contraction. When a muscle contracts concentrically, the force of contraction decreases as the speed of contraction increases. Instruct the patient to perform each muscle test movement at a moderate pace.

Type of Muscle Contraction. The ability to develop tension in a muscle varies depending on the type of muscle contraction (Fig. 1-55). More tension can be developed during an eccentric contraction than during an isometric contraction. A concentric contraction has the smallest tension capability. When assessing strength, the same type of contraction should be used on successive tests.

Joint Position (Fig. 1-55): Angle of Muscle Pull and Length–Tension Relations

- **Angle of Muscle Pull.** When a muscle contracts, it creates a force and causes the body segment in which it inserts to rotate around a particular axis of the joint that the muscle crosses. The turning effect produced by the muscle is called the torque and is the product of the muscle force and the perpendicular distance between the joint axis of rotation and the muscle force (Fig. 1-52). The position of the joint affects the angle of pull of a muscle and therefore changes the perpendicular distance between the joint axis of rotation and the muscle force and the torque. The optimal angle of muscle pull occurs when the muscle is pulling at a 90° angle or perpendicular to the bony segment. At this point, all of the muscle force is acting to rotate the segment and no force is wasted acting as a distracting or stabilizing force on the limb segment.

- **Length–Tension Relations.** The tension developed within a muscle depends on the initial length of the muscle. Regardless of the type of muscle contraction, a muscle contracts with more force when it is stretched than when it is shortened. The greatest amount of tension is developed when the muscle is stretched to the greatest length possible within the body, that is, if the muscle is in full outer range. Tension decreases as the muscle shortens until the muscle reaches less than 50% of its rest length, at which point it is not able to develop tension. When testing the strength of a two-joint muscle the nontest joint position is important to note. For example, the knee flexors (hamstrings) are able to develop greater tension and

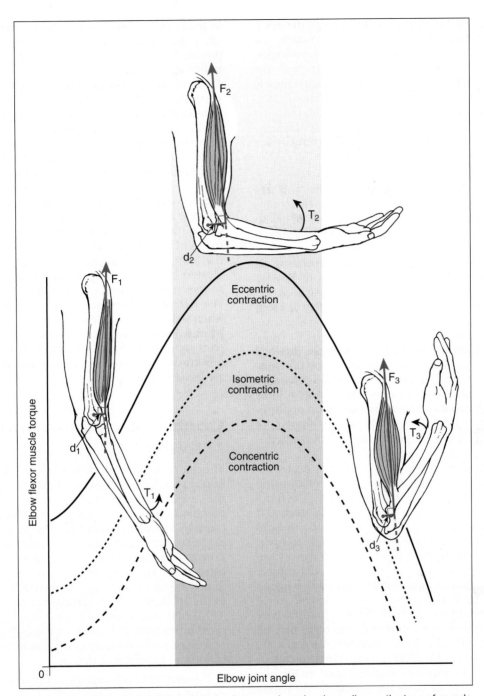

Figure 1-55 A. The ability to develop tension in a muscle varies depending on the type of muscle contraction, that is, eccentric > isometric > concentric. **B.** Changes in joint position change: muscle length that affects the ability of the muscle to develop force (*F*); and the angle of muscle pull that changes the perpendicular distance between the muscle force and the axis of joint rotation (*d*). The muscle torque (*T*) at different joint positions is determined by the interaction between changes in F and d.

demonstrate greater strength if the patient is tested in a position of hip flexion. This position places the muscles in a stretched position, as opposed to a position of hip extension, which places the muscles in a shortened position.

- **Angle of muscle pull and length–tension relations** interact to produce the muscle torque curve (Fig. 1-55). Most muscles demonstrate a decrease in force or strength from outer range into inner range, when

assessed using isometric contractions at different joint angles.[77] Not all strength curves illustrate a muscle developing maximal tension at the position of full stretch because the angle of pull of the muscle may be small at this point even though the muscle length is optimal for development of tension. Williams and Stutzman,[77] Kulig and coworkers,[78] and Williams and associates[79] give analyses of strength curves for different muscle groups. When testing muscle strength through range, strength patterns vary through the ROM; therefore, resistance must be varied to match the strength capability of the muscle at different joint angles, and enable the patient to move smoothly through the full ROM. When testing strength using isometric muscle contraction, if the muscle is tested in inner range, it may be graded much weaker than if tested in middle or outer ranges. When testing isometric strength, use the same joint position on successive tests to enable comparisons between tests to assess changes in strength.

Diurnal Variation[80,81]. Muscle strength is variable and this variability follows a regular cycle each day. Therefore, muscle strength should be assessed at the same time of day to accurately compare strength results and determine progress.

Temperature[82]. Strength of a muscle varies depending on the temperature of the muscle at the time of testing. Strength should be assessed when the muscle is at the same temperature on successive tests, preferably at room temperature.

Previous Training Effect. Strength performance depends on the ability of the nervous system to activate the muscle mass. Strength may increase as one becomes familiar with and learns the test situation. The therapist must instruct the patient well and give the patient an opportunity to move through or be passively moved through the test movement at least once before strength is assessed.

Fatigue. As the patient tires, muscle strength decreases. The therapist determines the strength of the muscle using as few repetitions as possible to avoid fatigue. The functional capability of a muscle is more accurately assessed if endurance is also considered when testing the muscle. After the therapist has determined the muscle strength, the patient remains in the test position and repeats the test movement against the same resistance the muscle was able to move according to the strength grade assigned to the muscle until the patient can no longer move through the ROM, that is, drops to the next lowest whole grade. The number of repetitions until this point may be recorded as a clinical indicator of endurance. Alternatively, the therapist may complete the muscle testing and then repeat only those movements requiring good endurance for ADL. The number of times the patient would repeat the movement in specific activities is an indicator of functional requirements.

The patient's level of motivation, level of pain, body type, occupation, and dominance are other factors that may affect strength. Consider the factors that affect strength to select the most appropriate method to use for the strength assessment and ensure consistency of application when performing MMT.

Joint Positions

Close-Packed Position. When a joint is in the close-packed position, the joint surfaces are fully congruent.[20]

In the close-packed position, there is maximal tension in the joint capsule and ligaments; the joint surfaces are pressed together firmly and the joint surfaces cannot be pulled apart using traction.[20]

Avoid the close-packed position when testing muscle strength. The patient can lock the joint and hold the joint in this position against resistance in the presence of a weak prime mover, resulting in an inaccurate assessment of muscle strength. Be especially careful of this positioning at the elbow, knee, and ankle joints. Close-packed joint positions are listed in Table 1-5.

Loose-Packed Position. The loose-packed position is any position of a joint other than the close-packed position, where the joint surfaces are not congruent and parts of the joint capsule are lax.[13] The position of least stress on the joint,[20] least congruency of joint surfaces, and the greatest laxity of the capsule and ligaments is the *resting position* or maximum loose-packed position of the joint.[13] The resting position may be used to prevent joint pain when testing isometric muscle strength in the region of a painful joint because of the decreased tension on the joint capsule and ligaments and decreased intra-articular pressure provided by this position. Resting joint positions are listed in Table 1-5.

Contraindications and Precautions

Muscle strength must not be assessed if any contraindications to this form of assessment exist. In special instances, the assessment techniques must be carried out with a modified approach. The same contraindications and precautions for assessing AROM or PROM apply when manually assessing muscle strength. Additional contraindications and precautions when assessing muscle strength are listed here. The contraindications and precautions presented are based on those described by Kisner and Colby[16] in the application of resistance exercise.

Manual assessment of muscle strength is contraindicated if this form of assessment could disrupt the healing process or result in injury or deterioration of the patient's condition. Examples of this are:

1. If inflammation is present in the region.
2. In the presence of inflammatory neuromuscular disease (e.g., Guillain-Barre, polymyositis, dermatomyositis).
3. For patients with severe cardiac or respiratory disease or disorders associated with acute symptoms.
4. In the presence of pain. Pain will inhibit muscle contraction and will not give an accurate indication of muscle strength. Testing muscle strength in the presence of pain may cause further injury.

Extra care must be taken where resisted movements might aggravate the condition, such as:

1. Following neurosurgery[16] or recent surgery of the abdomen, intervertebral disc, or eye[84]; in patients with intervertebral disc pathology,[16] or herniation of the

TABLE 1-5 Close-Packed and Loose-Packed Positions of Selected Joints[4,13,20,83]

Joint(s)	Close-Packed Position	Loose-Packed (Resting) Position
Facet (spine)	Extension	Midway between flexion and extension
Temporomandibular	Clenched teeth	Mouth slightly open
Glenohumeral (shoulder)	Abduction and external rotation	55°–70° abduction, 30° horizontal adduction, rotated so that the forearm is in the transverse plane
Acromioclavicular	Arm abducted to 90°	Arm resting by side, shoulder girdle in the physiological position*
Sternoclavicular	Maximum shoulder elevation	Arm resting by side, shoulder girdle in the physiological position*
Ulnohumeral (elbow)	Extension	70° elbow flexion, 10° forearm supination
Radiohumeral	Elbow flexed 90°, forearm supinated 5°	Full extension, full supination
Proximal radioulnar	5° supination	70° elbow flexion, 35° forearm supination
Distal radioulnar	5° supination	10° forearm supination
Radiocarpal (wrist)	Extension with radial deviation	Midway between flexion-extension (so that a straight line passes through the radius and third metacarpal) with slight ulnar deviation
Trapeziometacarpal	Full opposition	Midway between abduction-adduction and flexion-extension
Metacarpophalangeal (thumb)	Full opposition	Slight flexion
Metacarpophalangeal (fingers)	Full flexion	Slight flexion with slight ulnar deviation
Interphalangeal	Full extension	Slight flexion
Hip	Full extension, internal rotation and abduction	30° flexion, 30° abduction, and slight external rotation
Knee	Full extension and external rotation of the tibia	25° flexion
Talocrural (ankle)	Maximum dorsiflexion	10° plantarflexion, midway between maximum inversion and eversion
Subtalar	Full supination	Midway between extremes of inversion and eversion
Midtarsal	Full supination	Midway between extremes of ROM
Tarsometatarsal	Full supination	Midway between extremes of ROM
Metatarsophalangeal	Full extension	Neutral
Interphalangeal	Full extension	Slight flexion

*Physiological position[13] is the term given to the resting position of the shoulder girdle. The scapula is situated over the ribs two through seven and the vertebral border is 5 cm lateral to the spinous processes; the clavicle lies nearly in the horizontal plane. In the physiological position imaginary lines drawn through the long axis of the clavicle, along the plane of the scapula and along the midsagittal plane form the sides of an equilateral triangle having angles of 60°.

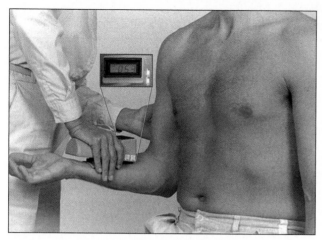

Figure 1-56 Isometric elbow flexor muscle strength assessment using a hand-held dynamometer (HHD) (i.e., the Nicholas Manual Muscle Tester). The digital display indicates the applied force (*inset*). If the patient is stronger than the therapist, the HHD measures the therapist's strength.

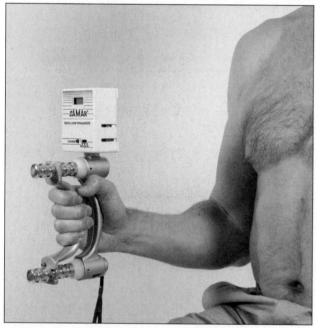

Figure 1-57 JAMAR hand grip dynamometer.

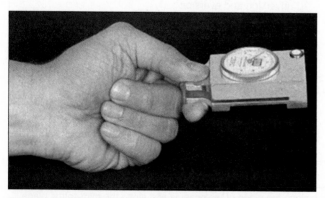

Figure 1-58 Lateral pinch strength measured using a pinch dynamometer.

abdominal wall; or in patients with a history of cardiovascular problems (e.g., aneurysm, fixed-rate pacemaker, arrhythmias, thrombophlebitis, recent embolus, marked obesity, hypertension, cardiopulmonary disease, angina pectoris, myocardial infarctions, and cerebrovascular disorders). Instruct these patients to avoid the *Valsalva maneuver* during the strength testing procedure.

Kisner and Colby[16] describe the sequence of events in the Valsalva maneuver, which consists of an expiratory effort against a closed glottis during a strenuous and prolonged effort. A deep breath is taken at the beginning of the effort and held by closing the glottis. The abdominal muscles contract, causing an increase in the intra-abdominal and intrathoracic pressures, and blood is forced from the heart, causing a temporary and abrupt rise in the arterial blood pressure. The abdominal muscle contraction may also put unsafe stress on the abdominal wall.

The Valsalva maneuver can be avoided by instructing the patient not to hold his or her breath during the assessment of AROM. Should this be difficult, instruct the patient to breathe out[17] or talk during the test.[16]

2. In situations in which fatigue may be detrimental to or exacerbate the patient's condition (e.g., extreme debility, malnutrition, malignancy, chronic obstructive pulmonary disease, cardiovascular disease, multiple sclerosis, poliomyelitis, postpoliomyelitis syndrome, myasthenia gravis, lower motor neuron disease, and intermittent claudication), strenuous testing should not be carried out. Signs of fatigue include complaints or observation of tiredness, pain, muscular spasm, a slow response to contraction, tremor, and a decreased ability to perform AROM.

3. In situations where overwork may be detrimental to the patient's condition (e.g., patients with certain neuromuscular diseases or systemic, metabolic, or inflammatory disease), care should be used to avoid fatigue or exhaustion.

Instrumentation

The instrument chosen to assess muscle strength depends on the degree of accuracy required in the measurement and the time and resources available to the clinician. The hand-held dynamometer (HHD) (Fig. 1-56), free weights, the use of the cable tensiometer, the handgrip dynamometer (Fig. 1-57), the pinch gauge (Fig. 1-58), or isokinetic dynamometers may give objective, valid, and reliable measures of muscle strength but are not always practical in the clinical environment. Instrumented means of assessing muscle strength have been in existence for many years and have "their own issues that await resolution."[85(p. 5)] Although MMT has issues too, it has still not been superseded by instruments. MMT remains the most practical method of assessing muscle strength in the clinical setting. When doing clinical research, the therapist is encouraged to investigate alternate instruments that will offer a more stringent assessment of muscle strength.

MMT Methods of Assessing Muscle Strength

Conventional and alternate methodologies of assessing and grading muscle strength are described in this text. Regardless of the method used when manually assessing muscle strength, a grade is assigned to indicate the strength of a muscle or muscle group. In conventional grading and some alternate grading methods, the grade indicates the strength of a voluntary muscle contraction and the AROM possible within the available PROM, previously assessed.

All methods of assessing muscle strength described are based on the principles of muscle testing that have evolved clinically over time. Lovett (cited in Daniels and Worthingham)[86] developed the concept of using gravity as a factor to assess the strength of a muscle. Wright[87] was the first to publish a method of classifying muscles according to the ability of the muscle to overcome the resistance of gravity or friction. Further developments have been documented by others including Brunnstrom,[88] Smith and colleagues,[89] Hines,[90] Daniels and Worthingham,[86] and Kendall and Kendall.[91]

Conventional Method

Manual grading of muscle strength is based on three factors[86]:

1. Evidence of contraction:
   - No palpable or observable muscle contraction (grade 0)
   - A palpable or observable muscle contraction and no joint motion (grade 1)
2. Gravity as a resistance—ability to move the part through the full available ROM:
   - Gravity eliminated (grade 2)
   - Against gravity (grade 3)
3. Amount of manual resistance—ability to move the part through the full available ROM against gravity and against:
   - Moderate manual resistance (grade 4)
   - Maximal manual resistance (grade 5).

In addition to the whole grades 0–5, more detailed grading of muscle strength is achieved by adding a plus or minus to the whole grade to denote variation in the ROM or the ability to move against minimal resistance. Numerals or letters are used to indicate grades of muscle strength. The numerical notation is not a precise graded quantitative determination of muscle strength.[64] Table 1-6 gives a description of each grade.

Beasley[92] found that a grade of 3 (fair) does not necessarily indicate 50% of the normal strength of the muscle or muscle group tested when compared with a standard normal reference. A grade of 3 is well below the 50% mark varying from being approximately 9% for some muscles and slightly greater than 30% for other muscles tested in the study. Therefore, there is a greater range between the grades of 3 and 5 (normal) than between the grades of 3 and 0.

Validity and Reliability

Validity

The therapist uses MMT to provide information about muscle strength, that is, the maximal amount of tension or force that a muscle or muscle group can voluntarily exert in one maximal effort.[66] Measurements must be accurate because the results, taken to be valid representations of muscle strength, are used to make a diagnosis, assess patient prognosis, plan treatment, determine treatment effectiveness, and evaluate functional status. There is a lack of evidence to demonstrate the validity of MMT. However, in an effort to establish criterion-related validity, MMT results have been compared to the measures obtained with HHD.[93–96] The close relationship between the measures obtained with MMT and the HHD measures suggest that muscle strength is measured by both techniques.

From the clinician's judgment, MMT seems to measure the torque-producing capability of the tested muscle(s)[97] and thus MMT appears to have content validity.

Reliability

It is important for the therapist to know that muscle strength can be evaluated consistently, so that results taken over time can be compared to evaluate treatment effectiveness and patient progress. If this is possible, then in comparing measures the similarity or difference between the measures can be relied on to indicate a true change in strength due to treatment or over time, and are not simply due to measurement error and lack of measurement consistency.

Most studies assessing the reliability of MMT are based on the use of isometric make or break testing techniques. Using a standardized procedure for testing, reliability of interrater MMT results with complete agreement of muscle grades is low.[98,99] Interrater and intrarater reliability within the range of one whole muscle grade[99–102] and interrater reliability within one half a grade (i.e., within a + or − grade)[94,98] is very high. Although this indicates a high level of consistency for MMT, a difference of one whole strength grade may not be adequate for clinical decision-making.[101]

Reliability and validity study results for MMT indicate the following:

1. Intratester reliability is better than intertester reliability; therefore, the same therapist should perform all MMTs when possible.[100,102,103]
2. MMT grading is limited by the strength of the examiner, especially in very strong patients when assessing grades of 5.[104]
3. MMT is not sensitive to strength changes in the higher grades of 4 and 5.[92,94–96,105,106]

TABLE 1-6 **Conventional Grading**

Numerals	Letters	Description
Against Gravity Tests		**The Patient is Able to Actively Move Through:**
5	N (normal)	The full available ROM against gravity and against maximal resistance
4	G (good)	The full available ROM against gravity and against moderate resistance
4–	G–	*If testing "through range"; grade n/a if testing "isometrically":* Greater than one half the available ROM against gravity and against moderate resistance
3+	F+	*If testing "through range":* Less than one half the available ROM against gravity and against moderate resistance *If testing "isometrically":* The full available ROM against gravity and against minimal resistance
3	F (fair)	The full available ROM against gravity
3–	F–	Greater than one half the available ROM against gravity
2+	P+	Less than one half the available ROM against gravity
Gravity Eliminated Tests		**The Patient is Able to Actively Move Through:**
2	P (poor)	The full available ROM gravity eliminated
2–	P–	Less than the full available ROM gravity eliminated
1	T (trace)	None of the available ROM gravity eliminated and there is a palpable or observable flicker of a muscle contraction
0	0 (zero)	None of the available ROM gravity eliminated and there is no palpable or observable muscle contraction

Note: When the patient cannot be positioned as required relative to gravity, or it is too tiring for the patient or too time consuming to change the patient's position, the therapist offers either assistance or resistance equal to the weight of the limb or limb segment to resemble the gravity eliminated situation or against gravity situation, respectively.

4. MMT scores tend to overestimate the patient's strength in the higher grades of 4 and 5.[92,94,104,107]

5. MMT scores are most sensitive in lower grades 0 to 3.[108]

6. It is suggested that MMT be supplemented with quantitative means of assessing strength (e.g., hand-held dynamometry, isokinetic dynamometry, and tensiometry) for grades that are greater than 3 and more subjective in nature.[101,105]

7. MMT grades are not equivalent to linear measurements,[98,109] for example, a grade 3 does not equal 50% muscle strength. Similarly, normal strength does not equal 100% strength and varies depending on the muscle group tested, for example, a grade 5 for the knee extensors equals 53%, the plantarflexors equals 34%, and the hip extensors equals 65% of the actual maximal strength of each muscle group.[92] It is estimated only 4% of the maximum strength of the elbow flexors represents a grade of 3.[110]

8. Training, practice, experience, and the use of strict standardized procedure are important for reliable MMT.[111]

To increase the reliability of the assessment of muscle strength, the MMT should be conducted:

• At the same time of day to avoid varying levels of fatigue.

• By the same therapist.

• In the same environment.

• Using the same patient position.

• Following a standard testing protocol, to allow for more accurate comparisons between tests and assessment of the patient's progress.

MMT is a convenient, versatile, quick to apply, and inexpensive means of assessing muscle strength. In weaker patients, it is not possible to use equipment such as an isokinetic testing device[112,113] or HHD[105,114] for testing lower grades (i.e., <3). Using MMT, specific stabilization, isolated testing of single muscle actions, and elimination of substitute action and movement are possible.

In the clinical setting, MMT is a common means of assessing strength. Although the validity and reliability of MMT appear to be less than ideal and further research is needed, there is merit in using MMT if the limitations are kept in mind.

Manual Assessment of Muscle Strength

Following the visual observation and assessment of AROM and PROM, perform the assessment of muscle strength.

Individual Versus Group Muscle Test

Muscles with a common action or actions are often tested as a group or a muscle is tested individually. For example, flexor carpi ulnaris and flexor carpi radialis are tested together as a group in the action of wrist flexion. Flexor carpi ulnaris is individually tested as the muscle contracts to simultaneously flex and ulnar deviate the wrist. Although it is not always possible to isolate a muscle completely, individual muscle tests are illustrated and described in this text.

Explanation and Instruction

• Briefly explain the manual muscle test assessment procedure to the patient.
• Explain and demonstrate the movement to be performed and/or passively move the patient's limb through the test movement.

Assessment of Normal Muscle Strength

• Initially assess and record the strength of the uninvolved limb to determine the patient's normal strength (i.e., grade 5) and to demonstrate the movement before assessing the strength of the involved side.
• If the contralateral limb cannot be used for comparison, rely on past experience to judge the patient's normal strength considering the factors that affect strength, such as the patient's age, gender, dominance, and occupation.

Assessment and Measurement Procedure

Patient Position

• Position the patient to isolate the muscle or muscle group to be tested in either a gravity eliminated or against gravity position.[115]
• Ensure the patient is comfortable and adequately supported.
• Place the muscle or muscle group being tested in full outer range, with only slight tension being placed on the muscle when testing strength through range. To test strength isometrically, place the muscle or muscle group being tested in the appropriate test position.

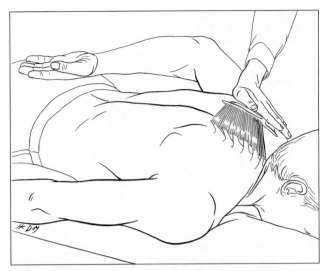

Figure 1-59 The weight of the trunk on the plinth serves to stabilize the spinal origins of the rhomboid muscles.

• When assessing muscle strength, "good control and specificity of body positions chosen during testing is essential to produce valid strength estimates."[116(p. 509)]

Stabilization. Stabilize the site of attachment of the origin of the muscle so that the muscle has a fixed point from which to pull. When testing a two- or multi-joint muscle, stabilize or fix the segment proximal to the joint where movement occurs to test the muscle action. Prevent substitute movements by making use of the following methods of stabilization:

1. The patient's body weight—use to help fix the shoulder girdle, pelvic girdle or trunk.
   Example:
   The weight of the trunk on the plinth serves to stabilize the spinal origin of the rhomboid muscles (Fig. 1-59).

2. The patient's normal muscles—have the patient use muscles that
   • would normally act as stabilizing or fixating synergists for the movement,
   Example:
   When strength testing the rhomboid muscles, instruct the patient to maintain an upright sitting position as the hand is moved directly off the contralateral buttock (Fig. 1-60).
   • are not normally used to perform the test movement,
   Example:
   • Instruct the patient to hold the edge of the plinth when the hip is flexed to assess the strength of the hip flexors (Fig. 1-61).

3. The patient's position:
   Example:
   When assessing hip abductor muscle strength in the side-lying position, instruct the patient to hold the nontest leg in maximal hip and knee flexion (Fig. 1-62). In this position, the posterior tilt of the pelvis acts to stabilize the pelvis and lumbar spine.

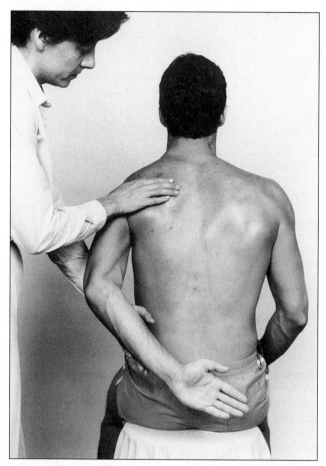

Figure 1-60 The patient contracts the trunk muscles to maintain the upright sitting position and stabilize the trunk when rhomboid muscle strength is tested.

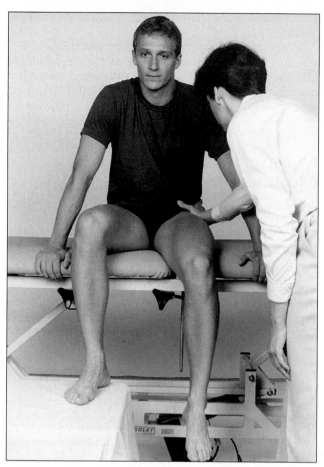

Figure 1-61 The patient holds the edge of the plinth to stabilize the spine and pelvis when the strength of the hip flexors is tested.

Example:

To assess the strength of the hip extensors (Fig. 1-63), instruct the patient to rest the weight of the trunk on the plinth, grasp the edge of the plinth, and position the contralateral hip in flexion with the foot flat on the floor. In this position, the pelvis and lumbar spine are stabilized.

4. External forces:

• Manually apply direct pressure

Example:

The radius and ulna are stabilized by the therapist when testing the wrist extensors (Fig. 1-64).

• Use devices such as belts and sandbags

Example:

A strap is used to stabilize the pelvis when testing the hip extensors (Fig. 1-65).

In stabilizing, ensure that manual contacts or devices avoid tender or painful regions; for example, in some viral diseases (i.e., poliomyelitis) muscle bellies may be tender. Ensure that manual contacts or devices do not exert too much force directly over the belly of the muscle being tested and inhibit contraction.[117]

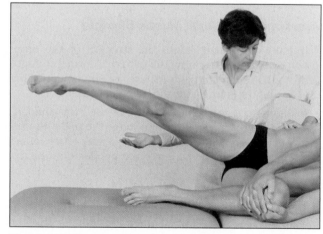

Figure 1-62 The patient holds the nontest leg in maximal hip and knee flexion to stabilize the pelvis, i.e., the origin of the hip abductor muscles.

Substitute Movements. When muscles are weak or paralyzed, other muscles may take over or gravity may be used to perform the movements normally carried out by the weak muscles.[118] These vicarious motions are called substitute movements.[72] The different types of substitute movements are listed below and are primarily based on

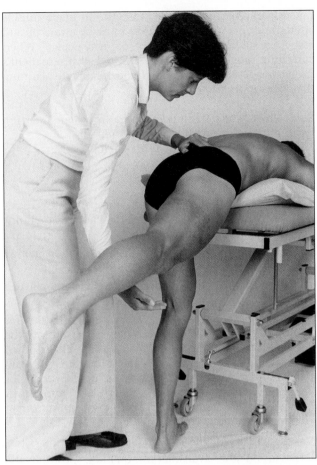

Figure 1-63 To assess the strength of the hip extensors, the patient is instructed to rest the weight of the trunk on the plinth, grasp the edge of the plinth, and position the contralateral hip in flexion and place the foot flat on the floor. In this position, the pelvis and lumbar spine and muscle origins are stabilized.

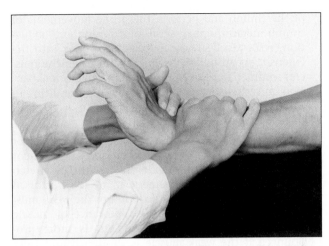

Figure 1-64 The therapist manually stabilizes the radius and ulna to assess wrist extensor muscle strength.

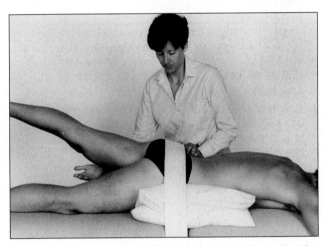

Figure 1-65 The pelvis is stabilized using a strap when testing the hip extensors.

the substitute movements described by Kendall and colleagues[72] and Wynn Parry.[118]

1. Direct or indirect substitution by:

   a. Another prime mover that may also result in deviation in the direction of the other actions performed by the substitute prime mover.

   Example:

   With weakness or absence of supinator, biceps brachii can contract to perform supination and elbow flexion may occur simultaneously.

   b. The fixator muscles producing movement that appears to have occurred through the site of origin of the weak agonist.

   Example:

   The lateral abdominals will contract to stabilize the pelvis during testing of the hip abductor muscles. If the hip abductors are weak, the lateral abdominals may elevate the pelvis and in turn move the lower extremity to give the appearance of hip abduction.

   c. Other favorably placed muscles in the region that may contract to position the joint so that other muscles by virtue of the new joint position can perform the test motion.

   Example:

   If the deltoid muscle is paralyzed, the external rotators externally rotate the humerus so that the long head of biceps brachii is positioned more laterally with respect to the shoulder joint, and is in a position to assist with shoulder abduction.

   d. Other muscles in the total limb pattern that may contract in an attempt to assist the weak muscles.

   Example:

   The shoulder flexes when the patient attempts to flex the elbow in the presence of elbow flexor muscle weakness.

2. Accessory insertion—The insertion of a muscle may be such that when the muscle contracts, it helps to perform the prime movement of the weak or paralyzed muscle.

   Example:

   The flexor pollicis brevis and abductor pollicis brevis muscles insert into the base of the proximal phalanx of the thumb and perform the prime movements of thumb metacarpophalangeal joint flexion and abduction, respectively. These muscles also insert into the extensor expansion of the thumb and when the muscles contract, tension is created on the extensor expansion and extensor pollicis longus tendon, resulting in extension of the thumb in the presence of extensor pollicis longus muscle paralysis.

3. Tendon action—When the antagonist to a weak or paralyzed muscle contracts, it produces movement that places the weaker muscle on stretch. The stretch will produce passive movement at the joints crossed by the weak muscle in the direction of the weak muscle's prime action, giving the appearance of muscle contraction. This passive movement is more pronounced if the weak muscle is shortened and lacks normal extensibility.

Example:

In the presence of flexor digitorum superficialis and profundus muscle paralysis, if the extensors of the wrist contract to produce wrist extension, the finger flexors are placed on stretch. The stretch on the finger flexors results in passive flexion of the fingers giving the appearance of contraction of the long finger flexors.

4. Rebound phenomenon—When an antagonist to a weak or paralyzed muscle contracts and then relaxes quickly, it will produce passive movement in the direction of the prime movement of the weak muscle. This gives the appearance of contraction of the weak muscle.

Example:

The interphalangeal joint of the thumb is positioned in extension to test the strength of the flexor pollicis longus muscle. In this position, the extensor pollicis longus may contract to pull the interphalangeal joint into further extension and then quickly relax. This sudden relaxation results in slight passive flexion of the interphalangeal joint that could be mistaken for movement performed by contraction of the flexor pollicis longus.

5. Gravity—The patient may shift the body part so that gravity may be used to perform the movement of the weak or paralyzed muscle.

Example:

In sitting with the shoulder abducted 90°, elbow flexed, and the upper limb resting on a table, the patient with a weak or paralyzed triceps may not be able to extend the elbow and move the forearm along the table top. The patient may attempt to extend the elbow by performing shoulder girdle depression and shoulder external rotation to position the forearm so that gravity assists the weak triceps.

Try to eliminate substitute movements through adequate explanation and instruction to the patient of the movement to be performed and the substitute movements that must be avoided, proper patient positioning, adequate stabilization of the muscle origin, palpation of the muscle(s) being tested to ensure contraction, and

practice in assessing muscle strength. To grade muscle strength accurately, the therapist must be aware of and recognize substitute movements that may occur.[99] When substitute movements are not recognized, the patient's problem will not be identified and treatment planning may be inappropriate.

Screen Test. A screen test is an arbitrarily assigned starting point in the assessment of muscle strength.

Use the screen test to perform the following:

- Streamline the muscle strength assessment.
- Avoid unnecessary testing.
- Avoid fatiguing or discouraging the patient by eliminating as many tests as possible the patient would not be able to successfully complete.

Screen the patient through the information gained from the following:

- Reading the patient's chart or previous muscle test results.
- Observing the patient perform functional activities; for example, shaking the patient's hand may indicate the strength of grasp (i.e., the finger flexors), sitting down and standing up may indicate lower limb strength, taking a shirt off overhead may indicate shoulder abductor and external rotator muscle strength, and lying down or getting up from lying may give an indication of abdominal muscle strength.
- Previous assessment of the patient's AROM.

Based on the available information, position the patient so that the assessment of strength begins at or near the patient's actual level of strength. Alternatively, screen the patient by:

- Beginning all muscle testing at a particular grade; this is usually a grade of 3. Instruct the patient to actively move the body part through the full ROM against gravity. Based on the results of the initial test, the muscle test is either stopped or it proceeds.

Grading Muscle Strength

Against Gravity

In the following chapters, the grade of 3 is normally used as the screen test to begin the illustration of MMT (Fig. 1-66A and B). To assess whether the muscle is at, below, or above a grade 3, position the patient so that the muscle is positioned in full outer range and gravity resists the prime movement(s) of the muscle or muscle group through as much of the ROM as possible. In most cases, it is not possible to move against gravity through the entire ROM as the bone moves from a horizontal to a vertical position or a vertical to a horizontal position. Therefore, the muscle has either little resistance from the pull of gravity at the start or end of motion, or the muscle has no resistance at the end of motion when gravity assists the movement and the antagonist contracts eccentrically to complete the ROM.[119]

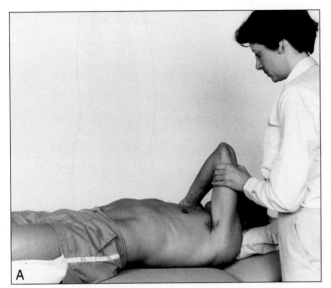

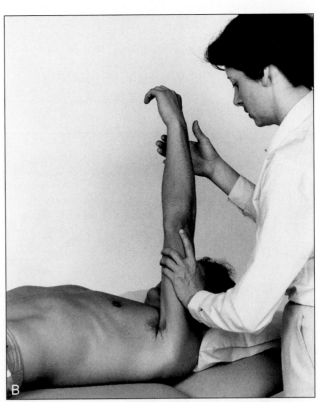

Figure 1-66 A. Manual muscle testing (MMT) start position **against gravity:** elbow extensors – triceps. **B.** Patient attempts to perform elbow extension against gravity. If a grade of 2+ or 3– is assigned, the MMT stops. If a grade 3 is assigned, repeat the test and apply manual resistance (Fig. 1-67). If unable to move against gravity, reposition the patient and test the movement gravity eliminated (Fig. 1-70).

The muscle force exerted during the muscle test can be influenced to a great extent by the instructions given to the patient.[69,120] The volume of the therapist's voice can influence voluntary muscle contraction. High-volume commands can elicit a stronger muscle contraction than low-volume commands.[121,122] During each test, give commands explicitly and consistently to elicit the strongest possible response from the patient. As the patient attempts to move at a moderate pace through the ROM, palpate the prime mover(s) to ensure contraction and rule out the possibility of substitute movements.

- If the patient moves through only part of the ROM against gravity, the muscle is given a grade of 2+ or 3– and this ends the muscle test.

- If the patient moves through the full ROM against gravity, the test is repeated against manual resistance to determine the grade (Fig. 1-67A and B). The grade of 3 is given if the patient cannot perform the test against manual resistance.

- If the patient can perform the test against manual resistance, a grade of greater than 3 is assigned depending on the magnitude of the resistance applied.

The patient is asked to relax at the end of each test movement and the therapist positions the limb for the next test movement.

Manual Resistance

To apply resistance, use a lumbrical grip, in which the metacarpophalangeal joints are flexed with the interpha-langeal joints held in extension and the thumb either adducted or relaxed in slight extension (Fig. 1-68). Add resistance gradually to allow the patient to "set" the muscles. Apply the resistance force at a 90° angle to the limb segment.

Apply the resistance force at the distal end of the segment into which the muscle(s) being tested is (are) inserted[11,85] (Fig. 1-69). Allowing a joint to come between the point of application of the resistance and the muscle insertion may increase the chance of substitution. Ensure resistance is not given distal to an unstable or weakly supported joint. Every attempt should be made to keep the length of the resistance arm (i.e., the distance between the axis of rotation of the joint and the point of application of the manual resistance) standard for each muscle test. *Note:* The longer the length of the resistance arm, the less the resistance force required to counteract the torque produced by the muscle.

Nicholas and coworkers[123] report that if the therapist gives an equal or greater resistance to the limb when testing muscle A but for a shorter period of time than when testing muscle B, it is possible that muscle A could be assessed as being weaker than muscle B. When applying resistance to test a muscle, the therapist mentally integrates the time taken to go through the ROM with the magnitude of the resistance force to arrive at a perception of the strength deficit and assign a grade.[123] Because of this and the force-velocity relationships, when performing comparable muscle tests, apply resistance over the same length of time, and if assessing muscle strength

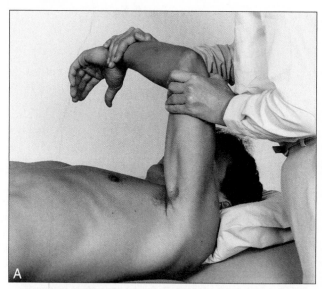

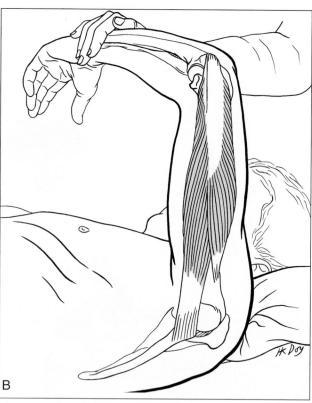

Figure 1-67 MMT elbow extensors – triceps. **A.** With the patient positioned against gravity apply **manual resistance** either through range, or isometrically, and grade the strength. **B.** Manual resistance is applied at the distal end of the segment the muscle inserts into, that is, the distal end of the radius and ulna.

through range, use the same velocity of movement to go through the ROM.

Resistance Applied to Test Strength "Through Range". When assessing muscle strength using concentric muscle contraction, the magnitude of the resistance force is based on the amount of resistance that can be applied and allow the patient to move smoothly through the full

ROM. The resistance force applied throughout the movement "should be just a little less than would stop the movement."[87(p. 568)] Modify the amount of resistance given throughout the ROM according to the patient's capabilities. If too much resistance is given, the patient will not be able to move through the ROM and this may lead to recruitment of other muscles to perform the movement.

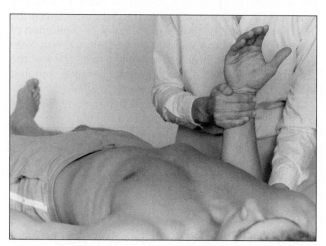

Figure 1-68 Manual resistance applied at a 90° angle to the limb segment using a lumbrical grip.

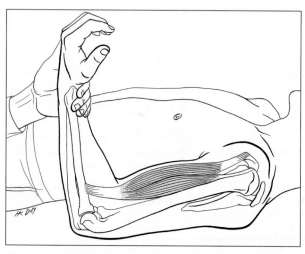

Figure 1-69 Apply manual resistance at the distal end of the segment the muscle(s) inserts into.

Testing strength through range requires considerable skill and experience.[85] For this reason, the results of testing strength through range may not be as certain as when performing MMT using isometric muscle contraction in selected part(s) of the ROM,[85] as is more commonly practiced now. This being said, it behooves the therapist to acquire the skill and experience to competently test strength through range. The most appropriate means of testing strength, either through range or at a selected joint position(s), is used based on the specific clinical requirement.

It may be advantageous to test muscle strength through range, for example, "to obtain a more specific clinical picture of a peripheral nerve lesion and its course of motor recovery".[103(p. 666)] When grading muscle strength, the ability of the patient to move through part or all of the ROM is more easily quantified than changes in the magnitude of the applied manual resistance.[96]

Resistance Applied to Test Strength "Isometrically" At Specific Joint Angles. When using isometric muscle contractions to test muscle strength, the strength needed to hold the test position is considered to be the same as the relative strength needed to move through the test movement,[11] although Wilson and Murphy[124] note, there is no research to suggest that force measured at any one point in the ROM is representative of muscle force throughout the entire movement. Strength varies throughout the ROM and a more accurate picture of the muscle's capabilities is attained if isometric muscle tests are performed with the muscle positioned in inner, middle, and outer ranges or better yet, the muscle test is performed through the ROM.

Koo and coworkers[125] studied the elbow muscle weakness of hemiplegic subjects using isometric testing. The study findings support the need to evaluate isometric muscle strength in multiple joint positions throughout range to provide a complete assessment of muscle weakness from a clinical and functional perspective.

To maintain reliability in testing when using isometric muscle contraction, the muscle should be tested in the same part(s) of the ROM each time.[86] Isometric testing is an accepted clinical method of assessing muscle strength,[126] but predicting dynamic work capabilities from isometric tests is generally not reliable.[69,124] Dynamic tests are superior to isometric tests in their relationship to dynamic activities.[124] It would be more appropriate to test a muscle or muscle group taking its normal function into account; that is, using isometric testing for muscles that function as stabilizers, such as the scapular muscles.

When using isometric contraction to grade muscle strength that is greater than a grade 3, the therapist positions the limb segment so the muscle will contract in either outer, middle, or inner range against gravity and then gradually takes away any support as the patient attempts to hold the position. Alternatively, the patient actively moves the limb segment into outer, middle, or inner range for the muscle being assessed. The position illustrated for most muscle tests in this textbook is inner range, as this position is often the weakest part of the range.

If the limb segment is held in the start position against gravity, the therapist gradually applies resistance and performs either of the following:

- *Make test*[127] in which the resistance must not "break" the muscle contraction so that the patient cannot hold the position.
- *Break test* in which the therapist gradually decreases the resistance as the limb segment is felt to fall toward the muscle's outer range. If the strength is considered to be a grade 5 or normal, the make test is used, and no effort is made to break the subject's hold.[11]

The break test is the most commonly used technique. Using either test method, the therapist has the patient maintain the contraction for about 4 seconds to allow time to establish a maximal isometric contraction.[128] The muscle is graded based on the maximal amount of resistance the muscle can hold against. The break test technique produces greater strength measurements than the make test technique.[129] To maintain reliability in testing, use the same test technique (i.e., make or break test) on subsequent testing, and record the technique used.

To assess strength if joint movement causes pain and no contraindications exist, it is extremely difficult if not impossible to perform a static contraction and produce a situation where absolutely no movement occurs at the joint crossed by the muscle. There is always some degree of joint movement, compression, and shearing even with static muscle contraction.[130] However, it may be possible to perform a pain-free isometric muscle test with the joint placed in the loose-packed (resting) position. Keep one hand immediately below the patient's limb so that no movement or only slight movement occurs if the patient is unable to hold the limb in any part of the ROM against gravity.

Based on the patient's condition and needs, the clinician must determine the efficacy of applying manual resistance through range, or at one or multiple joint positions in the joint ROM to assess muscle strength that is greater than a grade 3. The application of manual resistance through range and at a specified joint position are both described and illustrated in this text.

Gravity Eliminated

If the patient cannot move through any part of the ROM against gravity, position the patient so that the resistance of gravity is eliminated for the test movement (i.e., the patient performs the movement in the horizontal plane). In this case, it may be necessary to support the weight of the limb on a relatively friction-free surface or manually (Fig. 1-70). Stabilize the muscle origin and palpate the muscle(s) (Fig. 1-70B) during the test as the patient attempts to move through the ROM. During the actual test, give commands explicitly and consistently from one test to another. Commands should elicit the strongest response possible.

- If the patient moves through the full available ROM with gravity eliminated, the muscle is assigned a grade of 2.

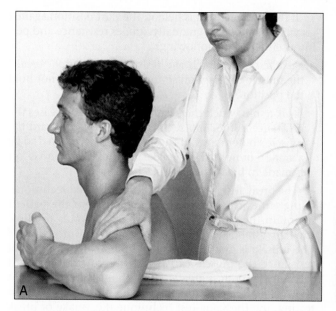

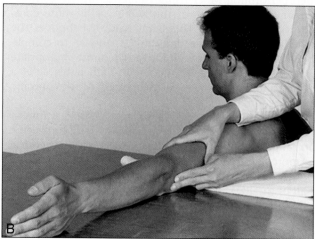

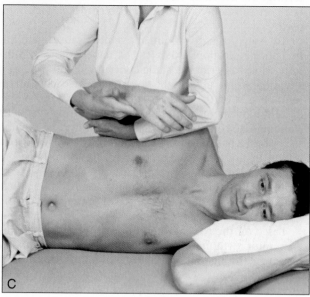

Figure 1-70 A. Manual muscle testing (MMT) start position **gravity eliminated:** elbow extensors. The weight of the limb rests on a powder board. **B.** Palpate and observe the muscle for contraction as the patient attempts to perform elbow extension through the full available range of motion (ROM) gravity eliminated. If able to move the limb, assign a grade 2 or 2– based on the magnitude of the ROM. If unable to move the limb, assign the muscle either a grade 1 or 0, based on **the presence or absence of muscle contraction. C.** In place of a powder board, manually support the arm and forearm as shown.

- If the patient is able to move through less than the full available ROM, then a grade of 2– is given.
- If no movement occurs, the therapist grades the muscle based on the presence or absence of a muscle contraction, grades 1 or 0, respectively.

The patient is asked to relax at the end of each test movement and the therapist positions the limb for the next test movement.

Palpation. Palpate a muscle near its tendon attachment or near a bony point using the pads of the index and middle fingers. Always palpate and observe the muscle(s) being tested when assessing grades of 0 through 3, because the muscle may be graded based on the quality of contraction when no movement is pos-

sible, or the lack of muscle tension with movement may indicate substitute movements. In cases of extreme weakness, a flicker of a contraction may be detected more easily by observing slight movement of the skin than by palpation.

When muscles are very weak, the strongest contraction possible from the muscle may be elicited by positioning and supporting the limb segment so the muscle will contract in inner range against gravity. Instruct the patient to hold this position and gradually withdraw support from the limb. Keep one hand just below the limb to control its fall if the patient is unable to hold the limb in any part of the ROM against gravity. This technique may elicit a minimal or prolonged firm contraction that can be palpated.

Number of Repetitions Used in Testing. Determine the strength after two to three repetitions of the test movement. Fatigue will become a factor with too many repetitions, resulting in erroneous recording and underestimating the patient's true strength because the grades of manual muscle strength assessment methods do not take endurance into account.

Other Assessment Procedures That Employ Isometric Muscle Contraction

Other clinical application for isometric muscle contractions are beyond the scope of this text and are only briefly discussed here. Aside from being used to assess muscle strength, isometric muscle contraction may also be used for the following:

1. To test for myotomal weakness (i.e., neurological weakness that originates from nerve root pathology). The joint is at or near the resting position and during the isometric contraction, the therapist notes whether the contraction is either weak or strong to determine if there is a deficiency in neural input to the muscle(s).

2. To selectively test the integrity of contractile tissue (i.e., muscle and tendon) by applying stress to the tissue by way of muscle contraction. The joint is in resting position and no movement occurs at the joint during the isometric contraction. Thus, stress is not placed on inert or noncontractile tissue (i.e., joint capsule, ligaments, and nerves). During the isometric contraction, the therapist notes whether pain is elicited and whether the contraction is weak or strong to determine if there is a muscular lesion.

Alternate Methods and Grading of Muscle Strength

Alternate methods and grading of muscle strength may be used in the following situations when:

- The weight of the part is so minimal that the effect of gravity is unimportant and need not be considered (i.e., muscles of the fingers, thumbs, and toes).
- It is not always practical or possible to palpate the muscle, apply resistance, or position the patient either against gravity or with gravity eliminated for the test movements (i.e., when testing facial muscles).
- The muscles require the resistance of body weight to be resisted maximally (i.e., gastrocnemius, soleus).

  The grading used when testing the facial muscles, muscles of the fingers, thumbs and toes, and the muscles requiring the resistance of body weight, will be described in the sections of this text that deal with the testing of these muscles.

Testing with a Two- or Multi-joint Muscle in the Region

When applying resistance to a two-joint muscle either directly or indirectly, take care to avoid positions of excessive shortening of the two-joint muscle because this may lead to painful cramping of the muscle.[72]

1. To test the strength of a one-joint muscle with a two-joint or multi-joint muscle in the region that performs the same action at the joint, the contribution of the two-joint or multi-joint muscle to the movement must be reduced or eliminated. To accomplish this, passively place the two-joint or multi-joint muscle in a shortened position at the nontest joint(s) to render it more actively insufficient before testing the one-joint muscle.

   Example:

   When testing the strength of coracobrachialis to flex and adduct the shoulder, the elbow and forearm are passively flexed and supinated, respectively, to place the biceps brachii muscle in a shortened position, thus rendering it more actively insufficient and reducing the contribution of the short head of biceps brachii to flex and adduct the shoulder.

2. To test a two- or multi-joint muscle at one joint, first place the nontest joint(s) in midposition to avoid active insufficiency of the muscle.

   Example:

   When testing the strength of the hamstrings to flex the knee, the hip is positioned in flexion.

3. To test a muscle at a joint where a two-joint or multi-joint muscle is the antagonist, place the two-joint or multi-joint muscle on slack at the nontest joint(s). This avoids stretching and creating a situation of passive insufficiency of the two-joint or multi-joint muscle during the muscle test that will decrease the ability of the prime mover to move the joint through full ROM.

   Example:

   When testing the strength of the iliopsoas to flex the hip, the knee is positioned in flexion to place the hamstring muscles on slack and prevent tightness of hamstrings from limiting hip flexion ROM (see Figs. 1-47 and 1-48).

Recording

Muscle strength assessment forms are used to record strength. See Figure 1-71 and Appendix B for examples of a muscle test recording form; Figure 1-71 gives examples of selected muscle strength recordings.

The inability to test a muscle accurately (e.g., due to the presence of pain or noncompliance of the patient) is indicated on the recording form using a question mark beside the grade;[89] for example, "3?". The question mark will prompt the therapist to retest the muscle at another time if appropriate. An explanation is given for the question mark under the comments or remarks section of the recording form.

Every space should include an entry on a recording form.[8] Enter "NT" (not tested) if the test was not performed, and a line may be drawn from the first such entry to the end of several adjacent entries so the NT does not have to be recorded in every space.[8]

Note any noncompliance of the patient, deviations from standard testing procedure, and other factors that may influence the results of a muscle test on the chart.

Manual Muscle Strength Assessment

Patient's Name *Connie Pearson*   Age   *54*

Diagnosis *Guillian Barre Syndrome*   Date of Onset *Oct 10/11*

Therapist Name *Sue Bart*

Signature *Sue Bart DPT*

Manual Muscle Testing (MMT) Method Used

Date of Assessment: *Oct 21/11*   MMT method used: *C*
Date of Assessment: *Nov 25/11*   MMT method used: *C*
Date of Assessment: *Dec 15/11*   MMT method used: *C*
Date of Assessment: _____   MMT method used: _____

Key: MMT Method Used.
C   Conventional "through range" grading
I   Conventional "Isometric" grading: **b** break test or **m** make test
        (eg: **Ib** indicates Conventional "Isometric" break test)

Left Side						Right Side		
SB	SB	SB	**Therapist Initials**			SB	SB	SB
Dec 15/11	Nov 25/11	Oct 21/11	**Date of Assessment**			Oct 21/11	Nov 25/11	Dec 15/11
			Motion	**Muscle**	**Nerve supply**			
			Scapula					
4	3+	3	Abduction Lateral rotation	Serratus anterior	Long Thoracic	3	3+	4
	3+	3	Elevation	Upper trapezius Levator scapulae	Accessory, CN XI Dorsal Scapular	3	3+	
	3+	NT	Adduction	Middle trapezius	Accessory, CN XI	NT	3+	
	3	NT	Adduction Medial rotation	Rhomboids	Dorsal Scapular	NT	3	
	3	NT	Depression	Lower trapezius	Accessory, CN XI	NT	3	
			Shoulder					
	3+	3-	Flexion	Anterior deltoid	Axillary	3-	3+	
			Hip					
4-	2	2	Flexion	Psoas major Illiacus	Lumar Femoral	2	2	4-
4-	2	1		Sartorius	Femoral	1	2	4-
3-	1	1	Extension	Gluteus maximus Biceps femoris Semitendinosus Semimembranosus	Gluteal Sciatic Sciatic Sciatic	1	1	3-
3-	2	1	Abduction	Gluteus medius Gluteus minimus	Gluteal Gluteal	1	2	3-
			Knee					
			Flexion	Biceps femoris	Sciatic			
3-	1	0		Semitendinosus Semimembranosus	Sciatic Sciatic	0	1	3-
4-	2	1	Extension	Quadriceps	Femoral	1	2	4-
			Ankle					
2	0	0	Dorsiflexion	Tibialis anterior	Peroneal	0	0	2
			Plantarflexion	Gastrocnemius	Tibial			
				Soleus	Tibial			
			Inversion	Tibialis posterior	Tibial			
				Extensor digitorum longus				

Remarks:

Figure 1-71 Example of recording muscle strength using a Manual Muscle Strength Assessment form.

Ensure that an appropriate legend of the muscle testing grading is noted on the chart.

A grade of 3 does not necessarily indicate a functional grade. Record grades of 3 or less for the upper extremity, trunk and neck, and grades of less than a 4 for the lower extremity so that they can be identified quickly on reading the chart as being nonfunctional grades or areas of major concern. Highlight these nonfunctional grades by placing the grade in brackets. Fatigue should be closely monitored and recorded to facilitate the application of strength tests to ADL.

FUNCTIONAL APPLICATION OF ASSESSMENT OF JOINT RANGE OF MOTION AND MANUAL MUSCLE TESTING

Evaluation of functional activities, through task analysis and observation of the patient's performance in activities, can guide the therapist in proceeding with a detailed assessment and provide objective and meaningful treatment goals. The therapist may ask the patient about his or her ability to perform activities. It is essential that the therapist observes the patient performing the functional activities.[131] The patient is observed performing functional activities such as dressing, sitting, or walking during the initial assessment.

On completion of the evaluation of ROM and muscle strength, the therapist must consider the impact of deficit on the patient's daily life. Knowledge of functional anatomy of the musculoskeletal system is required to integrate the assessment findings into meaningful and practical information. The knowledge of functional anatomy assists the therapist in gaining insight into the effect of joint ROM or strength limitations in the patient's daily life.

Outline of the Assessment Process

"An Outline of the Assessment Process", located on the inside back cover of this text, serves as an overview of the assessment process and a review of some of the main points presented in this chapter.

References

1. Basmajian JV. *Surface Anatomy: An Instructional Manual.* Baltimore: Williams & Wilkins; 1983.
2. Neumann DA. *Kinesiology of the Musculoskeletal System: Foundations for Rehabilitation.* St. Louis: Mosby Elsevier; 2010.
3. Hollis M. *Safer Lifting for Patient Care.* 2nd ed. Oxford, England: Blackwell Scientific Publications; 1985.
4. MacConaill MA, Basmajian JV. *Muscles and Movements: A Basis for Human Kinesiology.* 2nd ed. New York: Robert E. Krieger; 1977.
5. Kapandji AI. *The Physiology of the Joints. Vol. 1. The Upper Limb.* 6th ed. New York: Churchill Livingstone; 2007.
6. Standring S, ed. *Gray's Anatomy: The Anatomical Basis of Clinical Practice.* 39th ed. London: Elsevier Churchill Livingstone; 2005.
7. Stedman TL. *Stedman's Medical Dictionary for the Health Professions and Nursing.* 6th ed. Philadelphia: Lippincott Williams & Wilkins; 2008.
8. Duesterhaus Minor MA, Duesterhaus Minor S. *Patient Evaluation Methods for the Health Professional.* Reston, VA: Reston Publishing; 1985.
9. Soderberg GL. *Kinesiology: Application to Pathological Motion.* 2nd ed. Baltimore: Williams & Wilkins; 1997.
10. Perry J. Shoulder function for the activities of daily living. In: Matsen FA, Fu FH, Hawkins RJ, eds. *The Shoulder: A Balance of Mobility and Stability.* Rosemont, IL: American Academy of Orthopaedic Surgeons; 1993.
11. Kendall FP, McCreary EK, Provance PG, et al. *Muscles Testing and Function with Posture and Pain.* 5th ed. Baltimore: Lippincott Williams & Wilkins; 2005.
12. Gowitzke BA, Milner M. *Understanding the Scientific Bases of Human Movement.* 2nd ed. Baltimore: Williams & Wilkins; 1980.
13. Kaltenborn FM. *Mobilization of the Extremity Joints. Examination and Basic Treatment Techniques.* 3rd ed. Oslo: Olaf Norlis Bokhandel; 1985.
14. Lundon K, Hampson D. Acquired ectopic ossification of soft tissues: implications for physical therapy. *Can J Rehabil.* 1997;10:231–246.
15. Kisner C, Colby LA. *Therapeutic Exercise: Foundations and Techniques.* 5th ed. Philadelphia: FA Davis; 2007.
16. Hall CM, Brody LT. *Therapeutic Exercise: Moving Toward Function.* 2nd ed. Philadelphia: Lippincott Williams & Wilkins; 2005.
17. O' Connor P, Sforzo GA, Frye P. Effect of breathing instruction on blood pressure responses during isometric exercise. *Phys Ther.* 1989;69:55–59.
18. Cyriax J. *Textbook of Orthopaedic Medicine: Vol 1. Diagnosis of Soft Tissue Lesions.* 8th ed. London: Bailliere Tindall; 1982.
19. Norkin CC, White DJ. *Measurement of Joint Motion: A Guide to Goniometry.* 4th ed. Philadelphia: FA Davis; 2009.
20. Magee DJ. *Orthopedic Physical Assessment.* 5th ed. St. Louis: Saunders Elsevier; 2008.
21. Hayes KW, Petersen C, Falconer J. An examination of Cyriax's passive motion tests with patients having osteoarthritis of the knee. *Phys Ther.* 1994;74:697–707.
22. Klassbo M, Harms-Ringdahl K. Examination of passive ROM and capsular patterns in the hip. *Physiother Res Int.* 2003;8:1–12.
23. Mitsch J, Casey J, McKinnis R, Kegerreis S, Stikeleather J. Investigation of a consistent pattern of motion restriction in patients with adhesive capsulitis. *J Manual Manipulative Ther.* 2004;12:153–159.
24. Instruction Manual: OB Goniometer "Myrin." Available from OB Rehab, Solna, Sweden.
25. Performance Attainment Associates. *CROM Procedure Manual: Procedure for Measuring Neck Motion with the CROM.* St. Paul, MN: University of Minnesota; 1988.
26. Currier DP. *Elements of Research in Physical Therapy.* 3rd ed. Baltimore: Williams & Wilkins; 1990.
27. Sim J, Arnell P. Measurement validity in physical therapy research. *Phys Ther.* 1993;73:48–56.

28. Miller PJ. Assessment of joint motion. In: Rothstein JM, ed. *Measurement in Physical Therapy*. New York: Churchill Livingstone; 1985.

29. Gogia PP, Braatz JH, Rose SJ, Norton BJ. Reliability and validity of goniometric measurements at the knee. *Phys Ther*. 1987;67:192–195.

30. Enwemeka CS. Radiographic verification of knee goniometry. *Scand J Rehabil Med*. 1986;18:47–49.

31. Fish DR, Wingate L. Sources of goniometric error at the elbow. *Phys Ther*. 1985;65:1666–1670.

32. Youdas JW, Carey JR, Garrett TR. Reliability of measurements of cervical spine range of motion—comparison of three methods. *Phys Ther*. 1991;71:23–29.

33. Low J. The reliability of joint measurement. *Physiotherapy*. 1976;62:227–229.

34. Baldwin J, Cunningham K. Goniometry under attack: a clinical study involving physiotherapists. *Physiother Can*. 1974;26:74–76.

35. Watkins MA, Riddle DL, Lamb RL, Personius WJ. Reliability of goniometric measurements and visual estimates of knee range of motion obtained in a clinical setting. *Phys Ther*. 1991;71:15–22.

36. Banskota B, Lewis J, Hossain M, Irvine A, Jones MW. Estimation of the accuracy of joint mobility assessment in a group of health professionals. *Eur J Orthop Surg Traumatol*. 2008;18:287–289.

37. Lavernia C, D'Apuzzo M, Rossi MD, Lee D. Accuracy of knee range of motion assessment after total knee arthroplasty. *J Arthroplasty*. 2008;23(6):Suppl 1,85–91.

38. Rachkidi R, Ghanem I, Kalouche I, et al. Is visual estimation of passive range of motion in the pediatric lower limb valid and reliable? *BMC Musculoskelet Disord*. 2009;10:126–135.

39. Bovens AMPM, van Baak MA, Vrencken JGPM, et al. Variability and reliability of joint measurements. *Am J Sports Med*. 1990;18:58–63.

40. Pandya S, Florence JM, King WM, et al. Reliability of goniometric measurements in patients with Duchenne muscular dystrophy. *Phys Ther*. 1985;65:1339–1342.

41. Elveru RA, Rothstein JM, Lamb RL. Goniometric reliability in a clinical setting: subtalar and ankle joint measurements. *Phys Ther*. 1988;68:672–677.

42. Boone DC, Azen SP, Lin C-M, et al. Reliability of goniometric measurements. *Phys Ther*. 1978;58:1355–1360.

43. Dijkstra PU, deBont LGM, van der Weele LTh, Boering G. Joint mobility measurements: reliability of a standardized method. *J Craniomandibular Practice*. 1994;12:52–57.

44. Youdas JW, Bogard CL, Suman VJ. Reliability of goniometric measurements and visual estimates of ankle joint active range of motion obtained in a clinical setting. *Arch Phys Med Rehabil*. 1993;74:1113–1118.

45. Horger MM. The reliability of goniometric measurements of active and passive wrist motions. *Am J Occup Ther*. 1990;44:342–348.

46. Hellebrant FA, Duvall EN, Moore ML. The measurement of joint motion: Part III, reliability of goniometry. *Phys Ther Rev*. 1949;29:302–307.

47. Rothstein JM, Miller PJ, Roettger RF. Goniometric reliability in a clinical setting: elbow and knee measurements. *Phys Ther*. 1983;63:1611–1615.

48. Riddle DL, Rothstein JM, Lamb RL. Goniometric reliability in a clinical setting: shoulder measurements. *Phys Ther*. 1987;67:668–673.

49. Watkins B, Darrah J, Pain K. Reliability of passive ankle dorsiflexion measurements in children: comparison of universal and biplane goniometers. *Pediatr Phys Ther*. 1995;7: 3–8.

50. Kilgour G, McNair P, Stott NS. Intrarater reliability of lower limb sagittal range-of-motion measures in children with spastic diplegia. *Develop Med Child Neurol*. 2003;45:385–390.

51. Stuberg WA, Fuchs RH, Miedaner JA. Reliability of goniometric measurements of children with cerebral palsy. *Develop Med Child Neurol*. 1988;30:657–666.

52. Ashton B, Pickles B, Roll JW. Reliability of goniometric measurements of hip motion in spastic cerebral palsy. *Develop Med Child Neurol*. 1978;20:87–94.

53. Harris SR, Smith LH, Krukowski L. Goniometric reliability for a child with spastic quadriplegia. *J Pediatr Orthop*. 1985;5:348–351.

54. Mutlu A, Livanelioglu A, Gunel MK. Reliability of goniometric measurements in children with spastic cerebral palsy. *Med Sci Monit*. 2007;13(7):CR323–329.

55. McWhirk LB, Glanzman AM. Within-session inter-rater reliability of goniometric measures in patients with spastic cerebral palsy. *Pediatr Phys Ther*. 2006;18(4):262–265.

56. ten Berge SR, Habertsma JPK, Maathius PGM, Verheij NP, Dijkstra PU, Maathuis KGB. Reliability of popliteal angle measurement: A study in cerebral palsy patients and healthy controls. *J Paediatr Orthop*. 2007;27(6):648–652.

57. American Academy of Orthopaedic Surgeons. *Joint Motion: Method of Measuring and Recording*. Chicago: AAOS; 1965.

58. Berryman Reese N, Bandy WD. *Joint Range of Motion and Muscle Length Testing*. 2nd ed. St. Louis: Saunders Elsevier; 2010.

59. Moore ML. Clinical assessment of joint motion. In: Basmajian JV, ed. *Therapeutic Exercise*. 4th ed. Baltimore: Williams & Wilkins; 1984.

60. Ekstrand J, Wiktorsson M, Oberg B, Gillquist J. Lower extremity goniometric measurements: a study to determine their reliability. *Arch Phys Med Rehabil*. 1982;63:171–175.

61. Stratford P, Agostino V, Brazeau C, Gowitzke BA. Reliability of joint angle measurement: a discussion of methodology issues. *Physiother Can*. 1984;36:5–9.

62. Gerhardt JJ, Cocchiarella L, Randall LD. *The Practical Guide to Range of Motion Assessment*. Chicago: American Medical Association; 2002.

63. Wintz MM. Variations in current manual muscle testing. *Phys Ther Rev*. 1959;39:466–475.

64. Williams M. Manual muscle testing, development and current use. *Phys Ther Rev*. 1956;36:797–805.

65. Rothstein JM. Commentary. *Phys Ther*. 1989;69:61–66. In response to Bohannon RW. Is the measurement of muscle strength appropriate in patients with brain lesions? A special communication. *Phys Ther*. 1989;69:56–61 (Author's response: 66–67).

66. Fox EL, Mathews DK. *The Physiological Basis of Physical Education and Athletics*. 3rd ed. Philadelphia: Saunders College Publishing; 1981.

67. Knuttgen HG, ed. *Neuromuscular Mechanisms for Therapeutic and Conditioning Exercise*. Baltimore: University Park Press; 1976.

68. Lieber RL, Bodine-Fowler SC. Skeletal muscle mechanics: implications for rehabilitation. *Phys Ther*. 1993;73:25–37.

69. Kroemer KHE. Human strength: terminology, measurement, and interpretation of data. *Hum Factors*. 1970;12:297–313.

70. Smith LK, Weiss EL, Lehmkuhl LD. *Brunnstrom's Clinical Kinesiology*. 5th ed. Philadelphia: FA Davis; 1996.

71. Hollis M. *Practical Exercise Therapy*. 3rd ed. Oxford, England: Blackwell Scientific Publications; 1989.

72. Kendall FP, McCreary EK, Provance PG. *Muscles Testing and Function*. 4th ed. Baltimore: Williams & Wilkins; 1993.

73. Hamill J, Knutzen KM. *Biomechanical Basis of Human Movement.* 3rd ed. Philadelphia: Lippincott, Williams & Wilkins; 2009.
74. Brooks GA, Fahey TD. *Exercise Physiology: Human Bioenergetics and Its Application.* New York: John Wiley & Sons; 1984.
75. Oatis CA. *Kinesiology: The Mechanics and Pathomechanics of Human Movement.* 2nd ed. Philadelphia: Lippincott, Williams & Wilkins; 2009.
76. Laubach LL. Comparative muscular strength of men and women: a review of the literature. *Aviat Space Environ Med.* 1976;47:534–542.
77. Williams M, Stutzman L. Strength variation through the range of joint motion. *Phys Ther Rev.* 1959;39:145–152.
78. Kulig K, Andrews JG, Hay JG. Human strength curves. *Exerc Sport Sci Rev.* 1984;12:417–466.
79. Williams M, Tomberlin JA, Robertson KJ. Muscle force curves of school children. *J Am Phys Ther Assoc.* 1965;45:539–549.
80. Wyse JP, Mercer TH, Gleeson NP. Time-of-day dependence of isokinetic leg strength and associated interday variability. *Br J Sports Med.* 1994;28:167–170.
81. Gauthier A, Davenne D, Martin A, Cometti G, Van Hoecke J. Diurnal rhythm of the muscular performance of elbow flexors during isometric contractions. *Chronobiol Int.* 1996;13:135–146.
82. Holewijn M, Heus R. Effects of temperature on electromyogram and muscle function. *Eur J Appl Physiol.* 1992;65:541–545.
83. Hertling D, Kessler RM. *Management of Common Musculoskeletal Disorders: Physical Therapy Principles and Methods.* 4th ed. Philadelphia: Lippincott, Williams & Wilkins; 2006.
84. Sorenson EJ, Great Lakes ALS Study Group. A comparison of muscle strength testing techniques in amyotrophic lateral sclerosis. *Neurology.* 2003;61(11):1503–1507.
85. Hislop HJ, Montgomery J. *Daniels and Worthingham's Muscle Testing: Techniques of Manual Examination.* 8th ed. St. Louis: Saunders Elsevier; 2007.
86. Daniels L, Worthingham C. *Muscle Testing: Techniques of Manual Examination.* 5th ed. Philadelphia: WB Saunders; 1986.
87. Wright WG. Muscle training in the treatment of infantile paralysis. *Boston Med Surg J.* 1912;167:567–574.
88. Brunnstrom S. Muscle group testing. *Physiother Rev.* 1941;21:3–22.
89. Smith LK, Iddings DM, Spencer WA, Harrington PR. Muscle testing: Part 1. Description of a numerical index for clinical research. *Phys Ther Rev.* 1961;41:99–105.
90. Hines TF. Manual muscle examination. In: Licht S, ed. *Therapeutic Exercise.* 2nd ed. Baltimore: Waverly Press; 1965.
91. Kendall HO, Kendall FP. *Muscles Testing and Function.* Baltimore: Williams & Wilkins; 1949.
92. Beasley WC. Quantitative muscle testing: principles and applications to research and clinical services. *Arch Phys Med Rehabil.* 1961;42:398–425.
93. Bohannon RW. Manual muscle test scores and dynamometer test scores of knee extension strength. *Arch Phys Med Rehabil.* 1986;67:390–392.
94. Schwartz S, Cohen ME, Herbison GJ, Shah A. Relationship between two measures of upper extremity strength: manual muscle test compared to hand-held myometry. *Arch Phys Med Rehabil.* 1992;73:1063–1068.
95. Aitkens S, Lord J, Bernauer E, Fowler WM, Lieberman JS, Berck P. Relationship of manual muscle testing to objective strength measurements. *Muscle Nerve.* 1989;12:173–177.
96. Bohannon RW. Measuring knee extensor muscle strength. *Am J Phys Med Rehab.* 2001;80(1):13–18.
97. Lamb RL. Manual muscle testing. In: Rothstein JM, ed. *Measurement in Physical Therapy.* New York: Churchill Livingstone; 1985.
98. Silver M, McElroy A, Morrow L, Heafner BK. Further standardization of manual muscle test for clinical study: applied in chronic renal disease. *Phys Ther.* 1970;50:1456–1464.
99. Lilienfeld AM, Jacobs M, Willis M. A study of the reproducibility of muscle testing and certain other aspects of muscle scoring. *Phys Ther Rev.* 1954;34:279–289.
100. Iddings DM, Smith LK, Spencer WA. Muscle testing: Part 2. Reliability in clinical use. *Phys Ther Rev.* 1961;41:249–256.
101. Frese E, Brown M, Norton BJ. Clinical reliability of manual muscle testing. Middle trapezius and gluteus medius muscles. *Phys Ther.* 1987;67:1072–1076.
102. Florence JM, Pandya S, King WM, et al. Clinical trials in duchenne dystrophy: standardization and reliability of evaluation procedures. *Phys Ther.* 1984;64:41–45.
103. Paternostro-Sluga T, Grim-Stieger M, Posch M, et al. Reliability and validity of the Medical Research Council (MRC) scale and a modified scale for testing muscle strength in patients with radial palsy. *J Rehabil Med.* 2008;40:665–671.
104. Beasley WC. Influence of method on estimates of normal knee extensor force among normal and post-polio children. *Phys Ther Rev.* 1956;36:21–41.
105. Mahony K, Hunt A, Daley D, et al. Inter-tester reliability and precision of manual muscle testing and hand-held dynamometry in lower limb muscles of children with spina bifida. *Phys Occup Ther Pediatr.* 2009;29(1):44–59.
106. Bohannon RW, Corrigan D. A broad range of forces is encompassed by the maximum manual muscle test grade of five. *Percept Motor Skills.* 2000;90:747–750.
107. Hayes KW, Falconer J. Reliability of hand-held dynamometry and its relationship with manual muscle testing in patients with osteoarthritis in the knee. *J Orthop Sports Phys Ther.* 1992;16:145–149.
108. Bohannon RW. Nature, implications, and measurement of limb muscle strength in patients with orthopedic or neurological disorders. *Phys Ther Prac.* 1992;2:22–31.
109. Dvir Z. Grade 4 in manual muscle testing: the problem with submaximal strength assessment. *Clin Rehabil.* 1997;11:36–41.
110. MacAvoy MC, Green DP. Critical appraisal of medical research council muscle testing for elbow flexion. *J Hand Surg Am.* 2007;32(2):149–153.
111. Escolar DM, Henricson EK, Mayhew J, et al. Clinical evaluator reliability for quantitative and manual muscle testing measures of strength in children. *Muscle Nerve.* 2001;24:787–793.
112. Griffin JW, McClure MH, Bertorini TE. Sequential isokinetic and manual muscle testing in patients with neuromuscular disease. *Phys Ther.* 1986;66:32–35.
113. Rabin SI, Post M. A comparative study of clinical muscle testing and Cybex evaluation after shoulder operations. *Clin Orthop Rel Res.* 1990;258:147–156.
114. Wadsworth CT, Krishnan R, Sear M, Harrold J, Nielsen DH. Intrarater reliability of manual muscle testing and hand-held dynametric muscle testing. *Phys Ther.* 1987;67:1342–1347.
115. Donaldson R. The importance of position in the examination of muscles and in exercise. *Physiother Rev.* 1927;7:22–24.
116. Chaffin DB. Ergonomics guide for the assessment of human static strength. *Am Ind Hyg Assoc J.* 1975;36:505–511.
117. Brown T, Galea V, McComas A. Loss of twitch torque following muscle compression. *Muscle Nerve.* 1997;20:167–171.

118. Wynn Parry CB. Vicarious motions (trick movements). In: Basmajian JV, ed. *Therapeutic Exercise*. 4th ed. Baltimore: Williams & Wilkins; 1984.

119. Kendall FP, McCreary EK. *Muscles Testing and Function*. 3rd ed. Baltimore: Williams & Wilkins; 1983.

120. Christ CB, Boileau RA, Slaughter MH, Stillman RJ, Cameron J. The effect of test protocol instructions on measurement of muscle function in adult men. *J Orthop Sports Phys Ther*. 1993;18:502–510.

121. Johansson CA, Kent BE, Shepard KF. Relationship between verbal command volume and magnitude of muscle contraction. *Phys Ther*. 1983;63:1260–1265.

122. McNair PJ, Depledge J, Brettkelly M, Stanley SN. Verbal encouragement: effects on maximum effort voluntary muscle action. *Br J Sports Med*. 1996;30:243–245.

123. Nicholas JA, Sapega A, Kraus H, Webb JN. Factors influencing manual muscle tests in physical therapy: the magnitude and duration of the force applied. *J Bone Joint Surg [Am]*. 1978;60:186–190.

124. Wilson GJ, Murphy AJ. The use of isometric tests of muscular function in athletic assessment. *Sports Med*. 1996;22:19–37.

125. Koo TK, Mak AF, Hung LK, et al. Joint position dependence of weakness during maximum isometric voluntary contractions in subjects with hemiparesis. *Arch Phys Med Rehabil*. 2003;84:1380–1386.

126. McGarvey SR, Morrey BF, Askew LJ, Kai-Nan A. Reliability of isometric strength testing: temporal factors and strength variation. *Clin Orthop*. 1984;185:301–305.

127. Bohannon RW. Make tests and break tests of elbow flexor muscle strength. *Phys Ther*. 1988;68:193–194.

128. Velsher E. Factors affecting higher force readings: a survey of the literature on isometric exercise. *Physiother Can*. 1977;29:141–147.

129. Burns SP, Breuninger A, Kaplan C, et al. Hand-held dynamometry in persons with tetraplegia: Comparison of make- versus break-testing techniques. *Am J Phys Med Rehab*. 2005;84(1):22–29.

130. Lamb DW. A review of manual therapy for spinal pain. In: Boyling JD, Palastanga N, eds. *Grieve's Modern Manual Therapy: The Vertebral Column*. 2nd ed. London: Churchill Livingstone; 1994.

131. Smith LK. Functional tests. *Phys Ther Rev*. 1954;34:19–21.

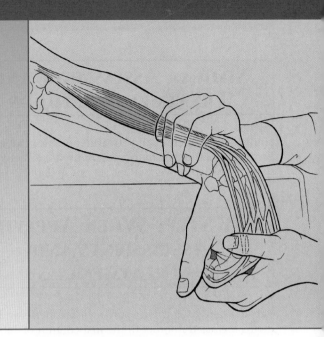

Chapter 2

Relating Assessment to Treatment

Chapter Rationale

- Although the guidelines for diagnosis and treatment protocols are beyond the scope of this text, this chapter links the techniques used to assess active range of motion (AROM), passive range of motion (PROM), muscle length, and muscle strength with the techniques used for treatment.

- Through illustration and description, the reader is provided with an overview of the similarities and differences between clinical assessments presented in this textbook and complementary treatments.

- Knowing the similarities between assessment and treatment, and using the knowledge and skills for assessing AROM, PROM, muscle length, and muscle strength, the reader will be able to utilize similar techniques for treatments using active, passive, or resisted movement.

- Understanding the link between assessment and treatment is essential for the reader to be able to integrate patient assessment and treatment in the clinical setting.

Optional learning approach: Should the reader prefer to learn the assessment techniques presented in this text prior to considering how assessment and treatment techniques are related, then this chapter would be considered the final chapter of this text.

SIMILAR ASSESSMENT AND TREATMENT METHODS

Similar assessments and treatments are categorized according to the type of movement used (i.e., active, passive, or resisted movement) as set out in Table 2-1.

KEY STEPS WHEN APPLYING ASSESSMENTS AND TREATMENTS

The key steps used when applying assessments and treatments are listed in order in the first column of Table 2-1. These steps are set out in detail for assessment in Chapter 1 and are summarized here and in Table 2-1 to compare with those for treatment.

Purpose

The therapist performs an assessment to evaluate how an injury or disease affects the patient's status. Treatment, if appropriate, is then used to eliminate or lessen the effects of an injury or disease. Assessment is repeated as required to evaluate the outcome of treatment.

Common Technique

Technique is the same when using active, passive, or resisted movement for similar assessment and treatment.

Explanation and Instruction

Before carrying out an assessment or treatment, explain the assessment or treatment to the patient and obtain the patient's informed consent. When applying a specific assessment or treatment for the first time, explain and/or demonstrate the movement to be performed and/or ask the patient to relax and passively move the patient's limb through the movement.

Expose Region

For assessment and treatment, expose the area to be assessed or treated and drape the patient as required.

Start Position

For assessment and treatment, ensure that the patient is in a safe, comfortable position and is adequately supported. When positioning the patient, the effect of gravity on the movement may be relevant.

Stabilization

For assessment and treatment, provide adequate stabilization to ensure that only the required movement occurs. For assessment and treatment, perform either of the following:

(a) The proximal joint segment or site of attachment of the origin of the muscle(s) is(are) stabilized.

(b) The distal joint segment or site of insertion of the muscle(s) is(are) stabilized.

Movement

For assessment and treatment, either of the following should be performed:

(a) The distal joint segment or site of attachment of the insertion of the muscle(s) is(are) moved.

(b) The proximal joint segment or site of origin of the muscle(s) is(are) moved.

Assistance/Resistance

For passive movements used in assessment and treatment, assistance is normally applied at the distal end of either the distal joint segment or the segment into which the muscle(s) is(are) inserted. For resisted movements used in assessment and treatment, resistance is normally applied at the distal end of the segment into which the muscle(s) is(are) inserted.

End Position

For assessment and treatment, either instruct the patient to move the body segment(s) (for active movement) or passively move the limb segment(s) (for passive movement) through either a selected part of or the full ROM possible. For prolonged passive stretch, the therapist passively moves the body segment(s) to the point in the ROM that provides maximal stretch of the muscle(s). When using resisted movement, the patient is instructed to either move through the ROM (for a concentric contraction), or maintain/hold a specified position (for an isometric contraction) against the therapist's manual resistance.

Substitute Movement

For assessment and treatment, ensure that there are no substitute movements that may exaggerate the actual joint ROM and/or muscle strength, or interfere with the patient's capacity to perform an exercise. To avoid unwanted movements, explain/demonstrate to the patient how the movement is to be performed and the substitute movements to be avoided. Pay attention to positioning and stabilizing the patient. Experience and careful observation enables the therapist to prevent substitute movements and detect any that may occur.

TABLE 2-1　Comparing of Assessment and Treatment

Key Steps	Active Movement		Passive Movement				Resisted Movement	
	Assessment	Treatment	Assessment	Treatment	Assessment	Treatment	Assessment	Treatment
	Active ROM (AROM)	*Active Exercise*	*Passive ROM (PROM)*	*Relaxed Passive Movement*	*Muscle Length*	*Prolonged Passive Stretch*	*Muscle Strength*	*Resisted Exercise*
PURPOSE	Assessment of: • AROM • Muscle strength (grades 0 to 3) • Ability to perform ADL	Treatment to maintain/increase: • Joint ROM muscle strength • Ability to perform ADL	Assessment of: • Joint PROM • End feel	Treatment to maintain/increase: • Joint ROM	Assessment of: • Muscle length	Treatment to maintain/increase: • Muscle length	Assessment of: • Muscle strength (grades >3)	Treatment to maintain/increase: • Muscle strength
COMMON TECHNIQUE								
Explanation/ Instruction	← Verbal (clear, concise), demonstration and/or passive movement →							
Expose Area	← Expose area and drape as required →							
Start Position	• Safe, comfortable, adequate support • Consider effect of gravity		• Safe, comfortable, adequate support, relaxed				• Safe, comfortable, adequate support • Consider effect of gravity	
Stabilization*	• Proximal joint segment(s) • Muscle origins		• Proximal joint segment(s)		• Muscle origin(s)		• Muscle origin(s)	
Movement[a]	• Distal joint segment(s)		• Distal joint segment(s)		• Joint(s) crossed by muscle(s)		• At joint(s) crossed by muscle(s), or none if resist isometric contraction	
Assistance/ Resistance	n/a		• Assistance applied at distal end of distal joint segment(s)		• Assistance applied at distal end of segment muscle(s) inserts into		• Resistance applied at distal end of segment muscle(s) inserts into	
End Position	• End of full or available AROM		• End of full available PROM		• Muscle(s) on full stretch		• End of full available ROM, or • Start position if isometric contraction	
Substitute Movement	← Ensure no substitute movement →							
PURPOSE-SPECIFIC PROCEDURE	• Estimate and/or measure AROM	• Active movement performed according to exercise prescription	• Observe and/or measure joint PROM • Note end feel	• Passive movement performed according to treatment prescription	• Visually observe and/or measure joint position at maximum stretch of muscle	• Joint held at position of maximal muscle stretch for prescribed length of time	• Determine the amount of resistance that can be applied and allow patient to move through movement, or hold position	• Resisted movement performed or position held against resistance according to exercise prescription

(continues)

TABLE 2-1 *Continued*

Key Steps	Active Movement		Passive Movement				Resisted Movement	
	Assessment	Treatment	Assessment	Treatment	Assessment	Treatment	Assessment	Treatment
	Active ROM (AROM)	*Active Exercise*	*Passive ROM (PROM)*	*Relaxed Passive Movement*	*Muscle Length*	*Prolonged Passive Stretch*	*Muscle Strength*	*Resisted Exercise*
CHARTING	• Joint AROM • MMT grade	• Describe exercise prescribed • Note any change in patient's condition	• Joint PROM • End feel	• Describe treatment prescribed • Note any change in patient's condition	• Joint position • End feel	• Describe position and duration of stretch • Note any change in patient's condition	• MMT grade	• Describe exercise prescribed • Note any change in patient's condition

*For ease of explanation and understanding, the proximal joint segment or site of attachment of the muscle origin is stabilized and the distal joint segment or site of attachment of the muscle insertion is described as the moving segment.

ADL, activities of daily living; MMT, manual muscle testing.

NOTE: The area shaded in orange highlights COMMON TECHNIQUE that is the same for similar assessment and treatment.

Purpose-Specific Procedure

After applying the common technique, specific procedure is used to provide outcomes that meet the specific purpose of the assessment or treatment. Purpose-specific procedures include measuring AROM, PROM, noting the end feel, grading muscle strength, changing the number of times a movement is performed, changing the length of time a position is held, and/or changing the magnitude of the resistance used.

Charting

For assessment, deviations from standardized testing procedure and the findings are noted in the chart. For treatment, details of the exercise or treatment prescription used and any change in the patient's condition are noted in the chart.

EXAMPLES OF SIMILAR ASSESSMENT AND TREATMENT METHODS

Specific joint movements and muscles are used as examples to illustrate similar assessments and treatments using active, passive, or resisted movement.

In the examples, note that for assessment and treatment which use a similar type of movement, the "Common Technique" is the same, but the "Purpose," "Purpose-Specific Procedure," and "Charting" are different.

In Table 2-1 and in these examples, for ease of explanation and understanding, the proximal joint segment or site of attachment of the origin of the muscle is stabilized and the distal joint segment or site of attachment of the insertion of the muscle is described as the moving segment.

Knee Extension*: Assess Active Range of Motion (AROM) Assessment and Treatment Using Active Exercise

Assessment
AROM

Treatment
Active Exercise

PURPOSE
To assess AROM, quadriceps muscle strength, and determine the ability to perform ADL.

PURPOSE
To maintain or increase AROM, quadriceps muscle strength, and the ability to perform ADL.

COMMON TECHNIQUE

Explanation/Instruction. The therapist explains, demonstrates, and/or passively moves the limb through knee extension. The therapist instructs the patient to straighten the knee as far as possible.

Expose Region. The patient wears shorts.

Start Position. The patient is sitting, grasps the edge of the plinth, and has the nontest foot supported on a stool (Fig. 2-1).

Stabilization. The patient is instructed to maintain the thigh in the start position or the therapist may stabilize the thigh.

Movement. The patient performs knee extension.

End Position. The knee is extended as far as possible through the ROM (Fig. 2-2). The hamstrings may restrict knee extension in this position.

Substitute Movement. The patient leans back to posteriorly tilt the pelvis and extend the hip joint.

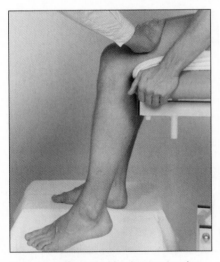

Figure 2-1 Start position knee extension: AROM assessment and active exercise.

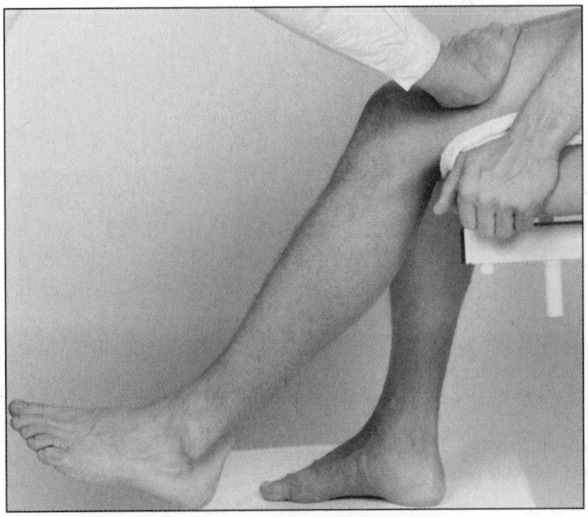

Figure 2-2 End position: AROM assessment and active exercise. The therapist may stabilize the femur and/or palpate for contraction of the knee extensors.

PURPOSE-SPECIFIC PROCEDURE
AROM is visually assessed or measured using the universal goniometer. Following the assessment of PROM, the therapist grades the strength of the knee extensors using AROM.

CHARTING
Knee extension AROM is recorded in degrees and/or the knee extensors are assigned a grade for strength.

PURPOSE-SPECIFIC PROCEDURE
Knee extension is performed actively by the patient a predetermined number of times according to the exercise prescription.

CHARTING
The prescribed exercise is described, and any change in the patient's condition is noted.

*To show an example of movement performed against gravity.
Note: Movement performed with gravity eliminated could also be used to illustrate the similarity between AROM assessment and active exercise.

Hip Flexion: Passive Range of Motion (PROM) Assessment and Treatment Using Relaxed Passive Movement

Assessment PROM	Treatment Relaxed Passive Movement

PURPOSE
To assess hip flexion PROM and determine an end feel.

PURPOSE
To maintain or increase hip flexion ROM.

COMMON TECHNIQUE

Explanation/Instruction. The therapist explains, demonstrates, and/or passively moves the limb through hip flexion. The therapist instructs the patient to relax as the movement is performed.

Expose Region. The patient wears shorts and is draped as required.

Start Position. The patient is supine. The hip and knee on the test side are in the neutral position. The other hip is extended on the plinth (Fig. 2-3).

Stabilization. The therapist stabilizes the pelvis. The trunk is stabilized through body positioning.

Movement. The therapist raises the lower extremity off the plinth and moves the femur anteriorly to flex the hip.

End Position. The femur is moved to the limit of hip flexion (Fig. 2-4).

Substitute Movement. Posterior pelvic tilt and flexion of the lumbar spine.

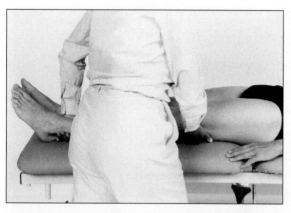

Figure 2-3 Start position hip flexion: PROM assessment and relaxed passive movement.

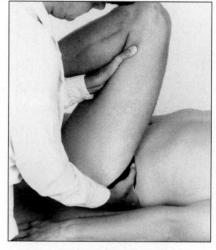

Figure 2-4 End position hip flexion: PROM assessment and relaxed passive movement.

PURPOSE-SPECIFIC PROCEDURE
The therapist applies slight overpressure at the end of the PROM to identify the end feel. The therapist observes and measures the joint PROM.

PURPOSE-SPECIFIC PROCEDURE
The hip is passively moved into flexion a predetermined number of times according to the treatment prescription.

CHARTING
The end feel and number of degrees of hip flexion PROM are recorded.

CHARTING
The prescribed treatment is described, and any change in the patient's condition is noted.

Long Finger Extensors: Muscle Length Assessment and Treatment Using Prolonged Passive Stretch

Assessment Muscle Length	Treatment Prolonged Passive Stretch

PURPOSE
To assess the length of the long finger extensor muscles.

PURPOSE
To maintain or increase the length of the long finger extensor muscles.

COMMON TECHNIQUE

Explanation/Instruction. The therapist explains, demonstrates, and/or passively positions the patient in the stretch position. The therapist instructs the patient to relax as the movement is performed and held.

Expose Region. The patient wears short-sleeved shirt.

Start Position. The patient is sitting. The elbow is extended, the forearm is pronated, and the fingers are flexed (Fig. 2-5).

Stabilization. The therapist stabilizes the radius and ulna.

Movement. The therapist flexes the wrist.

End Position. The wrist is flexed to the limit of motion so that the long finger extensors are fully stretched (Figs. 2-6 and 2-7).

Substitute Movement. Finger extension.

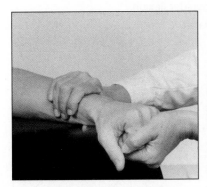

Figure 2-5 Start position long finger extensors: muscle length assessment and prolonged passive stretch.

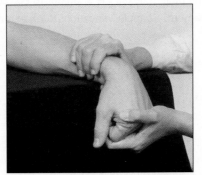

Figure 2-6 End position long finger extensors on stretch: muscle length assessment and prolonged passive stretch.

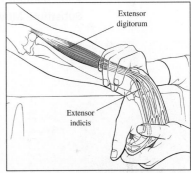

Figure 2-7 Long finger extensors on stretch.

PURPOSE-SPECIFIC PROCEDURE
With the long finger extensors on full stretch, the angle of wrist flexion is observed and/or measured, and the therapist identifies the end feel.

PURPOSE-SPECIFIC PROCEDURE
The position of maximum wrist flexion is maintained so that the long finger extensors are placed on full stretch for a prescribed length of time, and the therapist identifies the end feel.

CHARTING
The long finger extensors may be described as being shortened, and the angle of wrist flexion may be recorded. The end feel is noted.

CHARTING
The stretch position and the length of time the stretch is applied to the long finger extensors are recorded. Any change in the patient's condition is noted.

Anterior Fibers Deltoid*: Muscle Strength Assessment and Treatment Using Resisted Exercise

Assessment Muscle Strength	Treatment Resisted Exercise

PURPOSE
To assess the strength of the anterior fibers deltoid.

PURPOSE
To maintain or increase the strength of the anterior fibers deltoid.

COMMON TECHNIQUE

Explanation/Instruction. The therapist explains, demonstrates, and/or passively moves the patient through 90° shoulder flexion, with slight adduction and internal rotation. The therapist instructs the patient to work as hard as possible to raise the arm toward the ceiling as the therapist resists the movement.

Expose Region. The patient's shirt is removed. The patient is draped as required.

Start Position. The patient is sitting. The arm is at the side, with the shoulder in slight abduction and the palm facing medially (Fig. 2-8).

Stabilization. The therapist stabilizes the scapula and clavicle.

Movement. The patient flexes the shoulder, simultaneously slightly adducting and internally rotating the shoulder joint (Figs. 2-9 and 2-10).

Resistance Location. Applied on the anteromedial aspect of the arm just proximal to the elbow joint.

End Position. The patient flexes the shoulder to 90° shoulder flexion.

Substitute Movement. Scapular elevation, trunk extension.

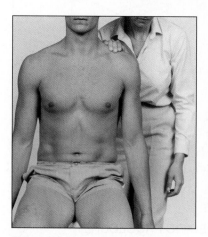

Figure 2-8 Start position for anterior fibers deltoid: manual muscle testing (MMT) and resisted exercise.

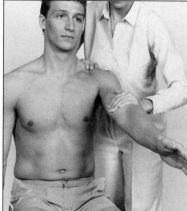

Figure 2-9 End position: for manual muscle testing (MMT) anterior fibers deltoid and resisted exercise to strengthen anterior fibers deltoid.

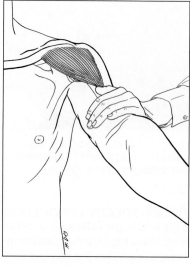

Figure 2-10 Anterior fibers deltoid.

PURPOSE-SPECIFIC PROCEDURE
The therapist assesses the amount of manual resistance that can be applied and allow the patient to move smoothly through the movement (i.e., shoulder flexion to 90°).

PURPOSE-SPECIFIC PROCEDURE
The anterior fibers of the deltoid are required to contract through the ROM against a predetermined resistance load a predetermined number of times according to the treatment prescription.

CHARTING
A grade of strength for the anterior fibers deltoid is recorded.

CHARTING
The prescribed exercise is described and any change in the patient's condition noted.

*Concentric muscle contraction is used in this example to show the similarity between muscle strength assessment and resisted exercise.
Note: isometric muscle contraction could also be used to show this similarity.

SECTION II
Regional Evaluation Techniques

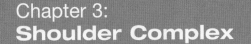

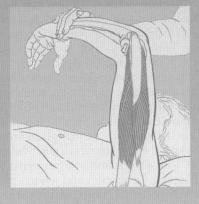

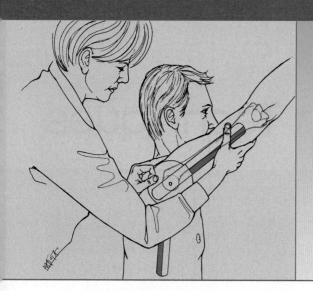

Chapter 3

Shoulder Complex

ARTICULATIONS AND MOVEMENTS

The *shoulder complex* is a related group of articulations. This group of articulations (Fig. 3-1) includes the sternoclavicular, acromioclavicular, scapulothoracic, and glenohumeral joints. The shoulder complex can be subdivided into two main components:

a. The *shoulder girdle,* which includes the sternoclavicular, acromioclavicular, and scapulothoracic joints

b. The shoulder joint, that is, the *glenohumeral joint*

The Shoulder Girdle

The shoulder girdle is connected directly to the trunk via the *sternoclavicular joint.* The medial end of the clavicle forms the lateral sternoclavicular joint surface and the lateral aspect of the manubrium sternum and adjacent superior surface of the first costal cartilage make up the medial joint surface. An articular disc lies between the articular surfaces. Categorized as a saddle joint, the clavicular surface of the joint is convex vertically and concave horizontally, and articulates with the reciprocal surfaces on the medial aspect of the joint.[1]

Movements at the sternoclavicular joint include elevation, depression, protraction, retraction, and rotation of the clavicle. During elevation and depression, the lateral end of the clavicle moves superiorly and inferiorly, respectively, in the frontal plane around a sagittal axis. The lateral end of the clavicle moves in an anterior direction with protraction and in a posterior direction with retraction. Protraction and retraction movements of the clavicle occur in a horizontal plane about a vertical axis. Rotation of the clavicle takes place in a sagittal plane around a frontal axis (i.e., an axis that passes along the long axis of the clavicle). Mobility at the sternoclavicular joint is requisite for the clavicular and scapular motion essential to the normal performance of shoulder elevation (i.e., movement of the arm above shoulder level to a vertical position alongside the head).

The *acromioclavicular joint,* linking the clavicle and scapula, is classified as a plane joint formed by the relatively flat articular surfaces of the lateral end of the clavicle and the acromion process of the scapula. In some instances, the joint surfaces are partially separated by an articular disc.[1] At the acromioclavicular joint, limited gliding motions between the clavicle and scapula during shoulder girdle movement allow scapular motion independent of clavicular motion, and alignment of the scapula against the chest wall.[2]

A physiological or functional joint, the *scapulothoracic joint* consists of flexible soft tissues (i.e., subscapularis and serratus anterior) sandwiched between the scapula and the chest wall that allow the scapula to move over the thorax. Scapular motions are accompanied by movement of the clavicle via the acromioclavicular joint.

Scapular motions include elevation, depression, retraction, protraction, lateral (upward) rotation, and medial (downward) rotation. Movement of the scapula in a cranial direction is called elevation and is accompanied by elevation of the clavicle. The scapula and clavicle move in a caudal direction with scapular depression. Scapular retraction and protraction occur in the horizontal plane around a vertical axis as the medial border of the scapula moves either toward (retraction) or away from (protraction) the vertebral column. Scapular retraction and protraction are accompanied by retraction and protraction of the clavicle, respectively. The scapula also rotates laterally and medially, with reference to the movement of the inferior angle, so that the glenoid cavity moves in either an upward (cranial) or a downward (caudal) direction, respectively (Fig. 3-2).

In the clinical setting, motion at the sternoclavicular joint and scapula is not easily measured, and it is not possible to measure motion at the acromioclavicular joint. Therefore, scapular and clavicular motions are normally assessed by visual observation of active movement and through passive movement.

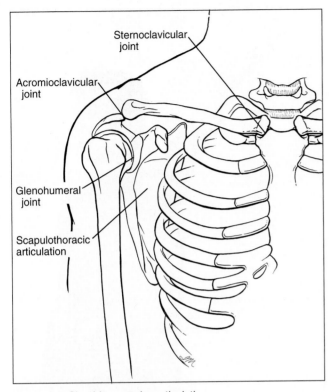

Figure 3-1 Shoulder complex articulations.

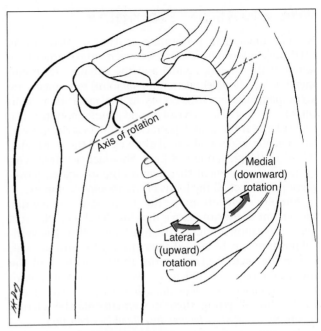

Figure 3-2 Scapular axis of rotation.

The Glenohumeral Joint

The *glenohumeral or shoulder joint* is a ball-and-socket joint formed medially by the concave surface of the scapular glenoid cavity and laterally by the convex surface of the head of the humerus. The axes around which glenohumeral joint motions occur are illustrated in Figures 3-3 and 3-4. In Figure 3-4, from the anatomical position, the glenohumeral joint may be flexed and extended in the sagittal plane with movement occurring around a frontal axis. The movements of shoulder abduction and adduction occur in the frontal plane around a sagittal axis. In Figure 3-3, the shoulder is positioned in 90° abduction for the purpose of illustrating the vertical axis around which the movements of shoulder horizontal adduction and abduction occur in the transverse plane. With the shoulder in 90° abduction, shoulder internal rotation and external rotation takes place in a sagittal plane about the longitudinal axis of the humerus (Fig. 3-3). However, with the arm at the side in anatomical position, internal and external rotation takes place in a horizontal plane about the longitudinal axis of the humerus.

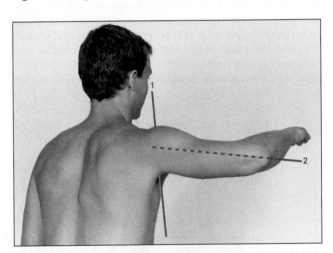

Figure 3-3 Glenohumeral axes: *(1)* horizontal abduction-adduction; *(2)* internal-external rotation.

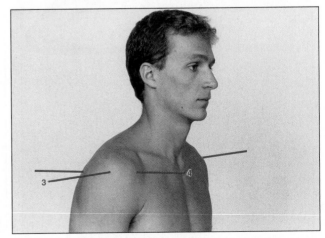

Figure 3-4 Glenohumeral axes: *(3)* flexion-extension; *(4)* abduction-adduction.

The Shoulder Complex

Normal function in performing activities of daily living (ADL) depends on the integrated movement patterns of the joints of the shoulder girdle and the shoulder (glenohumeral) joint. Shoulder (glenohumeral joint) movements are accompanied at varying points in the range of motion (ROM) by scapular, clavicular, and trunk motions. The movements at the scapulothoracic, acromioclavicular, sternoclavicular, and spinal articulations extend the ROM capabilities of the glenohumeral joint. Shoulder elevation is an example of movement that requires the integrated movement patterns of all the joints of the shoulder complex.

Shoulder elevation: is the term used to describe movement of the arm above shoulder level (i.e., 90°) to a vertical position alongside the head (i.e., 180°). The vertical position may be arrived at by moving the arm through either the sagittal plane or the frontal plane, and the movements are referred to as *shoulder elevation through flexion* or *shoulder elevation through abduction,* respectively. In the clinical setting, these movements may be referred to simply as *shoulder flexion* and *shoulder abduction.*

Moving the arm through other vertical planes located between the sagittal and frontal planes will also bring the arm to the vertical position alongside the head. The plane of the scapula lies 30° to 45° anterior to the frontal plane.[3] The scapular plane is the plane of reference for diagonal movements of shoulder elevation and is the plane often used when the arm is raised to perform overhead activities. This midplane elevation is called *scaption*[4] (Fig. 3-5).

Figures 3-6A and 3-7A illustrate the integrated movement patterns of the joints of the shoulder complex

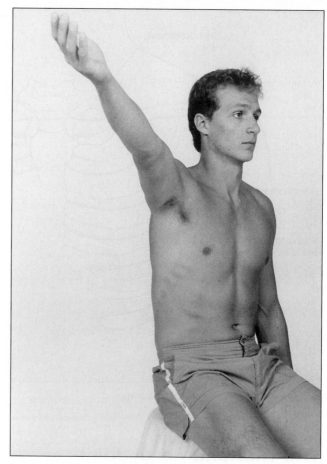

Figure 3-5 Elevation: plane of the scapula.

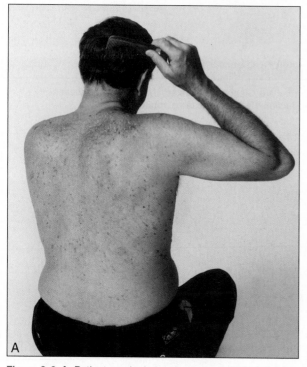

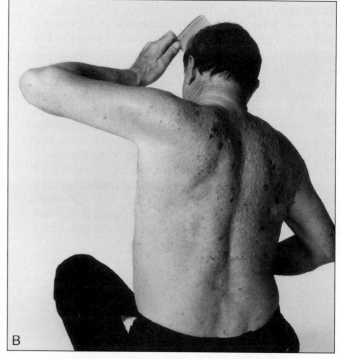

Figure 3-6 A. Patient combs hair using normal right upper extremity. **B.** Patient attempts to comb hair using left upper extremity with restricted glenohumeral joint movement. Substitute motions are observed at the left shoulder girdle and more distant joints.

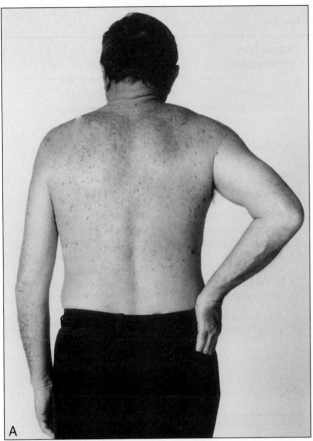 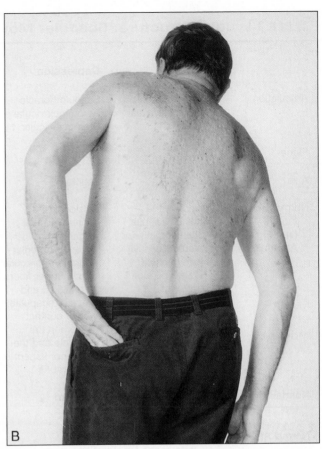

Figure 3-7 A. Patient reaches into back pocket using normal right upper extremity. **B.** Patient attempts to reach into back pocket using left upper extremity with restricted glenohumeral joint movement. Substitute motions are observed at the left shoulder girdle and more distant joints.

during the normal performance of two ADL, combing ones hair and reaching into a back pocket. Figures 3-6B and 3-7B illustrate the changes that occur in the integrated movement patterns when motion is restricted at one of the joints of the shoulder complex, in this case the glenohumeral joint. Observe how increased movement

(i.e., substitute motion) of the scapula and trunk is used to compensate for the loss of motion at the glenohumeral joint. The completion of the two ADL would not be possible without employing the substitute motions.

The joints and movements of the shoulder complex are summarized in Tables 3-1 to 3-3.

TABLE 3-1 Joint Structure: Scapular Movements

	Elevation	Depression	Abduction (Protraction)	Abduction (Retraction)
Articulation[1,5]	Scapulothoracic Acromioclavicular Sternoclavicular	Scapulothoracic Acromioclavicular Sternoclavicular	Scapulothoracic Acromioclavicular Sternoclavicular	Scapulothoracic Acromioclavicular Sternoclavicular
Plane	Frontal	Frontal	Horizontal	Horizontal
Axis	Sagittal	Sagittal	Vertical	Vertical
Normal limiting factors[5-9]* (see Fig. 3-8 A and B)	Tension in the costoclavicular ligament, inferior sternoclavicular joint capsule, lower fibers of trapezius, pectoralis minor, and subclavius	Tension in the interclavicular ligament, sternoclavicular ligament, articular disk, upper fibers of trapezius, and levator scapulae; bony contact between the clavicle and the superior aspect of the first rib	Tension in the trapezoid ligament, posterior sternoclavicular ligament, posterior lamina of the costoclavicular ligament, trapezius, and rhomboids	Tension in the conoid ligament, anterior lamina of the costoclavicular ligament, anterior sternoclavicular ligament, pectoralis minor, and serratus anterior
Normal end feel[6,10]	Firm	Firm/hard	Firm	Firm
Normal AROM[5]†	10–12 cm (total range for elevation—depression)		10–12 cm (total range for abduction—adduction)	

	Medial Rotation (Downward Rotation)	Lateral Rotation (Upward Rotation)		
Articulation[1,5]	Scapulothoracic Acromioclavicular Sternoclavicular	Scapulothoracic Acromioclavicular Sternoclavicular		
Plane	Frontal	Frontal		
Axis	Sagittal	Sagittal		
Normal limiting factors[5-9]* (see Fig. 3-8 A and B)	Tension in the conoid ligament and serratus anterior	Tension in the trapezoid ligament, the rhomboid muscles and the levator scapulae		
Normal end Feel[6,10]	Firm	Firm		
Normal AROM[5]	45–60° (total range for medial-lateral rotation)			

Note: Medial and lateral rotations of the scapula are associated with extension and/or adduction, and flexion and/or abduction of the shoulder, respectively.

*There is a paucity of definitive research that identifies the normal limiting factors (NLF) of joint motion. The NLF and end feels listed here are based on knowledge of anatomy, clinical experience, and available references.

†AROM, active range of motion.

TABLE 3-2   Joint Structure: Glenohumeral Joint Movements

	Extension	Internal Rotation	External Rotation	Horizontal Abduction	Horizontal Adduction
Articulation[1,5]	Glenohumeral	Glenohumeral	Glenohumeral	Glenohumeral	Glenohumeral
Plane	Sagittal	Horizontal	Horizontal	Horizontal	Horizontal
Axis	Frontal	Longitudinal	Longitudinal	Vertical	Vertical
Normal limiting factors[5–9]* (see Fig. 3-8B)	Tension in the anterior band of the coracohumeral ligament, the anterior joint capsule, and clavicular fibers of pectoralis major	Tension in the posterior joint capsule, infraspinatus, and teres minor	Tension in all bands of the glenohumeral ligament, coracohumeral ligament, the anterior joint capsule, subscapularis, pectoralis major, teres major, and latissimus dorsi	Tension in the anterior joint capsule, the glenohumeral ligament, and pectoralis major	Tension in the posterior joint capsule Soft tissue apposition
Normal end feel[6,10]	Firm	Firm	Firm	Firm	Firm/soft
Normal AROM[11] (AROM[12])	0–60° (0–60°)	0–70° (0–70°)	0–90° (0–90°)	0–45° (−)	0–135° (−)

*There is a paucity of definitive research that identifies the normal limiting factors (NLF) of joint motion. The NLF and end feels listed here are based on knowledge of anatomy, clinical experience, and available references.

TABLE 3-3   Joint Structure: Shoulder Complex Movements

	Elevation Through Flexion	Elevation Through Abduction
Articulation[1,5]	Glenohumeral Acromioclavicular Sternoclavicular Scapulothoracic	Glenohumeral Acromioclavicular Sternoclavicular Scapulothoracic Subdeltoid[1]
Plane	Sagittal	Frontal
Axis	Frontal	Sagittal
Normal limiting factors[5–9]* (see Fig. 3-8B)	Tension in the posterior band of the coracohumeral ligament, posterior joint capsule, shoulder extensors, and external rotators; scapular movement limited by tension in rhomboids, levator scapulae, and the trapezoid ligament	Tension in the middle and inferior bands of the glenohumeral ligament, inferior joint capsule, shoulder adductors; greater tuberosity of the humerus contacting the upper portion of the glenoid and glenoid labrum or the lateral surface of the acromion; scapular movement limited by tension in rhomboids, levator scapulae, and the trapezoid ligament
Normal end feel[6,10]	Firm	Firm/hard
Normal AROM[1,5,11] (AROM[12])	0–180° (0–165°) 0–60°, glenohumeral 60–180°, glenohumeral, scapular movement, and trunk movement	0–180° (0–165°) 0–30°, glenohumeral 30–180°, glenohumeral, scapular movement, and trunk movement
Capsular pattern[10,13]	Glenohumeral: external rotation, abduction (only through 90–120° range), internal rotation Sternoclavicular/acromioclavicular: pain at extreme range of motion notably horizontal adduction and full elevation	

*There is a paucity of definitive research that identifies the normal limiting factors (NLF) of joint motion. The NLF and end feels listed here are based on knowledge of anatomy, clinical experience, and available references.

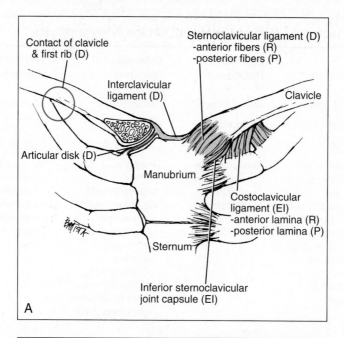

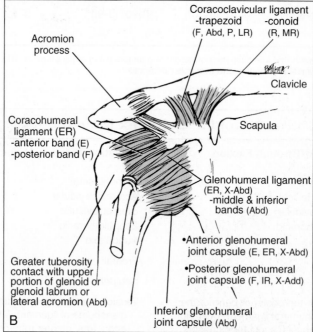

Figure 3-8 **Normal Limiting Factors. A.** Anterior view of sternoclavicular joints showing noncontractile structures that normally limit motion. **B.** Anterior view of the shoulder showing noncontractile structures that normally limit motion.*

*Motion limited by structure is identified in brackets, using the following abbreviations for (1) Scapular movements, (2) Glenohumeral joint movements, and (3) shoulder complex movements:
(1) Scapular movements:
El, elevation;   P, protraction;
D, depression;   R, retraction;
MR, medial (downward) rotation;   LR, lateral (upward) rotation.
(2) Glenohumeral joint movements:
E, extension;   X-Add, horizontal adduction;
IR, internal rotation;   X-Abd, horizontal abduction.
ER, external rotation;
(3) Shoulder complex movements:
F, elevation through flexion;   Abd, elevation through abduction.
Muscles normally limiting motion are not illustrated.

SURFACE ANATOMY (Figs. 3-9 through 3-14)

Structure	Location
1. Inion	Dome-shaped process that marks the center of the superior nuchal line.
2. Vertebral border of the scapula	Approximately 5–6 cm lateral to the thoracic spinous processes covering ribs 2–7.
3. Inferior angle of the scapula	At the inferior aspect of the vertebral border of the scapula.
4. Spine of the scapula	The bony ridge running obliquely across the upper four-fifths of the scapula.
5. Acromion process	Lateral aspect of the spine of the scapula at the tip of the shoulder.
6. Clavicle	Prominent S-shaped bone on the anterosuperior aspect of the thorax.
7. Coracoid process	Approximately 2 cm distal to the junction of the middle and lateral thirds of the clavicle in the deltopectoral triangle. Press firmly upward and laterally, deep to the anterior fibers of the deltoid.
8. Brachial pulse	Palpate pulse on the medial, proximal aspect of the upper arm posterior to the coracobrachialis.
9. Lateral epicondyle of the humerus	Lateral projection at the distal end of the humerus.
10. Olecranon process of the ulna	Posterior aspect of the elbow at the proximal end of the shaft of the ulna.
11. T12 spinous process	The most distal thoracic spinous process slightly above the level of the olecranon process of the ulna when the body is in the anatomical position.
12. Sternum	Flat bone surface along the midline of the anterior aspect of the thorax.

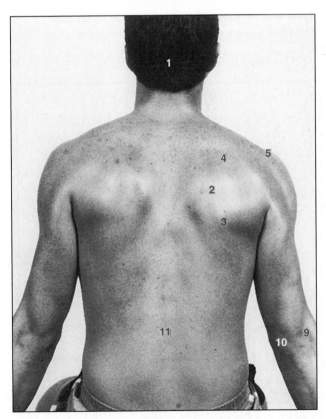

Figure 3-9 Posterior aspect of the shoulder complex.

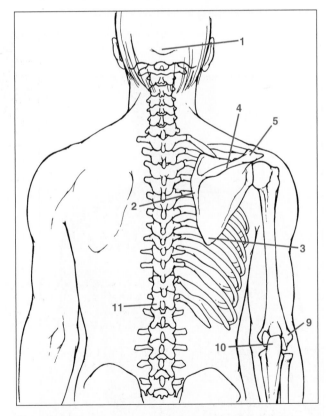

Figure 3-10 Bony anatomy, posterior aspect of the shoulder complex.

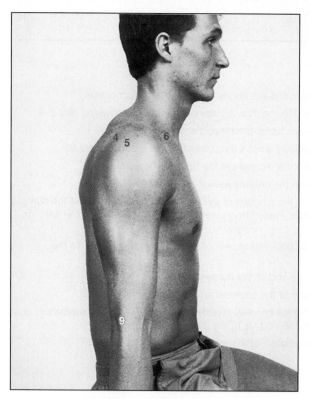

Figure 3-11 Lateral aspect of the shoulder complex.

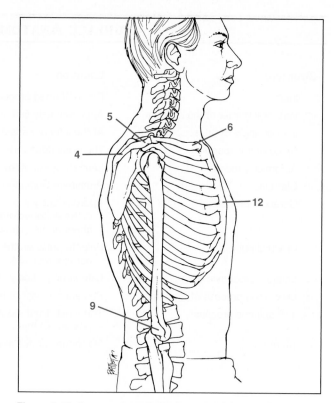

Figure 3-12 Bony anatomy, lateral aspect of the shoulder complex.

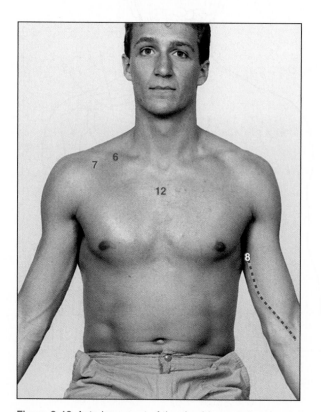

Figure 3-13 Anterior aspect of the shoulder complex.

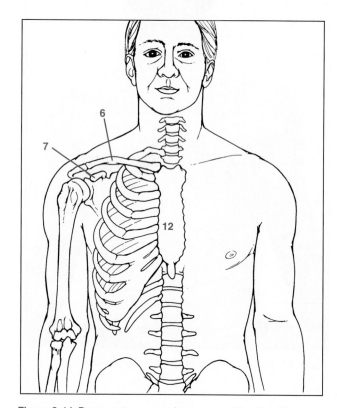

Figure 3-14 Bony anatomy, anterior aspect of the shoulder complex.

RANGE OF MOTION ASSESSMENT AND MEASUREMENT

Practice Makes Perfect

To aid you in practicing the skills covered in this section, or for a handy review, use the practical testing forms found at http://thepoint.lww.com/Clarkson3e.

Normal function of the shoulder complex depends on the integrated movement patterns of all joints that are a part of the shoulder complex. Therefore, a complete evaluation of ROM of the shoulder complex must include evaluation of scapular and glenohumeral joint active and passive ROM. Evaluation of scapular, glenohumeral, and integrated shoulder complex movement is presented.

General Scan: Upper Extremity Active Range of Motion

Scan the **active range of motion** (AROM) of the upper extremity joints, starting with the patient in the sitting or standing position with the arms at the sides (Fig. 3-15).

Instruct the patient to place the left hand behind the neck, and reach down the spine as far as possible (Fig. 3-16A). Observe the ROM of scapular abduction and lateral (upward) rotation, shoulder elevation and external rotation, elbow flexion, forearm supination, wrist radial deviation, and finger extension.

Instruct the patient to place the right hand on the low back (Fig. 3-16A), and reach up the spine as far as possible. Observe the ROM of scapular adduction and medial (downward) rotation, shoulder extension and internal rotation, elbow flexion, forearm pronation, wrist radial deviation, and finger extension.

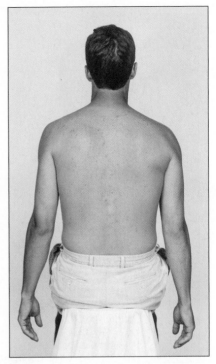

Figure 3-15 Start position: scan of AROM of the upper extremities.

The vertebral levels reached at the levels of the tips of the middle fingers as the patient reaches behind the neck or up the back may be used as a general measure of AROM of the upper extremity joints.

Instruct the patient to return to the start position and repeat the movements on the contralateral sides (see Fig. 3-16B).

As observed in Figure 3-16, there is often an appreciable difference in the ROM between sides that can be considered normal.

Figure 3-17 illustrates a general scan of the upper extremity AROM in the presence of normal right and decreased left glenohumeral joint ROM. As the patient attempts to perform the test movements, substitute movements at the left shoulder girdle and more distant joints are used to compensate for the restricted left shoulder joint ROM.

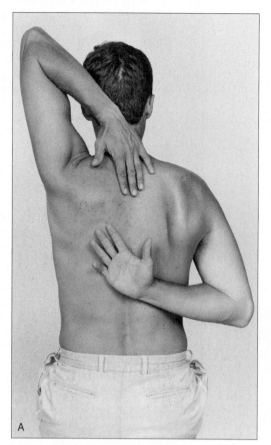
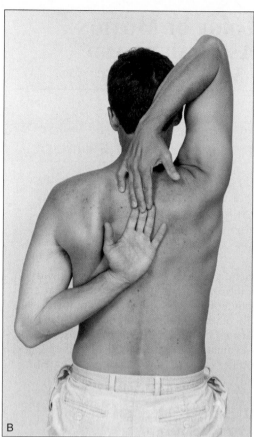

Figure 3-16 **A** and **B.** End positions: scan of AROM of the upper extremities.

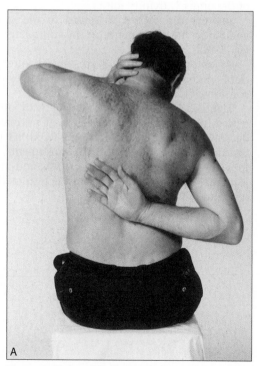
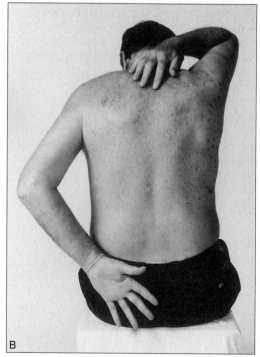

Figure 3-17 **A** and **B.** End positions: scan of AROM of the upper extremities with decreased left glenohumeral joint mobility. Substitute motions are observed at the left shoulder girdle and more distant joints.

Scapular Movements

Normal ROM at the sternoclavicular and acromioclavicular joints (i.e., clavicular motion) is required for normal scapular motion. In the clinical setting, motion at the sternoclavicular joint and scapula is not easily measured, and it is not possible to measure motion at the acromioclavicular joint.

Scapular movement (see Table 3-1) is assessed by visual observation of the AROM and the evaluation of passive movement. The ROM is estimated as either "full" or "restricted." In the presence of decreased scapular ROM, the motion at the sternoclavicular and acromioclavicular joints is assessed; however, these assessment techniques are beyond the scope of this text.

AROM Assessment

Start Position. The patient is sitting and assumes a relaxed, anatomical posture (Fig. 3-18). In this posture, the scapula normally lies between the second and seventh ribs and the vertebral border lays approximately 5 to 6 cm lateral to the spine. The therapist stands behind the patient to observe the scapular movements.

Scapular Elevation
Movement. The patient moves the shoulders toward the ears in an upward or cranial direction (Fig. 3-19).

Scapular Depression
Movement. The patient moves the shoulders toward the waist in a downward or caudal direction (Fig. 3-20).

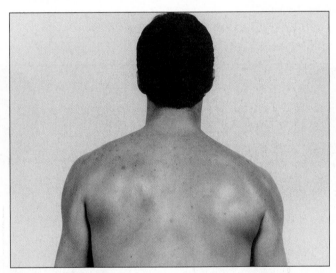

Figure 3-18 Start position for all active scapular movements.

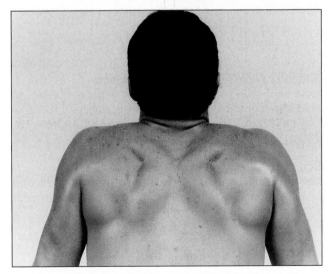

Figure 3-19 Active movement: scapular elevation.

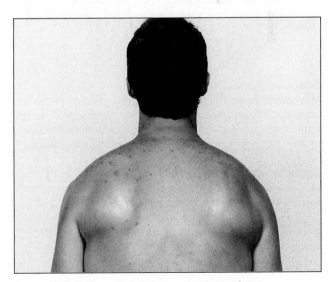

Figure 3-20 Active movement: scapular depression.

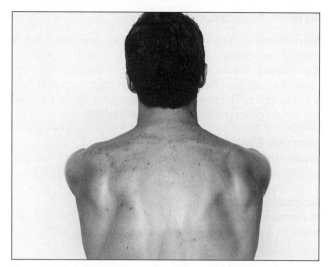

Figure 3-21 Active movement: scapular abduction.

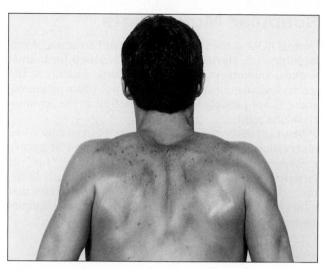

Figure 3-22 Active movement: scapular adduction.

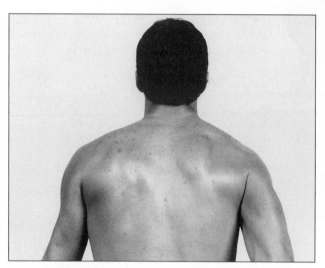

Figure 3-23 Active movement: scapular medial (downward) rotation.

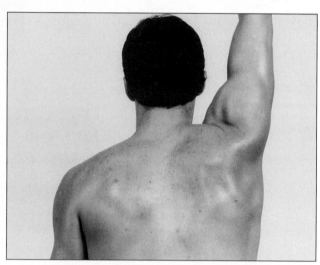

Figure 3-24 Active movement: scapular lateral (upward) rotation.

Scapular Abduction

Movement. From the start position, the patient flexes the arms to 90°, and scapular abduction is observed as the patient reaches forward (Fig. 3-21). The vertebral borders of the scapulae move away from the vertebral column.

Scapular Adduction

Movement. The patient moves the scapulae horizontally toward the vertebral column (Fig. 3-22).

Scapular Medial (Downward) Rotation

Movement. The patient extends and adducts the arm to place the hand across the small of the back and the inferior angle of the scapula moves in a medial direction (Fig. 3-23).

Scapular Lateral (Upward) Rotation

Movement. The patient elevates the arm through flexion or abduction (Fig. 3-24). During elevation, the inferior angle of the scapula moves in a lateral direction.

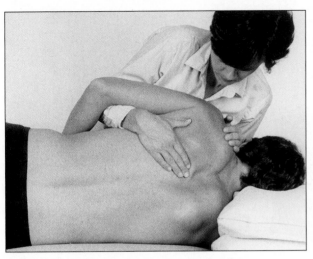

Figure 3-25 Passive movement: scapular elevation.

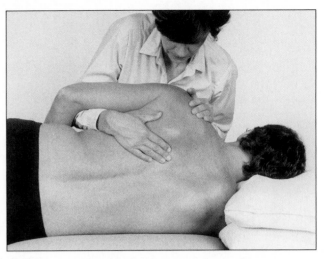

Figure 3-26 Passive movement: scapular depression.

PROM Assessment

Forms 3-1 to 3-4

Start Position. The patient is in a side-lying position with the hips and knees flexed, the head relaxed and supported on a pillow. This position remains unchanged for all scapular movements.

Stabilization. The weight of the trunk stabilizes the thorax.

Scapular Elevation
Procedure. The therapist cups the inferior angle of the scapula with one hand and elevates the scapula, while controlling the direction of movement with the other hand (Fig. 3-25).

End Feel. Firm.

Joint Glides. *Scapular elevation*—the scapula glides in a cranial direction on the thorax. *Sternoclavicular joint:* elevation of the clavicle—the convex medial end of the clavicle glides inferiorly on the fixed concave surface of the manubrium. *Acromioclavicular joint*—gliding.

Scapular Depression
Procedure. The therapist places one hand on the top of the shoulder girdle to depress the scapula. The therapist's other hand cups the inferior angle of the scapula to control the direction of movement (Fig. 3-26).

End Feel. Firm/hard.

Joint Glides. *Scapular depression*—the scapula glides in a caudal direction on the thorax. *Sternoclavicular joint:* depression of the clavicle—the convex medial end of the clavicle glides superiorly on the fixed concave surface of the manubrium. *Acromioclavicular joint*—gliding.

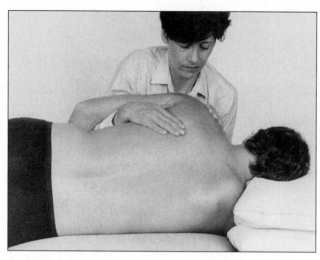

Figure 3-27 Passive movement: scapular abduction.

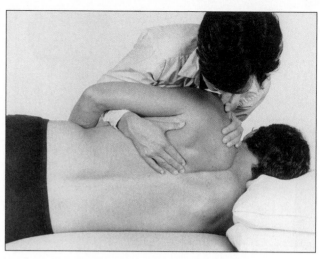

Figure 3-28 Passive movement: scapular adduction.

Scapular Abduction

Procedure. The therapist grasps the vertebral border and inferior angle of the scapula using the thumb and index finger of one hand and abducts the scapula. The therapist's other hand is placed on top of the shoulder girdle to assist in abduction (Fig. 3-27).

End Feel. Firm.

Joint Glides. *Scapular abduction*—the scapula glides laterally on the thorax. *Sternoclavicular joint:* protraction of the clavicle—the concave medial end of the clavicle glides anteriorly on the fixed convex surface of the manubrium. *Acromioclavicular joint*—gliding.

Scapular Adduction

Procedure. The therapist grasps the axillary border and inferior angle of the scapula using the thumb and index finger of one hand and adducts the scapula. The therapist's other hand is placed on top of the shoulder girdle to assist in adduction (Fig. 3-28).

End Feel. Firm.

Joint Glides. *Scapular adduction*—the scapula glides medially on the thorax. *Sternoclavicular joint:* retraction of the clavicle—the concave medial end of the clavicle glides posteriorly on the fixed convex surface of the manubrium. *Acromioclavicular joint*—gliding.

Shoulder Complex— Movements

Shoulder elevation depends on full ROM at the sternoclavicular, acromioclavicular, scapular, and glenohumeral joints (Tables 3-2 and 3-3). In the presence of decreased shoulder elevation ROM, the therapist must identify which joint(s) of the shoulder complex lack full ROM to effectively plan treatment to restore full ROM. The PROM at the shoulder girdle (i.e., scapular and clavicular motion) is evaluated independent of the PROM at the glenohumeral joint. To isolate the glenohumeral joint PROM, the therapist must stabilize the scapula and clavicle. To ensure adequate stabilization when measuring glenohumeral joint PROM, a second therapist may assist to align the goniometer. To assess and measure movements that require motion at all articulations of the shoulder complex, the trunk is stabilized.

Shoulder Elevation Through Flexion (Glenohumeral Joint, Scapular and Clavicular Motion)

AROM Assessment

Substitute Movement. Trunk extension and shoulder abduction.

PROM Assessment

Form 3-5

Start Position. The patient is in a crook-lying (Fig. 3-29) or a sitting position. The arm is at the side with the palm facing medially.

Stabilization. The weight of the trunk. The therapist stabilizes the thorax.

Therapist's Distal Hand Placement. The therapist grasps the distal humerus.

End Position. The therapist moves the humerus anteriorly and upward to the limit of motion for shoulder elevation through flexion (Fig. 3-30). The elbow is maintained in extension to prevent restriction of shoulder flexion ROM due to passive insufficiency of the two-joint triceps muscle.[14]

End Feel. Firm.

Joint Glides/Spin. Shoulder elevation through flexion:

Scapular lateral (upward) rotation—the inferior angle of the scapula rotates in a lateral direction on the thorax.

Sternoclavicular joint: (a) elevation of the clavicle—the convex medial end of the clavicle glides inferiorly on the fixed concave surface of the manubrium, and (b) posterior rotation of the clavicle—the clavicle spins on the fixed surfaces of the manubrium.

Acromioclavicular joint—gliding.

Glenohumeral joint flexion—the convex humeral head spins (i.e., rotates around a fixed point) on the fixed concave glenoid cavity.

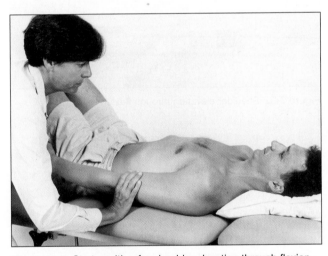

Figure 3-29 Start position for shoulder elevation through flexion.

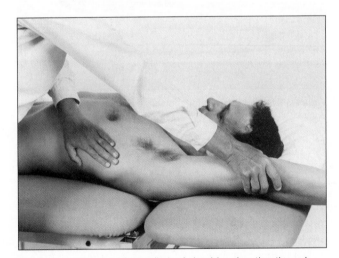

Figure 3-30 Firm end feel at limit of shoulder elevation through flexion.

Measurement: Universal Goniometer

Start Position. The patient is in a crook-lying position (Fig. 3-31) or sitting. The arm is at the side, with the palm facing medially.

Stabilization. The weight of the trunk. The scapula is left free to move.

Goniometer Axis. The axis is placed at the lateral aspect of the center of the humeral head. In anatomical position, the center of the humeral head is located about 2.5 cm inferior to the lateral aspect of the acromion process (see Figs. 3-31 and 3-36).

Stationary Arm. Parallel to the lateral midline of the trunk.

Movable Arm. Parallel to the longitudinal axis of the humerus.

End Position. The humerus is moved in an anterior and upward direction to the limit of motion (shoulder elevation 180°). This movement represents scapular, clavicular, and glenohumeral motion (Fig. 3-32).

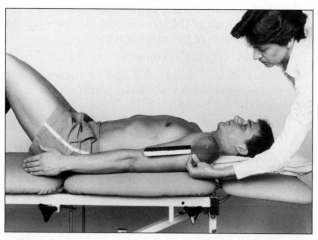

Figure 3-31 Start position for shoulder elevation through flexion: supine.

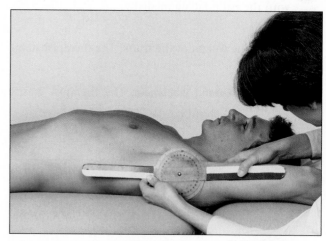

Figure 3-32 Shoulder elevation through flexion.

Glenohumeral Joint (Shoulder) Flexion

AROM Assessment

The patient cannot perform isolated glenohumeral joint flexion ROM without the scapula being stabilized.

PROM Assessment

Form 3-6

Start Position. The patient is in a crook-lying or a sitting position. The arm is at the side with the palm facing medially.

Stabilization. The therapist places one hand on the axillary border of the scapula to stabilize the scapula.

Therapist's Distal Hand Placement. The therapist grasps the distal humerus.

End Position. While stabilizing the scapula, the therapist moves the humerus anteriorly and upward to the limit of motion to assess glenohumeral joint motion (Fig. 3-33).

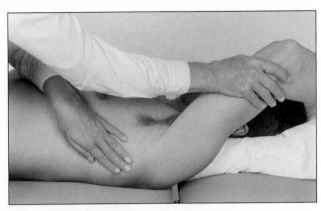

Figure 3-33 Firm end feel at limit of glenohumeral joint flexion.

End Feel. Firm.

Joint Spin. *Glenohumeral joint flexion*—the convex humeral head spins on the fixed concave glenoid cavity.

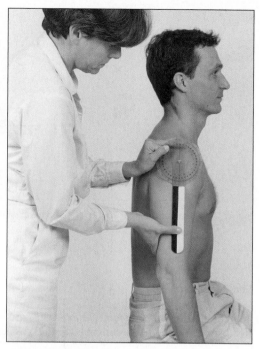

Figure 3-34 Start position for shoulder elevation through flexion: sitting.

Measurement: Universal Goniometer

Start Position. The patient is in sitting (Fig. 3-34) or crook-lying position. The arm is at the side, with the palm facing medially.

Stabilization. The therapist stabilizes the scapula.

Goniometer Axis. The axis is placed at the lateral aspect of the center of the humeral head about 2.5 cm inferior to the lateral aspect of the acromion process when in anatomical position (see Figs. 3-34 and 3-36).

Stationary Arm. Parallel to the lateral midline of the trunk.

Movable Arm. Parallel to the longitudinal axis of the humerus.

End Position. The humerus is moved in an anterior and upward direction to the limit of motion (glenohumeral joint flexion 120°)[8] (Figs. 3-35 and 3-36).

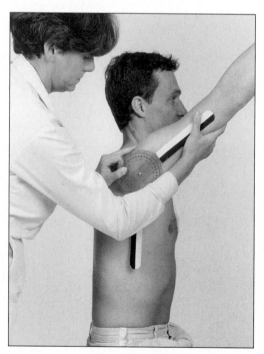

Figure 3-35 Goniometer alignment: shoulder elevation through flexion, glenohumeral joint flexion, and extension.

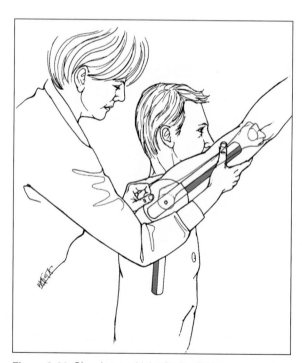

Figure 3-36 Glenohumeral joint flexion ROM.

Shoulder Extension

AROM Assessment

Substitute Movement. Scapular anterior tilting, scapular elevation, and shoulder abduction. In sitting, the patient may flex and ipsilaterally rotate the trunk.

PROM Assessment

Start Position. The patient is prone (Fig. 3-37) or sitting. The arm is at the side, with the palm facing medially.

Form 3-7

Stabilization. The therapist stabilizes the scapula to isolate and assess glenohumeral joint motion.

Therapist's Distal Hand Placement. The therapist grasps the distal humerus.

End Position. The therapist moves the humerus posteriorly until the scapula begins to move (Fig. 3-38). The elbow is flexed to prevent restriction of shoulder extension ROM due to passive insufficiency of the two-joint biceps brachii muscle.[14]

End Feel. Firm.

Joint Spin. *Glenohumeral joint extension*—the convex humeral head spins on the fixed concave glenoid cavity.

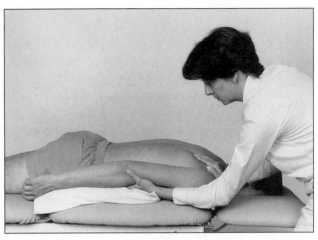

Figure 3-37 Start position for glenohumeral joint extension.

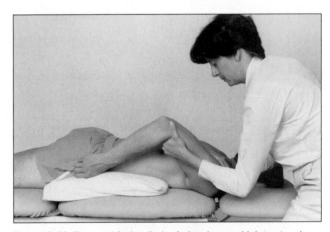

Figure 3-38 Firm end feel at limit of glenohumeral joint extension.

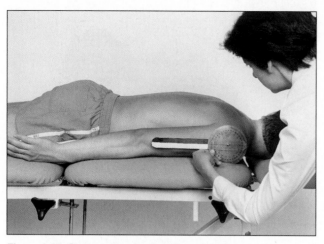

Figure 3-39 Start position for shoulder extension.

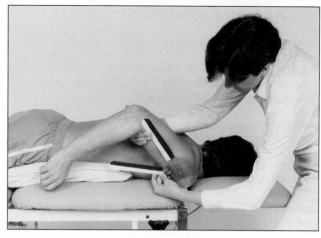

Figure 3-40 Shoulder extension: prone.

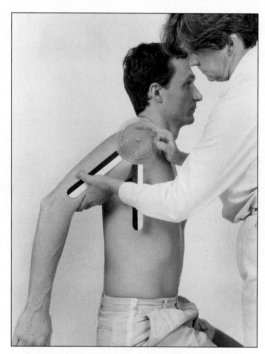

Figure 3-41 Shoulder extension: sitting.

Measurement: Universal Goniometer

Start Position. The patient is prone (Fig. 3-39) or sitting. The arm is at the side, with the palm facing medially.

Stabilization. The therapist's forearm may be used to stabilize the scapula.

Goniometer Axis. The axis is placed at the lateral aspect of the center of the humeral head about 2.5 cm inferior to the lateral aspect of the acromion process when in anatomical position (see Figs. 3-36 and 3-39).

Stationary Arm. Parallel to the lateral midline of the trunk.

Movable Arm. Parallel to the longitudinal axis of the humerus, pointing toward the lateral epicondyle of the humerus.

End Position. The humerus is moved posteriorly to the limit of motion in (shoulder extension 60°) (Figs. 3-40 and 3-41).

Shoulder Elevation Through Abduction (Glenohumeral Joint, Scapular and Clavicular Motion)

AROM Assessment

Substitute Movement. Contralateral trunk lateral flexion, scapular elevation, and shoulder flexion.

PROM Assessment

Form 3-8

The humerus is externally rotated when performing shoulder elevation through abduction to allow the greater tuberosity of the humerus to clear the acromion process. Prior to testing elevation through abduction, ensure the patient is capable of full shoulder external rotation.

Start Position. The patient is supine (Fig. 3-42) or sitting. The arm is at the side with the shoulder in external rotation. Ensure the patient sits in an upright posture, as the slouched sitting posture has been shown[15] to result in decreased shoulder abduction ROM.

Stabilization. The therapist stabilizes the trunk.

Therapist's Distal Hand Placement. The therapist grasps the distal humerus.

End Position. The therapist moves the humerus laterally and upward to the limit of motion for elevation through abduction (Fig. 3-43).

End Feel. Firm.

Joint Glides. Shoulder elevation through abduction:

Scapular lateral (upward) rotation—the inferior angle of the scapula rotates in a lateral direction on the thorax.

Sternoclavicular joint: (a) elevation of the clavicle—the convex medial end of the clavicle glides inferiorly on the fixed concave surface of the manubrium, and (b) posterior rotation of the clavicle—the clavicle spins on the fixed surface of the manubrium.

Acromioclavicular joint—gliding.

Glenohumeral joint abduction—the convex humeral head glides inferiorly on the fixed concave glenoid cavity.

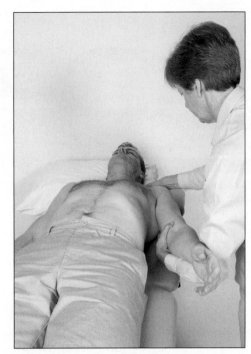

Figure 3-42 Start position for shoulder elevation through abduction.

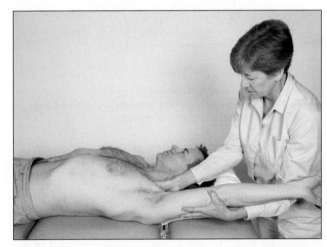

Figure 3-43 Firm end feel at limit of shoulder elevation through abduction.

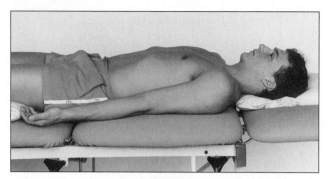

Figure 3-44 Start position for shoulder elevation through abduction.

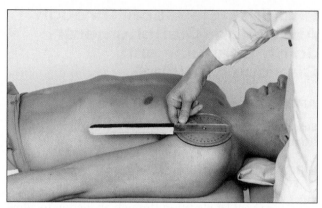

Figure 3-45 Goniometer placement for shoulder elevation through abduction.

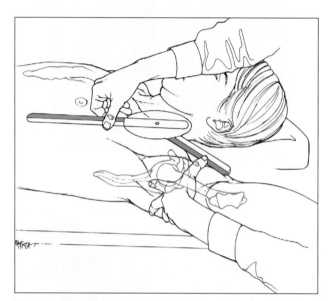

Figure 3-46 Goniometer alignment: shoulder elevation through abduction and glenohumeral joint abduction.

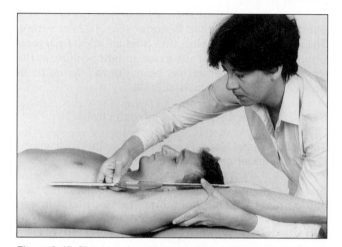

Figure 3-47 Shoulder elevation through abduction.

Measurement: Universal Goniometer

Start Position. The patient is supine (Fig. 3-44) or sitting. The arm is at the side in adduction and external rotation.

Stabilization. The weight of the trunk.

Goniometer Axis. The axis is placed at the midpoint of the anterior or posterior aspect of the glenohumeral joint, about 1.3 cm inferior and lateral to the coracoid process (Figs. 3-45 and 3-46).

Stationary Arm. Parallel to the sternum.

Movable Arm. Parallel to the longitudinal axis of the humerus.

End Position. The humerus is moved laterally and upward to the limit of motion (shoulder elevation 180°) (Fig. 3-47). This movement represents scapular and glenohumeral movement. The posterior aspect may be preferred for measurement of shoulder elevation through abduction range in women because the breast may interfere with the goniometer placement anteriorly (Fig. 3-48).

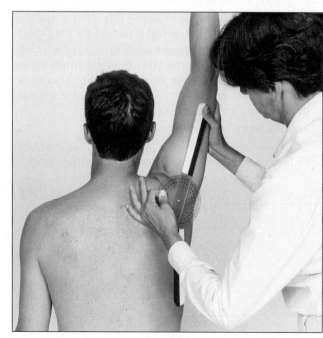

Figure 3-48 Shoulder elevation through abduction: sitting.

Glenohumeral Joint (Shoulder) Abduction

AROM Assessment

The patient cannot perform isolated glenohumeral joint abduction ROM without the scapula being stabilized.

PROM Assessment

Form 3-9

Start Position. The patient is supine (Fig. 3-49) or sitting. The arm is at the side with the elbow flexed to 90°.

Stabilization. The therapist stabilizes the scapula and clavicle.

Therapist's Distal Hand Placement. The therapist grasps the distal humerus.

End Position. The therapist moves the humerus laterally and upward to the limit of motion of glenohumeral joint abduction (Fig. 3-50).

End Feel. Firm or hard.

Joint Glide. *Glenohumeral joint abduction*—the convex humeral head glides inferiorly on the fixed concave glenoid cavity.

Measurement: Universal Goniometer (not shown)

Start Position. The patient is supine or sitting. The arm is at the side with the elbow flexed to 90° (see Fig. 3-49).

Goniometer Placement. The goniometer is placed the same as for shoulder elevation through abduction (see Figs. 3-45 and 3-46).

Stabilization. The therapist stabilizes the scapula and clavicle to isolate and measure glenohumeral joint abduction.

End Position. The humerus is moved laterally and upward to the limit of motion (glenohumeral joint abduction 90–120°)[8] to measure glenohumeral joint abduction.

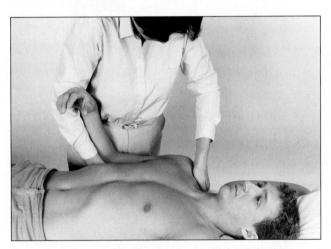

Figure 3-49 Start position for glenohumeral joint abduction.

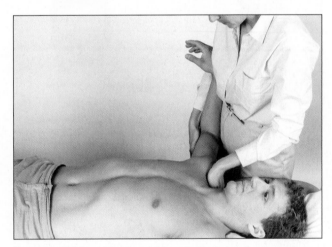

Figure 3-50 Firm or hard end feel at limit of glenohumeral joint abduction.

Shoulder Horizontal Abduction and Adduction

AROM Assessment

Substitute Movement. Scapular retraction (horizontal abduction), scapular protraction (horizontal adduction), and trunk rotation.

PROM Assessment

Forms
3-10, 3-11

Start Position. The patient is sitting. The shoulder is in 90° of abduction and neutral rotation. The elbow is flexed and the forearm is in midposition (Fig. 3-51).

Stabilization. The therapist stabilizes the trunk and scapula to isolate and assess glenohumeral joint motion.

Therapist's Distal Hand Placement. The therapist supports the arm in abduction and grasps the distal humerus.

End Position. The therapist moves the humerus posteriorly to the limit of motion for horizontal abduction (Fig. 3-52) and anteriorly to the limit of motion for horizontal adduction (Fig. 3-53).

End Feels. *Horizontal abduction—firm; horizontal adduction—firm/soft.*

Joint Glides. *Glenohumeral joint horizontal abduction—the convex humeral head glides anteriorly on the fixed concave glenoid cavity. Glenohumeral joint horizontal adduction—the convex humeral head glides posteriorly on the fixed concave glenoid cavity.*

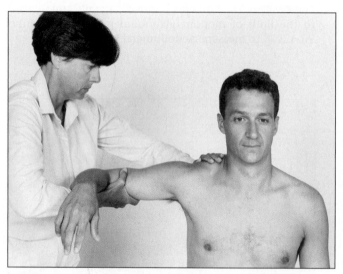

Figure 3-51 Start position for shoulder horizontal abduction and horizontal adduction.

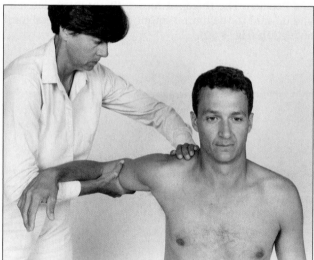

Figure 3-52 Firm end feel at limit of shoulder horizontal abduction.

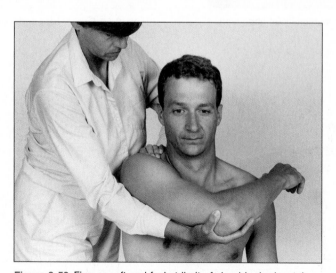

Figure 3-53 Firm or soft end feel at limit of shoulder horizontal adduction.

Measurement: Universal Goniometer

Start Position. The patient is sitting. The shoulder is in 90° of abduction and neutral rotation. The elbow is flexed and the forearm is in midposition (Fig. 3-54). An alternate start position has the shoulder in 90° of flexion, the

elbow is flexed, and the forearm is in midposition (Fig. 3-58). The start position of the shoulder should be recorded.

Stabilization. The therapist stabilizes the trunk and scapula.

Goniometer Axis. The axis is placed on top of the acromion process (Figs. 3-55 and 3-56).

Stationary Arm. Perpendicular to the trunk.

Movable Arm. Parallel to the longitudinal axis of the humerus.

End Position. The therapist supports the arm in abduction. The therapist moves the humerus anteriorly across the chest to the limit of motion (shoulder horizontal adduction 135°) (Figs. 3-55 and 3-56) and posteriorly to the limit of motion (shoulder horizontal abduction 45°) (Fig. 3-57).

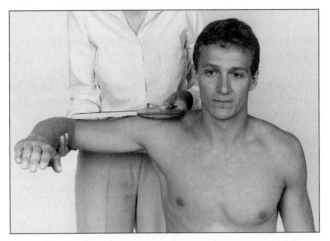

Figure 3-54 Start position for horizontal abduction and adduction.

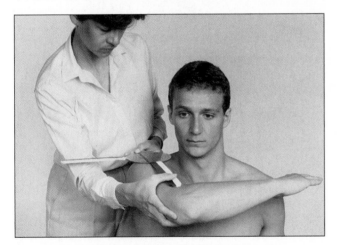

Figure 3-55 Shoulder horizontal adduction.

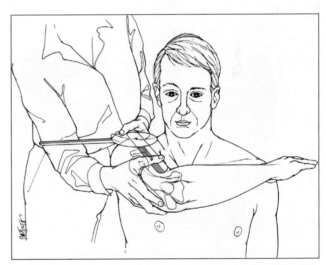

Figure 3-56 Goniometer alignment: shoulder horizontal adduction.

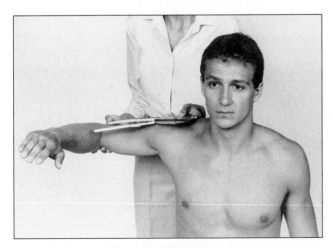

Figure 3-57 Shoulder horizontal abduction.

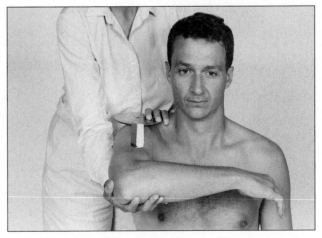

Figure 3-58 Alternate start position for horizontal abduction and adduction.

Shoulder Internal Rotation

AROM Assessment

Substitute Movement. In *prone* with the shoulder in 90° abduction: scapular elevation, shoulder abduction, and elbow extension. In *supine* with the shoulder in 90° abduction: scapular elevation, protraction and anterior tilt, shoulder abduction, and elbow extension. In *sitting* with the arm at the side: scapular elevation, shoulder abduction, and trunk rotation.

PROM Assessment

Form 3-12

Start Position. The patient is prone or supine. In prone, the shoulder is in 90° of abduction, the elbow is flexed to 90°, and the forearm is in midposition (Fig. 3-59). A towel is placed under the humerus to achieve the abducted position. This start position is contraindicated if the patient has a history of posterior dislocation of the glenohumeral joint.

Stabilization. The therapist stabilizes the scapula and maintains the position of the humerus, without restricting movement. In prone, the plinth limits scapular protraction and anterior tilt. When assessing internal rotation ROM in supine with the shoulder in 90° of abduction, Boon and Smith[16] recommend the therapist place one hand over the clavicle and coracoid process to stabilize the scapula for more reliable and reproducible results.

Therapist's Distal Hand Placement. The therapist grasps the distal radius and the ulna.

End Position. The therapist moves the palm of the hand toward the ceiling to the limit of internal rotation (Fig. 3-60)—that is, when scapular movement first occurs.

End Feel. Firm.

Joint Glide. *Glenohumeral joint internal rotation*—with the shoulder in the anatomical position, the convex humeral head glides posteriorly on the fixed concave glenoid cavity.

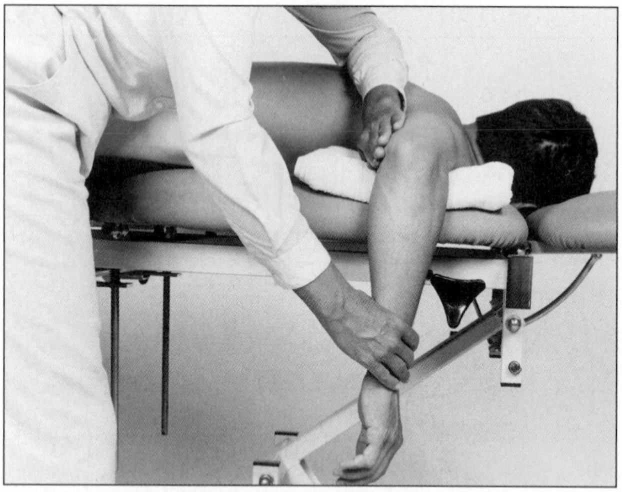

Figure 3-59 Start position for shoulder internal rotation.

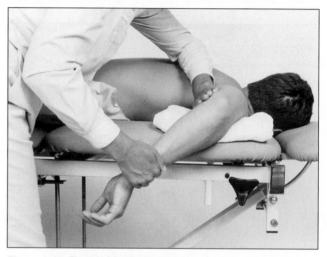

Figure 3-60 Firm end feel at limit of shoulder internal rotation.

Measurement: Universal Goniometer

Start Position. The patient is prone or supine. The shoulder is in 90° of abduction, the elbow is flexed to 90°, and the forearm is in midposition (Fig. 3-61). A towel is placed under the humerus to achieve the abducted position. This start position is contraindicated if the patient has a history of posterior dislocation of the glenohumeral joint.

Goniometer Axis. The axis is placed on the olecranon process of the ulna (Figs. 3-62 and 3-63).

Stationary Arm. Perpendicular to the floor.

Movable Arm. Parallel to the longitudinal axis of the ulna, pointing toward the ulnar styloid process.

End Position. The palm of the hand is moved toward the ceiling to the limit of motion (shoulder internal rotation 70°) (Figs. 3-63 and 3-64).

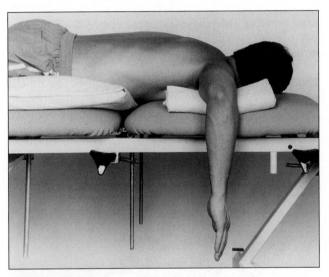

Figure 3-61 Start position for shoulder internal rotation.

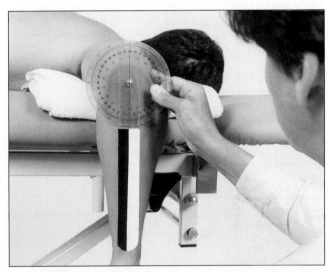

Figure 3-62 Goniometer placement for shoulder internal rotation.

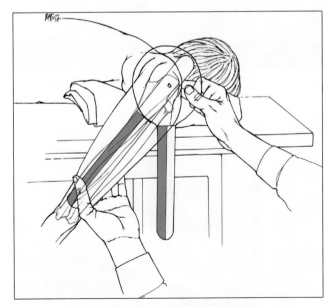

Figure 3-63 Shoulder internal rotation.

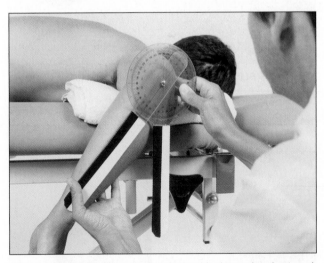

Figure 3-64 Goniometer alignment: shoulder internal and external rotation.

Shoulder External Rotation

AROM Assessment

Substitute Movement. In *supine* with the shoulder in 90° abduction: elbow extension, scapular depression, and shoulder adduction. In *sitting* with the arm at the side: scapular depression, shoulder adduction, and trunk rotation.

PROM Assessment

Form 3-13

Start Position. The patient is supine. The shoulder is in 90° of abduction, the elbow is flexed to 90°, and the forearm is in midposition (Fig. 3-65). A towel is placed under the humerus to achieve the abducted position. This start position is contraindicated if the patient has a history of anterior dislocation of the glenohumeral joint.

Stabilization. The weight of the trunk. The therapist stabilizes the scapula.

Therapist's Distal Hand Placement. The therapist grasps the distal radius and the ulna.

End Position. The therapist moves the dorsum of the hand toward the floor to the limit of external rotation (Fig. 3-66)—that is, when scapular movement first occurs.

End Feel. Firm.

Joint Glide. *Glenohumeral joint external rotation*—with the shoulder in the anatomical position, the convex humeral head glides anteriorly on the fixed concave glenoid cavity.

Measurement: Universal Goniometer

The measurement process is similar to that for internal rotation with the following exceptions.

Start Position. The patient is supine (Fig. 3-67). This start position is contraindicated if the patient has a history of anterior dislocation of the glenohumeral joint.

End Position. The dorsum of the hand moves toward the floor to the limit of motion (shoulder external rotation 90°) (Fig. 3-68).

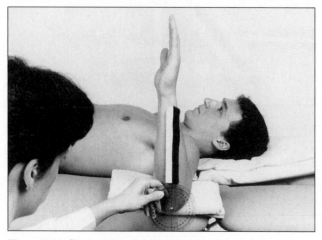

Figure 3-65 Start position for shoulder external rotation.

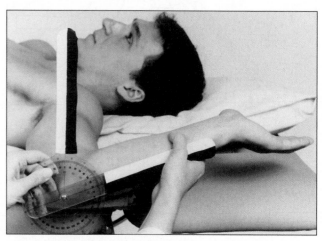

Figure 3-66 Firm end feel at limit of shoulder external rotation.

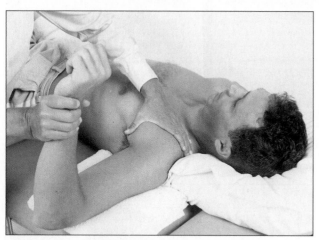

Figure 3-67 Start position for shoulder external rotation.

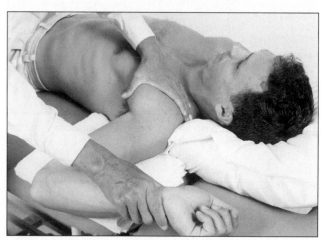

Figure 3-68 Shoulder external rotation.

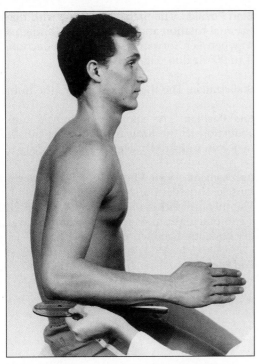

Figure 3-69 Alternate start position for shoulder internal rotation.

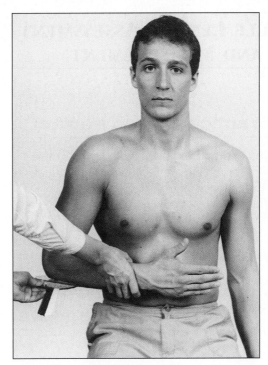

Figure 3-70 Shoulder internal rotation.

Alternate Assessment and Measurement: Internal/External Rotation

If the patient cannot achieve 90° of shoulder abduction, the end feel can be assessed (not shown) and the measurement can be taken while the patient is sitting. The starting position should be documented.

Start Position. The patient is sitting. To measure shoulder internal rotation, the shoulder is abducted to about 15°, the elbow is flexed to 90°, and the forearm is in midposition (Fig. 3-69). To measure external rotation (not shown), the arm is at the side in adduction, the elbow is flexed to 90°, and the forearm is in midposition.

Goniometer Axis. The axis is placed under the olecranon process.

Stationary Arm. Perpendicular to the trunk.

Movable Arm. Parallel to the longitudinal axis of the ulna.

End Positions. The palm of the hand is moved toward the abdomen to the limit of shoulder internal rotation (Fig. 3-70). The therapist moves the hand away from the abdomen to the limit of external rotation (not shown).

MUSCLE LENGTH ASSESSMENT AND MEASUREMENT

 Practice Makes Perfect

To aid you in practicing the skills covered in this section, or for a handy review, use the practical testing forms found at http://thepoint.lww.com/Clarkson3e.

Pectoralis Major

 This muscle length assessment technique is contraindicated if the patient has a history of anterior dislocation of the glenohumeral joint.

Form 3-14

Start Position. The patient is supine with the shoulder in external rotation and 90° elevation through a plane midway between forward flexion and abduction. The elbow is in 90° flexion (Fig. 3-71).

Stabilization. The therapist stabilizes the trunk.

End Position. The shoulder is moved into horizontal abduction to the limit of motion, to put the pectoralis major on full stretch (Figs. 3-72 and 3-73).

Assessment. With shortness of the pectoralis major muscle, shoulder horizontal abduction will be restricted. The therapist either observes the available PROM or uses a goniometer to measure and record the available shoulder horizontal abduction PROM.

End Feel. Pectoralis major on stretch—firm.

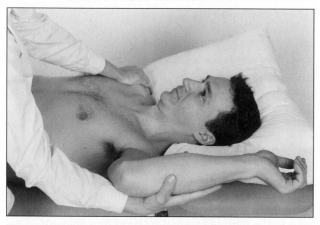

Figure 3-71 Start position: length of pectoralis major.

Origin[1]	Insertion[1]
Pectoralis Major	
a. Clavicular head: anterior border of the sternal half of the clavicle.	Lateral lip of the intertubercular groove of the humerus.
b. Sternal head: ipsilateral half of the anterior surface of the sternum; cartilage of the first 6 or 7 ribs; sternal end of the 6th rib; aponeurosis of the external abdominal oblique.	

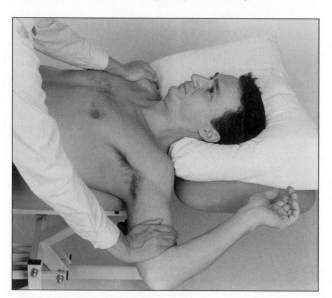

Figure 3-72 Pectoralis major on stretch.

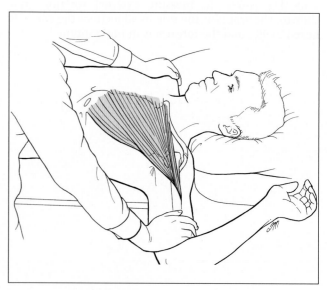

Figure 3-73 Pectoralis major.

Pectoralis Minor[17]

This muscle length assessment technique is contra-indicated if the patient has a history of posterior dislocation of the glenohumeral joint.

Form
3-15

Start Position. The patient is supine with the scapula over the side of the plinth, with the shoulder in external rotation and about 80° flexion. The elbow is flexed (Fig. 3-74).

Stabilization. The weight of the trunk.

End Position. The therapist applies force through the long axis of the shaft of the humerus to move the shoulder girdle in a cranial and dorsal direction to put the pectoralis minor on full stretch (Figs. 3-75 and 3-76).

Assessment. The therapist observes decreased scapular retraction ROM in the presence of a shortened length of pectoralis minor.

End Feel. Pectoralis minor on stretch—firm.

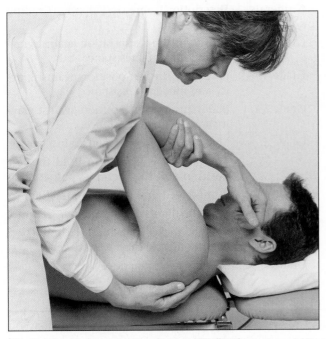

Figure 3-74 Start position: length of pectoralis minor.

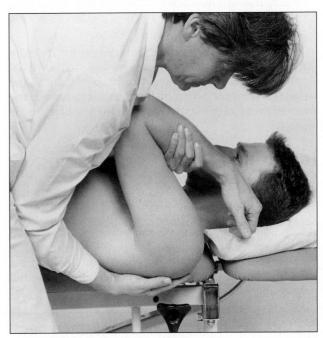

Figure 3-75 Pectoralis minor on stretch.

Origin[1]	Insertion[1]
Pectoralis Minor	
Outer surfaces of ribs 2 to 4 or 3 to 5 near the costal cartilages; fascia over corresponding external intercostals.	Medial border and upper surface of the coracoid process of the scapula.

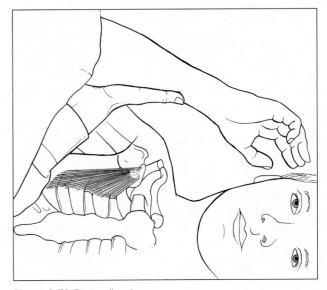

Figure 3-76 Pectoralis minor.

MUSCLE STRENGTH ASSESSMENT (TABLE 3-4)

 Practice Makes Perfect

To aid you in practicing the skills covered in this section, or for a handy review, use the practical testing forms found at http://thepoint.lww.com/Clarkson3e.

The strength of the muscles that connect the shoulder girdle to the trunk may be tested using Conventional Grading (either "through range" or "isometrically"). The weight of the upper extremity is often used to provide the necessary resistance to effectively test the scapular muscle strength.

Isometric/Palpation Grading (Scapular Muscles)

Isometric/palpation grading may be preferred to assess strength of the scapular muscles as these muscles function primarily as stabilizers, and effect relatively small scapular ranges of movement. When the patient cannot be positioned in a gravity eliminated test position for weak muscles that are less than a grade 2, the isometric/palpation grading can be used.

To employ isometric/palpation grading, the therapist positions the limb segment so the muscle contracts in inner range against gravity and grades the strength according to: the ability of the muscle to maintain the test position against gravity (grade 3) or against gravity and manual resistance (grades 3+ to 5), or the quality of the muscle contraction while the patient attempts to hold the test position (grades 0 to 2).

If the patient is unable to hold the limb in any part of the ROM against gravity, for grades 0 to 2, one of the therapist's hands remains just below the limb to control its fall, and palpates the muscle to grade the strength according to the feel of the muscle contraction.

Numerals	Description Isometric/Palpation Grading The patient:
Grade 5:	Maintains the test position against gravity and maximal resistance.
Grade 4:	Maintains the test position against gravity and moderate resistance.
Grade 3+:	Maintains the test position against gravity and minimal resistance.
Grade 3:	Maintains the test position against gravity.
	The patient is unable to hold the test position and the therapist palpates:
Grade 2:	A prolonged firm muscle contraction.
Grade 2-:	A minimal muscle contraction.
Grade 1:	A slight flicker of a muscle contraction and the muscle can be felt to relax.
Grade 0:	No muscle contraction.

TABLE 3-4 Muscle Actions, Attachments, and Nerve Supply: The Shoulder Girdle[18]

Muscle	Primary Muscle Action	Muscle Origin	Muscle Insertion	Peripheral Nerve	Nerve Root
Serratus anterior	Scapular abduction Scapular lateral rotation	Outer surfaces and superior borders of the upper 8, 9, or 10 ribs; fascia covering corresponding intercostal muscles	Costal surface of the medial border of the scapula including the superior angle and the inferior angle	Long thoracic	C567
Levator scapulae	Scapular elevation Scapular medial rotation	Transverse processes of the upper 4 cervical vertebrae	Medial border of the scapula between the superior angle and the root of the spine	Third and fourth cervical; dorsal scapular	C345
Trapezius a. Upper fibers	Scapular elevation	Medial one-third of the superior nuchal line of the occipital bone; external occipital protuberance; ligamentum nuchae	Posterior border of the lateral one-third of the clavicle	Spinal accessory	C34

(continued)

TABLE 3-4 *Continued*

Muscle	Primary Muscle Action	Muscle Origin	Muscle Insertion	Peripheral Nerve	Nerve Root
b. Middle fibers	Scapular adduction	Spinous processes of T1 to T5 and the corresponding supraspinous ligament	Medial border of the acromion process and the superior border of the rest of the spine of the scapula	Spinal accessory	C34
c. Lower fibers	Scapular depression Scapular adduction	Spinous processes of T6 to T12 and the corresponding supraspinous ligament	Tubercle at the apex of the triangular surface at the medial end of the spine of the scapula	Spinal accessory	C34
Rhomboid minor	Scapular adduction Scapular medial rotation	Inferior portion of the ligamentum nuchae; spinous processes of C7 and T1 and the corresponding supraspinous ligament	Base of the smooth triangular region at the root of the spine of the scapula	Dorsal scapular	C45
Rhomboid major	Scapular adduction Scapular medial rotation	Spinous processes of T2 to T5 and the corresponding supraspinous ligament	Medial border of the scapula between the root of the spine and inferior angle	Dorsal scapular	C45
Deltoid					
a. Anterior fibers	Shoulder flexion Shoulder internal rotation	Anterior border of the lateral one-third of the clavicle	Deltoid tuberosity on the lateral aspect of the humeral shaft	Axillary	C56
b. Middle fibers	Shoulder abduction	Lateral border and superior surface of the acromion process	Deltoid tuberosity on the lateral aspect of the humeral shaft	Axillary	C56
c. Posterior fibers	Shoulder extension Shoulder external rotation	Inferior lip of the crest of the spine of the scapula	Deltoid tuberosity on the lateral aspect of the humeral shaft	Axillary	C56
Supraspinatus	Shoulder abduction	Medial two-thirds of the supraspinous fossa	Superior facet of the greater tuberosity of the humerus	Suprascapular	C56
Coracobrachialis	Shoulder flexion and adduction	Tip of the coracoid process	Middle of the medial aspect of the shaft of the humerus	Musculocutaneous	C567
Pectoralis major	Shoulder horizontal adduction Shoulder internal rotation	a. Clavicular head: anterior border of the medial third of the clavicle	Lateral lip of the intertubercular groove of the humerus	Medial and lateral pectoral	C56

(continued)

TABLE 3-4   *Continued*

Muscle	Primary Muscle Action	Muscle Origin	Muscle Insertion	Peripheral Nerve	Nerve Root
		b. Sternal head: medial half of the anterior surface of the sternum; cartilage of the first 6 or 7 ribs; aponeurosis of the external abdominal oblique		Medial and lateral pectoral	C678T1
Pectoralis minor	Scapular protraction Scapular medial rotation	Outer surfaces of ribs 2–4 or 3–5 near the costal cartilages; fascia over corresponding external intercostals	Medial border and upper surface of the coracoid process of the scapula	Medial and lateral pectoral	C5678T1
Subscapularis	Shoulder internal rotation	Medial two-thirds of the subscapular fossa of the scapula	Lesser tuberosity of the humerus; anterior aspect shoulder joint capsule	Upper and lower subscapular	C56
Infraspinatus	Shoulder external rotation	Medial two-thirds of the infraspinous fossa	Middle facet of the greater tuberosity of the humerus	Suprascapular	C56
Teres minor	Shoulder external rotation	Upper two-thirds of the lateral aspect of the dorsal surface of the scapula, adjacent to the lateral border of the scapula	Inferior facet of the greater tuberosity of the humerus	Axillary	C56
Teres major	Shoulder extension Shoulder internal rotation	Posterior surface of the inferior angle of the scapula	Medial lip of the intertubercular groove of the humerus	Lower subscapular	C567
Latissimus dorsi	Shoulder extension Shoulder adduction Shoulder internal rotation	Posterior layer of the thoracolumbar fascia that takes attachment from the lumbar and sacral spinous processes, the corresponding supraspinous ligament, and the posterior aspect of the crest of the ilium; spines of the lower 6 thoracic vertebrae anterior to the attachment of trapezius; lower 3 or 4 ribs; inferior angle of the scapula	Floor of the intertubercular groove of the humerus	Thoracodorsal	C678

Scapular Abduction and Lateral Rotation

Against Gravity: Serratus Anterior

Accessory muscles: trapezius (lateral rotation) and pectoralis minor (abduction).

Form 3-16

Start Position. The patient is supine. The shoulder is flexed to 90° with slight horizontal adduction (i.e., 15° medial to the sagittal plane), and the elbow is extended (Fig. 3-77). This position is an optimal test position for serratus anterior while decreasing the participation of pectoralis major.[19]

Stabilization. The weight of the trunk.

Movement. The patient abducts (protracts) the scapula through full ROM (Fig. 3-78).

Palpation. Midaxillary line over the thorax.

Substitute Movement. Pectoralis major, pectoralis minor.

Resistance Location. Applied on the distal end of the humerus (Figs. 3-79 and 3-80).

Resistance Direction. Scapular adduction.

Figure 3-77 Start position: serratus anterior.

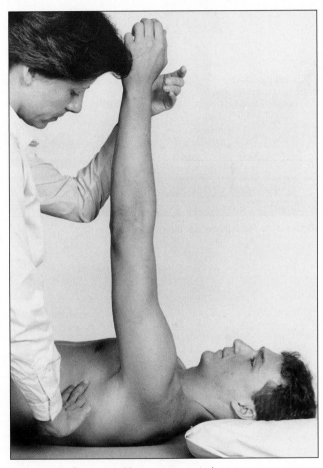

Figure 3-78 Screen position: serratus anterior.

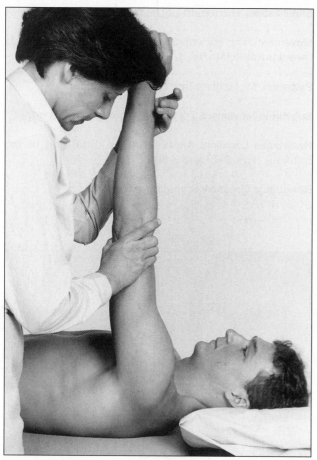

Figure 3-79 Resistance: serratus anterior.

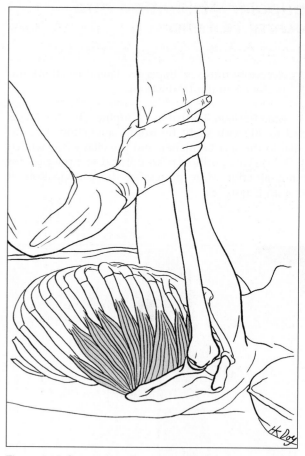

Figure 3-80 Serratus anterior.

Gravity Eliminated: Serratus Anterior

Start Position. The patient is sitting. The shoulder is flexed to 90° with slight horizontal adduction, and the elbow is extended (Fig. 3-81). The therapist supports the weight of the upper extremity.

Stabilization. The patient is instructed to avoid trunk rotation.

End Position. The patient abducts the scapula through full ROM (Fig. 3-82).

Substitute Movement. Pectoralis major and minor, upper and lower fibers of trapezius, and contralateral trunk rotation.

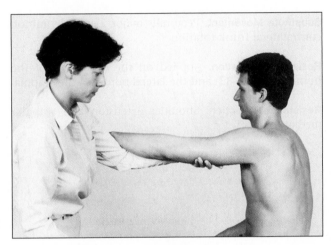

Figure 3-81 Start position: serratus anterior.

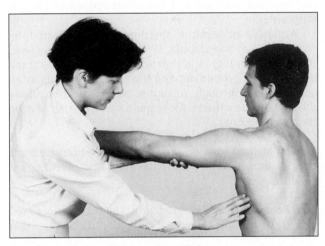

Figure 3-82 End position: serratus anterior.

Alternate Test

Against Gravity: Serratus Anterior

The patient must have adequate shoulder flexor muscle strength to perform this test.

Serratus anterior muscle activity is increased when the lateral (upward) rotation action of the muscle is stressed along with the straight scapular abduction action of the muscle.[20] This alternate test emphasizes the scapular lateral (upward) rotation and abduction actions of the serratus anterior.

Weakness of serratus anterior is demonstrated by "winging"[21] of the scapula. When "winging" is present, the medial border and inferior angle of the scapula become more prominent, and the scapula remains in an adducted and medially rotated position. This test allows the therapist to observe the scapula for "winging" during the test procedure.

Grading Method. This alternate test for Serratus Anterior is only performed against gravity using Isometric/Palpation Grading.

Start Position. The patient is sitting. The shoulder is flexed to 120° with slight horizontal adduction (i.e., 15° medial to the sagittal plane), and the elbow in extension (Fig. 3-83).

Stabilization. The patient may hold onto the plinth with the nontest hand.

Movement. The patient holds the test position.

Palpation. Midaxillary line over the thorax anterior to the lateral border of the scapula (Fig. 3-84).

Substitute Movement. Pectoralis major, pectoralis minor, contralateral trunk rotation.

Resistance Location. Applied on the distal end of the humerus (Fig. 3-83) and the lateral border of the scapula.

Resistance Direction. Shoulder extension and scapular medial rotation.

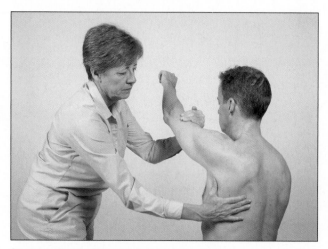

Figure 3-83 Alternate test: isometric grading of serratus anterior.

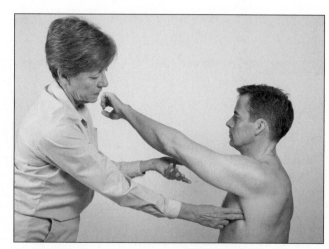

Figure 3-84 Alternate test: palpation grading of serratus anterior.

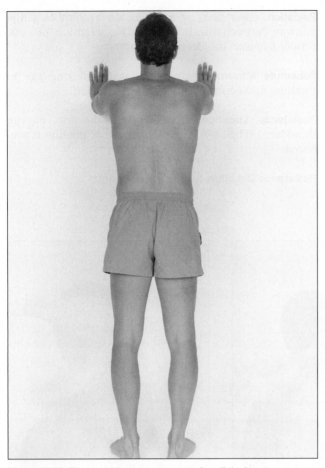

Figure 3-85 Start position: serratus anterior clinical test.

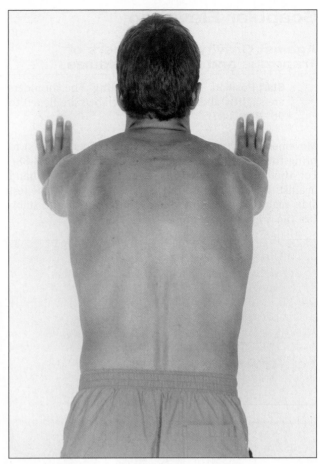

Figure 3-86 End position: serratus anterior clinical test.

Clinical Test: Serratus Anterior

This is a quick clinical test used to assess whether the serratus anterior muscle is strong or weak. A specific grade cannot be assigned.

Start Position. The patient is standing and facing a wall. The hands are placed on the wall at shoulder level, the shoulders are in slight horizontal abduction, and the elbows are extended (Fig. 3-85). The thorax is allowed to sag toward the wall so that the scapulae are adducted.

Movement. The patient pushes the thorax away from the wall so that the scapulae abduct (Fig. 3-86).

Observation. Weakness is demonstrated by "winging"[21] of the scapula. The medial border and inferior angle of the scapula become more prominent, and the scapula remains in an adducted and medially rotated position.

Scapular Elevation

Against Gravity: Upper Fibers of Trapezius and Levator Scapulae

Form 3-17

Start Position. The patient is sitting. The shoulders are slightly abducted, and the elbows are flexed to 90° (Fig. 3-87).

Movement. The patient elevates the shoulder girdle(s) to bring the acromion process closer to the ear (Fig. 3-88). For the unilateral test, the therapist places the hand against the lateral aspect of the patient's head on the test side, maintaining the head in a neutral position to stabilize the origins of the muscles (Fig. 3-89).

Palpation. *Upper fibers of trapezius:* on a point of a line midway between the inion and the acromion process. *Levator scapulae:* too deep to palpate.

Substitute Movement. Unilateral test: lowering ear to shoulder and contralateral trunk side flexion.

Resistance Location. Applied over the top of the shoulder(s) (Figs. 3-90 to 3-92). Isometric grading is preferred.

Resistance Direction. Scapular depression.

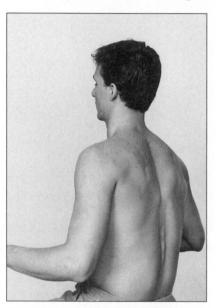

Figure 3-87 Start position: upper fibers of trapezius and levator scapulae.

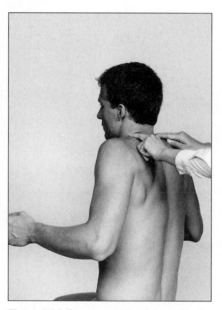

Figure 3-88 Screen position: bilateral test for upper fibers of trapezius and levator scapulae.

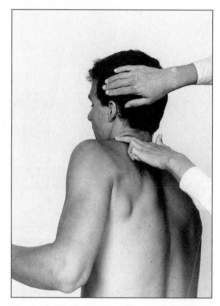

Figure 3-89 Screen position: unilateral test for upper fibers of trapezius and levator scapulae.

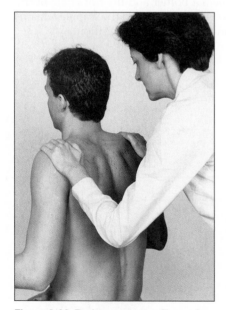

Figure 3-90 Resistance: upper fibers of trapezius and levator scapulae.

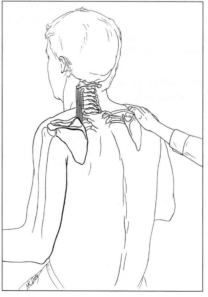

Figure 3-91 Levator scapulae.

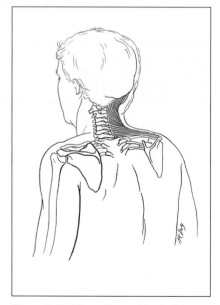

Figure 3-92 Upper fibers of trapezius.

Gravity Eliminated: Upper Fibers of Trapezius and Levator Scapulae

Start Position. The patient is prone. The arm is at the side, and the shoulder is in neutral rotation (Fig. 3-93). The therapist supports the weight of the upper extremity to reduce the resistance of friction between the plinth and the upper extremity.

Stabilization. The weight of the head.

End Position. The patient elevates the scapula through full ROM (Fig. 3-94).

Substitute Movement. Contralateral trunk side flexion.

Alternate Test. If the patient is unable to assume a prone position, these muscles can be tested in the against gravity position of sitting using Isometric/Palpation Grading to assess the muscle strength for grades 2 or less. The therapist positions the shoulder girdle in elevation and palpates for the quality of muscle contraction while the patient attempts to hold the position.

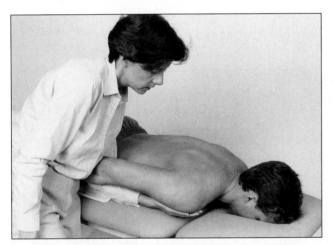

Figure 3-93 Start position: upper fibers of trapezius and levator scapulae.

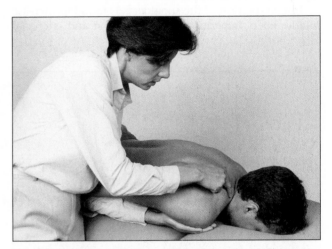

Figure 3-94 End position: upper fibers of trapezius and levator scapulae.

Scapular Adduction

Against Gravity: Middle Fibers of Trapezius

Form 3-18

Accessory muscles: trapezius (upper and lower fibers).

The patient must have adequate shoulder horizontal abduction muscle strength to perform this test.

Start Position[22]. The patient is prone. The shoulder is abducted to 90° and laterally rotated so the thumb points toward the ceiling. The elbow is extended (Fig. 3-95). Ekstrom and colleagues[20] confirm this to be an excellent position for activating middle fibers trapezius.

Lateral rotation of the shoulder was found to increase middle fibers trapezius muscle activation and is crucial when testing the muscle.[23] The laterally rotated position places teres major on stretch and subsequently exerts a pull on the lateral border of the scapula moving the scapula into a position of lateral rotation.[22] Positioning the scapula in lateral rotation favors testing of middle fibers trapezius as scapular adductors, as opposed to rhomboids that adduct the scapula with the scapula in medial rotation.[22]

Stabilization. The weight of the trunk. The therapist stabilizes the contralateral thorax as required, to prevent lifting of the trunk.

Movement. The patient raises the arm toward the ceiling and adducts the scapula toward the midline (Fig. 3-96).

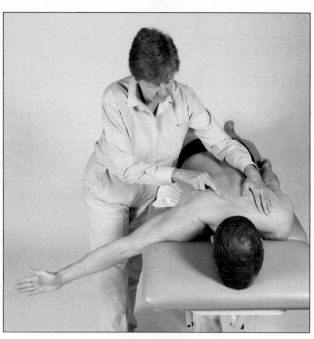

Figure 3-95 Start position: middle fibers of trapezius.

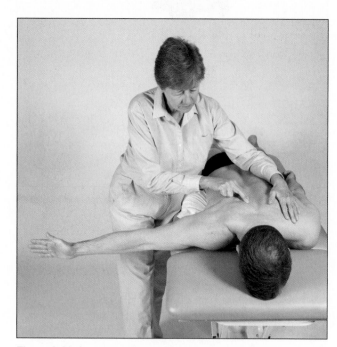

Figure 3-96 Screen position: middle fibers of trapezius.

Palpation. Between the medial (vertebral) border of the scapula and the vertebrae, above the spine of the scapula.

Substitute Movement. Rhomboid major, rhomboid minor, ipsilateral trunk rotation, and shoulder horizontal abduction.

Resistance Location. Applied at the distal forearm[22] (Fig. 3-97). In the presence of posterior deltoid muscle weakness, the arm hangs vertically over the edge of the plinth in 90° shoulder flexion and resistance is applied over the scapula (Fig. 3-98) and resistance location recorded. Isometric grading is preferred.

Resistance Direction. Scapular abduction.

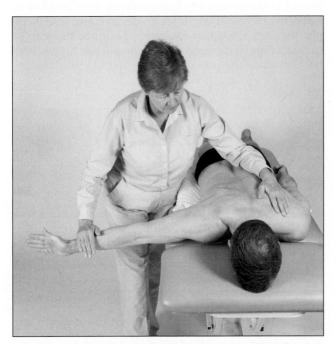

Figure 3-97 Resistance applied at distal forearm: middle fibers of trapezius.

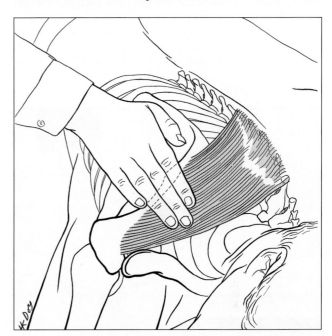

Figure 3-98 Resistance applied over scapula: middle fibers of trapezius.

Gravity Eliminated: Middle Fibers of Trapezius

Start Position. The patient is sitting. The shoulder is abducted to 90° and laterally rotated. The elbow is extended (Fig. 3-99). The arm is supported by the therapist or on a powder board.

Stabilization. The therapist instructs the patient to avoid trunk rotation.

End Position. The patient adducts the scapula through full ROM (Fig. 3-100).

Substitute Movement. Shoulder horizontal abduction, and ipsilateral trunk rotation.

Alternate Test. If the patient cannot assume a sitting posture, this muscle can be tested in the against gravity position of prone-lying using Isometric/Palpation Grading to assess the muscle strength for grades 2 or less. The therapist supports the upper extremity, positions the scapula in adduction, and palpates for the quality of muscle contraction while the patient attempts to hold the position.

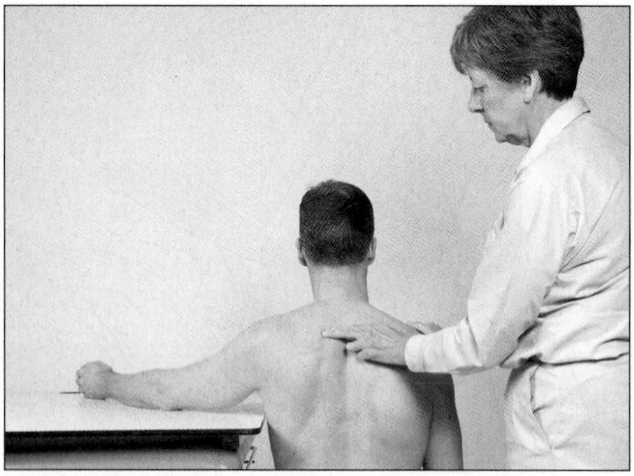

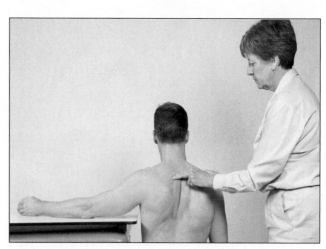

Figure 3-99 Start position: middle fibers of trapezius.

Figure 3-100 End position: middle fibers of trapezius.

Scapular Adduction and Medial Rotation

Against Gravity: Rhomboid Major and Rhomboid Minor

 Accessory muscles: levator scapulae, middle fibers of trapezius.

Form 3-19 **Start Position.** The patient is prone. The dorsum of the hand is placed over the buttock of the nontest side, and the shoulders remain relaxed (Fig. 3-101).

Stabilization. The weight of the trunk.

Movement. The patient raises the arm away from the back. The weight of the raised upper extremity provides resistance to the scapular test motion (Fig. 3-102).
Note: Inability to lift the hand off the buttock may be due to shoulder muscle weakness, notably subscapularis, not rhomboid muscle weakness. Ensure that the hand is maintained over the nontest side buttock and that the patient adducts and medially rotates the scapula during the test.

Palpation. On a point of an oblique line between the vertebral border of the scapula and C7 to T5. Rhomboid major can be palpated medial to the vertebral border of the scapula lateral to the lower fibers of trapezius, near the inferior angle of the scapula.

Substitute Movement. Tipping the scapula forward through pectoralis minor.[21]

Resistance Location. Applied over the scapula (Figs. 3-103 and 3-104). Ensure that resistance is not applied over the humerus. Isometric grading is preferred.

Resistance Direction. Scapular abduction and lateral rotation.

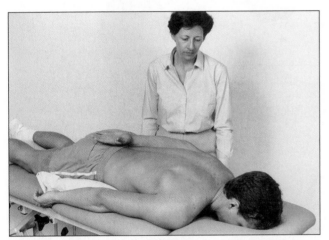

Figure 3-101 Start position: rhomboids.

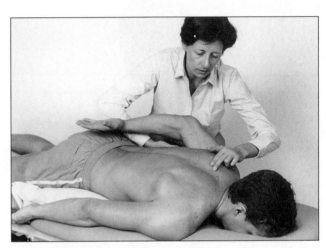

Figure 3-102 Screen position: rhomboids.

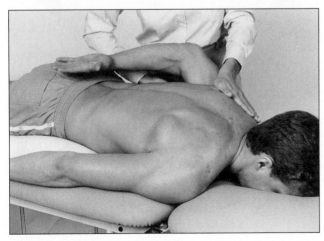

Figure 3-103 Resistance: rhomboids.

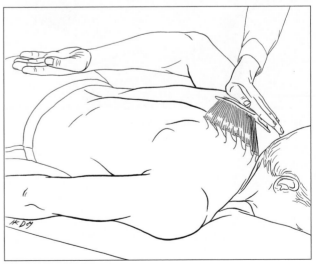

Figure 3-104 Rhomboids.

Gravity Eliminated: Rhomboid Major and Rhomboid Minor

Start Position. The patient is sitting. The dorsum of the hand is placed over the nontest side buttock, and the shoulders remain relaxed (Fig. 3-105).

Stabilization. The therapist instructs the patient to avoid trunk forward flexion and/or ipsilateral trunk rotation.

End Position. The patient adducts and medially rotates the scapula by moving the arm away from the back while maintaining the hand over the buttock (Fig. 3-106).

Substitute Movement. Ipsilateral trunk rotation and/or trunk forward flexion, and tipping the scapula forward.

Alternate Test. If the patient cannot assume a sitting posture, this muscle can be tested in the against gravity position of prone-lying, using Isometric/Palpation Grading to assess the muscle strength for grades 2 or less. The therapist supports the upper extremity away from the back while maintaining the hand over the buttock to position the scapula in adduction and medial rotation, and palpates for the quality of muscle contraction while the patient attempts to hold the position.

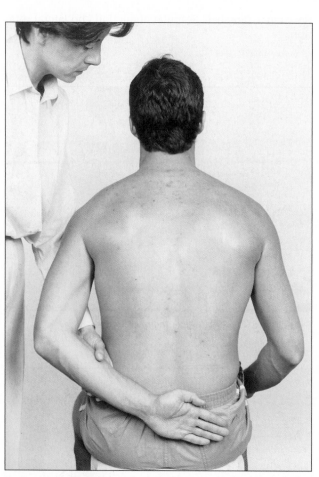

Figure 3-105 Start position: rhomboids.

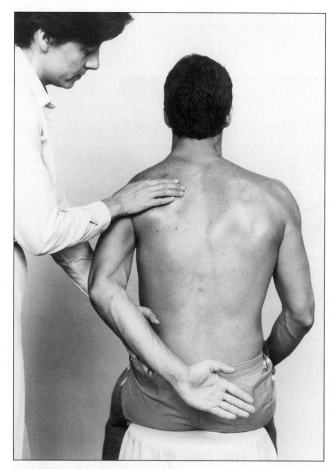

Figure 3-106 End position: rhomboids.

Alternate Test Against Gravity: Rhomboid Major and Rhomboid Minor

Accessory muscles: levator scapulae, middle fibers of trapezius.

This test utilizes Kendall's[22] against gravity testing of rhomboids and levator scapulae.

Start Position. The patient is prone. The shoulder is adducted 0°, the elbow is flexed and the forearm pronated (Fig. 3-107).

Stabilization. The weight of the trunk.

Movement. The patient raises the elbow upward and inward toward the opposite shoulder to extend and adduct the shoulder (Fig. 3-108).

Palpation. On a point of an oblique line between the vertebral border of the scapula and C7 to T5. Rhomboid major can be palpated medial to the vertebral border of the scapula lateral to the lower fibers of trapezius, near the inferior angle of the scapula.

Substitute Movement. Tipping the scapula forward using pectoralis minor.

Resistance Location. Applied proximal to the elbow joint on the posteromedial aspect of the humerus (Figs. 3-109).

Resistance Direction. Shoulder abduction and flexion.

For grades 2 or less. Isometric/Palpation Grading is used to assess the muscle strength. The therapist supports the humerus in extension and adduction and palpates rhomboid major for the quality of muscle contraction while the patient attempts to hold the position.

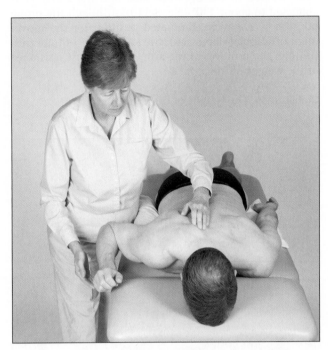

Figure 3-107 Start position: rhomboids.

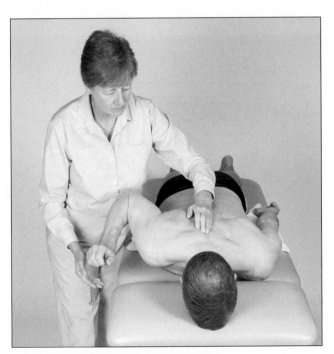

Figure 3-108 Screen position: rhomboids.

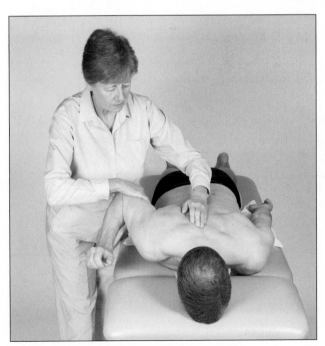

Figure 3-109 Resistance: rhomboids.

Scapular Depression and Adduction

Against Gravity: Lower Fibers of Trapezius

Accessory muscle: middle fibers of trapezius.

Form 3-20 **Start Position.** The patient is prone. The head is rotated to the opposite side, and the shoulder is abducted to about 130° (Fig. 3-110). Although the prone position is a gravity eliminated position for the movement of scapular depression, the lower fibers of trapezius, through the position of the arm, work against resistance of the weight of the arm.

Stabilization. The weight of the trunk.

Movement. The patient raises the arm to produce depression and adduction of the scapula (Fig. 3-111).

Palpation. Medial to the inferior angle of the scapula along a line between the root of the spine of the scapula and the T12 spinous process.

Substitute Movement. Trunk extension, middle fibers of trapezius.

Resistance Location. Isometric grading is preferred, and the resistance is applied over the scapula (Figs. 3-112 and 3-113).

Resistance Direction. Scapular elevation and abduction.

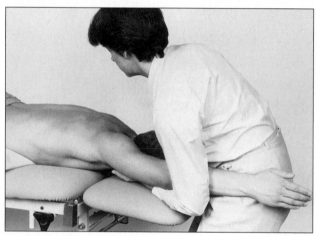

Figure 3-110 Start position: lower fibers of trapezius.

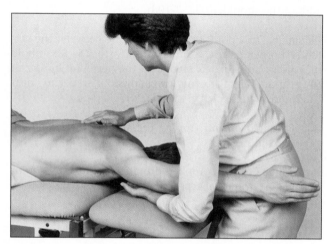

Figure 3-111 Screen position: lower fibers of trapezius.

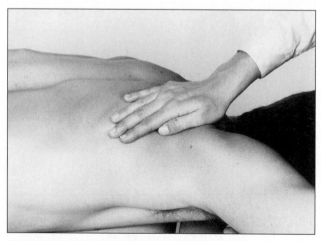

Figure 3-112 Resistance: lower fibers of trapezius.

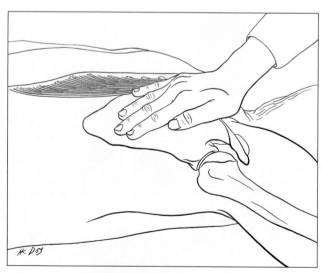

Figure 3-113 Lower fibers of trapezius.

Gravity Eliminated: Lower Fibers of Trapezius

Start Position. The patient is prone with the arms by the sides (Fig. 3-114). The therapist supports the arm through range, to reduce the resistance of friction between the plinth and the upper extremity.

Stabilization. The weight of the trunk.

End Position. The patient depresses and adducts the scapula through full ROM (Fig. 3-115).

Substitute Movement. Ipsilateral trunk side flexion and middle fibers of trapezius.

Alternate Test. If the patient cannot assume a sitting posture, this muscle can be tested in the against gravity position of prone-lying using Isometric/Palpation Grading to assess the muscle strength for grades 2 or less.

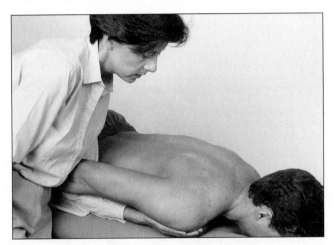

Figure 3-114 Start position: lower fibers of trapezius.

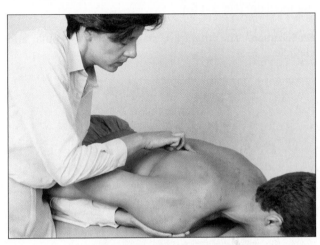

Figure 3-115 End position: lower fibers of trapezius.

Shoulder Flexion to 90°

Against Gravity: Anterior Fibers of Deltoid

Form 3-21

Accessory muscles: coracobrachialis, middle fibers of deltoid, clavicular fibers of pectoralis major, biceps brachii, upper and lower fibers of trapezius, and serratus anterior.

Start Position. The patient is sitting. The arm is at the side, with the shoulder in slight abduction and the palm facing medially (Fig. 3-116).

Stabilization. The therapist stabilizes the scapula and clavicle.

Movement. The patient flexes the shoulder to 90°, simultaneously slightly adducting and internally rotating the shoulder joint (Fig. 3-117).

Palpation. Anterior aspect of the shoulder joint just distal to the lateral one-third of the clavicle.

Resistance Location. Applied on the anteromedial aspect of the arm just proximal to the elbow joint (Figs. 3-118 and 3-119).

Resistance Direction. Shoulder extension, slight abduction and external rotation.

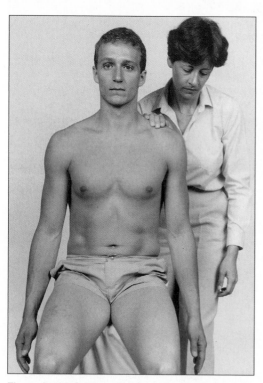

Figure 3-116 Start position: anterior fibers of deltoid.

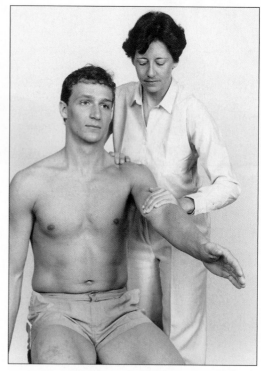

Figure 3-118 Resistance: anterior fibers of deltoid.

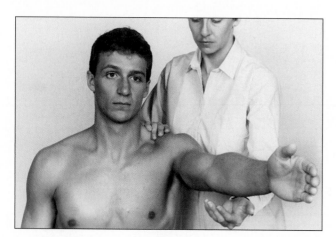

Figure 3-117 Screen position: anterior fibers of deltoid.

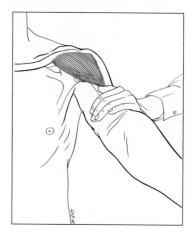

Figure 3-119 Anterior fibers of deltoid.

Gravity Eliminated: Anterior Fibers of Deltoid

Start Position. The patient is in a side-lying position on the nontest side. The arm is at the side, with the shoulder in slight abduction and neutral rotation (Fig. 3-120). The therapist supports the weight of the limb.

Stabilization. The therapist stabilizes the scapula and clavicle.

End Position. The patient flexes the shoulder to 90°, simultaneously slightly adducting and internally rotating the shoulder joint (Fig. 3-121).

Substitute Movement. Scapular elevation and trunk extension.

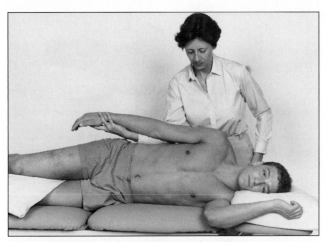

Figure 3-120 Start position: anterior fibers of deltoid.

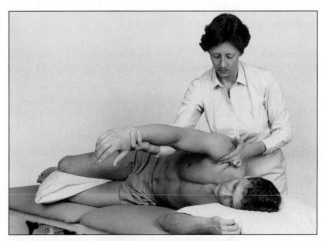

Figure 3-121 End position: anterior fibers of deltoid.

Shoulder Flexion and Adduction

Against Gravity: Coracobrachialis

 Form 3-22

Accessory muscles: anterior fibers of deltoid, clavicular fibers of pectoralis major, and the short head of biceps brachii.

Start Position. The patient is supine. The shoulder is in slight abduction and external rotation; the elbow is flexed with the forearm in supination (Fig. 3-122).

Stabilization. The weight of the trunk.

Movement. The patient flexes and adducts the shoulder while maintaining the shoulder in external rotation (Fig. 3-123).

Palpation. Proximal one-third of the anteromedial aspect of the arm, just anterior to the brachial pulse (Fig. 3-124).

Substitute Movement. Scapular elevation.

Resistance Location. Applied on the anteromedial aspect of the distal humerus (Figs. 3-125 and 3-126).

Resistance Direction. Shoulder abduction and extension.

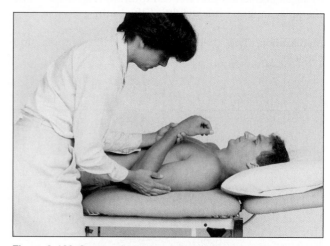

Figure 3-122 Start position: coracobrachialis.

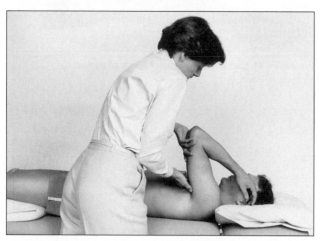

Figure 3-123 Screen position: coracobrachialis.

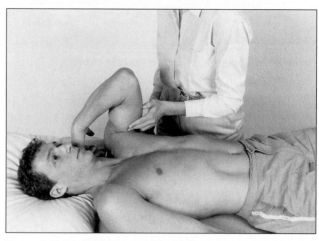

Figure 3-124 Palpation: coracobrachialis.

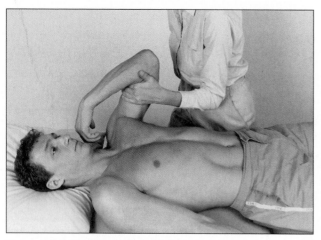

Figure 3-125 Resistance: coracobrachialis.

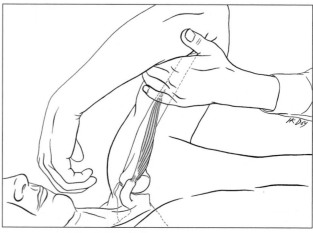

Figure 3-126 Coracobrachialis.

Gravity Eliminated: Coracobrachialis

Start Position. The patient is in a side-lying position on the nontest side. The arm is at the side, with the shoulder in slight abduction and external rotation and the elbow fully flexed with the forearm supinated (Fig. 3-127). The therapist supports the weight of the arm.

Stabilization. The therapist stabilizes the scapula.

End Position. The patient flexes and adducts the shoulder through full ROM (Fig. 3-128).

Substitute Movement. Scapular elevation.

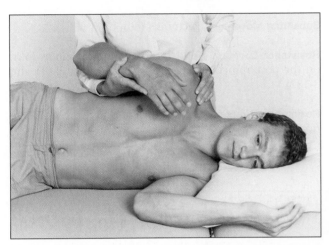

Figure 3-127 Start position: coracobrachialis.

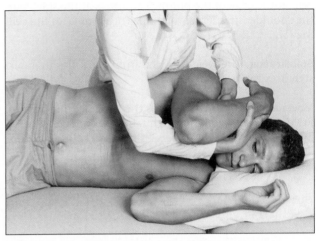

Figure 3-128 End position: coracobrachialis.

Shoulder Extension

Against Gravity: Latissimus Dorsi and Teres Major

 Accessory muscles: posterior fibers of deltoid, triceps, and teres minor.

Form 3-23 **Start Position.** The patient is in a prone-lying position at the edge of the plinth. The arm is at the side, with the shoulder in internal rotation. The palm faces the ceiling (Fig. 3-129).

Stabilization. The weight of the trunk, and the therapist stabilizes the scapula.

Movement. The patient extends the shoulder through full ROM while maintaining slight shoulder adduction (Fig. 3-130A). The posterior fibers of deltoid are essential for full shoulder extension.[24] In the event of deltoid paralysis, this test motion may be restricted to approximately one-third of the full shoulder extension ROM.

Palpation. *Latissimus dorsi:* lateral to the inferior angle of the scapula or at the posterior wall of the axilla (Fig. 3-130B) (inferior and lateral to palpation for teres major). *Teres major:* posterior wall of the axilla lateral to the axillary border of the scapula.

Substitute Movement. Pectoralis minor.

Resistance Location. Applied proximal to the elbow joint on the posteromedial aspect of the arm (Figs. 3-131 and 3-132).

Resistance Direction. Shoulder flexion and slight abduction.

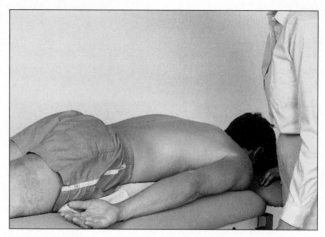

Figure 3-129 Start position: latissimus dorsi and teres major.

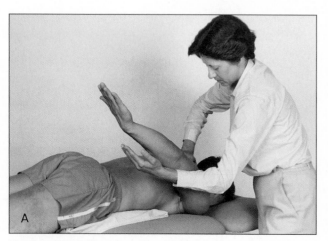

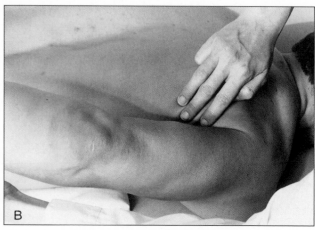

Figure 3-130 **A.** Screen position: latissimus dorsi and teres major. **B.** Palpation: latissimus dorsi.

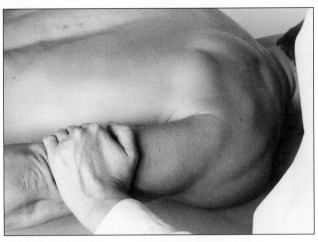

Figure 3-131 Resistance: latissimus dorsi and teres major.

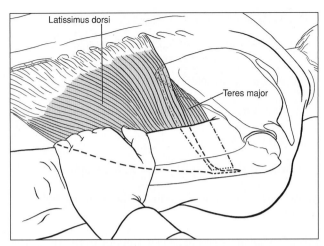

Figure 3-132 Latissimus dorsi and teres major.

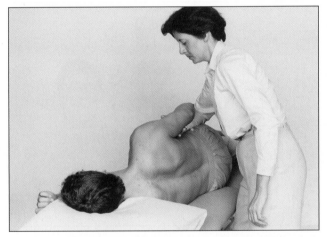

Figure 3-133 Start position: latissimus dorsi and teres major.

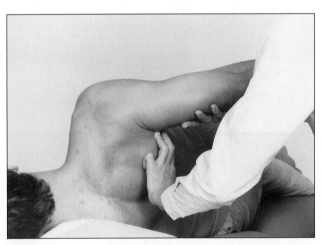

Figure 3-134 End position: latissimus dorsi and teres major.

Gravity Eliminated: Latissimus Dorsi and Teres Major

Start Position. The patient is in a side-lying position on the nontest side, with the arm at the side and the shoulder in internal rotation. The hips and knees are flexed (Fig. 3-133). The therapist supports the weight of the arm.

Stabilization. The weight of the trunk, and the therapist stabilizes the scapula.

End Position. The patient extends the shoulder while maintaining shoulder adduction (Fig. 3-134).

Substitute Movement. Pectoralis minor.

Shoulder Abduction to 90°

Against Gravity: Middle Fibers of Deltoid and Supraspinatus

Accessory muscles: none.

Form 3-24 **Start Position.** The patient is sitting. The test arm is at the side in neutral rotation, and the elbow is extended (Fig. 3-135).

Stabilization. The therapist stabilizes the scapula.

Movement. The patient abducts the arm to 90° (Fig. 3-136).

Palpation. *Middle fibers of deltoid:* inferior to the tip of the acromion process. *Supraspinatus:* too deep to palpate.

Substitute Movement. Upper fibers of trapezius (shoulder elevation), long head of biceps (shoulder external rotation), and contralateral or ipsilateral trunk side flexion.

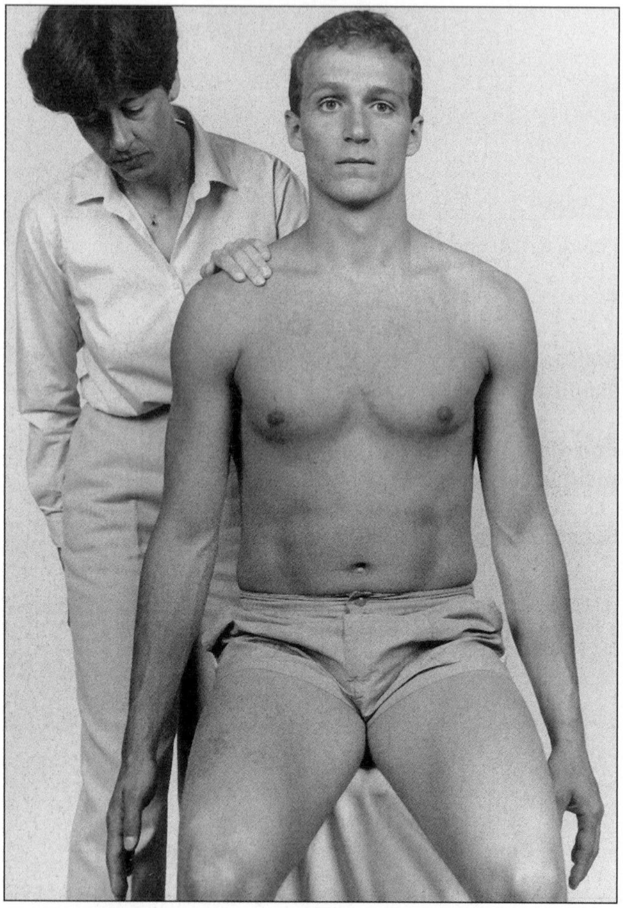

Resistance Location. Applied proximal to the elbow joint on the lateral aspect of the arm (Figs. 3-137 to 3-139).

Resistance Direction. Shoulder adduction.

Alternate Test (not shown). This test may also be performed abducting the arm in the plane of the scapula (Fig. 3-140). The scapular plane lies 30° to 45° anterior to the frontal plane.[3] Although there appears to be no difference in the strength of the shoulder abductors when tested in the frontal or scapular planes of motion[25], assessment in the plane of the scapula may be preferred. Movement performed in the scapular plane is a more functional plane of motion and produces less stress on the capsuloligamentous structures of the glenohumeral joint. The plane of motion used should be recorded.

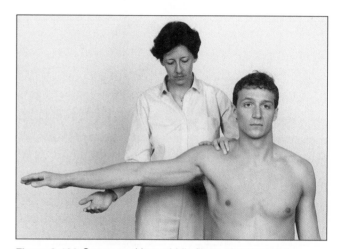

Figure 3-136 Screen position: middle fibers of deltoid and supraspinatus.

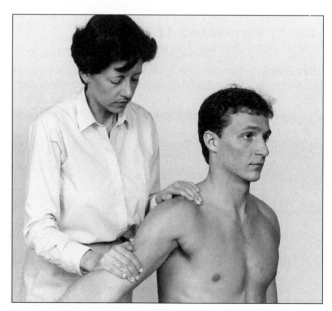

Figure 3-137 Resistance: middle fibers of deltoid and supraspinatus.

Figure 3-135 Start position: middle fibers of deltoid and supraspinatus.

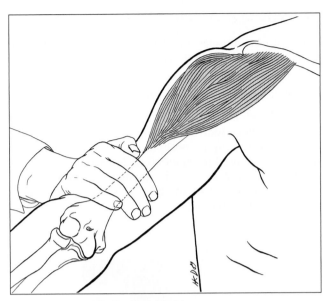

Figure 3-138 Middle fibers of deltoid.

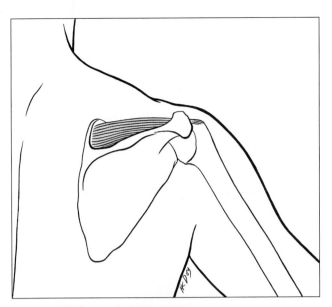

Figure 3-139 Supraspinatus.

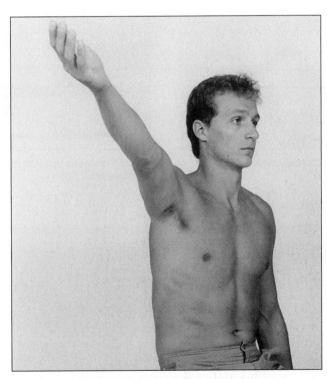

Figure 3-140 Shoulder abduction in the scapular plane.

Gravity Eliminated: Middle Fibers of Deltoid and Supraspinatus

Start Position. The patient is supine. The test arm is at the side in neutral rotation with the elbow extended (Fig. 3-141). The therapist supports the weight of the arm.

Stabilization. The therapist stabilizes the scapula.

End Position. The patient abducts the shoulder to 90° (Fig. 3-142).

Substitute Movement. Upper fibers of trapezius (shoulder elevation), long head of biceps (shoulder external rotation), and contralateral trunk side flexion.

Shoulder Adduction

The primary muscles involved in this movement are tested in the following movements:

Pectoralis major: shoulder horizontal adduction

Latissimus dorsi: shoulder extension

Teres major: shoulder extension.

The shoulder adductors can be tested as a group with the patient in a supine position. The conventional grading method is used for grades 0 to 2. For testing strength greater than a grade 2, the therapist offers resistance equal to the weight of the limb to simulate an against gravity testing situation.

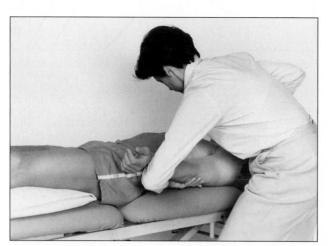

Figure 3-141 Start position: middle fibers of deltoid and supraspinatus.

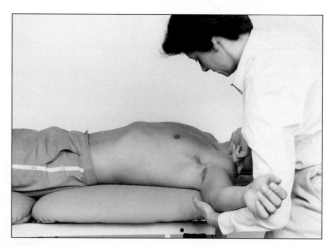

Figure 3-142 End position: middle fibers of deltoid and supraspinatus.

Shoulder Horizontal Adduction

Against Gravity: Pectoralis Major (Sternal and Clavicular Heads)

Accessory muscle: anterior fibers of deltoid.

Form 3-25 **Start Position.** The patient is supine. The shoulder is abducted to 90°, and the elbow is flexed to 90° (Fig. 3-143).

Stabilization. The weight of the trunk, and the therapist stabilizes over the contralateral shoulder as required to prevent lifting of the trunk.

Movement. The patient horizontally adducts the shoulder through full ROM (Fig. 3-144).

Palpation. *Pectoralis major sternal head:* anterior border of the axilla. *Pectoralis major clavicular head:* inferior to the middle of the anterior border of the clavicle.

Substitute Movement. Trunk rotation.

Resistance Location. Applied on the anterior aspect of the arm proximal to the elbow joint (Figs. 3-145 and 3-146).

Resistance Direction. Shoulder horizontal abduction.

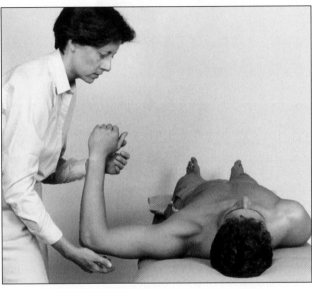

Figure 3-143 Start position: pectoralis major.

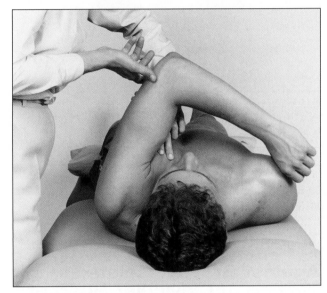

Figure 3-144 Screen position: pectoralis major.

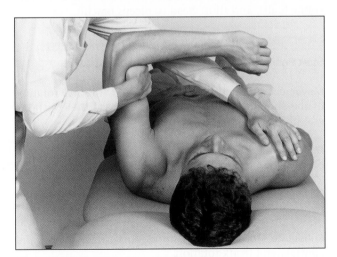

Figure 3-145 Resistance: pectoralis major.

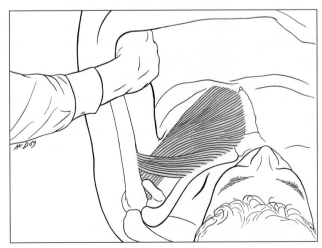

Figure 3-146 Pectoralis major.

Gravity Eliminated: Pectoralis Major (Sternal and Clavicular Heads)

Start Position. The patient is sitting. The shoulder is abducted to 90°, the elbow is flexed to 90°, and the arm is supported by the therapist (Fig. 3-147).

Stabilization. The therapist stabilizes the scapula and trunk by placing the hand on top of the shoulder.

End Position. The patient horizontally adducts the shoulder through full ROM (Fig. 3-148).

Substitute Movement. Contralateral trunk rotation.

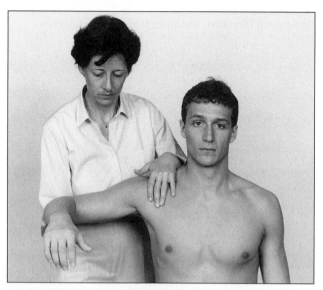

Figure 3-147 Start position: pectoralis major.

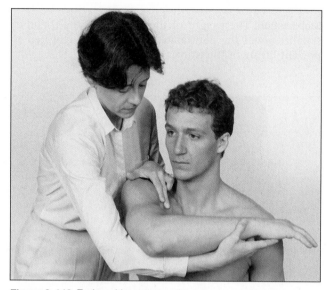

Figure 3-148 End position: pectoralis major.

Against Gravity: Isolated Testing of Clavicular Head of Pectoralis Major, and Sternal Head of Pectoralis Major

If there is weakness noted during testing of both heads of the pectoralis major, specific testing (not shown) of the sternal and clavicular heads should be performed because each head has a separate innervation. The patient is positioned so that the humerus is aligned with the direct line of pull of each segment of the muscle. The patient is in the against gravity position of supine-lying. For grades 0 to 2, the therapist offers assistance equal to the weight of the limb to simulate a gravity eliminated testing situation.

Clavicular Head

Start Position. Shoulder abducted to about 70° to 75°.

Movement. Adduction, forward flexion, and internal rotation of the shoulder (the hand reaches to a point above the contralateral shoulder).

Resistance Location. Applied on the anteromedial aspect of the arm, proximal to the elbow joint.

Resistance Direction. Abduction, extension, and slight external rotation of the shoulder.

Substitute Movement. Contralateral trunk rotation, coracobrachialis, and short head of biceps brachii.

Sternal Head

Start Position. Shoulder abducted to about 135°.

Movement. Adduction, extension, and internal rotation of the shoulder (the hand reaches toward the contralateral hip).

Resistance Location. Applied on the anteromedial aspect of the arm, proximal to the elbow joint.

Resistance Direction. Abduction, flexion, and slight external rotation of the shoulder.

Substitute Movement. Latissimus dorsi, teres major, and contralateral trunk rotation.

Shoulder Horizontal Abduction

Against Gravity: Posterior Fibers of Deltoid

Accessory muscles: infraspinatus and teres minor.

Form 3-26

Start Position. The patient is prone. The shoulder is abducted to about 75°, the elbow is flexed to 90°, and the forearm is hanging vertically over the edge of the plinth (Fig. 3-149).

Stabilization. The therapist stabilizes the scapula.

Movement. The patient horizontally abducts and slightly externally rotates the shoulder (Fig. 3-150).

Palpation. Inferior to the lateral aspect of the spine of the scapula.

Substitute Movement. Rhomboids, middle fibers of trapezius, and ipsilateral trunk rotation.

Resistance Location. Applied on the posterolateral aspect of the arm proximal to the elbow joint (Figs. 3-151 and 3-152).

Resistance Direction. Shoulder horizontal adduction and slight internal rotation.

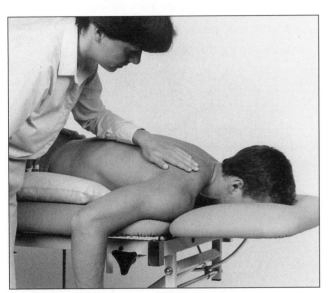

Figure 3-149 Start position: posterior fibers of deltoid.

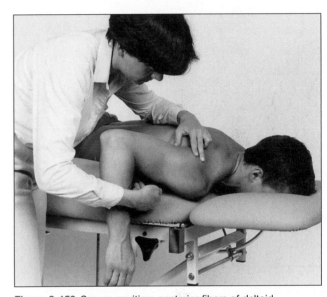

Figure 3-150 Screen position: posterior fibers of deltoid.

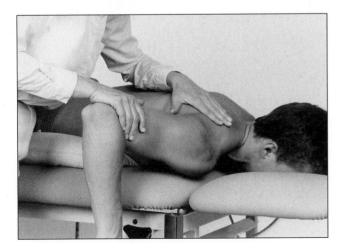

Figure 3-151 Resistance: posterior fibers of deltoid.

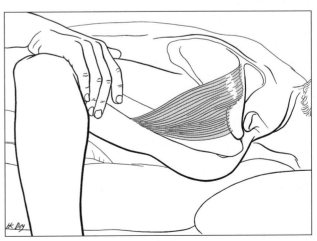

Figure 3-152 Posterior fibers of deltoid.

Gravity Eliminated: Posterior Fibers of Deltoid

Start Position. The patient is sitting. The shoulder is abducted to about 75° (Fig. 3-153). The upper extremity is supported by the therapist.

Stabilization. The therapist stabilizes the scapula.

End Position. The patient horizontally abducts and slightly externally rotates the shoulder (Fig. 3-154).

Substitute Movement. Rhomboids, middle fibers of trapezius, and ipsilateral trunk rotation.

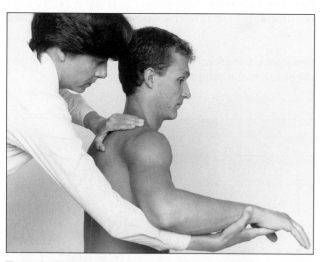

Figure 3-153 Start position: posterior fibers of deltoid.

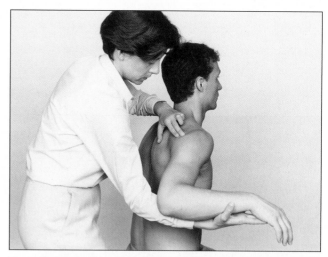

Figure 3-154 End position: posterior fibers of deltoid.

Shoulder Internal Rotation

Against Gravity: Subscapularis

Accessory muscles: teres major, pectoralis major, latissimus dorsi, and anterior fibers of deltoid.

Form 3-27

Start Position. The patient is prone. The shoulder is abducted to 90°, the elbow is flexed to 90°, the arm proximal to the elbow is resting on the plinth (Fig. 3-155).

Stabilization. The therapist stabilizes the humerus to prevent shoulder adduction.

Movement. The patient internally rotates the shoulder by moving the palm of the hand toward the ceiling (Fig. 3-156).

Palpation. Subscapularis is too deep to palpate.

Substitute Movement. Triceps (elbow extension) and pectoralis minor (scapular protraction).

Alternate Test. If the patient has a history of posterior dislocation of the glenohumeral joint and/or is unable to assume the prone position or achieve 90° of shoulder abduction, the gravity eliminated position of sitting is assumed (Fig. 3-158), and the therapist offers resistance equal to the weight of the limb to simulate an against gravity testing situation.

Resistance Location. Applied proximal to the wrist joint (Figs. 3-157 to 3-159). Application of resistance stresses the shoulder and elbow joints, and caution should be exercised.

Resistance Direction. Shoulder external rotation.

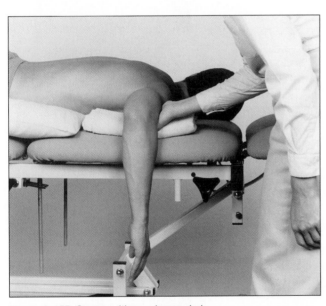

Figure 3-155 Start position: subscapularis.

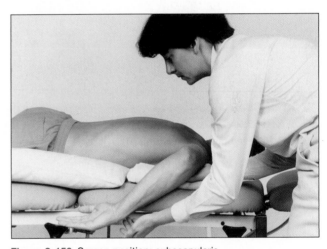

Figure 3-156 Screen position: subscapularis.

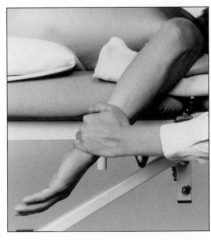

Figure 3-157 Resistance: subscapularis.

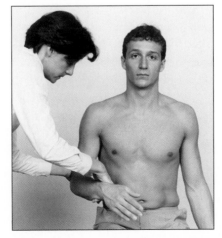

Figure 3-158 Alternate position: subscapularis.

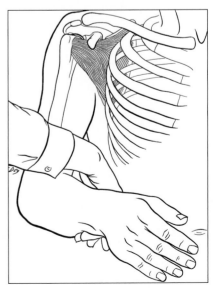

Figure 3-159 Subscapularis.

Gravity Eliminated: Subscapularis

Start Position. The patient is sitting. The shoulder is slightly abducted in neutral rotation and the elbow is flexed to 90° with the forearm in midposition (Fig. 3-160).

Stabilization. The therapist stabilizes the humerus to prevent shoulder abduction.

End Position. The patient internally rotates the shoulder by bringing the palm of the hand toward the abdomen (Fig. 3-161).

Substitute Movement. Triceps (elbow extension), shoulder abduction, and pronation of the forearm.

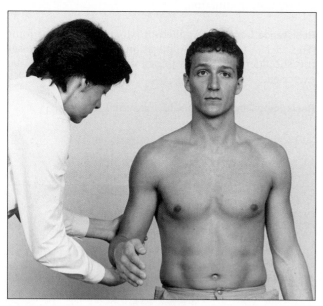

Figure 3-160 Start position: subscapularis.

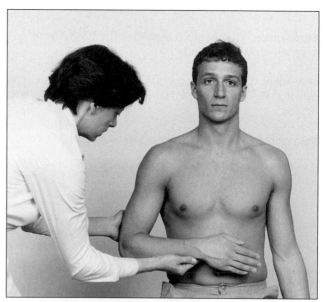

Figure 3-161 End position: subscapularis.

Subscapularis Alternate Test. The patient must have full shoulder internal rotation ROM to assume this test position. This test maximizes the activity of subscapularis and minimizes the activity of the accessory muscles: latissimus dorsi, pectoralis major,[26,27] and teres major.[26]

Start Position. The patient is sitting. The shoulder is internally rotated and the dorsum of the hand is placed over the midlumbar spine (Fig. 3-162).

Stabilization. The therapist instructs the patient to avoid trunk forward flexion and/or ipsilateral trunk rotation.

End Position (not shown). The patient moves the hand away from the back.

Palpation. Subscapularis is too deep to palpate.

Substitute Movement. Ipsilateral trunk rotation and/or trunk forward flexion, and scapular anterior tilt, retraction, medial rotation, and elevation.

Resistance Location (not shown). Applied proximal to the wrist joint. Application of resistance stresses the shoulder and elbow joints, and caution should be exercised.

Resistance Direction. Shoulder external rotation. The isometric test is preferred.

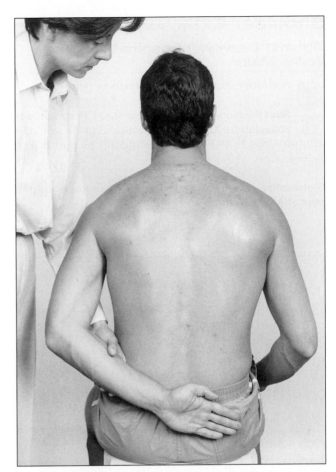

Figure 3-162 Alternate test start position: subscapularis.

Shoulder External Rotation

Against Gravity: Infraspinatus and Teres Minor

Accessory muscle: posterior fibers of deltoid.

Form 3-28 **Start Position.** The patient is prone. The shoulder is abducted to 90°, the elbow is flexed to 90°, and the arm proximal to the elbow is resting on the plinth (Fig. 3-163).

Stabilization. The therapist stabilizes the humerus to prevent shoulder adduction.

Movement. The patient externally rotates the shoulder by moving the dorsum of the hand toward the ceiling (Fig. 3-164).

Palpation. *Infraspinatus:* over the body of the scapula just inferior to the spine of the scapula. *Teres minor:* not palpable.

Substitute Movement. Triceps (elbow extension) and lower fibers of trapezius (scapular depression).

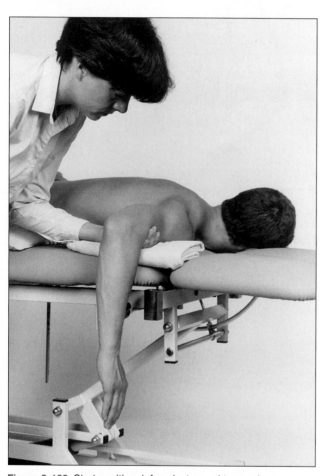

Figure 3-163 Start position: infraspinatus and teres minor.

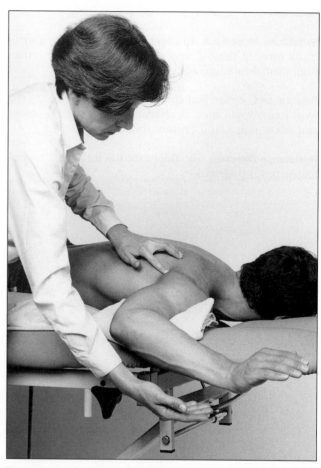

Figure 3-164 Screen position: infraspinatus and teres minor.

Alternate Test. If the patient has a history of anterior dislocation of the glenohumeral joint and/or is unable to assume the prone position or achieve 90° of shoulder abduction, the gravity eliminated position in sitting is assumed and the resisted gravity eliminated methodology is used (Fig. 3-166).

Resistance Location. Applied proximal to the wrist joint on the posterior aspect of the forearm (Figs. 3-165 to 3-167). Application of resistance stresses the elbow and shoulder joints, and caution should be exercised.

Resistance Direction. Shoulder internal rotation.

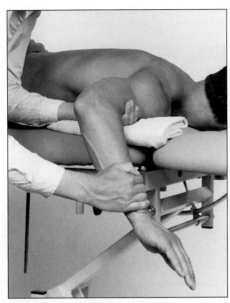

Figure 3-165 Resistance: infraspinatus and teres minor.

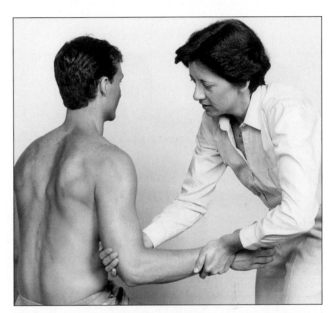

Figure 3-166 Alternate position: infraspinatus and teres minor.

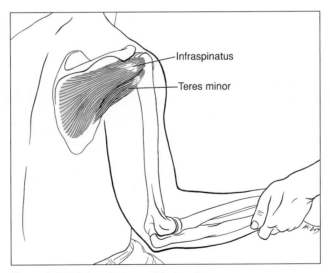

Figure 3-167 Infraspinatus and teres minor.

Gravity Eliminated: Infraspinatus and Teres Minor

Start Position. The patient is sitting. The arm is at the side, with the shoulder adducted in neutral rotation, and the elbow is flexed to 90° with the forearm in midposition (Fig. 3-168).

Stabilization. The therapist stabilizes the humerus.

End Position. The patient externally rotates the shoulder by taking the hand away from the body (Fig. 3-169).

Substitute Movement. Triceps (elbow extension), lower fibers of trapezius (scapular depression), and forearm supination.

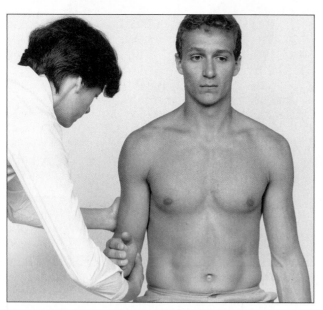

Figure 3-168 Start position: infraspinatus and teres minor.

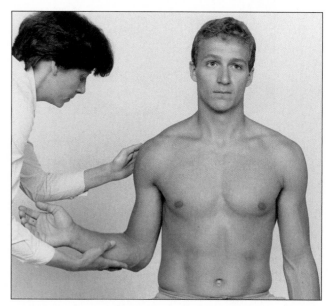

Figure 3-169 End position: infraspinatus and teres minor.

FUNCTIONAL APPLICATION

Joint Function

The function of the shoulder complex is to position or move the arm in space for the purpose of hand function. The shoulder complex is the most mobile joint complex in the body, providing a ROM that exceeds that of any other joint. Because of this mobility, stability is sacrificed.[8,28–32]

Functional Range of Motion

The glenohumeral joint may be abducted and adducted, flexed and extended, and internally and externally rotated. In the performance of functional activities, the glenohumeral movements are accompanied at varying points in the ROM by scapular, clavicular, and trunk motion. These motions extend the functional range capabilities of the shoulder joint, and without their contribution, movement of the upper limbs would be severely restricted.[29,31,32] The functional movements of the shoulder complex are described to emphasize the interdependence of the components of the shoulder complex and trunk throughout movement.

Elevation of the Arm over the Head

This functional motion of elevation to between 170° and 180° may be achieved through forward flexion in the sagittal plane or abduction in the frontal plane. Owing to the position of the scapula, which lies 30° to 45° anterior to the frontal plane,[3] many daily functional activities are performed in the plane of the scapula. The plane of the scapula is the plane of reference for diagonal movements of shoulder elevation (Fig. 3-5). *Scaption*[4] is the term given to this midplane elevation. The plane used by an individual depends on the motion requirements of the activity and the position of the hand required for the task (Table 3-5).

To attain the full 180° of elevation through flexion or abduction, movement of the glenohumeral joint is accompanied by movement at the sternoclavicular, acromioclavicular, and scapulothoracic joints. The final degrees of motion can be achieved only through contribution of the spinal movement of trunk extension and/or contralateral lateral flexion.[3,5,28] The total shoulder complex functions in a coordinated way to provide smooth movement and to gain a large excursion of movement for the upper extremity. The coordinated movement pattern achieved through scapulothoracic and glenohumeral movement is described as a "scapulohumeral rhythm".[3,8,28,30]

There are individual variations as to the contribution of all joints to the movement of elevating the arm overhead. Variation depends on the plane of elevation, the arc of elevation, the amount of load on the arm, and individual anatomical differences.[32] Recognizing these variations, it is generally noted that the range of glenohumeral to scapular motion throughout elevation is in the ratio of 2:1; that is, 2° of glenohumeral motion to every 1° of scapular motion.[8,30,31,34] The scapulohumeral rhythm is described for elevation through flexion and for elevation through abduction. An understanding of the scapulohumeral rhythm is essential in understanding the significance of limitations in joint range of motion at the shoulder complex.

Scapulohumeral Rhythm

During the initial 60° of shoulder flexion in the sagittal plane or the initial 30° of abduction in the frontal plane, there is an inconsistent scapulohumeral rhythm. It is

TABLE 3-5 Shoulder Horizontal Adduction/Abduction and Other Shoulder ROM* Required for Selected Functional Activities[33]

Activity	Horizontal Adduction ROM (degrees)[†]	Other Shoulder ROM (degrees)	
Washing axilla	104 ± 12	flexion	52 ± 14
Eating	87 ± 29	flexion	52 ± 8
Combing hair	54 ± 27	abduction	112 ± 10
	Horizontal Abduction ROM (degrees)[†]		
Reaching maximally up back	69 ± 11	extension	56 ± 13
Reaching perineum	86 ± 13	extension	38 ± 10

*Values are mean ± SD for eight normal subjects.

[†]The 0° start position for establishing the degrees of horizontal adduction and horizontal abduction is 90° shoulder abduction (see Fig. 3-51).

during this phase that the scapula is seeking stability in relationship to the humerus.[34–36] The scapula is in a setting phase where it may remain stationary, or it may slightly medially (downward) or laterally (upward) rotate[34] (Fig. 3-170). The glenohumeral joint is the main contributor to movement in this phase. Feeding activities that are performed within this phase of shoulder elevation include using a spoon or a fork and drinking from a cup. These activities are carried out within the ranges of 5° to 45° shoulder flexion and 5° to 30° shoulder abduction.[37]

Following the setting phase, there is a predictable scapulohumeral rhythm throughout the remaining arc of movement to 170° (Fig. 3-171). For every 15° of movement between 30° abduction or 60° flexion and 170° of abduction/flexion, 10° occurs at the glenohumeral joint and 5° occurs at the scapulothoracic joint. Movement of the scapula following the setting phase consists of the primary scapular movement of lateral (upward) rotation, accompanied by secondary rotations of posterior tilting (sagittal plane) and posterior rotation (transverse plane)

as the humeral angle is increased with elevation of the arm in the scapular plane.[38]

Range to 170° through abduction depends on a normal scapulohumeral rhythm and the ability to externally rotate the humerus fully through elevation. When the abducted arm reaches a position of 90°, movement through full range of elevation cannot continue because the greater tuberosity of the humerus contacts the superior margin of the glenoid fossa and the coracoacromial arch.[5,36,39] External rotation of the humerus (in the range of approximately 25° to 50°[2]) places the greater tuberosity posteriorly, allowing the humerus to move freely under the coracoacromial arch. Full shoulder elevation through flexion depends on scapulohumeral rhythm and the ability to rotate the humerus internally through range.[40]

The final degrees of elevation are achieved through contralateral trunk lateral flexion (Fig. 3-172) and/or trunk extension. From the discussion of scapulohumeral rhythm, it becomes apparent that restriction in movement at any of the joints of the shoulder complex will limit the ability to position the hand for function.

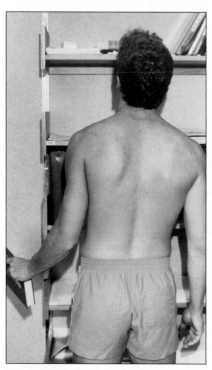

Figure 3-170 Setting phase of the scapula during elevation of the arm through abduction. The scapula remains stationary.

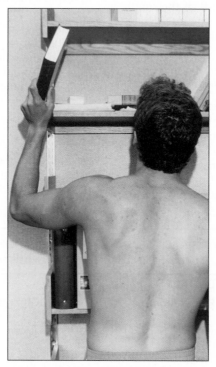

Figure 3-171 Scapulohumeral rhythm: during elevation beyond 60° of flexion or 30° of abduction, the scapula abducts and laterally (upward) rotates.

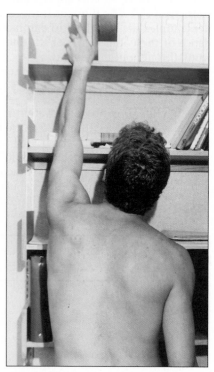

Figure 3-172 Full elevation through abduction: full range is achieved through contralateral trunk lateral flexion.

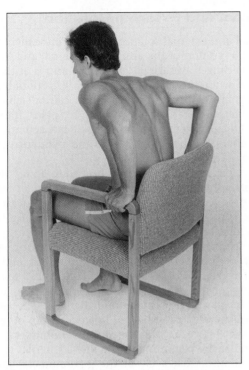

Figure 3-173 Shoulder extension accompanied by scapular adduction and medial (downward) rotation.

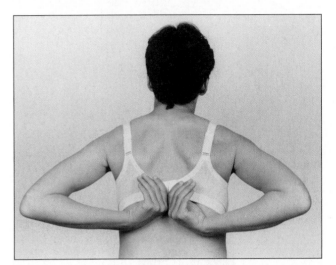

Figure 3-174 Functional extension and internal rotation of the shoulders.

Shoulder Extension

The range of 60° of shoulder extension is primarily obtained through the glenohumeral joint.[39] In the performance of functional activities, extension is often accompanied by adduction and medial (downward) rotation of the scapula (Fig. 3-173). A consistent scapulohumeral rhythm is not present in this movement.

Forty-three degrees to 69° of shoulder extension is required to reach maximally up the back[33] (e.g., when hooking a bra; see Fig. 3-174), and 28° to 48° shoulder extension is necessary to reach the perineum[33] when performing toilet hygiene.

Horizontal Adduction and Abduction

The movements of horizontal adduction and abduction allow the arm to be moved around the body at shoulder level for such activities as washing the axilla or the back (Fig. 3-175), writing on a blackboard (Fig. 3-176), and sliding a window horizontally open or closed. Although by definition horizontal adduction and abduction movements take place in the transverse plane, many ADL require similar motions in planes located above or below shoulder level. These movements may also be referred to as horizontal adduction and abduction until the frontal plane is approached; the movements are then referred to as either adduction or abduction. Table 3-5 provides examples of the ROM required for selected ADL, to bring the arm in front of the body (horizontal adduction) or behind the body (horizontal abduction) and position the arm for other shoulder movements needed to perform these activities.

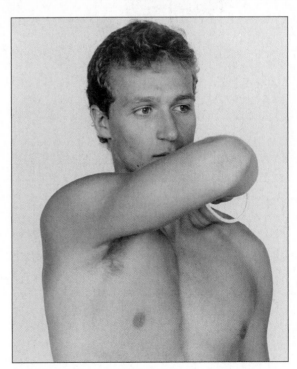

Figure 3-175 Horizontal adduction – pectoralis major function.

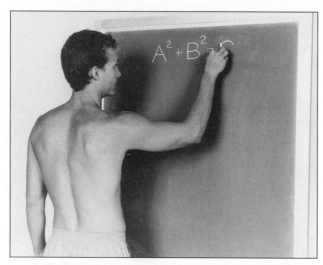

Figure 3-176 Horizontal abduction.

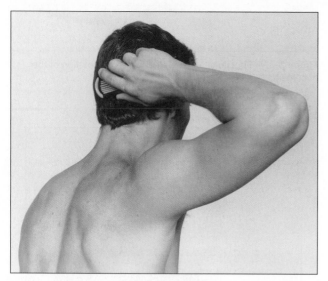

Figure 3-177 Full shoulder external rotation.

Internal and External Rotation

Internal and external rotation range of movement varies with the position of the arm. Both internal and external rotation ranges average 68° when the arm is at the side, whereas when the arm is abducted to 90°, 70° of internal rotation and 90° of external rotation can be achieved.[11] Full external rotation is required to place the hand behind the neck when performing self-care activities such as combing the hair (Fig. 3-177) and manipulating the clasp of a necklace.

Shoulder internal rotation is needed to do up the buttons on a shirt. Five degrees to 25° of shoulder internal rotation is required to use a spoon or fork and to drink from a cup.[37] Full glenohumeral joint internal rotation, augmented by scapulothoracic and elbow joint motion, positions the hand behind the back to reach into a back pocket, perform toilet hygiene, tuck in a shirt, and hook a bra (see Fig. 3-174). Mallon and colleagues[41] analyzed joint motions that occurred at the shoulder complex and elbow in placing the arm behind the back. The analysis revealed the presence of a coordinated pattern of motion occurring between scapular and glenohumeral joint motion. At the beginning of the ROM, internal rotation occurs almost exclusively at the glenohumeral joint as the hand is brought across in front of the body and to a position alongside the ipsilateral hip. As the movement continues and the hand is brought behind the low back, motion at the scapulothoracic joint augments glenohumeral joint internal rotation. The elbow is then flexed to reach up the spine to the level of the thorax.

Shoulder rotations have a functional link with forearm rotation.[28] When the arm is away from the side, rotation at both joints is concerned with turning the palm to face either the floor or the ceiling. Shoulder internal rotation is linked with pronation of the forearm, as both actions occur simultaneously with performance of many activities and pronation can be amplified by internal rotation of the shoulder (Fig. 3-178). Shoulder external rotation has a functional link with supination of the forearm when the elbow is extended. Examples of activities that illustrate this combined action are inserting a light bulb into a ceiling socket, releasing a bowling ball from the extended arm, and manipulating the foot into a shoe (Fig. 3-179).

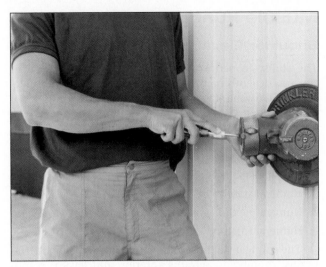

Figure 3-178 Functional association: shoulder internal rotation and forearm pronation.

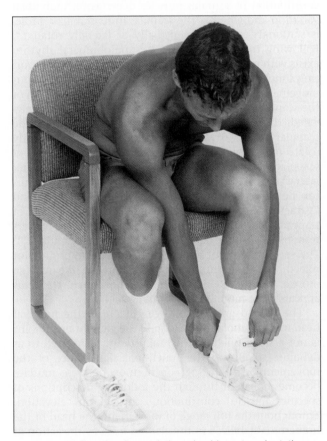

Figure 3-179 Functional association: shoulder external rotation and forearm supination.

Muscle Function

Shoulder Elevation

The ability to perform activities involving elevation of the arm depends on joint integrity for freedom of movement and on the strength and function of the muscles of the shoulder girdle that produce and control movement.[42] The muscles responsible for the smooth, coordinated action involved in elevation can be divided into four functional groups:

1. Scapular stabilizers and motivators
2. Humeral stabilizers
3. Humeral flexors or abductors
4. Humeral rotators

The scapular stabilizers and motivators include the trapezius, rhomboids, serratus anterior, and levator scapulae. During the setting phase of the scapula there is minimal activity in these muscles (Fig. 3-170). The specific contribution of scapular muscles depends on individual variation and whether the scapula, in its stabilizing role, is stationary, or slightly medially or laterally rotated.[34] Following the setting phase, a scapulohumeral rhythm exists with movements of the scapula and humerus occurring simultaneously. The setting phase and simultaneous movement can be visualized by observing the position of the scapula in Figures 3-170 and 3-171. As the arm is elevated, there is a gradual increase in the activity of the scapular muscles to full range[34] as these muscles primarily rotate the scapula laterally or upward. The purpose of scapular rotation is to place the glenoid fossa and other lateral parts of the scapula in positions where the humerus can be raised without limitation imposed by bony and ligamentous structures.[43] The upper and lower fibers of trapezius and the serratus anterior are the prime movers responsible for the lateral rotation of the scapula.[3,38,44] The serratus anterior appears to play a more prominent role in elevation through flexion, drawing the scapula more anteriorly around the chest wall, while the trapezius appears to be more important in abduction.[42]

The second group of muscles stabilizes the humeral head in the glenoid fossa. Because the glenohumeral joint is not a static fulcrum, this stabilization is referred to as dynamic stability.[45] The functional significance of the movement or stabilizing contribution of these muscles becomes apparent through the following descriptions of specific muscle contribution throughout elevation. Throughout the full range of movement, the head of the humerus is stabilized in the glenoid fossa by the action of subscapularis, supraspinatus, infraspinatus, the upper half of teres minor,[45,46] and the long head of biceps.[47] Through electromyographic studies, Saha[45] found that in abduction, the subscapularis and infraspinatus stabilize in the range of 0° to 150° and the infraspinatus is the primary stabilizer throughout the remainder of range. Supraspinatus provides stabilization in the pendant arm position.[30,46]

The third group of muscles acts to move the humerus in the sagittal or frontal plane. These muscles are active throughout a range of movement of 0° to 180°. These muscles proximally attach on the scapula and distally attach on the humerus and include the shoulder abductors and shoulder flexors. The middle fibers of the deltoid and supraspinatus elevate the humerus through abduction; the anterior fibers of deltoid and the clavicular portion of pectoralis major and coracobrachialis elevate the humerus through flexion.

As the shoulder muscles contract to flex or abduct the arm, the rotator cuff muscles stabilize or dynamically "fix" the head of the humerus in the glenoid fossa, thus creating a fulcrum or "fixed point" around which the humerus moves in abduction or flexion. This stabilization checks or prevents the occurrence of other, unwanted movements of the humerus that would be created by the contraction forces of the shoulder abductor or flexor muscles during elevation.

The purpose of the fourth group is to rotate the humerus externally or internally. Elevation through abduction is accompanied by external rotation of the humerus.[5,28,36,39] The anterior fibers of deltoid function to rotate the humerus internally[48], as flexion is accompanied by internal rotation.[40]

The function of elevation of the shoulder is to position and move the arm in space for the purpose of hand function. Hand activity places additional demands on the muscles of the shoulder girdle responsible for elevation. Sporrong and coworkers[49] evaluated activity in four muscles of the shoulder girdle, a scapular stabilizer and motivator (trapezius), the humeral stabilizers (supraspinatus, infraspinatus), and a humeral motivator (deltoid), with a small load, similar in weight to an industrial handtool, held in the hand in elevated arm positions while sitting. When increased hand-grip forces were applied to the load, muscle activity increased in the shoulder girdle muscles, most notably in the humeral stabilizers.

Shoulder Adduction and Extension

From elevation of the arm through flexion or abduction the arm is brought down to the side of the body through extension or adduction. When quick movement or force is required for an activity such as closing a window, climbing a ladder, or serving the ball in tennis (Fig. 3-180), the latissimus dorsi and teres major adduct and extend the humerus. Although latissimus dorsi functions with or without resistance as a factor, teres major is only active in activities where resistance is a factor.[46] In this instance, teres major is accompanied by the action of rhomboids, functioning to rotate the scapula medially.[5,46] When the arm is taken posteriorly from the side, in a sagittal plane, the latissimus dorsi and teres major are assisted by the posterior fibers of deltoid.

The functional significance of the latissimus dorsi, through its attachment on the crest of the ilium, is apparent in activities that require weight bearing with the hands.[28] In activities such as crutch walking or rising from a sitting position (Fig. 3-173), the latissimus dorsi depresses the shoulder girdle to raise the trunk and pelvis. The sternal fibers of pectoralis major assist latissimus dorsi to elevate the trunk on the fixed humerus as in performing a weight relief raise[50] or during depression transfers[51] for patients with low-level paraplegia.

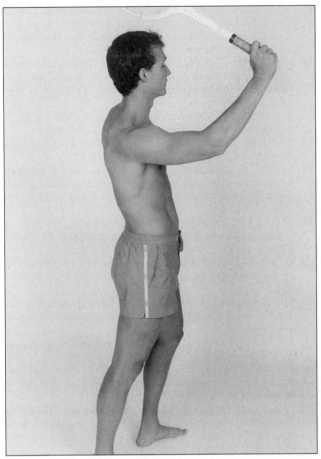

Figure 3-180 Shoulder extension – latissimus dorsi and teres major function.

Flexion and Adduction

Pectoralis major is a flexor and adductor of the arm. The functional significance of its integrity is illustrated in self-care activities where the arm is flexed and adducted. This pattern of movement is evident in many self-care activities, including dressing, bathing (Fig. 3-175), and hygiene tasks.

Internal Rotation

The subscapularis is the only pure internal rotator of the shoulder.[52] The teres major, latissimus dorsi, pectoralis major, and the anterior deltoid combine internal rotation with other movements previously described. Subscapularis internally rotates the humerus when the arm is positioned in front of or behind the body. The muscle plays a major role in lifting the hand away from the region of the midlumbar spine[26], for example, as one positions a pillow behind the back when sitting.

Internal rotation has a functional link with pronation of the forearm, as both actions occur simultaneously with performance of many activities[28] and pronation can be amplified by internal rotation of the shoulder (Fig. 3-178).

External Rotation

This movement is achieved through the action of infraspinatus, teres minor, and posterior deltoid. External rotation has a functional link with the supinators of the forearm when the elbow is extended.[28] Both muscle groups are concerned with turning the palm to face the ceiling. Examples of activities that illustrate this combined action are inserting a light bulb into a ceiling socket, releasing a bowling ball from the extended arm, and manipulating the foot into a shoe (Fig. 3-179).

References

1. Standring S, ed. *Gray's Anatomy: The Anatomical Basis of Clinical Practice.* 39th ed. London: Elsevier Churchill Livingstone; 2005.
2. Neumann DA. *Kinesiology of the Musculoskeletal System: Foundations for Rehabilitation.* 2nd ed. St Louis: Mosby Elsevier; 2010.
3. Soderberg GL. *Kinesiology: Application to Pathological Motion.* 2nd ed. Baltimore: Williams & Wilkins; 1997.
4. Perry J. Shoulder function for the activities of daily living. In: Matsen FA, Fu FH, Hawkins RJ, eds. *The Shoulder: A Balance of Mobility and Stability.* Rosemont, IL: American Academy of Orthopaedic Surgeons; 1993.
5. Kapandji IA. *The Physiology of the Joints. Vol. 1. The Upper Limb.* 6th ed. New York: Churchill Livingstone Elsevier; 2007.
6. Norkin CC, White DJ. *Measurement of Joint Motion: A Guide to Goniometry.* 4th ed. Philadelphia: FA Davis; 2009.
7. Daniels L, Worthingham C. *Muscle Testing: Techniques of Manual Examination.* 5th ed. Philadelphia: WB Saunders; 1986.
8. Levangie PK, Norkin CC. *Joint Structure & Function: A Comprehensive Analysis.* 3rd ed. Philadelphia: FA Davis; 2001.
9. Woodburne RT. *Essentials of Human Anatomy.* 5th ed. London: Oxford University Press; 1973.
10. Magee DJ. *Orthopedic Physical Assessment.* 5th ed. St Louis: Saunders Elsevier; 2008.
11. American Academy of Orthopaedic Surgeons. *Joint Motion: Method of Measuring and Recording.* Chicago: AAOS; 1965.
12. Berryman Reese N, Bandy WD. *Joint Range of Motion and Muscle Length Testing.* Philadelphia: WB Saunders; 2002.
13. Cyriax J. *Textbook of Orthopaedic Medicine, Vol. 1. Diagnosis of Soft Tissue Lesions.* 8th ed. London: Bailliere Tindall; 1982.
14. Gajdosik RL, Hallett JP, Slaughter LL. Passive insufficiency of two-joint shoulder muscles. *Clin Biomech.* 1994;9:377–378.
15. Kebaetse M, McClure P, Pratt NA. Thoracic position effect on shoulder range of motion, strength, and three-dimensional scapular kinematics. *Arch Phys Med Rehabil.* 1999;80:945–950.
16. Boon AJ, Smith J. Manual scapular stabilization: its effect on shoulder rotational range of motion. *Arch Phys Med Rehabil.* 2000;81:978–983.
17. Evjenth O, Hamberg J. *Muscle Stretching in Manual Therapy A Clinical Manual: The Extremities.* Vol. 1. Alfta, Sweden: *Alfta Rehab Forlag;* 1984.
18. Soames RW, ed. Skeletal system. In: Salmons S, ed. Muscle. *Gray's Anatomy.* 38th ed. New York: Churchill Livingstone; 1995.
19. Wang SS, Normile SO, Lawshe BT. Reliability and smallest detectable change determination for serratus anterior muscle strength and endurance tests. *Physiother Theor Pract.* 2006;22(1):33–42.

20. Ekstrom RA, Donatelli RA, Soderberg GL. Surface electromyographic analysis of exercises for the trapezius and serratus anterior muscles. *J Orthop Sports Phys Ther.* 2003; 33(5):247–258.

21. Brunnstrom MA. Muscle testing around the shoulder girdle. *J Bone Joint Surg [Am].* 1941;23:263–272.

22. Kendall FP, McCreary EK, Provance PG, Rodgers MM, Romani WA. *Muscles Testing and Function with Posture and Pain.* 5th ed. Philadelphia: Lippincott Williams & Wilkins; 2005.

23. Robel SJ, Mills MM, Terpstra L, Vardaxis V. Middle and lower trapezius manual muscle testing. *J Orthop Sports Phys Ther.* 2009;39:A79–A79.

24. Nishijima N, Yamamuro T, Fujio K, Ohba M. The swallowtail sign: a test of deltoid function. *J Bone Joint Surg [Br].* 1994; 77:152–153.

25. Whitcomb LJ, Kelley MJ, Leiper CI. A comparison of torque production during dynamic strength testing of shoulder abduction in the coronal plane and the plane of the scapula. *J Orthop Sports Phys Ther.* 1995;21:227–232.

26. Greis PE, Kuhn JE, Schultheis J, Hintermeister R, Hawkins R. Validation of the lift-off test and analysis of subscapularis activity during maximal internal rotation. *Am J Sports Med.* 1996;24:589–593.

27. Kelly BT, Kadrmas WR, Speer KP. The manual muscle examination for rotator cuff strength. *Am J Sports Med.* 1996;24: 581–588.

28. Smith LK, Lawrence Weiss E, Lehmkuhl LD. *Brunnstrom's Clinical Kinesiology.* 5th ed. Philadelphia: FA Davis; 1996.

29. MacConaill MA, Basmajian JV. *Muscles and Movements.* 2nd ed. New York: RE Kreiger; 1977.

30. Cailliet R. *Shoulder Pain.* 3rd ed. Philadelphia: FA Davis; 1991.

31. Rosse C. The shoulder region and the brachial plexus. In: Rosse C, Clawson DK, eds. *The Musculoskeletal System in Health and Disease.* New York: Harper & Row; 1980.

32. Zuckerman JD, Matsen FA. Biomechanics of the shoulder. In: Nordin M, Frankel VM, eds. *Basic Biomechanics of the Musculoskeletal System.* 2nd ed. Philadelphia: Lea & Febiger; 1989.

33. Matsen FA, Lippitt SB, Sidles JA, Harryman DT. *Practical Evaluation and Management of the Shoulder.* Philadelphia: WB Saunders; 1994.

34. Inman VT, Saunders M, Abbot LC. Observations on the function of the shoulder joint. *J Bone Joint Surg.* 1944;26:1–30.

35. Dvir Z, Berme N. The shoulder complex in elevation of the arm: a mechanism approach. *J Biomech.* 1978;11:219–225.

36. Kent BE. Functional anatomy of the shoulder complex: a review. *Phys Ther.* 1971;51:867–888.

37. Safaee-Rad R, Shwedyk E, Quanbury AO, Cooper JE. Normal functional range of motion of upper limb joints during performance of three feeding activities. *Arch Phys Med Rehabil.* 1990;71:505–509.

38. Ludewig PM, Cook TM, Nawoczenski DA. Three-dimensional scapular orientation and muscle activity at selected positions of humeral elevation. *J Orthop Sports Phys Ther.* 1996;24:57–65.

39. Peat M. The shoulder complex: a review of some aspects of functional anatomy. *Physiother Can.* 1977;29:241–246.

40. Blakey RL, Palmer ML. Analysis of rotation accompanying shoulder flexion. *Phys Ther.* 1984;64:1214–1216.

41. Mallon WJ, Herring CL, Sallay PI, et al. Use of vertebral levels to measure presumed internal rotation at the shoulder: a radiologic analysis. *J Shoulder Elbow Surg.* 1996;5:299–306.

42. Norkin CC, Levangie PK. *Joint Structure & Function: A Comprehensive Analysis.* 2nd ed. Philadelphia: FA Davis; 1992.

43. Duvall EN. Critical analysis of divergent views of movement of the shoulder joint. *Arch Phys Med Rehabil.* 1955;36:149–153.

44. Johnson G, Bogduk N, Nowitzke A, House D. Anatomy and actions of the trapezius muscle. *Clin Biomechanics.* 1994;9:44–50.

45. Saha AK. Dynamic stability of the glenohumeral joint. *Acta Orthop Scand.* 1971;42:491–505.

46. Basmajian JV, DeLuca CJ. *Muscles Alive: Their Functions Revealed by Electromyography.* 5th ed. Baltimore: Williams & Wilkins; 1985.

47. Pagnani MJ, Deng X-H, Warren RF, Torzilli PA, O'Brien SJ. Role of the long head of the biceps brachii in glenohumeral stability: A biomechanical study in cadavers. *J Shoulder Elbow Surg.* 1996;5:255–262.

48. Moore KL. *Clinically Oriented Anatomy.* Baltimore: Williams & Wilkins; 1980.

49. Sporrong H, Palmerud G, Herberts P. Hand grip increases shoulder muscle activity: an EMG analysis with static hand contractions in 9 subjects. *Acta Orthop Scand.* 1996;67:485–490.

50. Reyes ML, Gronley JK, Newsam CJ, Mulroy SJ, Perry J. Electromyographic analysis of shoulder muscles of men with low-level paraplegia during a weight relief raise. *Arch Phys Med Rehabil.* 1995;76:433–439.

51. Perry J, Gronley JK, Newsam CJ, Reyes ML, Mulroy SJ. Electromyographic analysis of shoulder muscles during depression transfers in subjects with low-level paraplegia. *Arch Phys Med Rehabil.* 1996;77:350–355.

52. Lehmkuhl LD, Smith LK. *Brunnstrom's Clinical Kinesiology.* 4th ed. Philadelphia: FA Davis; 1983.

Chapter 4

Elbow and Forearm

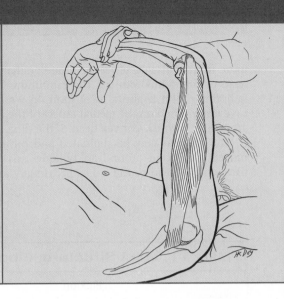

ARTICULATIONS AND MOVEMENTS

The elbow, a modified hinge joint (Fig. 4-1), is composed of the humeroulnar and humeroradial joints. The humeroulnar joint is formed proximally by the trochlea of the humerus, that is convex anteroposteriorly,[1] and articulates with the concave surface of the trochlear notch of the ulna. The convex surface of the capitulum of the humerus articulates with the concave proximal aspect of the radial head to form the humeroradial joint.

The elbow may be flexed and extended in the sagittal plane with movement occurring around a frontal axis (Fig. 4-2). The axis for elbow flexion and extension "passes through the center of the arcs formed by the trochlear sulcus and the capitellum"[2(p. 534)] of the humerus, except at the extremes of motion, when the axis is displaced anteriorly and posteriorly,[2] respectively.

The forearm articulations (Fig. 4-1) consist of the superior and inferior radioulnar joints and the syndesmosis formed by the interosseous membrane between the radius and the ulna. The superior radioulnar joint is contained within the capsule of the elbow joint[1] and is a pivot joint formed between the convex surface of the radial head and the concave radial notch on the radial aspect of the proximal ulna. The annular ligament, lined with articular cartilage, encompasses the rim of the radial head.[3] When motion occurs at the superior radioulnar

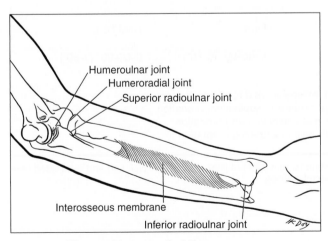

Figure 4-1 Elbow and forearm articulations.

Humeroulnar joint
Humeroradial joint
Superior radioulnar joint
Interosseous membrane
Inferior radioulnar joint

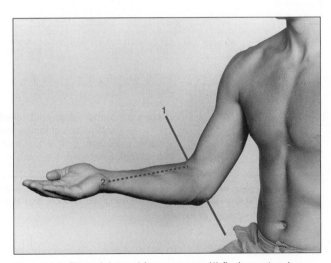

Figure 4-2 Elbow joint and forearm axes: (1) flexion–extension and (2) supination–pronation.

joint, motion also occurs at the humeroradial joint as the head of the radius spins on the capitulum. The inferior radioulnar joint is also a pivot joint, in which the concave ulnar notch on the medial aspect of the distal radius articulates with the convex head of the ulna.

The forearm may be supinated and pronated. These movements occur around an oblique axis that passes through the head of the radius proximally and through the head of the ulna distally[4,5] (Fig. 4-2). With the elbow in anatomical position, the movements of pronation and supination occur in the transverse plane around a longitudinal axis. In supination, the radius lies alongside the ulna (Fig. 4-3A). In pronation, the radius rotates around the relatively stationary ulna (Fig. 4-3B). The joints and movements of the elbow and forearm joints are described in Table 4-1.

TABLE 4-1 Joint Structure: Elbow and Forearm Movements

	Flexion	Extension	Supination	Pronation
Articulation[1,6]	Humeroulnar, Humeroradial	Humeroulnar, Humeroradial	Humeroradial, Superior radioulnar, Inferior radioulnar, Interosseous membrane	Humeroradial, Superior radioulnar, Inferior radioulnar, Interosseous membrane
Plane	Sagittal	Sagittal	Transverse	Transverse
Axis	Frontal	Frontal	Longitudinal	Longitudinal
Normal limiting factors[3,6–8]* (see Fig. 4-3A and B)	Soft tissue apposition of the anterior forearm and upper arm; coronoid process contacting the coronoid fossa and the radial head contacting the radial fossa; tension in the posterior capsule and triceps	Olecranon process contacting the olecranon fossa; tension in the elbow flexors and anterior joint capsule and medial collateral ligament	Tension in the pronator muscles, quadrate ligament, palmar radioulnar ligament of the inferior radioulnar joint, and oblique cord	Contact of the radius on the ulna; tension in the quadrate ligament, the dorsal radioulnar ligament of the inferior radioulnar joint, the distal tract of the interosseous membrane,[9] supinator, and biceps brachii muscles with elbow in extension
Normal end feel[7,10,11]*	Soft/hard/firm	Hard/firm	Firm	Hard/firm
Normal AROM[12]† (AROM[13])	0–150° (0–140°)	0° (0°)	0–80–90° (0–80°)	0–80–90° (0–80°)
Capsular pattern[10,11]	Elbow joint: humeroulnar joint - flexion, extension, and rotation full and painless radiohumeral joint - flexion, extension, supination, pronation Superior radioulnar joint: equal limitation of supination and pronation Inferior radioulnar joint: full rotation with pain at extremes of rotation			

*There is a paucity of definitive research that identifies the normal limiting factors (NLF) of joint motion. The NLF and end feels listed here are based on knowledge of anatomy, clinical experience, and available references.

†AROM, active range of motion.

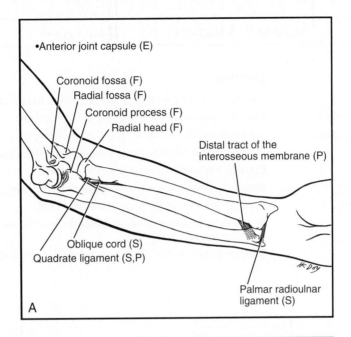

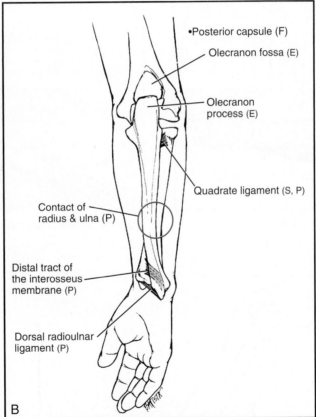

Figure 4-3 Normal limiting factors. A. Anteromedial view of elbow and supinated forearm showing noncontractile structures that normally limit motion. **B.** Posterior view of the elbow with forearm pronated showing noncontractile structures that normally limit motion. Motion limited by structure is identified in parentheses, using the following abbreviations: *F*, flexion; *E*, extension; *P*, pronation; *S*, supination. Muscles normally limiting motion are not illustrated.

SURFACE ANATOMY (Figs. 4-4, 4-5, and 4-6)

Structure	Location
1. Acromion process	Lateral aspect of the spine of the scapula at the tip of the shoulder.
2. Medial epicondyle of the humerus	Medial projection at the distal end of the humerus.
3. Lateral epicondyle of the humerus	Lateral projection at the distal end of the humerus.
4. Olecranon process	Posterior aspect of the elbow; proximal end of the shaft of the ulna.
5. Head of the radius	Distal to the lateral epicondyle of the humerus.
6. Styloid process of the radius	Bony prominence on the lateral aspect of the forearm at the distal end of the radius.
7. Head of the third metacarpal	Bony prominence at the base of the third digit.
8. Head of the ulna	Round bony prominence on the posteromedial aspect of the forearm at the distal end of the ulna.
9. Styloid process of the ulna	Bony projection on the posteromedial aspect of the distal end of the ulna.

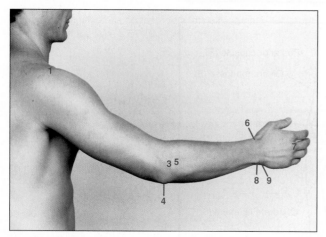

Figure 4-4 Posterolateral aspect of the arm.

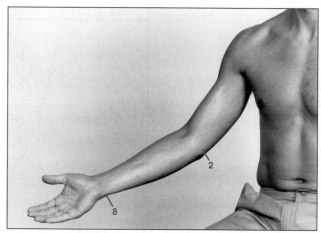

Figure 4-5 Anteromedial aspect of the arm.

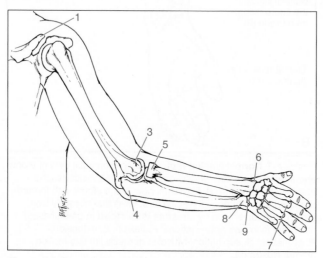

Figure 4-6 Bony anatomy, posterolateral aspect of the arm.

RANGE OF MOTION ASSESSMENT AND MEASUREMENT

 Practice Makes Perfect

To aid you in practicing the skills covered in this section, or for a handy review, use the practical testing forms found at http://thepoint.lww.com/Clarkson3e.

Elbow Flexion–Extension/ Hyperextension

AROM Assessment

Substitute Movement. *Flexion*—trunk extension, shoulder flexion, scapular depression, and wrist flexion. *Extension*—trunk flexion, shoulder extension, scapular elevation, and wrist extension.

PROM Assessment

Start Position. The patient is supine or sitting. The arm is in the anatomical position with the elbow in extension (Fig. 4-7). A towel is placed under the distal end of the humerus to accommodate the range of motion (ROM). Owing to biceps muscle tension, unusually muscular men may not be able to achieve 0°. Up to 15° of hyperextension is common in women[12,14,15] or children because the olecranon is smaller.[15]

Forms 4-1, 4-2

Stabilization. The therapist stabilizes the humerus.

Therapist's Distal Hand Placement. The therapist grasps the distal radius and the ulna.

End Positions. The therapist moves the forearm in an anterior direction, to the limit of motion of elbow flexion (Fig. 4-8). The therapist moves the forearm in a posterior direction, to the limit of motion of elbow extension/hyperextension (Fig. 4-9).

End Feels. *Flexion*—soft/hard/firm; *extension/hyperextension*—hard/firm.

Joint Glides. *Flexion*—concave trochlear notch and concave radial head glide anteriorly on the fixed convexities of the trochlea and capitulum, respectively. *Extension*—concave trochlear notch and concave radial head glide posteriorly on the fixed convexities of the trochlea and capitulum, respectively.

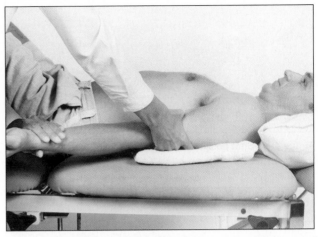

Figure 4-7 Start position for elbow flexion and extension/ hyperextension PROM.

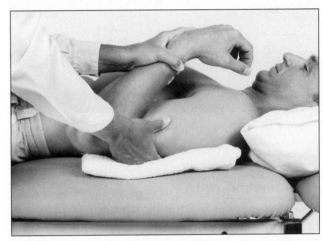

Figure 4-8 Soft, hard, or firm end feel at limit of elbow flexion.

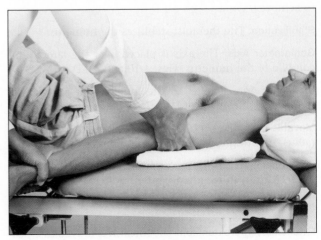

Figure 4-9 Hard or firm end feel at limit of elbow hyperextension.

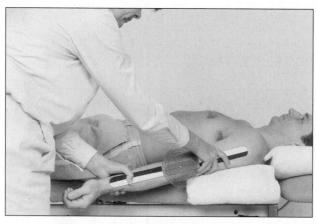

Figure 4-10 Start position for elbow flexion and extension.

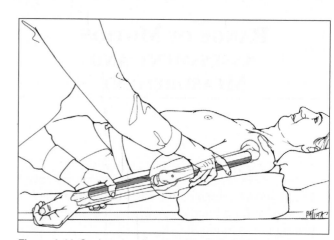

Figure 4-11 Goniometer alignment for elbow flexion and extension.

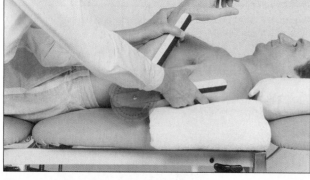

Figure 4-12 End position for elbow flexion.

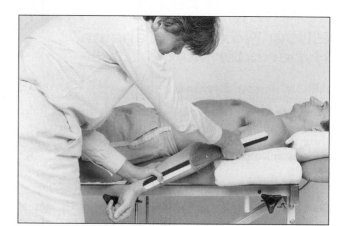

Figure 4-13 End position for elbow hyperextension.

Measurement: Universal Goniometer

Start Position. The patient is supine or sitting. The arm is in the anatomical position with the elbow in extension (0°) (Fig. 4-10). A towel is placed under the distal end of the humerus to accommodate the ROM. Owing to biceps muscle tension, unusually muscular men may not be able to achieve 0°.

Stabilization. The therapist stabilizes the humerus.

Goniometer Axis. The axis is placed over the lateral epicondyle of the humerus (Figs. 4-10 and 4-11).

Stationary Arm. Parallel to the longitudinal axis of the humerus, pointing toward the tip of the acromion process.

Movable Arm. Parallel to the longitudinal axis of the radius, pointing toward the styloid process of the radius.

End Position. From the start position of elbow extension, the forearm is moved in an anterior direction so that the hand approximates the shoulder to the limit of elbow flexion (150°) (Fig. 4-12).

Extension/Hyperextension. The forearm is moved in a posterior direction to the limit of elbow extension (0°)/ hyperextension (up to 15°) (Fig. 4-13).

Alternate Measurement

The patient is sitting (Figs. 4-14 and 4-15).

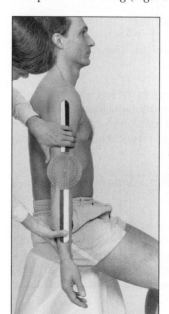

Figure 4-14 Elbow extension of 0°.

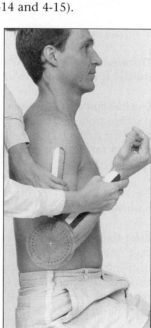

Figure 4-15 Elbow flexion.

Supination-Pronation

AROM Assessment

Substitute Movement. *Supination*—adduction and external rotation of the shoulder and ipsilateral trunk lateral flexion. *Pronation*—abduction and internal rotation of the shoulder and contralateral trunk lateral flexion.

PROM Assessment

Forms
4-3, 4-4

Start Position. The patient is sitting. The arm is at the side, and the elbow is flexed to 90° with the forearm in midposition (Fig. 4-16A).

Stabilization. The therapist stabilizes the humerus.

Therapist's Distal Hand Placement. The therapist grasps the distal radius and the ulna (see Fig. 4-16B).

End Positions. The forearm is rotated externally from midposition so that the palm faces upward and toward the ceiling to the limit of forearm supination (Fig. 4-17A and B). The forearm is rotated internally so that the palm faces downward and toward the floor to the limit of forearm pronation (Fig. 4-18A and B).

End Feels. *Supination*—firm; *pronation*—hard/firm.

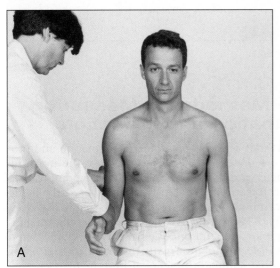
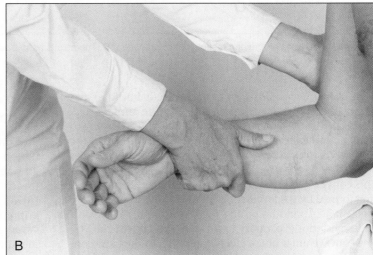

Figure 4-16 **A.** Start position for supination and pronation. **B.** Therapist's hand position for PROM.

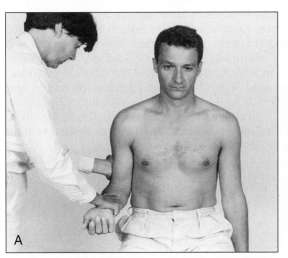
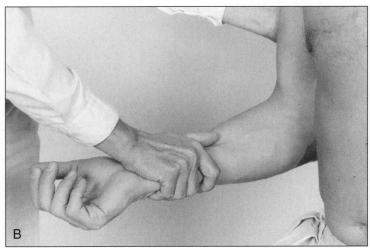

Figure 4-17 **A.** Firm end feel at limit of supination. **B.** Therapist's hand position.

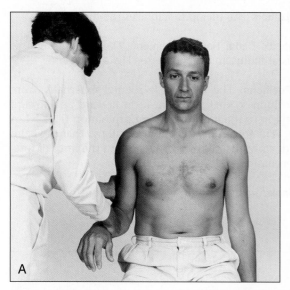
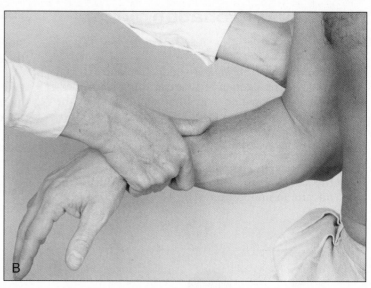

Figure 4-18 A. Hard or firm end feel at limit of pronation. **B.** Therapist's hand position.

Joint Glides. *Supination*—(1) The convex radial head rotates within the fibro-osseous ring formed by the annular ligament and the fixed concave radial notch[16] and according to Baeyens and colleagues,[17] glides anteriorly, contrary to the concave–convex rule. (2) The concave ulnar notch glides posteriorly on the fixed convex ulnar head.[16] *Pronation*—(1) The convex radial head rotates within the fibro-osseous ring formed by the annular ligament and the fixed concave radial notch[16] and according to Baeyens and colleagues[17] glides posteriorly, contrary to the concave–convex rule. (2) The concave ulnar notch glides anteriorly on the fixed convex ulnar head.[16] *Humeroradial joint*—the head of the radius spins on the fixed capitulum during supination and pronation.

Five Methods for Measuring Supination and Pronation

Five methods of measuring forearm supination and pronation are presented. Three methods use the universal goniometer and two use the OB "Myrin" goniometer to measure forearm ROM. Most activities of daily living (ADL) combine forearm rotation with hand use (e.g., gripping).[18] Two of the five methods (one using the universal goniometer and one the OB "Myrin" goniometer) measure forearm rotation with the hand in a gripping posture that simulates functional movements (see Figs. 4-19 and 4-29). The measurements performed using the universal goniometer (see Figs. 4-25 to 4-28) and the OB "Myrin" goniometer (see Fig. 4-32) positioned proximal to the wrist measure isolated forearm ROM.

Forearm supination and pronation ROM are affected by change in elbow joint position, that is, as the elbow is flexed, forearm supination ROM increases and forearm pronation ROM decreases, and as the elbow is extended, the converse occurs.[19] The total forearm pronation and supination ROM is greatest between 45° and 90° of elbow flexion.[19] It is therefore important to maintain the elbow in 90° flexion when measuring forearm supination and pronation ROM.

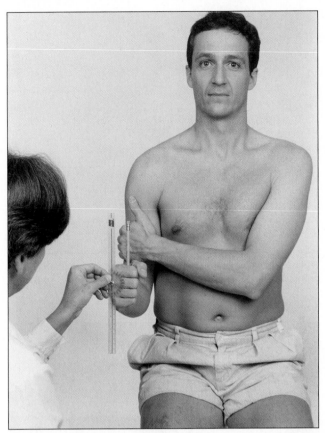

Figure 4-19 Functional measurement method: start position for supination and pronation.

Measurement: Universal Goniometer

Start Position. The patient is sitting. The arm is at the side, and the elbow is flexed to 90° with the forearm in midposition. A pencil is held in the tightly closed fist with the pencil protruding from the radial aspect of the hand,[14] and the wrist in the neutral position (Fig. 4-19). The fist is tightly closed to stabilize the fourth and fifth metacarpals, thus avoiding unwanted movement of the pencil as the test movements are performed.

Stabilization. The patient stabilizes the humerus using the nontest hand.

Goniometer Axis. The axis is placed over the head of the third metacarpal.

Stationary Arm. Perpendicular to the floor.

Movable Arm. Parallel to the pencil.

End Position. The forearm is rotated externally from midposition so that the palm faces upward and toward the ceiling to the limit of forearm supination (80° to 90° from midposition) (Fig. 4-20).

Substitute Movement. Altered grasp of the pencil if the fist is not tightly closed during testing, thumb touching and moving the pencil, wrist extension and/or radial deviation.

End Position. The forearm is rotated internally so that the palm faces downward and toward the floor to the limit of forearm pronation (80° to 90° from midposition) (Fig. 4-21).

Substitute Movement. Altered grasp of the pencil, wrist flexion and/or ulnar deviation.

High intratester[18,20] and intertester[18] reliability has been reported for the functional measurement method using the universal goniometer and the pencil held in the hand to measure active supination and pronation ROM.

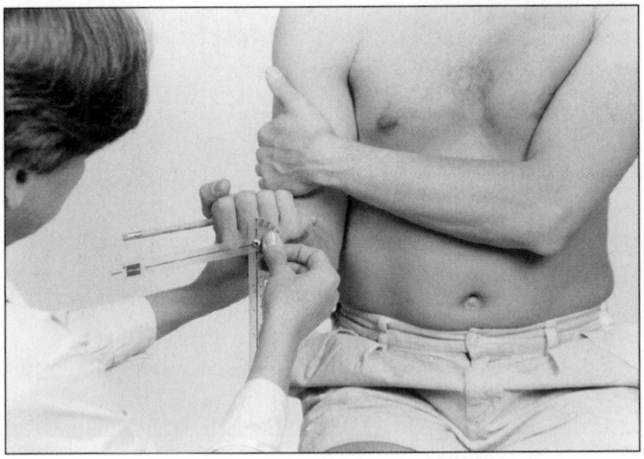

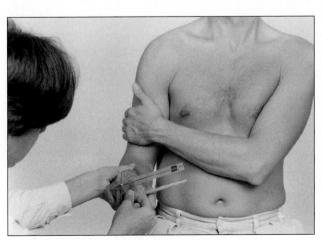

Figure 4-20 Supination.

Figure 4-21 Pronation.

Alternate Measurement: Universal Goniometer

This measurement is indicated if the patient cannot grasp a pencil.

Start Position. The arm is at the side, and the elbow is flexed to 90° with the forearm in midposition. The wrist is in neutral, and the fingers are extended (Fig. 4-22).

Stabilization. The patient stabilizes the humerus using the nontest hand.

Goniometer Axis. The axis is placed at the tip of the middle digit.

Stationary Arm. Perpendicular to the floor.

Movable Arm. Parallel to the tips of the four extended fingers.

End Position. The forearm is rotated externally so that the palm faces upward and toward the ceiling to the limit of forearm supination (80° to 90° from midposition) (Fig. 4-23).

Substitute Movement. Finger hyperextension, wrist extension, and wrist deviations.

End Position. The forearm is rotated internally so that the palm faces downward and toward the floor to the limit of forearm pronation (80° to 90° from midposition) (Fig. 4-24).

Substitute Movement. Finger flexion, wrist flexion, and wrist deviations.

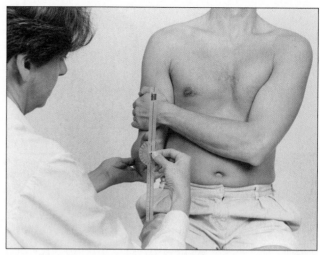

Figure 4-22 Alternate method: start position for supination and pronation.

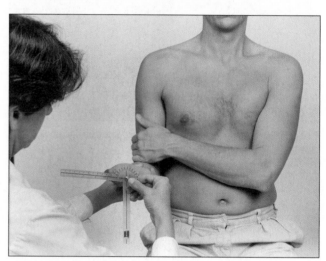

Figure 4-23 Supination.

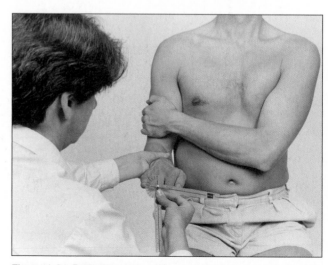

Figure 4-24 Pronation.

Alternate Measurement: Universal Goniometer Proximal to Wrist

This method eliminates joints distal to the forearm from influencing the measurement and can be used if the patient cannot grasp a pencil. Active range of motion (AROM) measured using this method demonstrated good intratester reliability with the stationary arm parallel to the midline of the humerus.[20]

Start Position. The arm is at the side, and the elbow is flexed to 90° with the forearm in midposition. The wrist is in neutral, and the fingers are relaxed (see Figs. 4-25 and 4-27).

Stabilization. The patient stabilizes the humerus using the nontest hand.

Goniometer Axis. The axis is placed in line with the ulnar styloid process.

Stationary Arm. Perpendicular to the floor.

Movable Arm. *Supination*—against the anterior aspect of the distal forearm in line with the ulnar styloid process (Fig. 4-25). *Pronation*—against the posterior aspect of the distal forearm in line with the ulnar styloid process (Fig. 4-27).

End Position. The forearm is rotated externally so that the palm faces upward and toward the ceiling to the limit of forearm supination (80° to 90° from midposition) (Fig. 4-26).

Substitute Movement. Shoulder adduction, shoulder external rotation, and ipsilateral trunk lateral flexion.

End Position. The forearm is rotated internally so that the palm faces downward and toward the floor to the limit of forearm pronation (80° to 90° from midposition) (Fig. 4-28).

Substitute Movement. Shoulder abduction, shoulder internal rotation, and contralateral trunk lateral flexion.

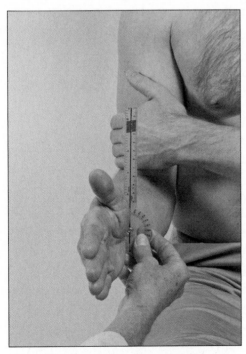

Figure 4-25 Start position for supination.

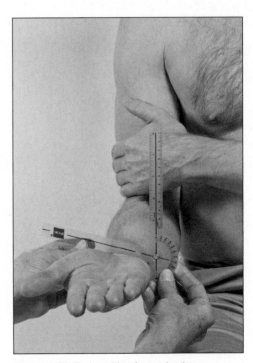

Figure 4-26 End position for supination.

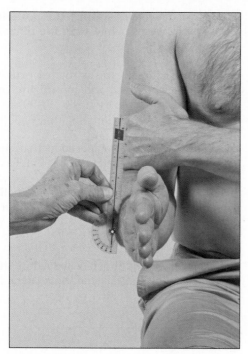

Figure 4-27 Start position for pronation.

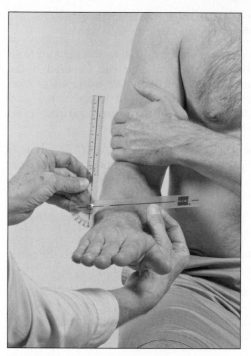

Figure 4-28 End position for pronation.

Measurement: OB "Myrin" Goniometer

Start Position. The patient is sitting. The shoulder is adducted, and the elbow is flexed to 90° with the forearm in midposition. The wrist is in neutral, and the fingers are flexed (Fig. 4-29).

Goniometer Placement. The dial is placed on the right-angled plate. The plate is held between the patient's index and middle fingers.

Stabilization. The therapist stabilizes the humerus.

End Position. The forearm is rotated externally from midposition to the limit of motion for supination (Fig. 4-30).

Substitute Movement. Wrist extension and deviations, shoulder adduction with external rotation, and ipsilateral trunk lateral flexion.

End Position. The forearm is rotated internally from midposition to the limit of motion for pronation (Fig. 4-31).

Substitute Movement. Wrist flexion and deviations, shoulder abduction with internal rotation, and contralateral trunk lateral flexion.

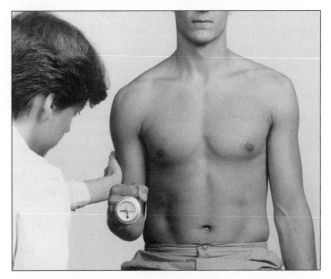

Figure 4-29 Start position for supination and pronation using the OB goniometer.

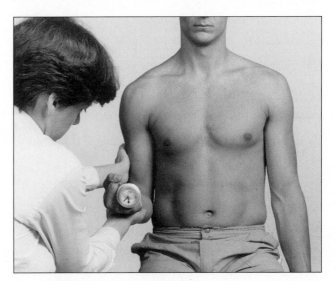

Figure 4-30 End position for supination.

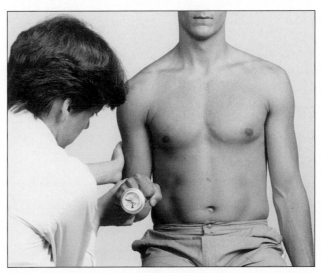

Figure 4-31 End position for pronation.

Alternate Placement: OB "Myrin" Goniometer Proximal to Wrist

The strap is placed around the distal forearm. The dial is placed on the right-angled plate and attached on the radial side of the forearm (Fig. 4-32). This goniometer placement measures isolated forearm rotation ROM.

Substitute Movement. Using this alternate goniometer placement, substitute movements for supination are limited to shoulder adduction, shoulder external rotation, and ipsilateral trunk lateral flexion. Substitute movements for pronation are limited to shoulder abduction, shoulder internal rotation, and contralateral trunk lateral flexion.

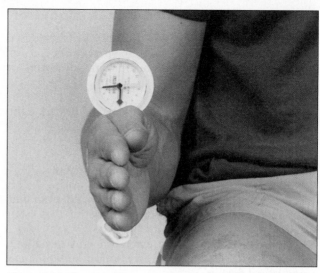

Figure 4-32 Alternate OB goniometer placement for supination and pronation.

MUSCLE LENGTH ASSESSMENT AND MEASUREMENT

 Practice Makes Perfect

To aid you in practicing the skills covered in this section, or for a handy review, use the practical testing forms found at http://thepoint.lww.com/Clarkson3e.

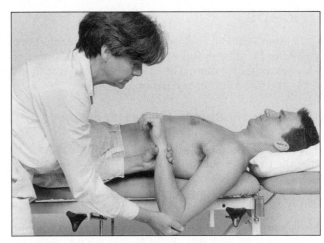

Figure 4-33 Start position: length of biceps brachii.

Biceps Brachii

Origin[1]	Insertion[1]
Biceps Brachii	
a. Short head: apex of the coracoid process of the scapula. b. Long head: supraglenoid tubercle of the scapula.	Posterior aspect of the radial tuberosity and via the bicipital aponeurosis fuses with the deep fascia covering the origins of the flexor muscles of the forearm.

 Start Position. The patient is supine with the shoulder in extension over the edge of the plinth, the elbow is flexed, and the forearm is pronated (Fig. 4-33).

Form 4-5

Stabilization. The therapist stabilizes the humerus.

End Position. The elbow is extended to the limit of motion so that the biceps brachii is put on full stretch (Figs. 4-34 and 4-35).

End Feel. Biceps brachii on stretch—firm.

Measurement. The therapist uses a goniometer to measure and record the available elbow extension PROM. If the biceps is shortened, elbow extension PROM will be restricted proportional to the decrease in muscle length.

Universal Goniometer Placement. The goniometer is placed the same as for elbow flexion–extension.

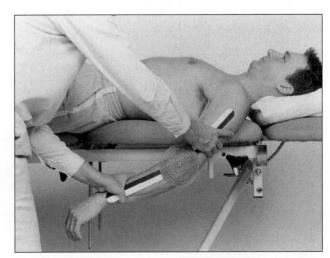

Figure 4-34 Goniometer measurement: length of biceps brachii.

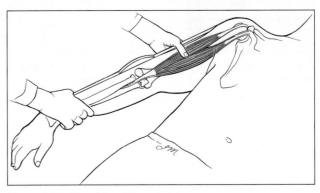

Figure 4-35 Biceps brachii on stretch.

Triceps

 Start Position. The patient is sitting with the shoulder in full elevation through forward flexion and external rotation. The elbow is in extension and the forearm is in supination (Fig. 4-36).

Form 4-6

Stabilization. The therapist stabilizes the humerus.

End Position. The elbow is flexed to the limit of motion so that the triceps is put on full stretch (Figs. 4-37 and 4-38).

End Feel. Triceps on stretch—firm.

Measurement. The therapist uses a goniometer to measure and record the available elbow flexion PROM. If the triceps is shortened, elbow flexion PROM will be restricted proportional to the decrease in muscle length.

Goniometer Placement. The goniometer is placed the same as for elbow flexion–extension.

Origin[1]	Insertion[1]
Triceps	
a. Long head: infraglenoid tubercle of the scapula. b. Lateral head: posterolateral surface of the humerus between the radial groove and the insertion of teres minor; lateral intermuscular septum. c. Medial head: posterior surface of the humerus below the radial groove between the trochlea of the humerus and the insertion of teres major; medial and lateral intermuscular septum.	Posteriorly, on the proximal surface of the olecranon; some fibers continue distally to blend with the antebrachial fascia.

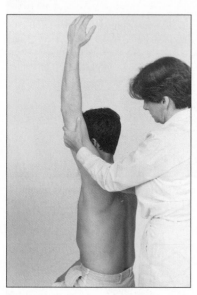

Figure 4-36 Start position: length of triceps.

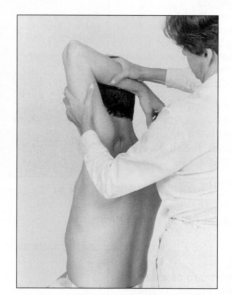

Figure 4-37 End position: triceps on stretch.

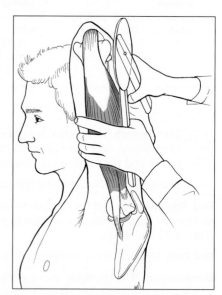

Figure 4-38 Goniometer measurement: length of triceps.

Alternate Measurement: Supine

This position is used if the patient has decreased shoulder flexion ROM.

Start Position. The patient is supine with the shoulder in 90° flexion and the elbow in extension (Fig. 4-39).

Stabilization. The therapist stabilizes the humerus.

End Position. The elbow is flexed to the limit of motion to put the triceps on stretch (Fig. 4-40).

Universal Goniometer Placement. The goniometer is placed the same as for elbow flexion–extension (see Fig. 4-38).

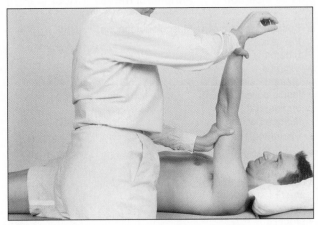

Figure 4-39 Alternate start position: triceps length.

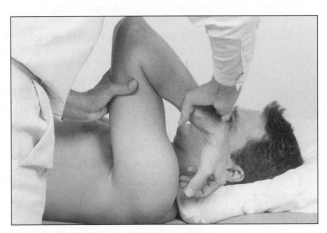

Figure 4-40 End position: triceps on stretch.

MUSCLE STRENGTH ASSESSMENT (TABLE 4-2)

TABLE 4-2	Muscle Actions, Attachments, and Nerve Supply: The Elbow and the Forearm[21]				
Muscle	**Primary Muscle Action**	**Muscle Origin**	**Muscle Insertion**	**Peripheral Nerve**	**Nerve Root**
Biceps brachii	Elbow flexion Forearm supination	a. Short head: apex of the coronoid process of the scapula b. Long head: supraglenoid tubercle of the scapula	a. Posterior aspect of the radial tuberosity b. Bicipital aponeurosis: deep fascia covering origins of the flexor muscles of the forearm	Musculocutaneous	C56
Brachialis	Elbow flexion	Distal one-half of the anterior aspect of the humerus; medial and lateral intermuscular septa	Tuberosity of the ulna; rough impression on the anterior surface of the coronoid process	Musculocutaneous, Radial	C56(7)
Brachioradialis	Elbow flexion	Proximal two-thirds of the lateral supracondylar ridge of the humerus; lateral intermuscular septum	Lateral side of the distal end of the radius, just proximal to the styloid process	Radial	C56
Triceps	Elbow extension	a. Long head: infraglenoid tubercle of the scapula b. Lateral head: posterolateral surface of the humerus between the radial groove and the insertion of teres minor; lateral intermuscular septum c. Medial head: posterior surface of the humerus below the radial groove between the trochlea of the humerus and the insertion of teres major; medial and lateral intermuscular septa	Posteriorly, on the proximal surface of the olecranon; some fibers continue distally to blend with the antebrachial fascia	Radial	C678

(continues)

TABLE 4-2 *Continued*

Muscle	Primary Muscle Action	Muscle Origin	Muscle Insertion	Peripheral Nerve	Nerve Root
Supinator	Forearm supination	Lateral epicondyle of the humerus; radial collateral ligament of the elbow joint; annular ligament of the superior radioulnar joint; from the supinator crest of the ulna and the posterior part of the depression anterior to it	Anterolateral and posterolateral surfaces of the proximal one-third of the radius	Posterior interosseous branch of radial	C67
Pronator teres	Forearm pronation	a. Humeral head: just proximal to the medial epicondyle; common forearm flexor muscle tendon b. Ulnar head: medial side of the coronoid process of the ulna	Midway along the lateral surface of the radial shaft	Median	C67
Pronator quadratus	Forearm pronation	Distal one-fourth of the anterior surface of the shaft of the ulna	Distal one-fourth of the anterior border and surface of the shaft of the radius; triangular area proximal to the ulnar notch of the radius	Anterior interosseous branch of median	C78

Practice Makes Perfect

To aid you in practicing the skills covered in this section, or for a handy review, use the practical testing forms found at http://thepoint.lww.com/Clarkson3e.

Elbow Flexion

Against Gravity: Biceps Brachii

Form 4-7

Accessory muscles: brachialis, brachioradialis, pronator teres,[21] and extensor carpi radialis longus and brevis.[22]

Start Position. The patient is supine or sitting. The arm is at the side, the elbow is extended, and the forearm is supinated (Fig. 4-41).

Stabilization. The therapist stabilizes the humerus.

Movement. The patient flexes the elbow through full ROM (Fig. 4-42).

Palpation. Anterior aspect of the antecubital fossa.

Substitute Movement. Brachialis may substitute for biceps brachii, because it is an elbow flexor, irrespective of forearm positioning.[23]

Resistance Location. Applied proximal to the wrist joint on the anterior aspect of the forearm (Figs. 4-43 and 4-44).

Resistance Direction. Forearm pronation and elbow extension.

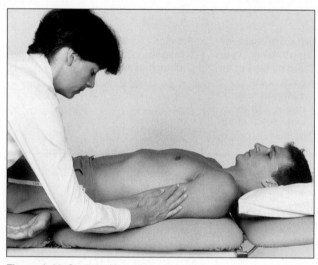

Figure 4-41 Start position: biceps brachii.

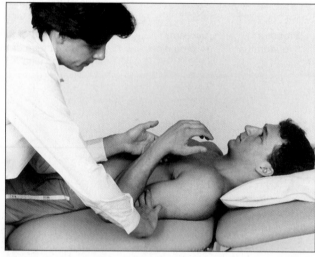

Figure 4-42 Screen position: biceps brachii.

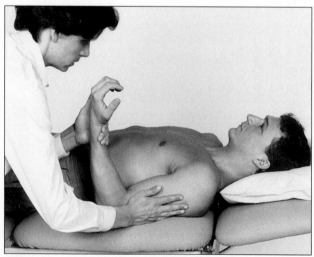

Figure 4-43 Resistance: biceps brachii.

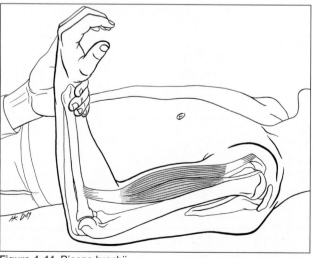

Figure 4-44 Biceps brachii.

Gravity Eliminated: Biceps Brachii

Start Position. The patient is sitting with the arm supported on a powder board. The shoulder is abducted to 90°, the elbow is extended, and the forearm is supinated (Fig. 4-45).

Alternate Start Position. The patient is in a side-lying position. The therapist supports the weight of the upper extremity (Fig. 4-46).

Stabilization. The therapist stabilizes the humerus.

End Position. The patient flexes the elbow through full ROM (Fig. 4-47).

Substitute Movement. Brachialis.

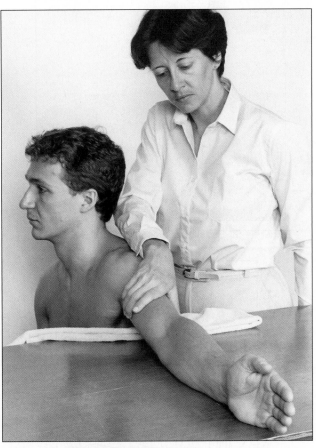

Figure 4-45 Start position: biceps brachii.

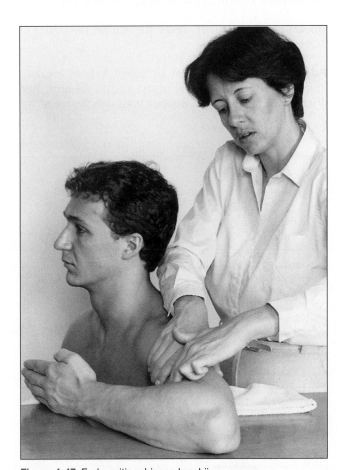

Figure 4-47 End position: biceps brachii.

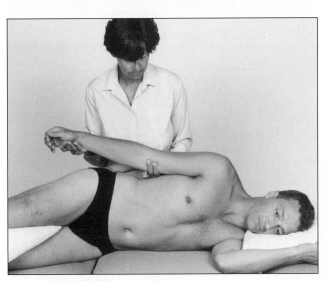

Figure 4-46 Alternate start position.

Against Gravity: Brachialis and Brachioradialis

 Accessory muscles: biceps brachii, pronator teres,[21] and extensor carpi radialis longus and brevis.[22]

Form 4-8

Start Position. The patient is supine or sitting. The arm is at the side, the elbow is extended, and the forearm is in pronation (Fig. 4-48).

Stabilization. The therapist stabilizes the humerus.

Movement. The patient flexes the elbow through full ROM (Fig. 4-49).

Palpation. *Brachialis:* medial to biceps brachii tendon. *Brachioradialis:* anterolateral aspect of the forearm, just distal to the elbow crease. Because both muscles are active when the forearm is pronated,[23] muscle contraction must be confirmed by palpation and/or observation.

Resistance Location. Applied proximal to the wrist joint on the posterior aspect of the forearm (Figs. 4-50, 4-51, and 4-52).

Resistance Direction. Elbow extension.

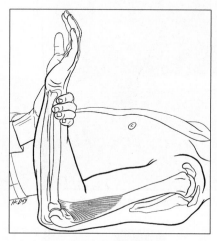

Figure 4-50 Resistance: brachialis and brachioradialis.

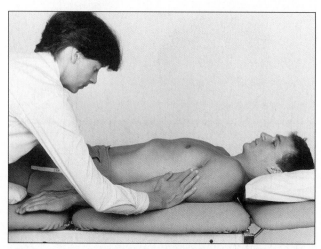

Figure 4-48 Start position: brachialis and brachioradialis.

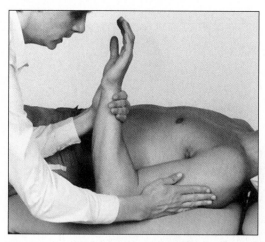

Figure 4-51 Brachialis.

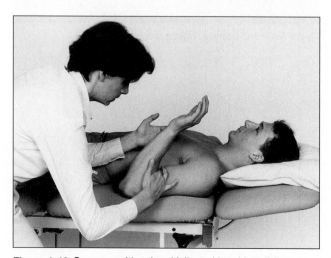

Figure 4-49 Screen position: brachialis and brachioradialis.

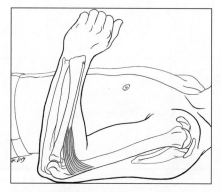

Figure 4-52 Brachioradialis.

Gravity Eliminated: Brachialis and Brachioradialis

Start Position. The patient is sitting with the arm supported on a powder board. The shoulder is abducted to 90°, the elbow is extended, and the forearm is pronated (Fig. 4-53). An alternate position is side-lying (not shown).

Stabilization. The therapist stabilizes the humerus.

End Position. The patient flexes the elbow through full ROM (Fig. 4-54).

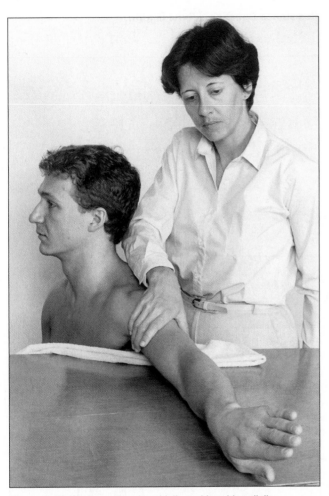

Figure 4-53 Start position: brachialis and brachioradialis.

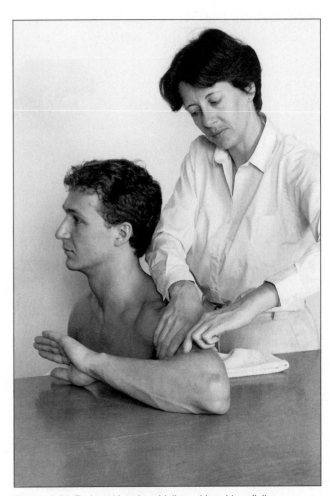

Figure 4-54 End position: brachialis and brachioradialis.

Elbow Extension

Against Gravity: Triceps

Accessory muscle: anconeus.

Form 4-9 **Start Position.** The patient is supine. The shoulder is internally rotated and flexed to 90°, the elbow is flexed, and the forearm is supinated (Fig. 4-55).

Stabilization. The therapist stabilizes the humerus.

Movement. The patient extends the elbow through full ROM (Fig. 4-56). Ensure the patient does not lock the elbow in full extension (i.e., the close-packed position).

Palpation. Just proximal to the olecranon process.

Resistance Location. Applied proximal to the wrist joint on the posterior aspect of the forearm (Figs. 4-57 and 4-58).

Resistance Direction. Elbow flexion.

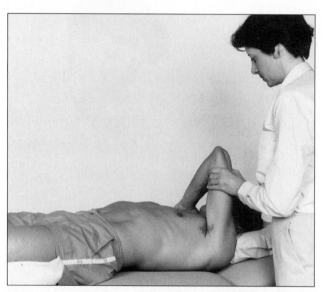

Figure 4-55 Start position: triceps.

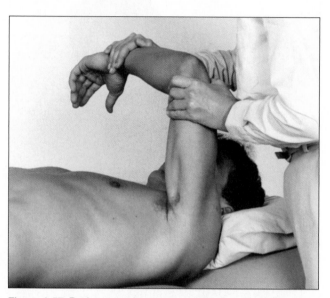

Figure 4-57 Resistance: triceps.

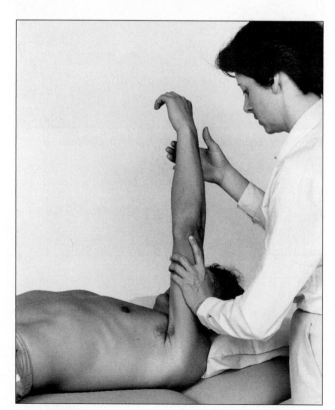

Figure 4-56 Screen position: triceps.

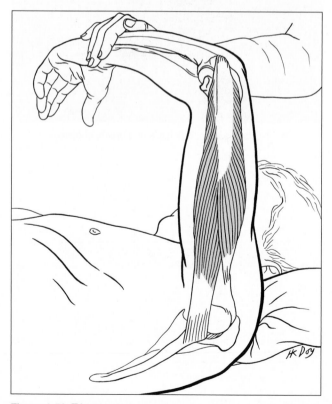

Figure 4-58 Triceps.

Gravity Eliminated: Triceps

Start Position. The patient is sitting with the arm supported on a powder board. The shoulder is abducted to 90°, the elbow is flexed, and the forearm is supinated (Fig. 4-59).

Alternate Start Position. The patient is in a side-lying position. The therapist supports the weight of the upper extremity (Fig. 4-60).

Stabilization. The therapist stabilizes the humerus.

End Position. The patient extends the elbow through full ROM, avoiding the close-packed position (Fig. 4-61).

Substitute Movement. Scapular depression and shoulder external rotation, permitting gravity to complete the ROM.

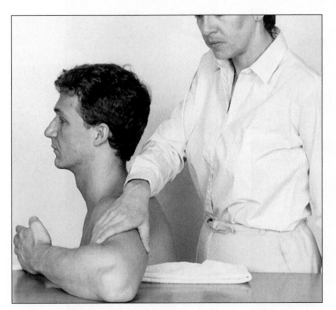

Figure 4-59 Start position: triceps.

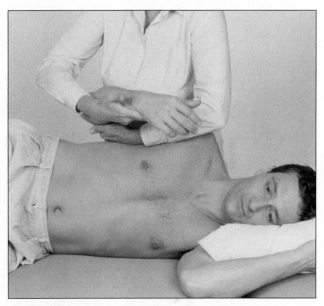

Figure 4-60 Alternate start position.

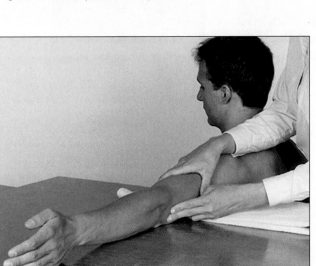

Figure 4-61 End position: triceps.

Alternate Against Gravity Assessment: Triceps

This test is indicated if the patient has shoulder muscle weakness.

The patient is prone. A towel is placed under the humerus for patient comfort during application of stabilization and resistance. The shoulder is abducted, and the elbow is flexed with the forearm and hand hanging vertically over the edge of the plinth (Fig. 4-62). The patient extends the elbow through the full ROM, avoiding the close-packed position (Fig. 4-63). Resistance is applied proximal to the wrist joint on the posterior aspect of the forearm (Fig. 4-64).

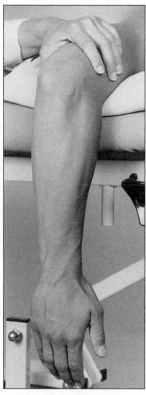

Figure 4-62 Start position: triceps.

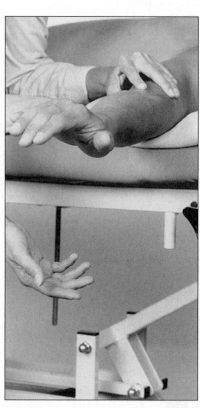

Figure 4-63 Screen position: triceps.

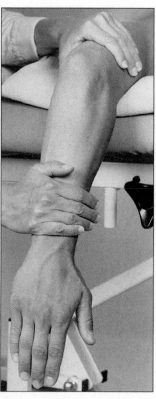

Figure 4-64 Resistance: triceps.

Supination

Against Gravity: Supinator and Biceps Brachii

Start Position. The patient is sitting. The arm is at the side, the elbow is flexed to 90°, and the forearm is pronated (Fig. 4-65).

Form 4-10

Stabilization. The therapist stabilizes the humerus.

Movement. The patient supinates the forearm through full ROM (Fig. 4-66). Because gravity assists supination beyond midposition, slight resistance, equal to the weight of the forearm, may be applied by the therapist.

Palpation. *Biceps brachii:* anterior aspect of the antecubital fossa. *Supinator:* posterior aspect of the forearm, distal to the head of the radius.

Substitute Movement. Shoulder external rotation, shoulder adduction, and ipsilateral trunk side flexion.

Resistance Location. Applied on the posterior surface of the distal end of the radius with counterpressure on the anterior aspect of the ulna (Figs. 4-67 and 4-68).

Resistance Direction. Forearm pronation.

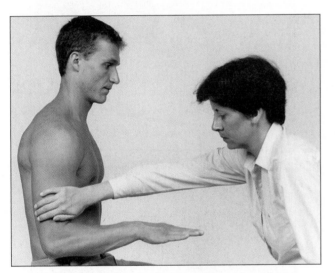

Figure 4-65 Start position: supinator and biceps brachii.

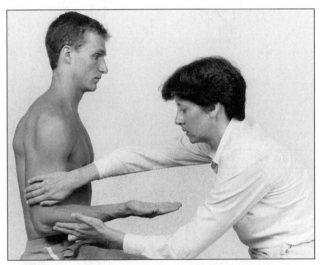

Figure 4-66 Screen position: supinator and biceps brachii.

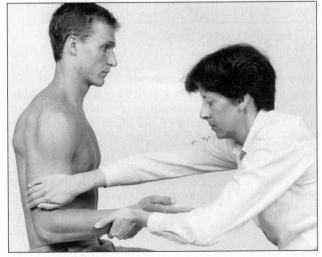

Figure 4-67 Resistance: supinator and biceps brachii.

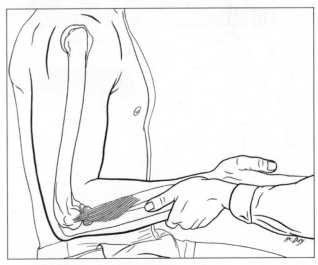

Figure 4-68 Supinator.

Gravity Eliminated: Supinator and Biceps Brachii

Start Position. The patient is supine with the arm at the side, the elbow flexed to 90°, and the forearm pronated (Fig. 4-69).

Alternate Start Position (not shown). The patient is sitting, the shoulder and the elbow are flexed to 90°, and the forearm is pronated.

Stabilization. The therapist stabilizes the humerus.

End Position. The patient supinates the forearm through full ROM (Fig. 4-70).

Substitute Movement. Shoulder adduction and external rotation.

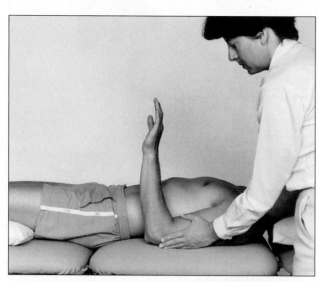

Figure 4-69 Start position: supinator and biceps brachii.

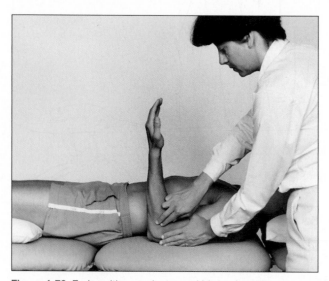

Figure 4-70 End position: supinator and biceps brachii.

Isolation of Supinator

The biceps brachii does not supinate the forearm when the elbow is in extension and the movement is performed slowly and without resistance.[3,23]

Start Position. The patient is sitting, the arm is at the side, the elbow extended, and the forearm is pronated.

Stabilization. The therapist stabilizes the humerus.

Movement. The patient supinates the forearm through full ROM. The therapist palpates supinator during the movement (Fig. 4-71).

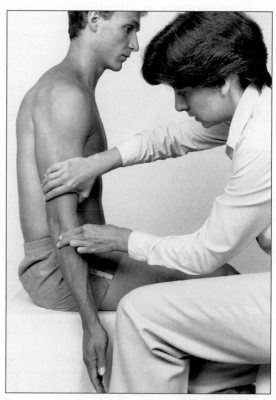

Figure 4-71 Clinical test for isolation of supinator.

Alternate Start Position (not shown). Using this test position, the biceps brachii is placed in a maximally shortened position, that is, a position of active insufficiency. In this position, the biceps is put on slack and no longer has the ability to develop effective tension, thus isolating supinator.

Start Position. The patient is supine, the shoulder is flexed 90°, the elbow is fully flexed, and the forearm pronated.

Stabilization. The therapist stabilizes the humerus.

Movement. The patient slowly supinates the forearm. The therapist palpates supinator during the movement.

In the presence of supinator muscle weakness, the patient will be unable to maintain the forearm in the fully supinated position using biceps alone.[24]

Pronation

Against Gravity: Pronator Teres and Pronator Quadratus

 Start Position. The patient is sitting. The arm is at the side, the elbow is flexed to 90°, and the forearm is supinated (Fig. 4-72).

Form 4-11 **Stabilization.** The therapist stabilizes the humerus.

Movement. The patient pronates the forearm through full ROM (Fig. 4-73). Because gravity assists pronation beyond midposition, slight resistance, equal to the weight of the forearm, may be applied by the therapist.

Palpation. *Pronator teres:* proximal one-third of the anterior surface of the forearm on a diagonal line from the medial epicondyle of the humerus to the middle of the lateral border of the radius. *Pronator quadratus:* too deep to palpate.

Substitute Movement. Shoulder abduction and internal rotation, and contralateral trunk side flexion.

Resistance Location. Applied on the anterior surface of the distal end of the radius with counterpressure on the posterior aspect of the ulna (Figs. 4-74, 4-75, and 4-76).

Resistance Direction. Forearm supination.

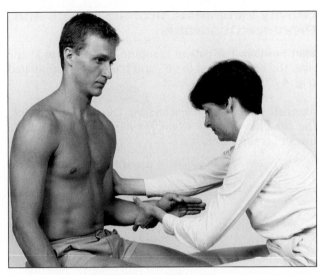

Figure 4-74 Resistance: pronator teres and pronator quadratus.

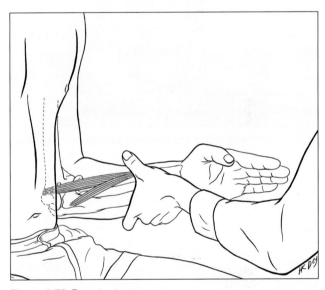

Figure 4-75 Pronator teres.

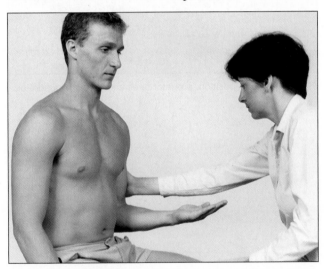

Figure 4-72 Start position: pronator teres and pronator quadratus.

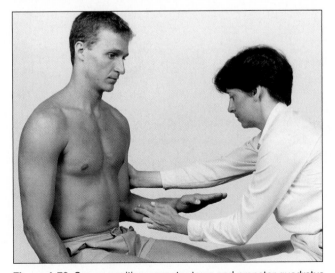

Figure 4-73 Screen position: pronator teres and pronator quadratus.

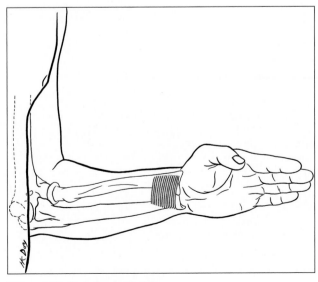

Figure 4-76 Pronator quadratus.

Gravity Eliminated: Pronator Teres and Pronator Quadratus

Start Position. The patient is supine with the arm at the side, the elbow flexed to 90°, and the forearm supinated (Fig. 4-77).

Alternate Start Position (not shown). The patient is sitting, the shoulder and the elbow are flexed to 90°, and the forearm is supinated.

Stabilization. The therapist stabilizes the humerus.

End Position. The patient pronates the forearm through full ROM (Fig. 4-78).

Substitute Movement. Shoulder abduction and internal rotation.

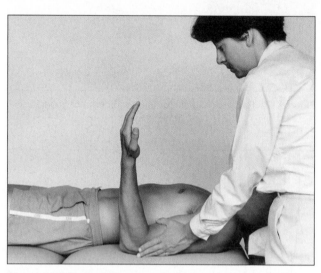

Figure 4-77 Start position: pronator teres and pronator quadratus.

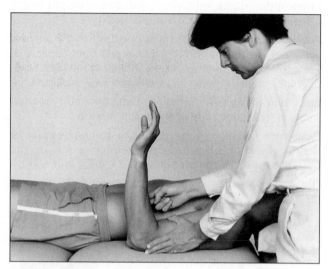

Figure 4-78 End position: pronator teres and pronator quadratus.

FUNCTIONAL APPLICATION

Joint Function

The function of the elbow complex is to serve the hand.[3,6,25] Movement at the elbow joint adjusts the overall functional length of the arm.[16] Elbow extension moves the hand away from the body; elbow flexion moves the hand toward the body. Hand orientation in space and hand mobility are enhanced through supination and pronation of the forearm. The elbow complex, including the forearm, contributes to many skilled and forceful hand movements involved in daily self-care, leisure, and work functions. The elbow complex also provides the power necessary to perform lifting activities[26] and activities involving raising and lowering of the body using the hands.[25]

The elbow and the forearm do not function in isolation, but link with the shoulder and wrist to enhance hand function.[3] When the elbow is extended, supination and pronation are functionally linked with shoulder external and internal rotations, respectively.[25] These linked movements occur simultaneously during activity. However, when the elbow is flexed, forearm rotation can be isolated from shoulder rotation.[25] This is illustrated in activities such as turning a door handle or using a screwdriver (Fig. 4-79).

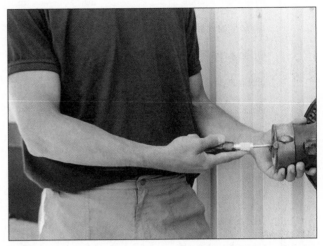

Figure 4-79 Elbow flexion isolates forearm rotation from shoulder rotation.

TABLE 4-3 Elbow and Forearm Range of Motion (ROM) Required for Selected Activities of Daily Living (ADL)[26-28,29,30,31]*

Activity	Flexion ROM (°)		Supination ROM (°)		Pronation ROM (°)	
	Min	Max	Start	End	Start	End
Read a newspaper[26]	78	104	—	—	7	49
Rise from a chair[26]	20	95	—	—	10	34
Sit to stand to sit[28]	15	100	—	—	—	—
Open a door[26]	24	57	—	23	35	—
Open a door[31]	—	—	—	77	—	—
Pour from a pitcher[26]	36	58	22	—	—	43
Pour water into a glass[30]	38	50	20	—	—	55
Drink from a cup[27]	72	129	3	31	—	—
Drink from a glass[30]	42	132	1	23	—	—
Use a telephone[26]	43	136	23	—	—	41
Use a telephone[28]	75	140	—	—	—	—
Use a telephone[30]	69	143	21	—	—	42
Use a telephone[31]	—	146	—	—	—	—
Use a cellular phone[31]	—	147	—	—	—	—
Type on a computer keyboard[31]	—	—	—	—	—	65
Cut with a knife[26]	89	107	—	—	27	42
Put fork to mouth[26]	85	128	—	52	10	—
Eat with a fork[27]	94	122	—	59	38	—
Eat with a spoon[27]	101	123	—	59	23	—
Eat with a spoon[28]	70	115	—	—	—	—
Eat with a spoon[30]	74	133	—	50	9	—
Comb the hair[29]	112	157	—	—	—	—
Wash axilla[29]	104	132	—	—	—	—
Perineal care[29]	35	100	—	—	—	—

*Mean values from original sources[26,27,30] rounded to the nearest degree. Median values from original source.[28] Minimal and maximal values from the original source[29,31] rounded to the nearest degree.

TABLE 4-4 Elbow and Forearm Positions* of Healthy Subjects Measured During Personal Care and Hygiene Activities[26]

Hand to:	Elbow Flexion (°)	Supination (°)	Pronation (°)
Head—vertex	119	47	—
Head—occiput	144	2	—
Waist	100	12	—
Chest	120	29	—
Neck	135	41	—
Sacrum	70	56	—
Shoe	16	—	19

*Mean values from original source[26] rounded to the nearest degree.

Functional Range of Motion

The normal AROM[12] at the elbow is from 0° of extension to 150° of flexion, 80° to 90° of forearm pronation, and 80° to 90° of forearm supination. However, many daily functions are performed with less than these ranges. The ROM required at the elbow and the forearm for selected ADL is shown in Table 4-3, as compiled from the works of Morrey,[26] Safaee-Rad,[27] Packer,[28] Magermans,[29] Raiss,[30] Sardelli,[31] and their colleagues. Positions of the elbow and the forearm required to touch different body parts for personal care and hygiene activities are shown in Table 4-4, as based on the work of Morrey and colleagues.[26] The ROM requirements for ADL are influenced by the design of furniture, the placement of utensils, and the patient's posture. In part, these factors could account for the difference in ROM findings between studies for similar ADL shown in Tables 4-3 and 4-4. Thus, the ROM values in Tables 4-3 and 4-4 should be used as a guide for ADL requirements.

Many self-care activities can be accomplished within the arc of movement from 30° to 130° of flexion and from 50° of pronation to 50° of supination.[26] Writing, pouring from a pitcher, reading a newspaper, and performing perineal hygiene are examples of activities performed within these ranges of motion. Feeding activities such as drinking from a cup, using a spoon or a fork, and cutting with a knife (Fig. 4-80) may be performed within an arc of movement from about 45° to 136° of flexion and from about 47° of pronation to 59° of supination.[26,28,32]

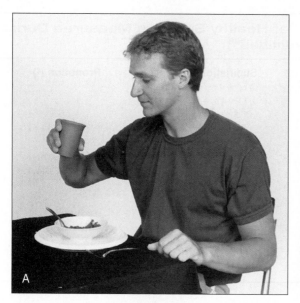

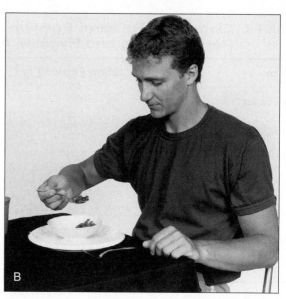

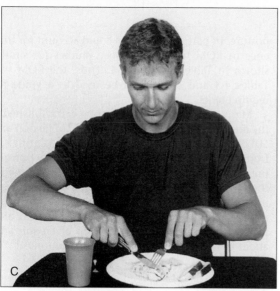

Figure 4-80 Elbow range within the arc of movement from about 45° to 136° of flexion and from about 47° of pronation to 59° of supination. **A.** Drinking from a cup. **B.** Eating using a spoon. **C.** Eating using a knife and a fork.

Daily functions that may involve extreme ranges of elbow motion include combing or washing the hair (flexion, pronation, and supination) (Fig. 4-81), reaching a back zipper at the neck level (flexion, pronation), using a standard or cellular telephone (approximately 135° to 145° flexion[26,28,30,31]) (Fig. 4-82), tying a shoe (16° flexion[26]) (Fig. 4-83), donning a pair of trousers (extension) (Fig. 4-84), throwing a ball (extension), walking with axillary crutches (extension), using the arms to elevate the body when getting up from a chair (15° flexion[28]), playing tennis (extension), and using a computer mouse or keyboard (65° pronation[31]) (Fig. 4-85).

Less elbow ROM is required to perform most upper extremity activities when elbow flexion and extension ROM is restricted and compensatory motions are allowed at normal adjacent joints. In this case, functional elbow ROM is from 75° to 120° flexion.[33] These compensatory motions occur at the thoracic and lumbar spines, shoulder (primarily scapulothoracic and clavicular joints), and wrist.[34] With the elbow in a fixed position of 90° flexion, although there are limitations in function, in most cases all personal care ADL (i.e., feeding and personal hygiene) can be performed.[33,35] This is supported by the findings of van Andel and colleagues[36] that a minimum of 85° elbow

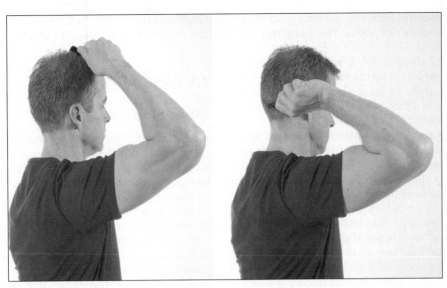

Figure 4-81 Combing hair requires elbow flexion and forearm supination and pronation.

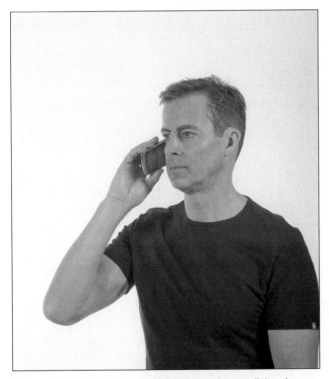

Figure 4-82 Elbow flexion required when using a cellular phone.

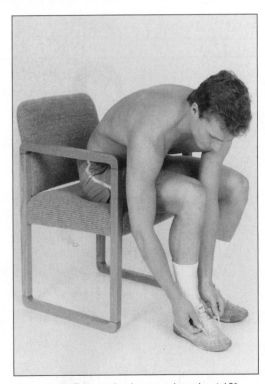

Figure 4-83 Tying a shoelace requires about 16° elbow flexion.

flexion is required to comb hair, reach a back pocket or the contralateral shoulder, or bring the hand to the mouth to drink.

With restriction of elbow ROM, loss of elbow flexion has a greater impact on loss of function than loss of elbow extension in a ratio of about 2:1.[37] Thus, the functional impact of a 5° loss of elbow flexion is approximately equivalent to a 10° loss of elbow extension ROM.

In the presence of restricted forearm ROM, Kasten and associates[38] identified the main compensatory motions at the shoulder and elbow to be shoulder internal/external rotation, followed by shoulder abduction/adduction and elbow flexion/extension, and to a lesser extent shoulder flexion/extension. Compensatory motion also occurs at the wrist joint in the presence of restricted forearm ROM.[39] Kasten and associates[38] concluded that with the forearm fixed in nearly neutral rotation, all of the following ADL tasks, that is, pouring water in a glass, drinking from a glass, eating with a spoon, answering the phone, drawing a large number "8" on a desk, using a keyboard, turning a page, turning a key in a keyhole, combing the hair, and cleaning genitals and buttocks, could be completed with the contribution of shoulder and elbow movements.

Muscle Function

Elbow Flexion

Biceps brachii, brachialis, and brachioradialis are the primary flexors of the elbow. The role of the flexors in functional activities is partially determined by the position of the elbow, forearm and adjacent joints, the magnitude of the resistance load, and the speed of movement.[3] Of clinical and functional significance is the electromyographic data that indicate a fine interplay between the action of the flexors during activity and a wide range of muscle response between individuals.[23] The movement combinations required for a specific task are an important consideration in specifying the contribution of each muscle to function and in analyzing movement compensation due to paralysis.

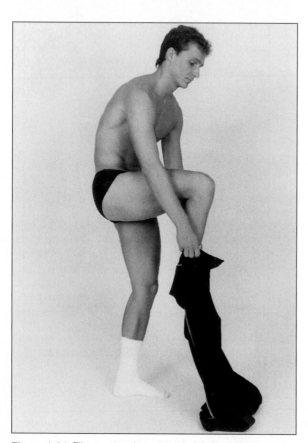

Figure 4-84 Elbow extension when donning a pair of trousers.

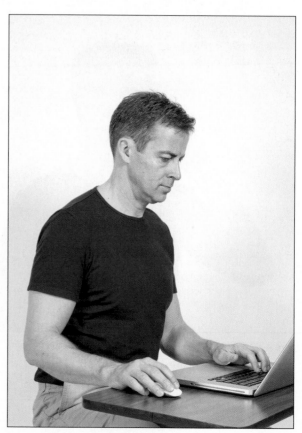

Figure 4-85 Forearm pronation is required when using a computer mouse or keyboard.

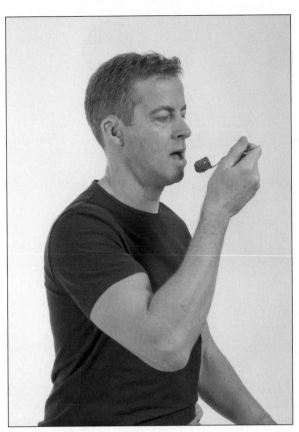

Figure 4-86 Biceps brachii functions to bring food to the mouth.

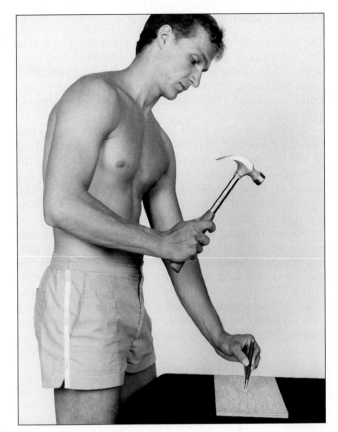

Figure 4-87 Brachialis and brachioradialis function.

Biceps Brachii

The biceps brachii acts as an elbow flexor and forearm supinator. This action is well illustrated in activities involving both movements, such as using a corkscrew, feeding utensil (Fig. 4-86), or screwdriver (see Fig. 4-79). Biceps functions most efficiently at 90° of elbow flexion.[6,22] The muscle does not contribute to supination when the elbow is extended, unless supination is strongly resisted, and does not function as an elbow flexor when the forearm is pronated.[23] Thus, the weakest elbow flexion strength is associated with forearm pronation.[40] The greatest elbow flexion strength occurs with the forearm in midposition.[22,40] Because the biceps brachii acts on three joints (i.e., the shoulder, elbow, and radioulnar), its efficiency is affected by the position of the shoulder.[22,25] The biceps brachii is more efficient when the shoulder is extended than when flexed. This efficiency can be illustrated in pulling activities that require shoulder extension and elbow flexion, such as rowing, playing tug-of-war games, pulling the beater of a loom, and sweeping the floor.

Brachialis

The brachialis has been labeled the servile muscle among the elbow flexors,[41] because it is active in all positions of the forearm, with and without resistance.[23] Because the attachments of the brachialis are at the proximal end of the ulna, and the distal end of the humerus, this muscle is unaffected by changes in the position of the forearm resulting from rotation of the radius and the position of the shoulder.[3] Although all flexors are recruited for a task such as hammering (Fig. 4-87), the brachialis is the ideal selection because its sole function is elbow flexion.

Brachioradialis

This elbow flexor functions as a reserve flexor muscle, contributing to elbow flexion when speed of movement and force are required in the semipronated or pronated forearm position.[23] Its action can be illustrated in activities such as drinking from a cup, hammering (see Fig. 4-87), typing, or playing a keyboard instrument.

Elbow Extension: Triceps

The triceps is the extensor muscle at the elbow. The role of the anconeus is controversial. The anconeus has been described as a muscle that is active in slow movements,[23] has a stabilizing function during supination and pronation,[23] assists in elbow extension,[3] and has negligible action in extension.[41]

Because the long head of triceps crosses two joints, the effectiveness of this muscle is affected by the position of the shoulder. The long head becomes stretched with the elbow and shoulder joints in flexion. Therefore, the triceps is more effective in elbow extension when the shoulder is flexed.[25] This is illustrated in activities such as pushing a broom or vacuum cleaner or sawing wood.

The medial head of triceps can be identified as the servile portion of the muscle because it is always active during elbow extension. The lateral and long heads are recruited when force is required.[23] The function of the triceps is illustrated in activities that involve elevation of the body, such as getting up from a chair (Fig. 4-88), walking with axillary crutches, performing push-ups, or other pushing activities such as pushing a door closed.

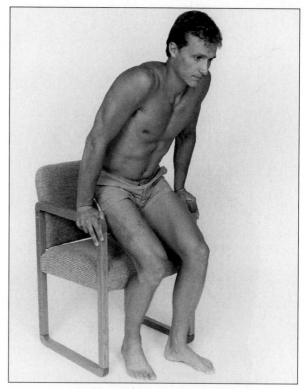

Figure 4-88 Triceps functions to elevate the body when getting up from a chair.

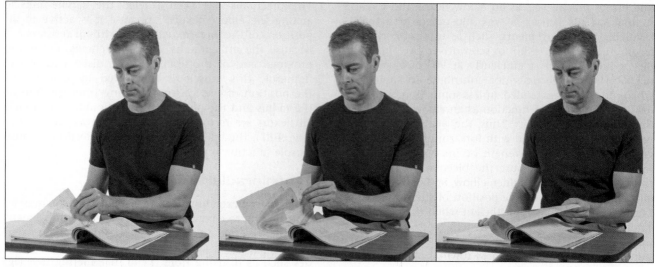

Figure 4-89 Supinator and biceps brachii function to supinate the forearm.

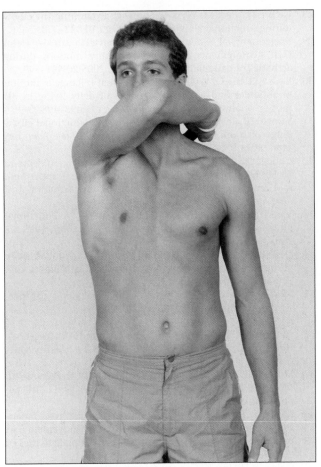

Figure 4-90 Pronator teres and pronator quadratus function.

Forearm Supination: Supinator and Biceps Brachii

The supinator, acting alone, produces supination in all positions of the elbow.[23,41] The biceps is recruited in elbow flexion when force and speed are demanded. The supination function of biceps is affected by elbow position and the muscle is most effective as a supinator with the elbow flexed at about 90°.[42] Most daily activities demand varying amounts of force and the combined movements of elbow flexion and forearm supination, for example, bringing food to the mouth and turning a page (Fig. 4-89). This combination functions to maintain or move the hand closer to the body and to rotate the hand so that the palm faces the ceiling. Brachioradialis also functions as a supinator through only a part of the ROM

to bring the forearm from a pronated position to midposition.[42]

The supinators and external rotators of the shoulder are functionally linked when the elbow is extended,[25] because supination and shoulder external rotation occur simultaneously during activity. Supination strength is greater when performed with the shoulder in external than internal rotation, possibly due to the position of the long head of biceps increasing the length of the muscle in external rotation and thus contributing greater force output.[43]

Forearm Pronation: Pronator Teres and Pronator Quadratus

The pronator teres and pronator quadratus muscles are active in pronation of the forearm. The pronator quadratus has been described as the most consistent muscle of the two, with the pronator teres being recruited for activities demanding fast or powerful movement,[23,41] such as using a screwdriver to remove a tight screw, pitching a ball, or playing racket sports. The pronators are recruited for many self-maintenance activities, including writing, washing one's body (Fig. 4-90), dressing, and hygiene tasks. Brachioradialis also functions as a pronator through only a part of the ROM to bring the forearm from a supinated position to midposition.[42] The pronators are functionally linked to the internal rotators of the shoulder,[25] because pronation and internal rotation of the shoulder occur simultaneously in many activities.

References

1. Standring S, ed. *Gray's Anatomy: The Anatomical Basis of Clinical Practice.* 39th ed. London: Elsevier Churchill Livingstone; 2005.
2. London JT. Kinematics of the elbow. *J Bone Joint Surg [Am].* 1981;63(4):529–535.
3. Levangie PK, Norkin CC. *Joint Structure and Function: A Comprehensive Analysis.* 4th ed. Philadelphia: FA Davis; 2005.
4. Steindler A. *Kinesiology of the Human Body Under Normal and Pathological Conditions.* Springfield: Charles C Thomas; 1955.
5. Nakamura T, Yabe Y, Horiuchi Y, Yamazaki N. In vivo motion analysis of forearm rotation utilizing magnetic resonance imaging. *Clin Biomech.* 1999;14:315–320.
6. Kapandji IA. *The Physiology of the Joints. Vol. 1. The Upper Limb.* 6th ed. New York: Churchill Livingstone Elsevier; 2007.
7. Norkin CC, White DJ. *Measurement of Joint Motion: A Guide to Goniometry.* 4th ed. Philadelphia: FA Davis; 2009.
8. Nordin M, Frankel VH. *Basic Biomechanics of the Musculoskeletal System.* 3rd ed. Philadelphia: Lippincott Williams & Wilkins; 2001.

9. Gabl M, Zimmermann R, Angermann P, et al. The interosseous membrane and its influence on the distal radioulnar joint. An anatomical investigation of the distal tract. *J Hand Surg [Br]*. 1998;23(2):179–182.

10. Cyriax J. *Textbook of Orthopaedic Medicine. Vol 1. Diagnosis of Soft Tissue Lesions*. 8th ed. London: Bailliere Tindall; 1982.

11. Magee DJ. *Orthopaedic Physical Assessment*. 5th ed. Philadelphia: Saunders Elsevier; 2008.

12. American Academy of Orthopaedic Surgeons. *Joint Motion: Method of Measuring and Recording*. Chicago: AAOS; 1965.

13. Berryman Reese N, Bandy WD. *Joint Range of Motion and Muscle Length Testing*. 2nd ed. Philadelphia: Saunders Elsevier; 2010.

14. Hoppenfeld S. *Physical Examination of the Spine and Extremities*. New York: Appleton-Century-Crofts; 1976.

15. Kaltenborn FM. *Mobilization of the Extremity Joints*. 3rd ed. Oslo: Olaf Norlis Bokhandel; 1985.

16. Neumann DA. *Kinesiology of the Musculoskeletal System: Foundations for Physical Rehabilitation*. 2nd ed. Philadelphia: Mosby Elsevier; 2010.

17. Baeyens J-P, Van Glabbeek F, Goossens M, Gielen J, Van Roy P, Clarys J-P. In vivo 3D arthrokinematics of the proximal and distal radioulnar joints during active pronation and supination. *Clin Biomech*. 2006;21:S9–S12.

18. Karagiannopoulos C, Sitler M, Michlovitz S. Reliability of 2 functional goniometric methods for measuring forearm pronation and supination active range of motion. *J Orthop Sports Phys Ther*. 2003;33(9):523–531.

19. Shaaban H, Pereira C, Williams R, Lees VC. The effect of elbow position on the range of supination and pronation of the forearm. *J Hand Surg Eur Vol*. 2008;33(1):3–8.

20. Gajdosik RL. Comparison and reliability of three goniometric methods for measuring forearm supination and pronation. *Percept Mot Skills*. 2001;93:353–355.

21. Soames RW, ed. Skeletal system. Salmons S, ed. Muscle. *Gray's Anatomy*. 38th ed. New York: Churchill Livingstone; 1995.

22. Soderberg GL. *Kinesiology: Application to Pathological Motion*. 2nd ed. Baltimore: Williams & Wilkins; 1997.

23. Basmajian JV, DeLuca CJ. *Muscles Alive: Their Function Revealed by Electromyography*. 5th ed. Baltimore: Williams & Wilkins; 1985.

24. Kendall FP, McCreary EK, Provance PG. *Muscles Testing and Function*. 4th ed. Baltimore: Williams & Wilkins; 1993.

25. Smith LK, Lawrence Weiss EL, Lehmkuhl LD. *Brunnstrom's Clinical Kinesiology*. 5th ed. Philadelphia: FA Davis; 1996.

26. Morrey BF, Askew LJ, An KN, Chao EY. A biomechanical study of normal functional elbow motion. *J Bone Joint Surg [Am]*. 1981;63:872–876.

27. Safaee-Rad R, Shwedyk E, Quanbury AO, Cooper JE. Normal functional range of motion of upper limb joints during performance of three feeding activities. *Arch Phys Med Rehabil*. 1990;71:505–509.

28. Packer TL, Peat M, Wyss U, Sorbie C. Examining the elbow during functional activities. *OTJR*. 1990;10:323–333.

29. Magermans DJ, Chadwick EKJ, Veeger HEJ, van der Helm FCT. Requirements for upper extremity motions during activities of daily living. *Clin Biomech*. 2005;20:591–599.

30. Raiss P, Rettig O, Wolf S, Loew M, Kasten P. Range of motion of shoulder and elbow in activities of daily living in 3D motion analysis. *Z Orthop Unfall*. 2007;145:493–498.

31. Sardelli M, Tashjian RZ, MacWilliams BA. Functional elbow range of motion for contemporary tasks. *J Bone Joint Surg [Am]*. 2011;93:471–477.

32. Cooper JE, Shwedyk E, Quanbury AO, Miller J, Hildebrand D. Elbow joint restriction: effect on functional upper limb motion during performance of three feeding activities. *Arch Phys Med Rehabil*. 1993;74:805–809.

33. Vasen AP, Lacey SH, Keith MW, Shaffer JW. Functional range of motion of the elbow. *J Hand Surg [Am]*. 1995;20:288–292.

34. O'Neill OR, Morrey BF, Tanaka S, An KN. Compensatory motion in the upper extremity after elbow arthrodesis. *Clin Orthop Relat Res*. 1992;281:89–96.

35. Nagy SM, Szabo RM, Sharkey NA. Unilateral elbow arthrodesis: the preferred position. *J Southern Orthop Assoc*. 1999;8(2):80–85.

36. van Andel CJ, Wolterbeek N, Doorenbosch CAM, Veeger D, Harlaar J. Complete 3D kinematics of upper extremity functional tasks. *Gait Posture*. 2008;27:120–127.

37. Morrey BF, An KN. Functional evaluation of the elbow. In: Morrey BF, ed. *The Elbow and Its Disorders*. 3rd ed. Philadelphia: WB Saunders; 2000.

38. Kasten P, Rettig O, Loew M, Wolf S, Raiss P. Three dimensional motion analysis of compensatory movements in patients with radioulnar synostosis performing activities of daily living. *J Orthop Sci*. 2009;14:307–312.

39. Ogino T, Hikino K. Congenital radio-ulnar synostosis: compensatory rotation around the wrist and rotation osteotomy. *J Hand Surg [Br]*. 1987;12(2):173–178.

40. Morrey BF, An KN, Chao EYS. Functional evaluation of the elbow. In: Morrey BF, ed. *The Elbow and Its Disorders*. 2nd ed. Toronto: WB Saunders; 1993.

41. Rosse C. The arm, forearm, and wrist. In: Rosse C, Clawson DK, eds. *The Musculoskeletal System in Health and Disease*. New York: Harper & Row; 1980.

42. Bremer AK, Sennwald GR, Favre P, Jacob HAC. Moment arms of forearm rotators. *Clin Biomech*. 2006;21:683–691.

43. Savva N, McAllen CJP, Giddins GEB. The relationship between the strength of supination of the forearm and rotation of the shoulder. *J Bone Joint Surg [Br]*. 2003;85:406–407.

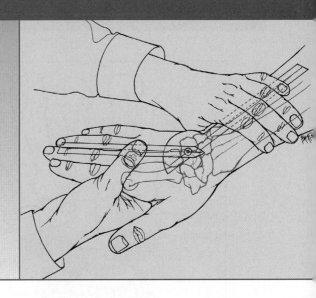

Chapter 5

Wrist and Hand

ARTICULATIONS AND MOVEMENTS

The articulations of the wrist and hand are illustrated in Figures 5-1 and 5-2. The movements of the wrist and hand are summarized in Tables 5-1, 5-2, and 5-3.

Located between the forearm and hand, the *wrist* is made up of eight small bones (Figs. 5-1 and 5-2A). These bones are arranged in a proximal row (the scaphoid, lunate, triquetrum, and pisiform) and a distal row (the trapezium, trapezoid, capitate, and hamate).

The proximal surface of the proximal row of carpal bones (excluding the pisiform, which articulates solely with the triquetrum) is convex (Fig. 5-2B). This convex surface articulates with the concave surface of the distal aspect of the radius and the articular disc of the inferior radioulnar joint to form the ellipsoidal, *radiocarpal joint.*[2]

The *midcarpal joint* is a compound articulation[2] formed between the proximal and distal rows of carpal bones. The proximal aspect of the distal row of carpal bones has a concave surface laterally, formed by the trapezium and trapezoid bones, and a convex surface medially, formed by the capitate and hamate (Fig. 5-2B). These surfaces articulate with the corresponding distal aspect of the proximal row of carpal bones that has a convex surface laterally, formed by the scaphoid bone, and a concave surface medially, formed by the scaphoid, lunate, and triquetrum.

In the clinical setting, it is not possible to independently measure the motion at the radiocarpal and midcarpal joints. Thus, wrist range of motion (ROM) measurements include the combined motion of both joints. Movement at the radiocarpal and midcarpal joints include wrist flexion, extension, radial deviation, and ulnar deviation. From the anatomical position, wrist flexion and extension occur in the sagittal plane around a frontal axis (Fig. 5-3). Wrist radial deviation and ulnar

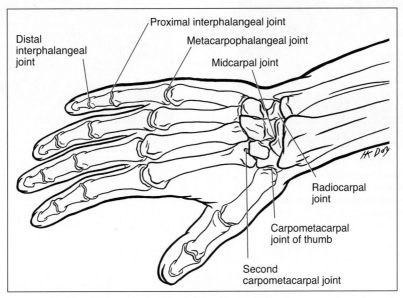

Figure 5-1 Wrist, finger, and thumb articulations.

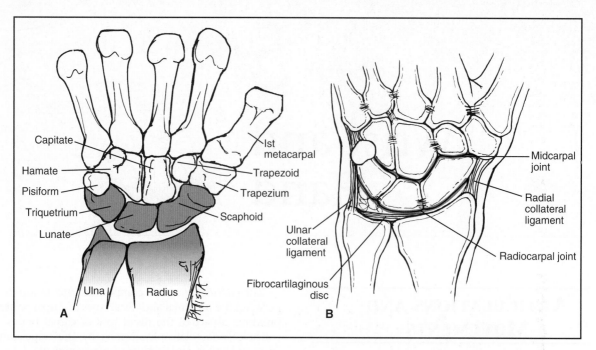

Figure 5-2 Anterior view of the wrist showing the **(A)** bony anatomy and **(B)** the concave-convex contours of the midcarpal and radiocarpal joints.

deviation occur in the frontal plane about a sagittal axis (Fig. 5-4). Maximal wrist flexion and extension active range of motion (AROM) occur with the wrist positioned near 0° radial and ulnar deviation and vice versa.[10]

Movement at the *carpometacarpal (CM) joints* (Fig. 5-1), formed between the distal surfaces of the distal row of carpal bones and the bases of the metacarpal bones, is essential for normal hand function. CM joint movement contributes to the flattening of the palm when the hand is opened fully (Fig. 5-5A), and the guttering of the palm when gripping or manipulating objects (Fig. 5-5B). The mobile peripheral metacarpals of the ring and little fingers and the thumb move around the fixed metacarpals of the index and middle fingers. The mobility of the thumb, fourth, and fifth metacarpals around the fixed metacarpals of the index and middle fingers is observed as the open hand is made into a relaxed fist and then into a clenched fist (Fig. 5-6). In the clinical setting, it is not

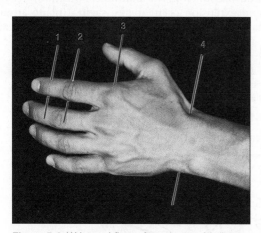

Figure 5-3 Wrist and finger frontal axes: *(1)* distal interphalangeal flexion–extension, *(2)* proximal interphalangeal flexion–extension, *(3)* metacarpophalangeal flexion–extension, and *(4)* wrist flexion–extension.

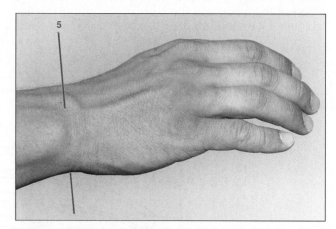

Figure 5-4 Wrist sagittal axis: *(5)* ulnar-radial deviation.

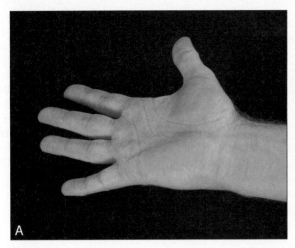
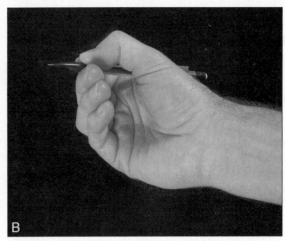

Figure 5-5 **A.** Flattening of the palm when hand is opened. **B.** Guttering of the palm when gripping or manipulating an object.

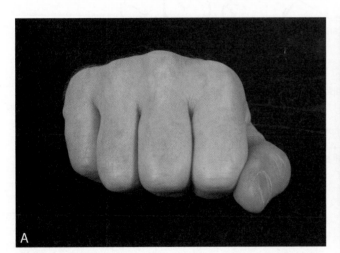
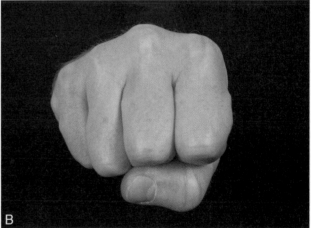

Figure 5-6 Mobility at the fourth and fifth carpometacarpal joints is observed when **(A)** the relaxed fist is compared to **(B)** the clenched fist.

possible to directly measure movements at the CM joints of the second through fifth metacarpals, but it is possible to measure movement at the CM joint of the thumb.

The *CM joint of the thumb* (Fig. 5-7) is a saddle joint formed between the distal surface of the trapezium, which is concave anteroposteriorly and convex mediolaterally, and the corresponding reciprocal surface of the base of the first metacarpal. The movements at the first CM joint include flexion, extension, abduction, adduction, rotation, and opposition. Flexion and extension occur in an oblique frontal plane about an oblique sagittal axis (Fig. 5-8). During flexion, the thumb is moved from anatomical position (Fig. 5-9A) across the palmar surface of the hand (Fig. 5-9B). Thumb extension (Fig.

5-9C) at the CM joint involves movement of the thumb laterally away from the anatomical position in the opposite direction to flexion. The thumb is abducted when moved from the anatomical position (Fig. 5-9D) in a direction perpendicular to the palm of the hand (Fig. 5-9E). Adduction of the thumb returns the thumb to the anatomical position from the abducted position. Abduction and adduction of the thumb occur in an oblique sagittal plane around an oblique frontal axis. Opposition (Fig. 5-9F) is a sequential movement incorporating abduction, flexion, and adduction of the first metacarpal, with simultaneous rotation.[11]

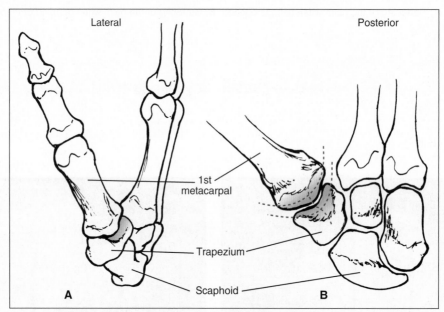

Figure 5-7 **(A)** Right thumb carpometacarpal joint with **(B)** articular surfaces exposed to show concave–convex contours.

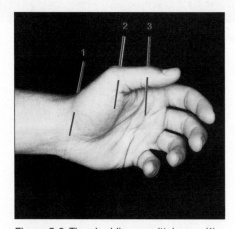

Figure 5-8 Thumb oblique sagittal axes: *(1)* carpometacarpal flexion–extension, *(2)* metacarpophalangeal flexion–extension, and *(3)* interphalangeal flexion–extension.

The *metacarpophalangeal (MCP) joints* of the hand are classified as ellipsoid joints,[2] each formed proximally by the convex head of the metatarsal articulating with the concave base of the adjacent proximal phalanx (Fig. 5-1). The movements at the MCP articulations include flexion, extension, abduction, adduction, and rotation. The movements that are measured in the clinical setting are flexion and extension, which occur in the sagittal plane around a frontal axis (see Fig. 5-3), and abduction and adduction, which occur in the frontal plane around a sagittal axis. It is not possible to measure rotation at the MCP joints in the clinical setting.

The *interphalangeal (IP) joints* of the thumb and fingers (see Fig. 5-1) are classified as hinge joints, formed by the convex head of the proximal phalanx articulating with the concave base of the adjacent distal phalanx. The IP joints allow flexion and extension movements of the fingers that occur in the sagittal plane around a frontal axis (Fig. 5-3) and the thumb that occur in the oblique frontal plane about an oblique sagittal axis (Fig. 5-8).

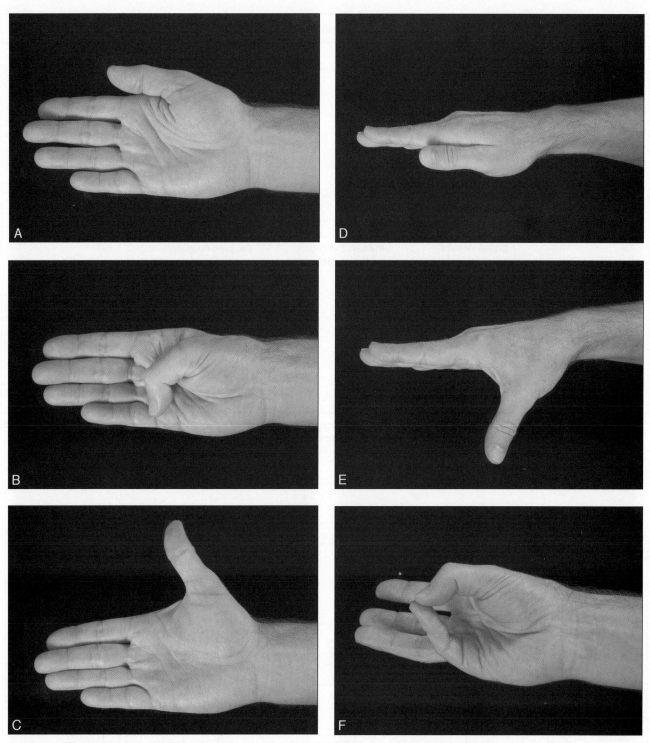

Figure 5-9 (A) Anterior view—thumb in anatomical position. Thumb **(B)** flexion and **(C)** extension. **(D)** Lateral view—thumb in anatomical position. Thumb **(E)** abduction, and **(F)** opposition.

TABLE 5-1   Joint Structure: Wrist Movements

	Flexion	Extension	Radial Deviation	Ulnar Deviation
Articulation[1,2]	Radiocarpal Midcarpal	Midcarpal Radiocarpal	Midcarpal Radiocarpal	Radiocarpal (predominant) Midcarpal
Plane	Sagittal	Sagittal	Frontal	Frontal
Axis	Frontal	Frontal	Sagittal	Sagittal
Normal limiting factors[1,3,4]* (see Fig. 5-10A and B)	Tension in the posterior radiocarpal ligament and posterior joint capsule	Tension in the anterior radiocarpal ligament and anterior joint capsule; contact between the radius and the carpal bones	Tension in the ulnar collateral ligament, ulnocarpal ligament, and ulnar portion of the joint capsule; contact between the radial styloid process and the scaphoid bone	Tension in the radial collateral ligament and radial portion of the joint capsule
Normal end feel[3,5]	Firm	Firm/hard	Firm/hard	Firm
Normal AROM[6] (AROM[7])	0–80° (0–80°)	0–70° (0–70°)	0–20° (0–20°)	0–30° (0–30°)
Capsular pattern[5,8]	Flexion and extension are equally restricted			

*There is a paucity of definitive research that identifies the normal limiting factors (NLF) of joint motion. The NLF and end feels listed here are based on knowledge of anatomy, clinical experience, and available references.

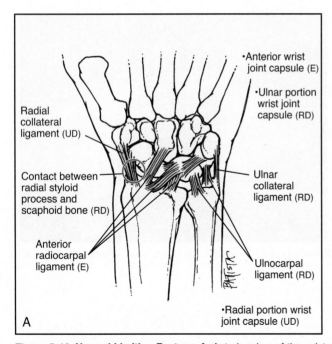

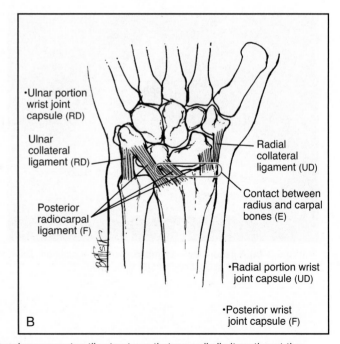

Figure 5-10 **Normal Limiting Factors. A.** Anterior view of the wrist showing noncontractile structures that normally limit motion at the wrist. **B.** Posterior view of the wrist showing noncontractile structures that normally limit motion at the wrist. Motion limited by structures is identified in brackets, using the following abbreviations: *F*, flexion; *E*, extension; *UD*, ulnar deviation; *RD*, radial deviation. Muscles normally limiting motion are not illustrated.

TABLE 5-2 Joint Structure: Finger Movements

	Flexion	Extension	Abduction	Adduction
Articulation[1,2]	Metacarpophalangeal (MCP) Proximal interphalangeal (PIP) Distal interphalangeal (DIP)	MCP PIP DIP	MCP	MCP
Plane	Sagittal	Sagittal	Frontal	Frontal
Axis	Frontal	Frontal	Sagittal	Sagittal
Normal limiting factors [1,3,4]* **(see Fig. 5-11)**	MCP: tension in the posterior joint capsule, collateral ligaments; contact between the proximal phalanx and the metacarpal; tension in extensor digitorum communis and extensor indicis (when the wrist is flexed)[9] PIP: contact between the middle and proximal phalanx; soft tissue apposition of the middle and proximal phalanges; tension in the posterior joint capsule, and collateral ligaments DIP: tension in the posterior joint capsule, collateral ligaments, and oblique retinacular ligament	MCP: Tension in the anterior joint capsule, palmar fibrocartilagenous plate (palmar ligament); tension in flexor digitorum profundus and flexor digitorum superficialis (when the wrist is extended)[9] PIP: tension in the anterior joint capsule, palmar ligament DIP: tension in the anterior joint capsule, palmar ligament	Tension in the collateral ligaments, fascia, and skin of the web spaces	Contact between adjacent fingers
Normal end feel[3,5]	MCP: firm/hard PIP: hard/soft/firm DIP: firm	MCP: firm PIP: firm DIP: firm	Firm	
Normal AROM[6] (AROM[7])	MCP: 0–90° (0–90°) PIP: 0–100° (0–100°) DIP: 0–90° (0–70°)	MCP: 0–45° (0–20°) PIP: 0° (0°) DIP: 0° (0°)		
Capsular pattern[5,8]	Metacarpophalangeal and interphalangeal joints: flexion, extension			

*There is a paucity of definitive research that identifies the normal limiting factors (NLF) of joint motion. The NLF and end feels listed here are based on knowledge of anatomy, clinical experience, and available references.

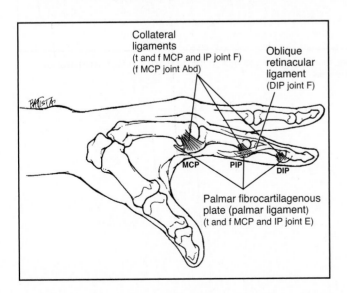

Collateral ligaments
(t and f MCP and IP joint F)
(f MCP joint Abd)

Oblique retinacular ligament
(DIP joint F)

MCP   PIP   DIP

Palmar fibrocartilagenous plate (palmar ligament)
(t and f MCP and IP joint E)

Figure 5-11 Normal Limiting Factors. Lateral view of the wrist and hand showing noncontractile structures that normally limit motion at the MCP and IP joints of the fingers (f) and thumb (t). Other noncontractile structures that normally limit motion at the MCP and IP joints and first CM joint are listed in Table 5-2. Motion limited by structures is identified in brackets, using the following abbreviations: *F*, flexion; *E*, extension; *Abd*, abduction. Muscles normally limiting motion are not illustrated.

TABLE 5-3   Joint Structure: Thumb Movements

	Flexion	Extension	Palmar Abduction	Adduction
Articulation[1,2]	Carpometacarpal (CM) Metacarpophalangeal (MCP) Interphalangeal (IP)	CM MCP IP	CM MCP	CM MCP
Plane	CM: oblique frontal MCP: frontal IP: frontal	CM: oblique frontal MCP: frontal IP: frontal	CM: oblique sagittal	CM: oblique sagittal
Axis	CM: oblique sagittal MCP: sagittal IP: sagittal	CM: oblique sagittal MCP: sagittal IP: sagittal	CM: oblique frontal	CM: oblique frontal
Normal limiting factors[1,3,4]* **(see Fig. 5-11)**	CM: soft tissue apposition between the thenar eminence and the palm; tension in the posterior joint capsule, extensor pollicis brevis, and abductor pollicis brevis MCP: contact between the first metacarpal and the proximal phalanx; tension in the posterior joint capsule, collateral ligaments, and extensor pollicis brevis IP: tension in the collateral ligaments, and posterior joint capsule; contact between the distal phalanx, fibrocartilagenous plate and the proximal phalanx	CM: tension in the anterior joint capsule, flexor pollicis brevis, and first dorsal interosseous MCP: tension in the anterior joint capsule, palmar ligament, and flexor pollicis brevis IP: tension in the anterior joint capsule, palmar ligament	Tension in the fascia and skin of the first web space, first dorsal interosseous, and adductor pollicis	Soft tissue apposition between the thumb and index finger
Normal end feel[3,5,8]	CM: soft/firm MCP: hard/firm IP: hard/firm	CM: firm MCP: firm IP: firm	Firm	Soft
Normal AROM[6] (AROM[7])	CM: 0–15° (0–15°) MCP: 0–50° (0–50°) IP: 0–80° (0–65°)	CM: 0–20° (0–20°) MCP: 0° (0°) IP: 0–20° (0–10 to 20°)	0–70° (0–70°)	0° (0°)
Capsular pattern[5,8]	CM joint: abduction, extension MCP and IP joints: flexion, extension			

*There is a paucity of definitive research that identifies the normal limiting factors (NLF) of joint motion. The NLF and end feels listed here are based on knowledge of anatomy, clinical experience, and available references.

SURFACE ANATOMY (Figs. 5-12, 5-13, and 5-14)

Structure

Location

1. Styloid process of the ulna — Bony prominence on the posteromedial aspect of the forearm at the distal end of the ulna.

2. Styloid process of the radius — Bony prominence on the lateral aspect of the forearm at the distal end of the radius.

3. Metacarpal bones — The bases and shafts are felt through the extensor tendons on the posterior surface of the wrist and hand. The heads are the bony prominences at the bases of the digits.

4. Capitate bone — In the small depression proximal to the base of the third metacarpal bone.

5. Pisiform bone — Medial bone of the proximal row of carpal bones; proximal to the base of the hypothenar eminence.

6. Thumb web space — The web of skin connecting the thumb to the hand.

7. Distal palmar crease — Transverse crease commencing on the medial side of the palm and extending laterally to the web between the index and middle fingers.

8. Proximal palmar crease — Transverse crease commencing on the lateral side of the palm, extending medially and fading out on the hypothenar eminence.

9. Thenar eminence — The pad on the palm of the hand at the base of the thumb; bound medially and distally by the longitudinal palmar crease.

10. Hypothenar eminence — The pad on the medial side of the base of the palm.

11. First CM joint — At the distal aspect of the anatomical snuffbox, the articulation between the base of the first metacarpal and the trapezium.
(*Anatomical snuffbox:* with the thumb held in extension, the triangular area on the posterolateral aspect of the wrist and hand outlined by the tendons of the extensor pollicis longus laterally and the extensor pollicis brevis medially.)

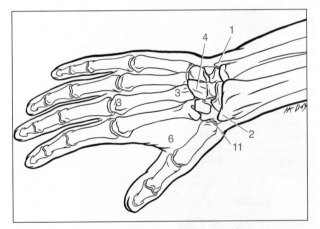

Figure 5-12 Bony anatomy, posterior aspect of the wrist and hand.

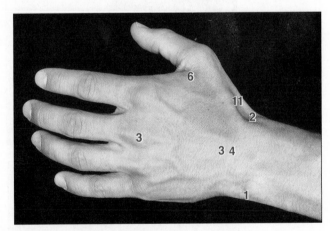

Figure 5-13 Posterior aspect of the wrist and hand.

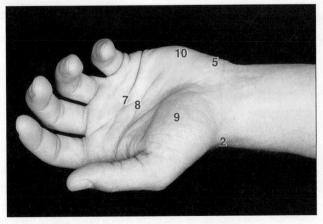

Figure 5-14 Anterior aspect of the wrist and hand.

RANGE OF MOTION ASSESSMENT AND MEASUREMENT

 Practice Makes Perfect

To aid you in practicing the skills covered in this section, or for a handy review, use the practical testing forms found at http://thepoint.lww.com/Clarkson3e.

General Scan: Wrist and Hand Active Range of Motion

The AROM of the wrist and hand is scanned to provide a general indication of the available ROM and/or muscle strength at the wrist and hand. With the patient sitting, the elbow flexed 90° and the forearm pronated, instruct the patient to:

- Make a fist (Fig. 5-15A). Observe the AROM of finger flexion, thumb flexion and abduction, and wrist extension.
- Open the hand, and maximally spread the fingers (Fig. 5-15B). Observe the AROM for finger extension and abduction, thumb extension, and wrist flexion.
- Supinate the forearm and touch the pad of the thumb to the pad of the fifth finger (Fig. 5-15C). Observe the AROM for opposition of the thumb and fifth finger.

The findings of the scan serve as a guide for detailed assessment of the region.

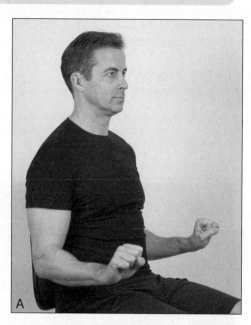

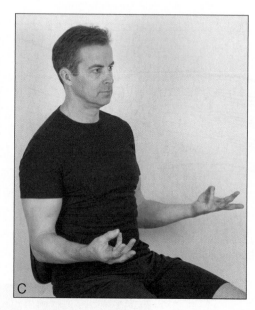

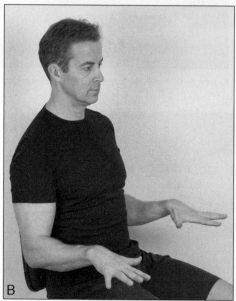

Figure 5-15 General scan of wrist and hand AROM — the patient **(A)** makes a fist, **(B)** opens the hand, and **(C)** supinates the forearm and touches the pad of the thumb to the pad of the little finger.

Wrist Flexion–Extension

AROM Assessment

Substitute Movement. Wrist ulnar or radial deviation.

PROM Assessment

Start Position. The patient is sitting. The elbow is flexed, the forearm is resting on a table in pronation, the wrist is in neutral position, the hand is over the end of the table, and the fingers are relaxed (Fig. 5-16). Finger position influences wrist ROM, therefore, wrist ROM should be assessed using consistently standardized finger position.[12]

Forms 5-1, 5-2

Stabilization. The therapist stabilizes the forearm.

Therapist's Distal Hand Placement. The therapist grasps the metacarpals.

End Position. The therapist moves the hand anteriorly to the limit of motion to assess wrist flexion (Fig. 5-17). The therapist moves the hand posteriorly to the limit of motion for wrist extension (Fig. 5-18). The fingers should be relaxed when assessing the end feels to avoid restriction of wrist flexion or extension due to stretch of the long finger extensors or flexors, respectively.

End Feels. *Wrist flexion*—firm; *wrist extension*—firm/hard.

Joint Glides. *Flexion. Radiocarpal joint*—the convex surface of the proximal row of carpal bones glides posteriorly on the fixed concave surface of the distal radius and articular disc of the inferior radioulnar joint. *Midcarpal joint*—the concave surface formed by the trapezium and trapezoid glides in an anterior direction on the fixed convex surface of the scaphoid; the convex surface formed by the capitate and hamate glides in a posterior direction on the fixed concave surface formed by the scaphoid, lunate, and triquetrum bones.

Extension. Radiocarpal joint—the convex surface of the proximal row of carpal bones glides anteriorly on the fixed concave surface of the distal radius and articular disc of the inferior radioulnar joint. *Midcarpal joint*—the

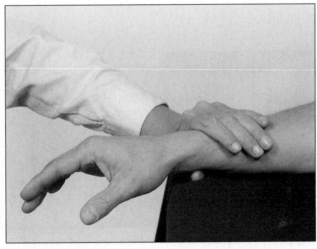

Figure 5-16 Start position for wrist flexion and extension.

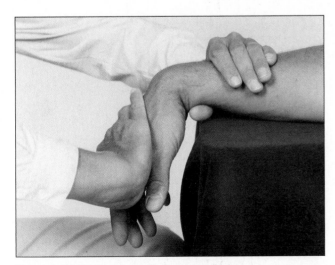

Figure 5-17 Firm end feel at limit of wrist flexion.

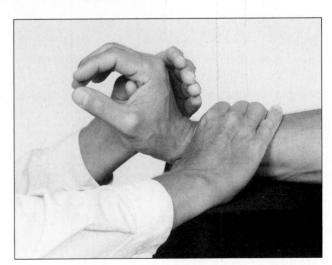

Figure 5-18 Firm or hard end feel at limit of wrist extension.

concave surface formed by the trapezium and trapezoid glides in a posterior direction on the fixed convex surface of the scaphoid; the convex surface formed by the capitate and hamate glides in an anterior direction on the fixed concave surface formed by the scaphoid, lunate, and triquetrum bones.

The above represents a simplified explanation of wrist arthrokinematics with application of the concave–convex rule during wrist movement.

Measurement: Universal Goniometer

Start Position. The patient is sitting. The elbow is flexed, the forearm is resting on a table in pronation, the wrist is in a neutral position, and the hand is over the end of the table (Fig. 5-19). The fingers are relaxed to avoid restriction of wrist flexion or extension due to stretch of the long finger extensors or flexors, respectively.

Stabilization. The therapist stabilizes the forearm.

Goniometer Axis. The axis is placed at the level of the ulnar styloid process (Fig. 5-20).

Stationary Arm. Parallel to the longitudinal axis of the ulna.

Movable Arm. Parallel to the longitudinal axis of the fifth metacarpal.

End Positions. The wrist is moved in an anterior direction to the limit of wrist flexion (80°) (Figs. 5-20 and 5-21). The wrist is moved in a posterior direction to the limit of wrist extension (70°) (Fig. 5-22). For both movements, ensure that the mobile fourth and fifth metacarpals are not moved away from the start position throughout the assessment procedure, and ensure that no wrist deviation occurs if full range cannot be obtained.

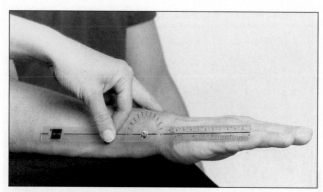

Figure 5-19 Start position for wrist flexion and extension.

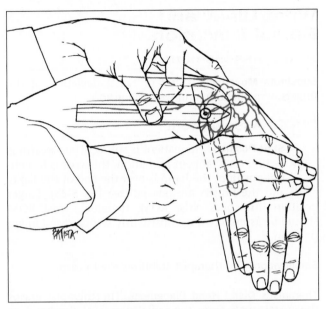

Figure 5-20 Goniometer alignment for wrist flexion and extension, illustrated at limit of wrist flexion.

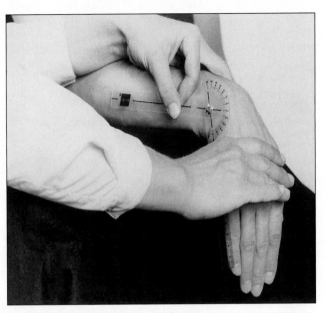

Figure 5-21 End position for wrist flexion.

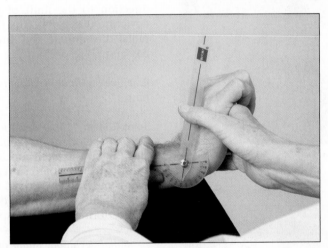

Figure 5-22 End position for wrist extension.

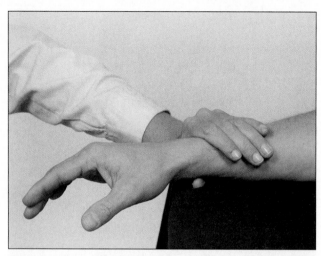

Figure 5-23 Start position for wrist ulnar and radial deviation.

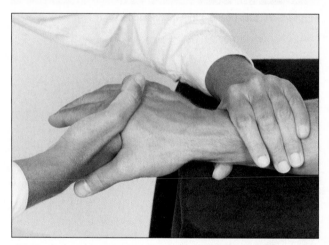

Figure 5-24 Firm end feel at limit of wrist ulnar deviation.

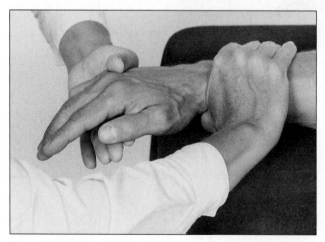

Figure 5-25 Firm or hard end feel at limit of wrist radial deviation.

Wrist Ulnar and Radial Deviation

AROM Assessment

Substitute Movement. Ulnar or radial deviation of the fingers, wrist flexion, and wrist extension.

PROM Assessment

Start Position. The patient is sitting. The forearm is resting on a table in pronation, the wrist is in neutral position, the hand is over the end of the table, and the fingers are relaxed (see Fig. 5-23). Finger position influences wrist ROM, therefore, wrist ROM should be assessed using consistently standardized finger position.[12]

Forms 5-3, 5-4

Stabilization. The therapist stabilizes the forearm.

Therapist's Distal Hand Placement. The therapist grasps the metacarpals from the radial aspect of the hand to assess wrist ulnar deviation. The therapist grasps the metacarpals from the ulnar aspect of the hand to assess wrist radial deviation.

End Positions. The therapist moves the hand in an ulnar direction to the limit of motion to assess wrist ulnar deviation (Fig. 5-24). The therapist moves the hand in a radial direction to the limit of motion for wrist radial deviation (Fig. 5-25).

End Feels. *Ulnar deviation*—firm; *radial deviation*—firm/hard.

Joint Glides.[13] *Ulnar deviation. Radiocarpal joint*—the convex surface of the proximal row of carpal bones glides laterally on the fixed concave surface of the distal radius and articular disc of the inferior radioulnar joint. *Midcarpal joint*—the convex surface formed by the capitate and hamate glides in a lateral direction on the fixed concave surface formed by the scaphoid, lunate, and triquetrum bones.

Radial deviation. Radiocarpal joint—the convex surface of the proximal row of carpal bones glides medially on the fixed concave surface of the distal radius and articular disc of the inferior radioulnar joint. *Midcarpal joint*—the convex surface formed by the capitate and hamate glides in a medial direction on the fixed concave surface formed by the scaphoid, lunate, and triquetrum bones.

The above represents a simplified explanation of wrist arthrokinematics with application of the concave–convex rule during wrist movement.

Measurement: Universal Goniometer

Start Position. The patient is sitting. The elbow is flexed, the forearm is pronated, and the palmar surface of the hand is resting lightly on a table. The wrist remains in a neutral position and the fingers are relaxed (Fig. 5-26) to avoid restriction of wrist ulnar deviation due to finger constraints.[12]

Stabilization. The therapist stabilizes the forearm.

Goniometer Axis. The axis is placed on the posterior aspect of the wrist joint over the capitate bone (Fig. 5-27).

Stationary Arm. Along the midline of the forearm.

Movable Arm. Parallel to the longitudinal axis of the shaft of the third metacarpal.

End Positions. Ulnar deviation (Figs. 5-27 and 5-28): the wrist is adducted to the ulnar side to the limit of ulnar deviation (30°). Radial deviation (Fig. 5-29): the wrist is abducted to the radial side to the limit of radial deviation (20°). Ensure the wrist is not moved into flexion or extension.

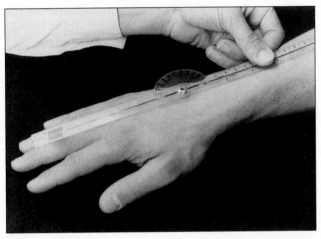

Figure 5-26 Start position for ulnar and radial deviation of the wrist.

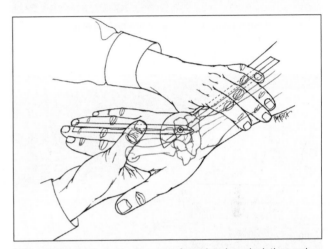

Figure 5-27 Goniometer alignment for wrist ulnar deviation and radial deviation, illustrated at limit of ulnar deviation.

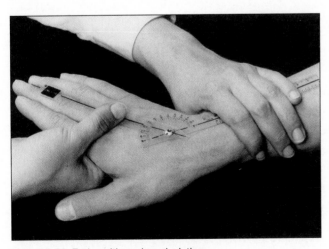

Figure 5-28 End position: ulnar deviation.

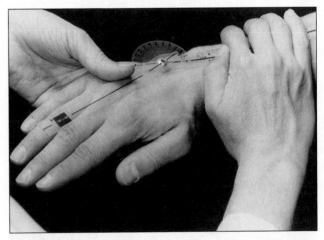

Figure 5-29 End position: radial deviation.

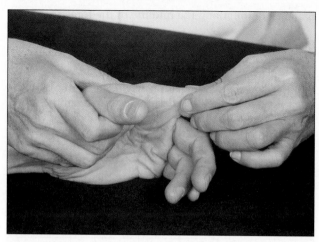

Figure 5-30 Start position: MCP joint flexion and extension.

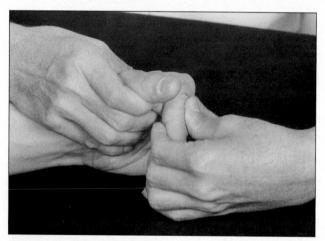

Figure 5-31 Firm or hard end feel at the limit of MCP flexion.

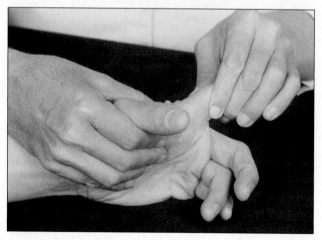

Figure 5-32 Firm end feel at the limit of MCP extension.

Finger MCP Flexion–Extension
PROM Assessment

Forms
5-5, 5-6

Start Position. The patient is sitting. The forearm is resting on a table in midposition, the wrist is in neutral position, and the fingers are relaxed (Fig. 5-30).

Stabilization. The therapist stabilizes the metacarpal.

Therapist's Distal Hand Placement. The therapist grasps the proximal phalanx.

End Positions. The therapist moves the proximal phalanx in an anterior direction to the limit of motion to assess MCP joint flexion (Fig. 5-31). The therapist moves the proximal phalanx in a posterior direction to the limit of motion for MCP joint extension (Fig. 5-32).

End Feels. *MCP joint flexion*—firm/hard; *MCP joint extension*—firm.

Joint Glides. *MCP joint flexion*—the concave base of the proximal phalanx glides in an anterior direction on the fixed convex head of the adjacent metacarpal. *MCP joint extension*—the concave base of the proximal phalanx glides in a posterior direction on the fixed convex head of the adjacent metacarpal.

Measurement: Universal Goniometer

Finger MCP Flexion

Start Position. The patient is sitting. The forearm is resting on a table, the elbow is flexed, the wrist is slightly extended, and the MCP joint of the finger being measured is in 0° of extension (Fig. 5-33).

Stabilization. The therapist stabilizes the metacarpal.

Goniometer Axis. The axis is placed on the posterior aspect of the MCP joint being measured.

Stationary Arm. Parallel to the longitudinal axis of the shaft of the metacarpal.

Movable Arm. Parallel to the longitudinal axis of the proximal phalanx.

End Position. All fingers are moved toward the palm to the limit of MCP joint flexion (90°) (Fig. 5-34). Range increases progressively from the index to the fifth finger.[1] The IP joints are allowed to extend so that flexion at the MCP joint is not restricted due to tension of the long finger extensor tendons.

Alternate Goniometer Placement. The index and fifth MCP joints may be measured on the lateral aspect of the joint (Figs. 5-35 and 5-36). Should joint enlargement prevent measurement on the posterior aspect, the index and fifth fingers may be measured and the range estimated for the middle and fourth fingers.[14]

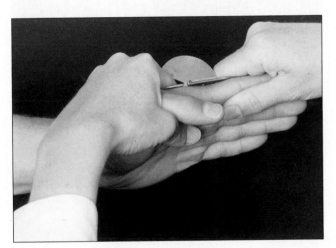

Figure 5-33 Start position for MCP flexion.

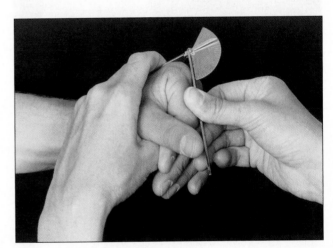

Figure 5-34 End position: MCP flexion.

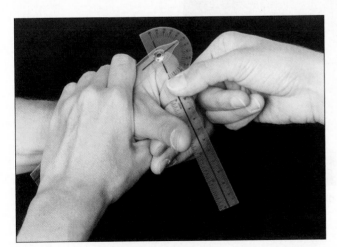

Figure 5-35 Alternate goniometer placement for MCP flexion.

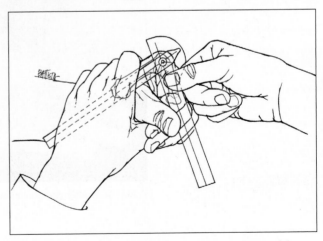

Figure 5-36 Goniometer alignment on the lateral aspect of the joint for MCP joint flexion and extension, illustrated with the MCP joint in flexion.

Measurement: Universal Goniometer

Finger MCP Extension

Start Position. The patient is sitting. The forearm is resting on a table, the elbow is flexed, the wrist is slightly flexed, and the MCP joint of the finger being measured is in 0° of extension (Fig. 5-37).

Stabilization. The therapist stabilizes the metacarpal.

Goniometer Axis. The axis is placed on the anterior surface of the MCP joint being measured.

Stationary Arm. Parallel to the longitudinal axis of the shaft of the metacarpal.

Movable Arm. Parallel to the longitudinal axis of the proximal phalanx.

End Position. The finger is moved in a posterior direction to the limit of MCP joint extension (45°) (Fig. 5-38). The IP joints are allowed to flex so that extension at the MCP joint is not restricted due to tension of the long finger flexor tendons.

Alternate Goniometer Placement. The index and fifth MCP joints may be measured on the lateral aspect of the MCP joint (Fig. 5-39).

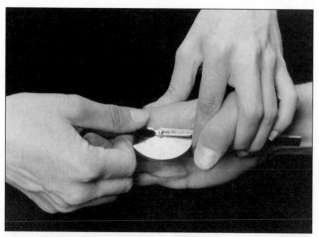

Figure 5-37 Start position for MCP extension.

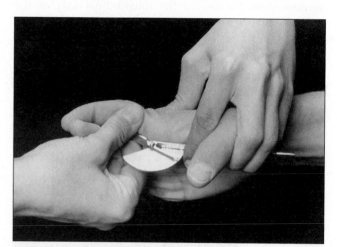

Figure 5-38 End position: MCP extension.

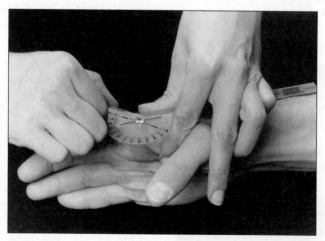

Figure 5-39 Alternate goniometer placement for MCP extension.

Finger MCP Abduction–Adduction

AROM Assessment

MCP Abduction

To gain a composite measure of finger spread and thumb web stretch, finger abduction and thumb extension can be measured in centimeters. A sheet of paper is placed under the patient's hand. The therapist stabilizes the wrist and metacarpals. The patient spreads all fingers and thumb and the therapist traces the contour of the hand (Fig. 5-40). The patient's hand is removed, and a linear measure of the distances between the midpoint of the tip of each finger and the index finger and thumb is recorded in centimeters (Fig. 5-41). *Note:* The ROM at the IP, MCP, and CM joints of the thumb influence the measurement of thumb extension ROM using this method.

PROM Assessment

MCP Abduction

Forms 5-7, 5-8

Start Position. The patient is sitting. The forearm is resting on a table, the wrist is in neutral position, and the fingers are in the anatomical position (Fig. 5-42).

Stabilization. The therapist stabilizes the metacarpal.

Therapist's Distal Hand Placement. The therapist grasps the sides of the proximal phalanx.

End Position. The therapist moves the proximal phalanx to the limit of motion to assess MCP joint abduction (Fig. 5-43).

End Feel. MCP joint abduction—firm.

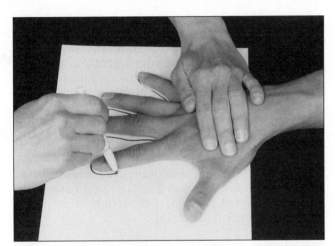

Figure 5-40 Alternate measurement: hand placement for MCP abduction and thumb extension.

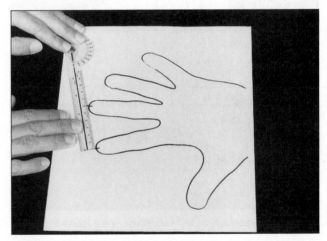

Figure 5-41 Ruler measurement: finger MCP abduction and thumb extension.

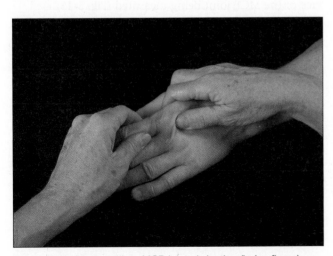

Figure 5-42 Start position: MCP joint abduction (index finger).

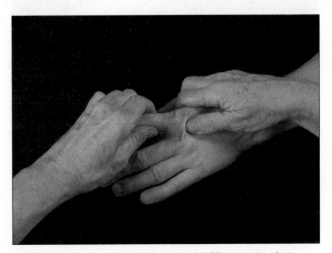

Figure 5-43 Firm end feel at the limit of MCP abduction (index finger).

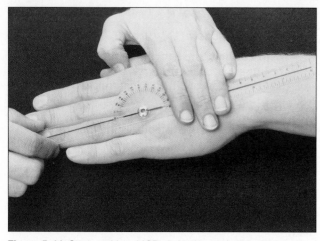

Figure 5-44 Start position: MCP abduction and adduction.

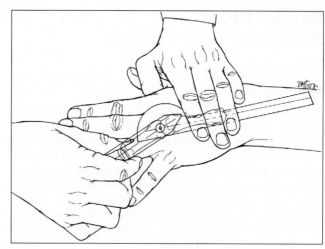

Figure 5-45 Goniometer alignment for MCP joint abduction/adduction, shown with the ring finger in abduction.

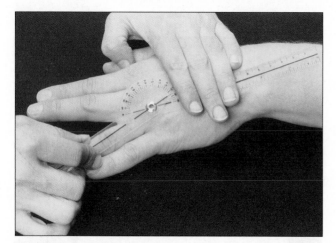

Figure 5-46 End position: MCP abduction of the fourth finger.

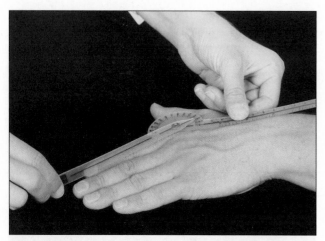

Figure 5-47 End position: MCP adduction of the index finger.

Joint Glides. *MCP joint abduction*—the concave base of the proximal phalanx moves on the fixed convex head of the corresponding metacarpal in the same direction of movement as the shaft of the proximal phalanx. *MCP joint adduction*—the concave base of the proximal phalanx moves on the fixed convex head of the corresponding metacarpal in the same direction of movement as the shaft of the proximal phalanx.

Measurement: Universal Goniometer

Start Position. The patient is sitting. The elbow is flexed to 90°, the forearm is pronated and resting on a table, the wrist is in neutral position, and the fingers are in the anatomical position (Fig. 5-44).

Stabilization. The therapist stabilizes the metacarpal bones.

Goniometer Axis. The axis is placed on the posterior surface of the MCP joint being measured (Fig. 5-45).

Stationary Arm. Parallel to the longitudinal axis of the shaft of the metacarpal.

Movable Arm. Parallel to the longitudinal axis of the proximal phalanx.

End Position. The finger is moved away from the midline of the hand to the limit of motion in abduction (Figs. 5-45 and 5-46). The finger is moved toward the midline of the hand to the limit of motion in adduction (Fig. 5-47). The remaining fingers are moved to allow full adduction.

Finger IP Flexion–Extension

PROM Assessment

Forms
5-9, 5-10

Start Position. The patient is sitting. The forearm is resting on a table, the wrist is in neutral position, and the fingers are relaxed.

Stabilization. The therapist stabilizes the proximal phalanx for assessment of the proximal interphalangeal (PIP) joint and the middle phalanx for the distal interphalangeal (DIP) joint.

Therapist's Distal Hand Placement. The therapist grasps the middle phalanx to assess the PIP joint and the distal phalanx to assess the DIP joint.

End Positions. The therapist moves the middle or distal phalanx in an anterior direction to the limit of motion to assess PIP (not shown) or DIP joint flexion (Fig. 5-48), respectively. The therapist moves the middle or distal phalanx in a posterior direction to the limit of motion for PIP joint (not shown) or DIP joint extension (Fig. 5-49), respectively.

End Feels. *PIP joint flexion*—hard/soft/firm; *DIP joint flexion*—firm; *PIP joint extension*—firm; *DIP joint extension*—firm.

Joint Glides. *IP joint flexion*—the concave base of the distal phalanx glides in an anterior direction on the fixed convex head of the adjacent proximal phalanx. *IP joint extension*—the concave base of the distal phalanx glides in a posterior direction on the fixed convex head of the adjacent proximal phalanx.

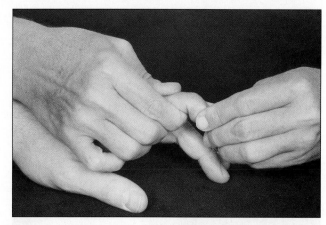
Figure 5-48 Firm end feel at limit of DIP joint flexion.

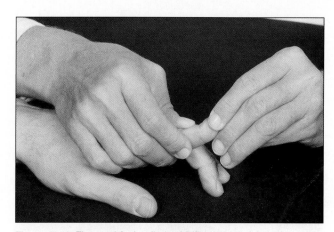
Figure 5-49 Firm end feel at limit of DIP joint extension.

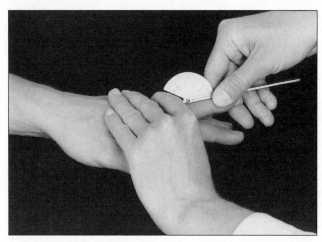

Figure 5-50 Start position: PIP joint flexion.

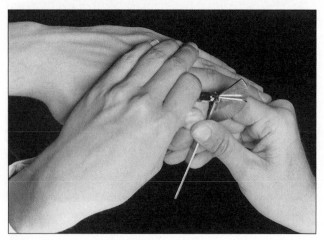

Figure 5-51 End position: PIP joint flexion.

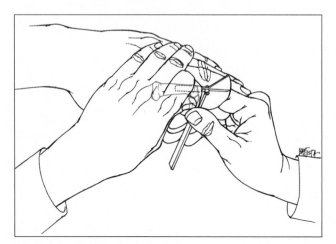

Figure 5-52 Goniometer alignment over posterior surface of PIP joint to assess flexion.

Measurement: Universal Goniometer

Start Position. The patient is sitting. The forearm is resting on a table in either midposition or pronation. The wrist and fingers are in the anatomical position (0° extension at the MCP and IP joints) (Fig. 5-50).

Stabilization. The therapist stabilizes the proximal phalanx for measurement of the PIP joint and the middle phalanx for the DIP joint.

Goniometer Axis. To measure IP joint flexion, use a goniometer with at least one short arm and place the axis over the posterior surface of the PIP (Figs. 5-50 and 5-51) or DIP joint being measured. To measure IP joint extension, the axis is placed over the anterior surface of the PIP or DIP joint being measured.

Kato and colleagues[15] studied the accuracy of goniometric measurements for PIP joint flexion ROM in cadaver hands using 3 types of goniometer. The researchers recommend use of goniometers with short arms when measuring the ROM with the goniometer placed over the dorsal aspect of the PIP joint.

Stationary Arm. PIP joint: parallel to the longitudinal axis of the proximal phalanx. DIP joint: parallel to the longitudinal axis of the middle phalanx.

Movable Arm. PIP joint: parallel to the longitudinal axis of the middle phalanx. DIP joint: parallel to the longitudinal axis of the distal phalanx.

End Positions. The PIP joint (Figs. 5-51 and 5-52) or DIP joint (not shown) is flexed to the limit of PIP or DIP joint flexion (100° or 90°, respectively). The PIP joint (Fig. 5-53) or DIP joint (not shown) is extended to the limit of PIP or DIP joint extension (0°).

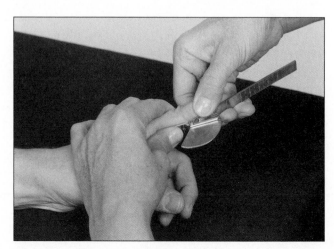

Figure 5-53 End position: PIP joint extension.

Finger MCP and IP Flexion

When evaluating impairment of hand function, a linear measurement of finger flexion should be used in conjunction with goniometry. This measure is particularly relevant in evaluating the extent of impairment[16] associated with grasp. The patient is sitting. The elbow is flexed and the forearm is resting on a table in supination. Two measurements are taken.

1. The patient flexes the IP joints while maintaining 0° of extension at the MCP joints (Fig. 5-54). A ruler measurement is taken from the pulp or tip of the middle finger to the distal palmar crease.

2. The patient flexes the MCP and IP joints (Fig. 5-55), and a ruler measurement is taken from the pulp of the finger to the proximal palmar crease.

Note: Long fingernails limit the flexion ROM at the finger joints (MCP joint flexion being the most affected) when the fingernails contact the palm.[17]

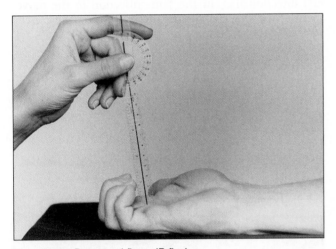

Figure 5-54 Decreased finger IP flexion.

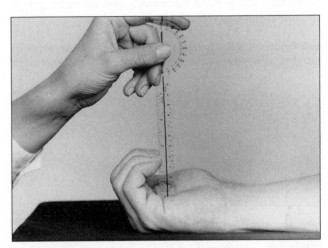

Figure 5-55 Decreased finger MCP and IP flexion.

Thumb CM Flexion–Extension

PROM Assessment

Start Position. The patient is sitting. The elbow is flexed with the forearm in midposition and resting on a table. The wrist is in neutral position, the fingers are relaxed, and the thumb is in the anatomical position.

Forms 5-11, 5-12

Stabilization. The therapist stabilizes the trapezium, wrist, and forearm (see Fig. 5-56).

Therapist's Distal Hand Placement. The therapist grasps the first metacarpal (Fig. 5-57).

End Positions. The therapist moves the first metacarpal in an ulnar direction to the limit of motion to assess thumb CM joint flexion (Fig. 5-58). The therapist moves the first metacarpal in a radial direction to the limit of motion for thumb CM joint extension (Fig. 5-59).

End Feels. *Thumb CM joint flexion*—soft/firm; *thumb CM joint extension*—firm.

Joint Glides[13]. *Thumb CM joint flexion*—the concave surface of the base of the first metacarpal glides in a medial direction (i.e., in the same direction to the movement of the shaft of the first metacarpal) on the convex surface of the trapezium. *Thumb CM joint extension*—the concave surface of the base of the first metacarpal glides in a lateral direction (i.e., in the same direction to the movement of the shaft of the first metacarpal) on the convex surface of the trapezium.

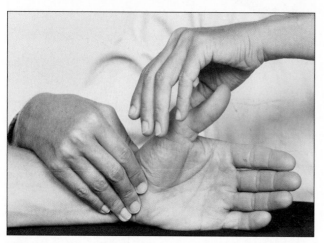

Figure 5-56 Start position: thumb CM flexion and extension. The therapist stabilizes the trapezium between the left thumb and index finger.

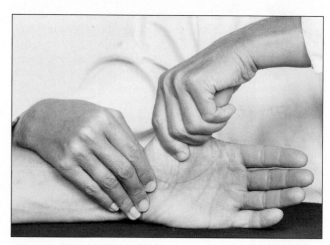

Figure 5-57 Therapist's distal hand grasps the first metacarpal.

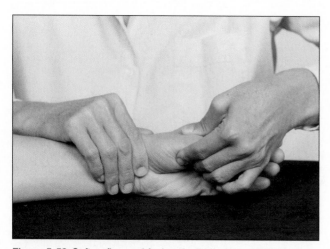

Figure 5-58 Soft or firm end feel at the limit of thumb CM flexion.

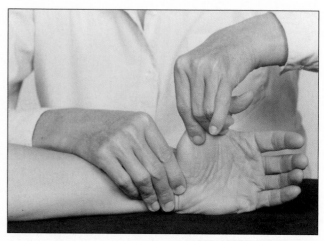

Figure 5-59 Firm end feel at the limit of thumb CM extension.

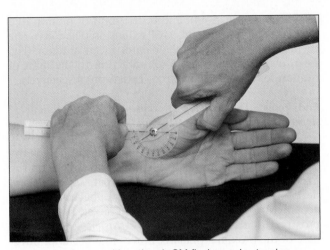

Figure 5-60 Start position: thumb CM flexion and extension.

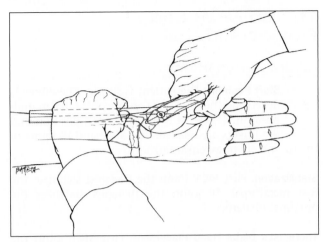

Figure 5-61 Goniometer alignment thumb CM joint flexion and extension.

Measurement: Universal Goniometer

Start Position. The patient is sitting. The elbow is flexed with the forearm in midposition and resting on a table. The wrist is in slight ulnar deviation, the fingers assume the anatomical position, and the thumb maintains contact with the metacarpal and proximal phalanx of the index finger (Fig. 5-60).

Stabilization. The therapist stabilizes the trapezium, wrist, and forearm.

Goniometer Axis. The axis is placed over the CM joint (Fig. 5-61).

Stationary Arm. Parallel to the longitudinal axis of the radius.

Movable Arm. Parallel to the longitudinal axis of the thumb metacarpal. *Note:* Although the goniometer arms are not aligned at 0° in this start position, this position is recorded as the 0° start position. The number of degrees the metacarpal is moved away from this 0° start position is recorded as the ROM for the movement. For example, if the goniometer read 30° at the start position for CM joint flexion/extension (see Fig. 5-60) and 15° at the end position for CM joint flexion (see Fig. 5-62), the CM joint flexion ROM would be 15°.

End Positions. Flexion (Fig. 5-62): the thumb is flexed across the palm to the limit of thumb CM joint flexion (15°). Extension (Fig. 5-63): the thumb is extended away from the palm to the limit of thumb CM joint extension (20°).

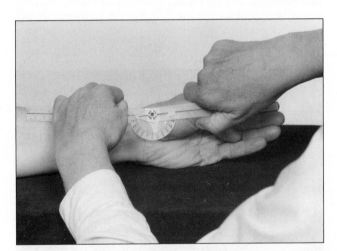

Figure 5-62 End position: thumb CM flexion.

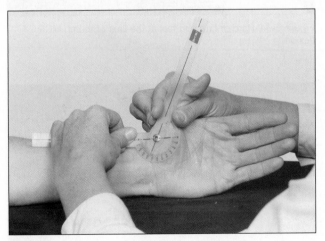

Figure 5-63 End position: thumb CM extension.

Thumb MCP and IP Flexion–Extension

PROM Assessment

Start Position. The patient is sitting. The elbow is flexed and the forearm is resting on a table in mid-position. The wrist is in the neutral position and the fingers are relaxed. The MCP and IP joints of the thumb are in extension (0°).

Forms 5-13–5-16

Stabilization. First MCP joint: the therapist stabilizes the first metacarpal. IP joint: the therapist stabilizes the proximal phalanx.

Therapist's Distal Hand Placement. First MCP joint: the therapist grasps the proximal phalanx. IP joint: the therapist grasps the distal phalanx.

End Positions. The therapist moves the proximal phalanx across the palm to the limit of motion to assess thumb MCP flexion (Fig. 5-64), and to the limit of motion in a radial direction for thumb MCP extension (Fig. 5-65). The therapist moves the distal phalanx in an anterior (Fig. 5-66) or a posterior (Fig. 5-67) direction to the limit of motion for thumb IP flexion or extension, respectively.

End Feels. *Thumb MCP flexion*—hard/firm; *thumb IP flexion*—hard/firm; *thumb MCP and IP extension*—firm.

Joint Glides. *Thumb MCP flexion*—the concave base of the proximal phalanx moves in an anterior direction on the fixed convex head of the first metacarpal. *Thumb IP joint flexion*—the concave base of the distal phalanx glides in an anterior direction on the fixed convex head of the proximal phalanx. *Thumb MCP extension*—the concave base of the proximal phalanx moves in a posterior direction on the fixed convex head of the first metacarpal. *Thumb IP joint extension*—the concave base of the distal phalanx glides in a posterior direction on the fixed convex head of the proximal phalanx.

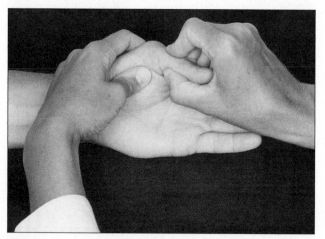

Figure 5-64 Hard or firm end feel at the limit of thumb MCP flexion.

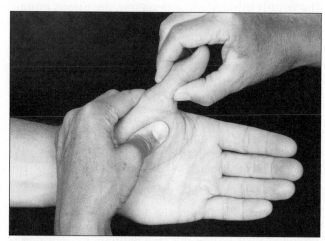

Figure 5-65 Firm end feel at the limit of thumb MCP extension.

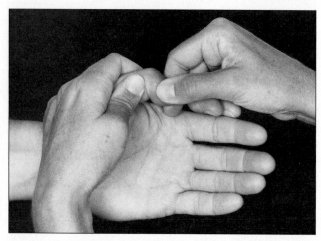

Figure 5-66 Hard or firm end feel at the limit of thumb IP flexion.

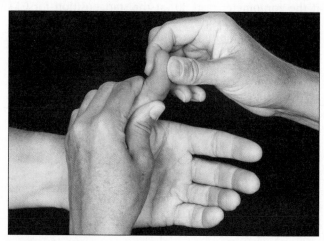

Figure 5-67 Firm end feel at the limit of thumb IP extension.

Measurement: Universal Goniometer

Start Position. The patient is sitting. The elbow is flexed and the forearm is resting on a table in midposition. The wrist and fingers are in the anatomical position. The MCP and IP joints are in extension (0°).

Stabilization. MCP joint: the therapist stabilizes the first metacarpal. IP joint: the therapist stabilizes the proximal phalanx.

Goniometer Axis. The axis is placed over the posterior or lateral aspect of the MCP joint (Fig. 5-68) or IP joint (Fig. 5-69) of the thumb.

Stationary Arm. MCP joint: parallel to the longitudinal axis of the shaft of the thumb metacarpal. IP joint: parallel to the longitudinal axis of the proximal phalanx.

Movable Arm. MCP joint: parallel to the longitudinal axis of the proximal phalanx. IP joint: parallel to the longitudinal axis of the distal phalanx.

End Positions. The MCP joint is flexed so that the thumb moves across the palm to the limit of thumb MCP joint flexion (50°) (Fig. 5-70). The IP joint is flexed to the limit of thumb IP joint flexion (80°) (Fig. 5-71). The goniometer is positioned on the lateral or anterior surface of the thumb to assess MCP and IP joint extension. The MCP joint is extended to the limit of thumb MCP joint extension (0°).

Hyperextension. Hyperextension of the IP joint of the thumb occurs beyond 0° of extension. The thumb IP joint can actively be hyperextended to 10° and passively to 30°[1] (Fig. 5-67).

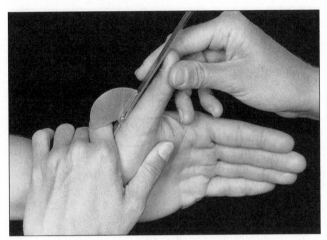

Figure 5-68 Start position: thumb MCP flexion.

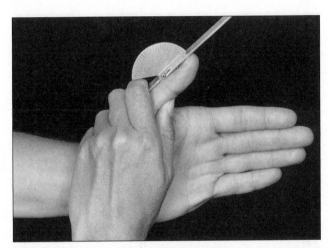

Figure 5-69 Start position: thumb IP flexion.

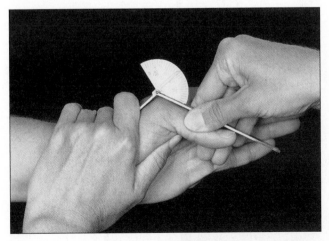

Figure 5-70 End position: thumb MCP flexion.

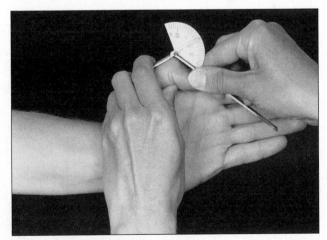

Figure 5-71 End position: thumb IP flexion.

Thumb CM Abduction

PROM Assessment

 Start Position. The patient is sitting. The forearm is in midposition resting on a table, the wrist is in neutral position, and the fingers and thumb are relaxed (Fig. 5-72).

Form 5-17

Stabilization. The therapist stabilizes the second metacarpal.

Therapist's Distal Hand Placement. The therapist grasps the first metacarpal.

End Position. The therapist moves the first metacarpal away from the second metacarpal in an anterior direction perpendicular to the plane of the palm to the limit of motion to assess CM joint abduction (Fig. 5-73).

End Feel. CM joint abduction—firm.

Joint Glide[13]. *CM joint abduction*—the convex surface of the base of the first metacarpal glides in a posterior direction (i.e., in the opposite direction as the shaft of the first metacarpal) on the fixed concave surface of the trapezium.

Measurement: Universal Goniometer

Start Position. The patient is sitting. The elbow is flexed and the forearm is resting on a table in midposition. The wrist and fingers are in the anatomical position. The thumb maintains contact with the metacarpal and proximal phalanx of the index finger (Fig. 5-74).

Stabilization. The therapist stabilizes the second metacarpal.

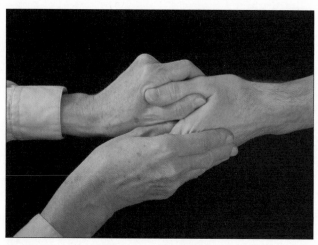

Figure 5-72 Start position: thumb abduction.

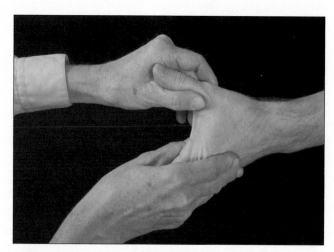

Figure 5-73 Firm end feel at the limit of thumb CM joint abduction.

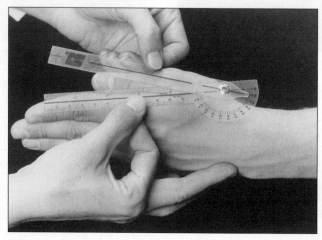

Figure 5-74 Start position: thumb abduction.

Goniometer Axis. The axis is placed at the junction of the bases of the first and second metacarpals (Fig. 5-75).

Stationary Arm. Parallel to the longitudinal axis of the second metacarpal.

Movable Arm. Parallel to the longitudinal axis of the first metacarpal. In the start position described, the goniometer will indicate 15°–20°. This is recorded as 0°.[14] For example, if the goniometer read 15° at the start position for CM joint abduction (see Fig. 5-74) and 60° at the end position for CM joint abduction (Fig. 5-76), the first CM joint abduction ROM would be 45°.

End Position. The thumb is abducted to the limit of thumb CM joint abduction (70°) so that the thumb column moves in the plane perpendicular to the palm (see Fig. 5-76).

Measurement: Ruler

As an alternate measurement to goniometry, thumb abduction may be measured by using a ruler or tape mea-sure. With the thumb in the abducted position, a ruler measurement is taken from the lateral aspect of the mid-point of the MCP joint of the index finger to the posterior aspect of the midpoint of the MCP joint of the thumb (Fig. 5-77).

Measurement: Caliper

As an alternate, more reliable measurement method to conventional goniometry, thumb abduction is assessed using calipers to measure the intermetacarpal distance (IMD method).[18] With the thumb in the abducted posi-tion, a caliper measurement (Fig. 5-78) is taken with the caliper points positioned on the mid-dorsal points marked on the heads of the first and second metacarpals and is recorded in millimeters. However, unlike angular measure-ments, the IMD method is affected by changes in hand size that may not permit results to be comparable either between patients or in children when hand size changes.[18]

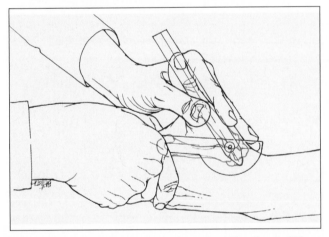

Figure 5-75 Goniometer alignment for end position thumb CM joint abduction.

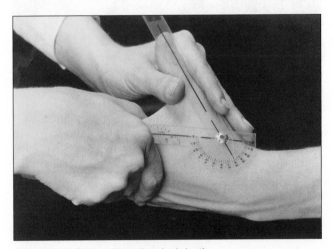

Figure 5-76 End position: thumb abduction.

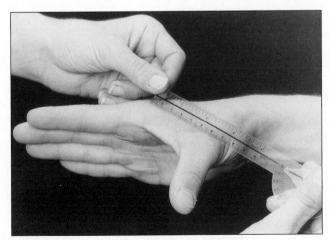

Figure 5-77 Ruler measurement: thumb abduction.

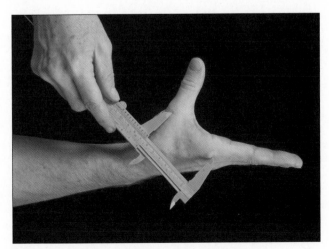

Figure 5-78 Caliper measurement: thumb abduction.

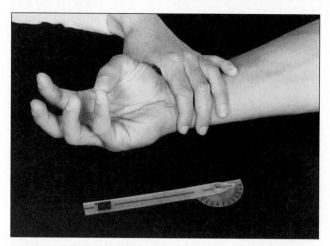

Figure 5-79 Full opposition ROM.

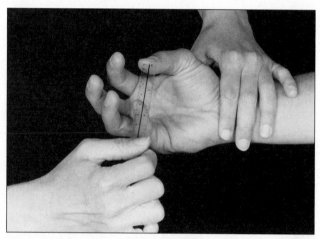

Figure 5-80 Opposition deficit.

Thumb Opposition

Measurement: Ruler

Form 5-18

On completion of full range of opposition between the thumb and fifth finger (Fig. 5-79), it is normally possible to place the pads of the thumb and fifth finger in the same plane.[19] An evaluation of a deficit in opposition (Fig. 5-80) can be obtained by taking a linear measurement between the center of the tip of the thumb pad and the center of the tip of the fifth finger pad.

MUSCLE LENGTH ASSESSMENT AND MEASUREMENT

Practice Makes Perfect

To aid you in practicing the skills covered in this section, or for a handy review, use the practical testing forms found at http://thepoint.lww.com/Clarkson3e.

Flexor Digitorum Superficialis, Flexor Digitorum Profundus, Flexor Digiti Minimi, and Palmaris Longus

Form 5-19

Start Position. The patient is in supine or sitting with the elbow in extension, the forearm supinated, wrist in neutral position, and the fingers extended (Fig. 5-81).

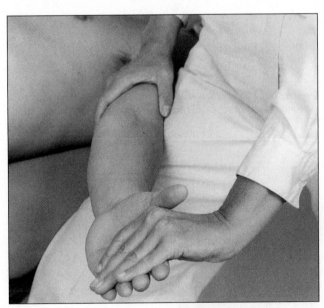

Figure 5-81 Start position: length of flexor digitorum superficialis, flexor digitorum profundus, and flexor digiti minimi.

Origin[2]	Insertion[2]
Flexor Digitorum Superficialis	
a. Humeroulnar head: common flexor origin on the medial epicondyle of the humerus, the anterior band of the ulnar collateral ligament, and the medial aspect to the coronoid process. b. Radial head: anterior border of the radius from the radial tuberosity to the insertion of pronator teres.	Anterior surface of the middle phalanges of the index, middle, ring, and little fingers.
Flexor Digitorum Profundus	
Upper three fourths of the anterior and medial aspects of the ulna; medial aspect of the coronoid process; by an aponeurosis on the upper three fourths of the posterior border of the ulna; anterior surface of the medial half of the interosseous membrane.	Palmar aspect of the bases of the distal phalanges of the index, middle, ring, and little fingers.
Flexor Digiti Minimi	
Hook of hamate; flexor retinaculum.	Ulnar aspect of the base of the proximal phalanx of the little finger.
Palmaris Longus (vestigial)	
Common flexor origin on the medial epicondyle of the humerus.	Palmar aspect of the flexor retinaculum; the palmar aponeurosis.

Stabilization. The therapist manually stabilizes the humerus. The radius and ulna are stabilized against the therapist's thigh.

End Position. The therapist maintains the fingers in extension and extends the wrist to the limit of motion so that the long finger flexors are put on full stretch (Figs. 5-82 and 5-83).

Assessment and Measurement. If the finger flexors are shortened, wrist extension ROM will be restricted proportional to the decrease in muscle length. The therapist either observes the available PROM or uses a goniometer (Fig. 5-84) to measure and record the available wrist extension PROM. A second therapist may be required to measure the ROM using a goniometer.

End Feel. Finger flexors on stretch—firm.

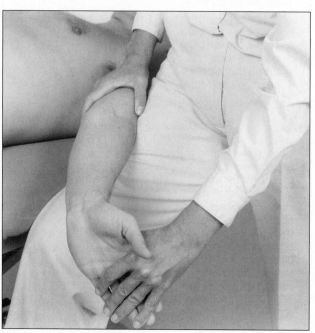

Figure 5-82 Flexor digitorum superficialis, flexor digitorum profundus, and flexor digiti minimi on stretch.

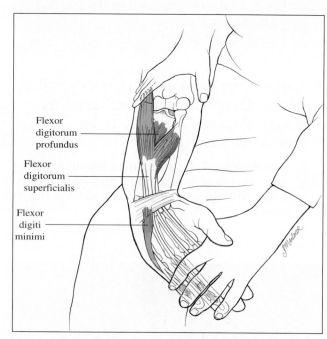

Flexor digitorum profundus

Flexor digitorum superficialis

Flexor digiti minimi

Figure 5-83 Flexor digitorum superficialis, flexor digitorum profundus, and flexor digiti minimi on stretch.

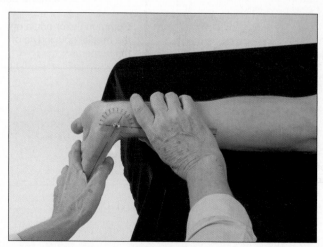

Figure 5-84 Goniometer measurement: length of long finger flexors.

Extensor Digitorum Communis, Extensor Indicis Proprius, and Extensor Digiti Minimi

Start Position. The patient is in supine or sitting. The elbow is extended, the forearm is pronated, the wrist is in the neutral position, and the fingers are flexed (Fig. 5-85).

Form 5-20

Stabilization. The therapist stabilizes the radius and ulna.

End Position. The therapist flexes the wrist to the limit of motion so that the long finger extensors are fully stretched (Figs. 5-86 and 5-87).

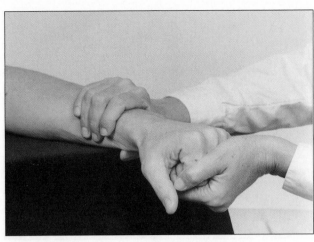

Figure 5-85 Start position: length of extensor digitorum communis, extensor indicis proprius, and extensor digiti minimi.

Origin[2]	Insertion[2]
Extensor Digitorum Communis	
Common extensor origin on the lateral epicondyle of the humerus.	Posterior surfaces of the bases of the distal and middle phalanges of the index, middle, ring, and little fingers.
Extensor Indicis Proprius	
Posterior surface of the ulna distal to the origin of extensor pollicis longus; posterior aspect of the interosseous membrane.	Ulnar side of the extensor digitorum tendon to the index finger at the level of the second metacarpal head.
Extensor Digiti Minimi	
Common extensor origin on the lateral epicondyle of the humerus.	Dorsal digital expansion of the fifth digit.

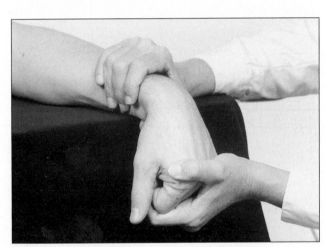

Figure 5-86 Extensor digitorum communis, extensor indicis proprius, and extensor digiti minimi on stretch.

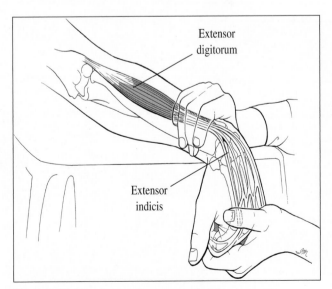

Extensor digitorum

Extensor indicis

Figure 5-87 Long finger extensors on stretch.

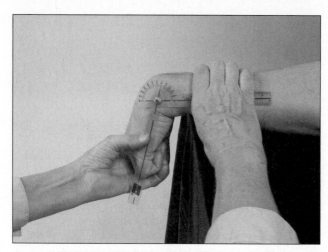

Figure 5-88 Goniometer measurement: length of long finger extensors.

Assessment and Measurement. If the finger extensors are shortened, wrist flexion PROM will be restricted proportional to the degree of muscle shortening. The therapist either observes the available PROM or uses a goniometer (Fig. 5-88) to measure and record the available wrist flexion PROM.

End Feel. Long finger extensors on stretch—firm.

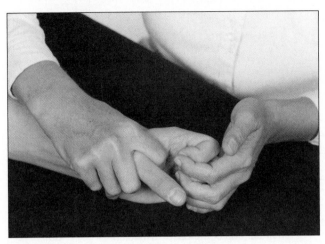

Figure 5-89 Start position: length of lumbricales.

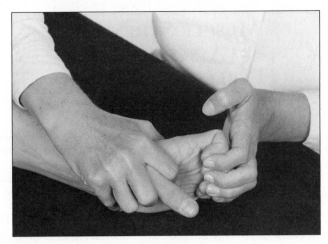

Figure 5-90 Lumbricales on stretch.

Lumbricales

Form 5-21

Start Position. The patient is in sitting or supine with the elbow flexed, forearm in midposition or supination, and the wrist in extension. The IP joints of the fingers are flexed (Fig. 5-89).

Stabilization. The therapist stabilizes the metacarpals.

End Position. The therapist simultaneously applies over-pressure to flex the IP joints and extends the MCP joints of the fingers to the limit of motion so that lumbricales are put on full stretch (Figs. 5-90 and 5-91). The lumbricales may be stretched as a group or individually.

Assessment and Measurement. If the lumbricales are shortened, MCP joint extension ROM will be restricted proportional to the degree of muscle shortness. The therapist either observes the available PROM or uses a goniometer (Fig. 5-92) to measure and record the available MCP joint extension PROM.

End Feel. Lumbricales on stretch—firm.

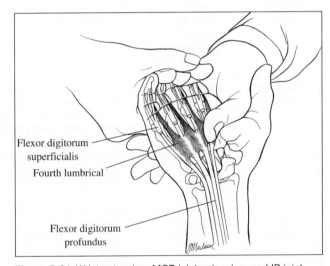

Flexor digitorum superficialis

Fourth lumbrical

Flexor digitorum profundus

Figure 5-91 Wrist extension, MCP joint extension, and IP joint flexion to place lumbricales on stretch.

Origin[2]	Insertion[2]
Lumbricales	
Tendons of flexor digitorum profundus:	Radial aspect of the dorsal digital expansion of the corresponding index, middle, ring, and little fingers.
a. First and second lumbricales: radial sides and palmar surfaces of the tendons of the index and middle fingers.	
b. Third: adjacent sides of the tendons of the middle and ring fingers.	
c. Fourth: adjacent sides of the tendons of the ring and little fingers.	

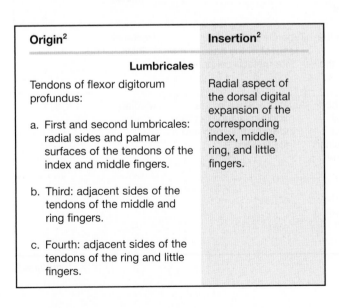

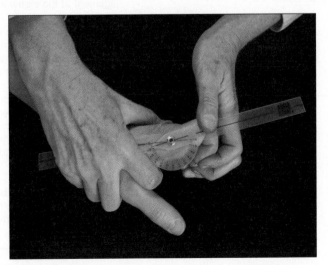

Figure 5-92 Goniometer measurement: length of lumbricales.

MUSCLE STRENGTH ASSESSMENT (TABLES 5-4 AND 5-5)

TABLE 5-4 Muscle Actions, Attachments, and Nerve Supply: The Wrist and Fingers[20]

Muscle	Primary Muscle Action	Muscle Origin	Muscle Insertion	Peripheral Nerve	Nerve Root
Flexor carpi radialis	Wrist flexion Wrist radial deviation	Common flexor origin on the medial epicondyle of the humerus	Palmar surface of the base of the second metacarpal and a slip to the base of the third metacarpal	Median	C67
Palmaris longus	Anchors palmar skin and fascia Wrist flexion	Common flexor origin on the medial epicondyle of the humerus	Distal palmar aspect of the flexor retinaculum; the palmar aponeurosis; skin and fascia of distal palm and webs of fingers	Median	C78
Flexor carpi ulnaris	Wrist flexion Wrist ulnar deviation	a. Humeral head: common flexor origin on the medial epicondyle of the humerus b. Ulnar head: medial margin of the olecranon process and by an aponeurosis on the upper two thirds of the posterior border of the ulna	Pisiform bone; sends slips to the hook of the hamate (pisohamate ligament), base of the fifth metacarpal (pisometacarpal ligament), and flexor retinaculum	Ulnar	C78T1
Extensor carpi radialis longus	Wrist extension Wrist radial deviation	Lower one third of the lateral supracondylar ridge of the humerus; common extensor origin on the lateral epicondyle of the humerus	Dorsal surface of the base of the second metacarpal bone	Radial	C67
Extensor carpi radialis brevis	Wrist extension Wrist radial deviation	Common extensor origin on the lateral epicondyle of the humerus; radial collateral ligament of the elbow joint	Dorsal surface of the base of the third metacarpal bone	Posterior interosseous (radial)	C78
Extensor carpi ulnaris	Wrist extension Wrist ulnar deviation	Common extensor origin on the lateral epicondyle of the humerus; aponeurosis on the posterior border of the ulna	Tubercle on the ulnar aspect of the base of the fifth metacarpal bone	Posterior interosseous	C78
Flexor digitorum superficialis	Finger PIP flexion	a. Humeroulnar head: common flexor origin on the medial epicondyle of the humerus, the anterior band of the ulnar collateral ligament, and the medial aspect of the coronoid process b. Radial head: anterior border of the radius from the radial tuberosity to the insertion of pronator teres	Anterior surface of the middle phalanges of the index, middle, ring and little fingers	Median	C8T1

(continued)

TABLE 5-4 *Continued*

Muscle	Primary Muscle Action	Muscle Origin	Muscle Insertion	Peripheral Nerve	Nerve Root
Flexor digitorum profundus	Finger DIP flexion	Upper three fourths of the anterior and medial aspects of the ulna; medial aspect of the coronoid process; by an aponeurosis on the upper three fourths of the posterior border of the ulna; anterior surface of the medial half of the interosseous membrane	Palmar aspect of the bases of the distal phalanges of the index, middle, ring, and little fingers	a. Lateral portion of muscle—anterior interosseus branch of median b. Medial portion of muscle—ulnar	C8T1
Extensor digitorum communis	Finger MCP extension	Common extensor origin on the lateral epicondyle of the humerus	Dorsal surfaces of the bases of the distal and middle phalanges of the index, middle, ring, and little fingers	Posterior interosseous	C78
Extensor indicis proprius	Index finger MCP extension	Posterior surface of the ulna distal to the origin of extensor pollicis longus; posterior aspect of the interosseous membrane	Ulnar side of the extensor digitorum tendon to the index finger at the level of the second metacarpal head	Posterior interosseous	C78
Extensor digiti minimi	Fifth finger MCP extension	Common extensor origin on the lateral epicondyle of the humerus	Dorsal digital expansion of the fifth digit	Posterior interosseous	C78
Interosseous a. Dorsal	Finger MCP abduction	a. First: adjacent sides of the first and second metacarpal bones b. Second: adjacent sides of the second and third metacarpal bones c. Third: adjacent sides of the third and fourth metacarpal bones d. Fourth: adjacent sides of the fourth and fifth metacarpal bones	All insert into the dorsal digital expansions of either the index, middle, or ring fingers a. First: radial aspect of the base of the proximal phalanx of the index finger b. Second and third: radial and ulnar aspects respectively, of the base of the proximal phalanx of the middle finger c. Fourth: ulnar aspect of the base of the proximal phalanx of the ring finger	Ulnar	C8T1
b. Palmar	Finger MCP adduction	a. First: ulnar side of the base of the first metacarpal bone b. Second: ulnar side of the palmar aspect of the second metacarpal bone c. Third: radial side of the palmar aspect of the fourth metacarpal bone d. Fourth: radial side of the palmar aspect of the fifth metacarpal bone	All insert into the dorsal digital expansions of either the thumb, index, ring, or little fingers The first also inserts into the sesamoid bone on the ulnar side of the base of the proximal phalanx of the thumb and into the phalanx The fourth also inserts into the radial side of the base of the proximal phalanx of the little finger	Ulnar	C8T1

(continued)

TABLE 5-4 *Continued*

Muscle	Primary Muscle Action	Muscle Origin	Muscle Insertion	Peripheral Nerve	Nerve Root
Lumbricales	Finger MCP flexion and IP extension	Tendons of flexor digitorum profundus: a. First and second lumbricales: radial sides and palmar surfaces of the tendons of the index and middle fingers b. Third: adjacent sides of the tendons of the middle and ring fingers c. Fourth: adjacent sides of the tendons of the ring and little fingers	Radial aspect of the dorsal digital expansion of the corresponding index, middle, ring, and little fingers	a. Medial two lumbricales—ulnar b. Lateral two lumbricales—median	C8T1 C8T1
Abductor digiti minimi	Little finger MCP abduction	Pisiform bone; pisohamate ligament; tendon of flexor carpi ulnaris	Ulnar aspect of the base of the proximal phalanx of the little finger; dorsal digital expansion of the little finger	Ulnar	C8T1
Opponens digiti minimi	Little finger opposition (flexion, and internal rotation of the 5th metacarpal bone)	Hook of hamate; flexor retinaculum	Ulnar and adjacent palmar surface of the fifth metacarpal bone	Ulnar	C8T1
Flexor digiti minimi	Little finger MCP flexion	Hook of hamate; flexor retinaculum	Ulnar aspect of the base of the proximal phalanx of the little finger	Ulnar	C8T1

TABLE 5-5   Muscle Actions, Attachments, and Nerve Supply: the Thumb[20]

Muscle	Primary Muscle Action	Muscle Origin	Muscle Insertion	Peripheral Nerve	Nerve Root
Flexor pollicis longus	Thumb IP joint flexion	Anterior surface of the radius between the bicipital tuberosity and the pronator quadratus; anterior surface of the lateral half of the interosseous membrane; lateral aspect of the coronoid process and the medial epicondyle of the humerus	Palmar aspect of the base of the distal phalanx of the thumb	Anterior interosseous branch of median	C78
Flexor pollicis brevis	Thumb MCP joint flexion	1. Superficial head: flexor retinaculum and the tubercle of the trapezium bone 2. Deep head: capitate and trapezoid bones and the palmar ligaments of the distal row of carpal bones	The radial side of the base of the proximal phalanx of the thumb	1. Superficial head— median 2. Deep head— ulnar	C8T1
Extensor pollicis longus	Thumb IP joint extension	Middle third of the posterolateral aspect of the ulna; posterior surface of the interosseous membrane	Dorsal aspect of the base of the distal phalanx of the thumb	Posterior interosseous	C78
Extensor pollicis brevis	Thumb MCP joint extension	Posterior aspect of the radius below the abductor pollicis longus; posterior surface of the interosseous membrane	Dorsal aspect of the base of the proximal phalanx of the thumb	Posterior interosseous	C78
Abductor pollicis longus	Thumb radial abduction	Posterior aspect of the shaft of the ulna distal to the insertion of anconeus; posterior aspect of the shaft of the radius distal to the insertion of supinator; posterior aspect of the interosseous membrane	Radial aspect of the base of the first metacarpal bone; the trapezium bone	Posterior interosseous	C78
Abductor pollicis brevis	Thumb palmar abduction	Flexor retinaculum; tubercles of the scaphoid and trapezium bones; tendon of abductor pollicis longus	Radial aspect of the base of the proximal phalanx of the thumb; dorsal digital expansion of the thumb	Median	C8T1
Adductor pollicis	Thumb adduction	1. Oblique head: capitate bone and the palmar surfaces of the bases of the second and third metacarpal bones 2. Transverse head: distal two thirds of the palmar surface of the shaft of the third metacarpal bone	Ulnar aspect of the base of the proximal phalanx of the thumb; dorsal digital expansion of the thumb	Ulnar	C8T1
Opponens pollicis	Thumb opposition (abduction, flexion, and internal rotation of the first metacarpal bone)	Flexor retinaculum; tubercle of the trapezium bone	Lateral surface and lateral aspect of the palmar surface of the first metacarpal bone	Median	C8T1

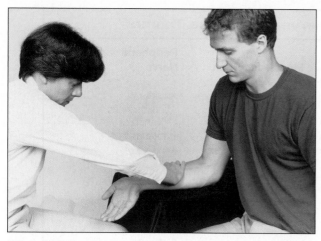

Figure 5-93 Start position: flexor carpi radialis.

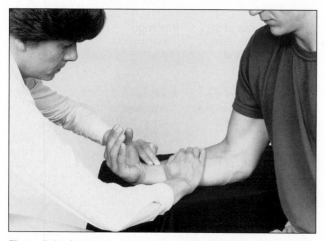

Figure 5-94 Screen position: flexor carpi radialis.

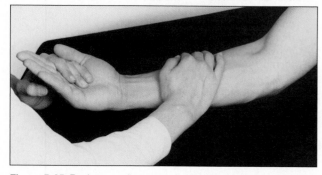

Figure 5-95 Resistance: flexor carpi radialis.

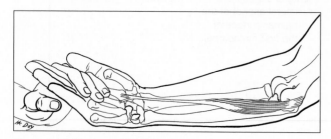

Figure 5-96 Flexor carpi radialis.

Practice Makes Perfect

To aid you in practicing the skills covered in this section, or for a handy review, use the practical testing forms found at
http://thepoint.lww.com/Clarkson3e.

Wrist Flexion and Radial Deviation

Against Gravity: Flexor Carpi Radialis

 Accessory muscles: flexor carpi ulnaris and palmaris longus.

Form 5-22 **Start Position.** The patient is sitting or supine. If sitting, the forearm is supinated and supported on a table. The wrist is extended and in ulnar deviation and the fingers and thumb are relaxed (Fig. 5-93).

Stabilization. The therapist stabilizes the forearm proximal to the wrist.

Movement. The patient flexes and radially deviates the wrist (Fig. 5-94). The patient should be instructed to keep the fingers and thumb relaxed.

Palpation. Anterolateral aspect of the wrist in line with the second web space, on the radial side of palmaris longus.

Substitute Movement. The patient may flex the wrist with palmaris longus and flexor carpi ulnaris. Using flexor carpi ulnaris alone, the patient will flex with ulnar deviation. If the patient flexes the fingers, the flexor digitorum superficialis and profundus may substitute for the wrist flexors when movement is initiated.[21]

Resistance Location. Applied distal to the wrist over the thenar eminence or the lateral aspect of the palm (Figs. 5-95 and 5-96).

Resistance Direction. Wrist extension and ulnar deviation.

Gravity Eliminated: Flexor Carpi Radialis

Start Position. The patient is sitting or supine. The forearm is in slight pronation and supported on a table or powder board. The wrist is extended and in ulnar deviation and the fingers and thumb are relaxed (Fig. 5-97).

Stabilization. The therapist stabilizes the forearm proximal to the wrist.

End Position. The patient flexes and radially deviates the wrist through full ROM (Fig. 5-98).

Substitute Movement. Flexor carpi ulnaris, palmaris longus, and flexor digitorum superficialis and profundus. As the patient flexes the wrist from the anatomical position, forearm pronation and thumb abduction through the action of abductor pollicis longus may be attempted.

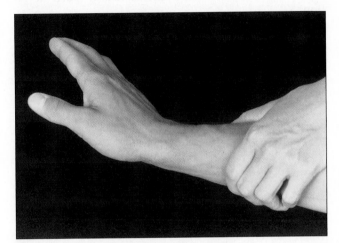

Figure 5-97 Start position: flexor carpi radialis.

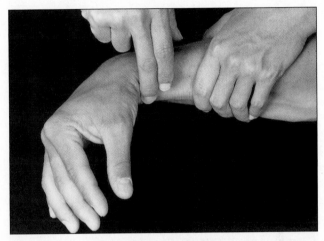

Figure 5-98 End position: flexor carpi radialis.

Wrist Flexion and Ulnar Deviation

Against Gravity: Flexor Carpi Ulnaris

 Accessory muscles: flexor carpi radialis and palmaris longus.

Form 5-23 **Start Position.** The patient is sitting or supine. If sitting, the forearm is supinated and supported on a table. The wrist is extended and in radial deviation, and the fingers and thumb are relaxed (Fig. 5-99).

Stabilization. The therapist stabilizes the forearm proximal to the wrist.

Movement. The patient flexes and ulnarly deviates the wrist through full ROM (Fig. 5-100).

Palpation. Anteromedial aspect of the wrist proximal to the pisiform bone.

Substitute Movement. Flexor carpi radialis, palmaris longus, and flexor digitorum superficialis and profundus. Using flexor carpi radialis alone, the patient will flex with radial deviation.

Resistance Location. Applied over the hypothenar eminence (Figs. 5-101 and 5-102).

Resistance Direction. Wrist extension and radial deviation.

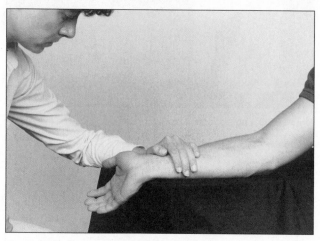

Figure 5-99 Start position: flexor carpi ulnaris.

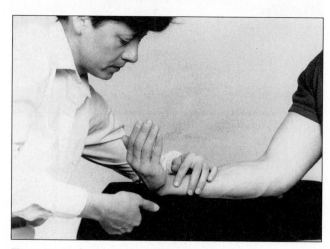

Figure 5-100 Screen position: flexor carpi ulnaris.

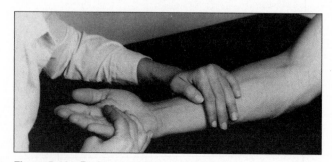

Figure 5-101 Resistance: flexor carpi ulnaris.

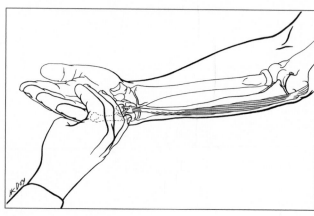

Figure 5-102 Flexor carpi ulnaris.

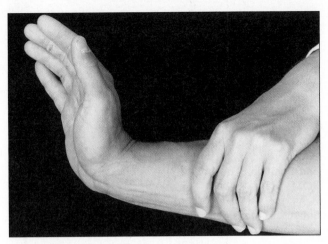

Figure 5-103 Start position: flexor carpi ulnaris.

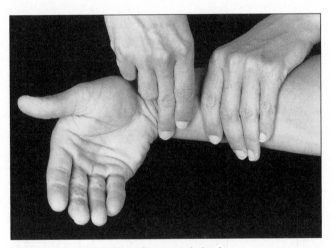

Figure 5-104 End position: flexor carpi ulnaris.

Gravity Eliminated: Flexor Carpi Ulnaris

Start Position. The patient is sitting or supine. The forearm is in slight supination and supported on a table or powder board. The wrist is extended and in radial deviation, and the fingers and thumb are relaxed (Fig. 5-103).

Stabilization. The therapist stabilizes the forearm proximal to the wrist.

End Position. The patient flexes the wrist with ulnar deviation through full ROM (Fig. 5-104).

Substitute Movement. Flexor carpi radialis, palmaris longus, and flexor digitorum superficialis and profundus.

Wrist Flexion (Not Shown)

Against Gravity: Flexor Carpi Radialis and Flexor Carpi Ulnaris

 Accessory muscle: palmaris longus.

Form 5-24 **Start Position.** The patient is sitting or supine. If sitting, the forearm is supinated and supported on a table. The wrist is extended and the fingers and thumb are relaxed.

Stabilization. The therapist stabilizes the forearm proximal to the wrist.

Movement. The patient flexes the wrist through full ROM.

Palpation. *Flexor carpi radialis:* Anterolateral aspect of the wrist in line with the second web space, on the radial side of palmaris longus. *Flexor carpi ulnaris:* anteromedial aspect of the wrist proximal to the pisiform bone.

Substitute Movement. Flexor digitorum superficialis and profundus.

Resistance Location. Applied over the palm of the hand.

Resistance Direction. Wrist extension.

Gravity Eliminated: Flexor Carpi Radialis and Flexor Carpi Ulnaris

Start Position. The patient is sitting or supine. The forearm is in midposition and supported on a table or powder board. The wrist is extended and the fingers and thumb are relaxed.

Stabilization. The therapist stabilizes the forearm proximal to the wrist.

End Position. The patient flexes the wrist through full ROM.

Substitute Movement. Flexor digitorum superficialis and profundus.

Palmaris Longus

Palmaris longus is a weak flexor of the wrist and is not isolated for individual muscle testing. It can be palpated on the midline of the anterior aspect of the wrist during testing of flexor carpi radialis and ulnaris.

The presence of palmaris longus can be established through flexing the wrist and cupping the fingers and palm of the hand (Figs. 5-105 and 5-106). The muscle tendon stands out boldly when present. However, palmaris longus is a vestigial muscle in about 13% of subjects.[22] A decrease of grip or pinch strength is not associated with the absence of palmaris longus.[23]

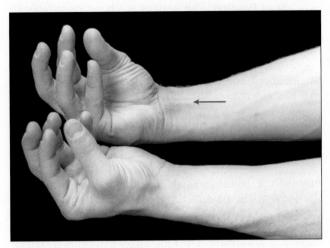

Figure 5-105 Palmaris longus: the muscle is present in the right arm (observe the tendon at the wrist). The muscle is absent in the left arm.

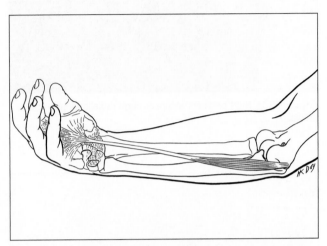

Figure 5-106 Palmaris longus.

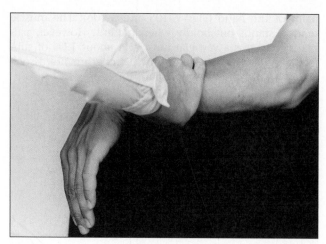

Figure 5-107 Start position: extensor carpi radialis longus and brevis.

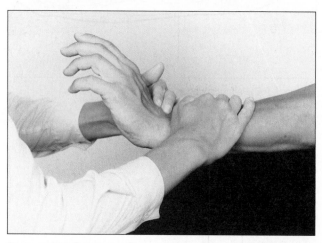

Figure 5-108 Screen position: extensor carpi radialis longus and brevis.

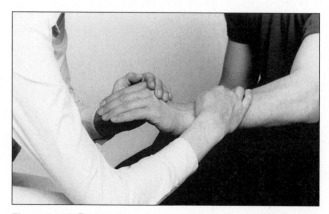

Figure 5-109 Resistance: extensor carpi radialis longus and brevis.

Wrist Extension and Radial Deviation

Against Gravity: Extensor Carpi Radialis Longus and Extensor Carpi Radialis Brevis

 Accessory muscle: extensor carpi ulnaris.

Form 5-25 **Start Position.** The patient is sitting or supine. In sitting, the forearm is pronated and supported on a table. The wrist is flexed and in ulnar deviation and the fingers and thumb are slightly flexed (Fig. 5-107).

Stabilization. The therapist stabilizes the forearm proximal to the wrist.

Movement. The patient extends and radially deviates the wrist through full ROM (Fig. 5-108). The patient should be instructed to keep the thumb and fingers relaxed.

Palpation. *Extensor carpi radialis longus:* dorsal aspect of the wrist at the base of the second metacarpal. *Extensor carpi radialis brevis:* base of the third metacarpal.

Substitute Movement. The long finger extensors (extensor digitorum communis, extensor indicis, extensor digiti minimi). The patient may extend using extensor carpi ulnaris. Using only this muscle, the patient will extend with ulnar deviation.

Resistance Location. Applied on the dorsal aspect of the hand over the second and third metacarpals (Figs. 5-109 and 5-110).

Resistance Direction. Wrist flexion and ulnar deviation.

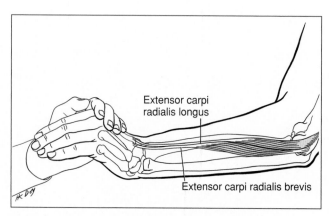

Figure 5-110 Extensor carpi radialis longus and brevis.

Gravity Eliminated: Extensor Carpi Radialis Longus and Extensor Carpi Radialis Brevis

Start Position. The patient is sitting or supine. The forearm is in slight supination and supported on a table or powder board. The wrist is flexed in ulnar deviation. The fingers and thumb are slightly flexed (Fig. 5-111).

Stabilization. The therapist stabilizes the forearm proximal to the wrist.

End Position. The patient extends the wrist with simultaneous radial deviation through full ROM (Fig. 5-112).

Substitute Movement. The long finger extensors (extensor digitorum communis, extensor indicis, and extensor digiti minimi). Extensor carpi ulnaris.

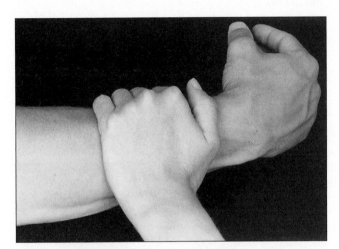

Figure 5-111 Start position: extensor carpi radialis longus and brevis.

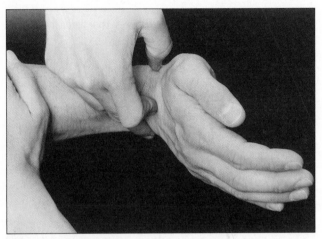

Figure 5-112 End position: extensor carpi radialis longus and brevis.

Wrist Extension and Ulnar Deviation

Against Gravity: Extensor Carpi Ulnaris

 Accessory muscles: extensor carpi radialis longus and brevis.

Form 5-26

Start Position. The patient is sitting or supine. If sitting, the forearm is pronated and supported on a table. The wrist is flexed and in radial deviation, and the fingers and thumb are slightly flexed (Fig. 5-113).

Stabilization. The therapist stabilizes the forearm proximal to the wrist.

Movement. The patient extends and ulnarly deviates the wrist through full ROM (Fig. 5-114). The patient should be instructed to keep the fingers relaxed.

Palpation. On the dorsal aspect of the wrist proximal to the fifth metacarpal and distal to the ulnar styloid process.

Substitute Movement. The long finger extensors (extensor digitorum communis, extensor indicis, extensor digiti minimi). The patient may extend and radially deviate the wrist through the action of extensor carpi radialis longus and brevis.

Resistance Location. Applied on the dorsal aspect of the hand over the fourth and fifth metacarpals (Figs. 5-115 and 5-116).

Resistance Direction. Wrist flexion and radial deviation.

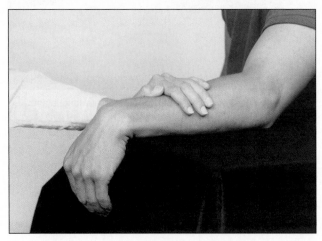

Figure 5-113 Start position: extensor carpi ulnaris.

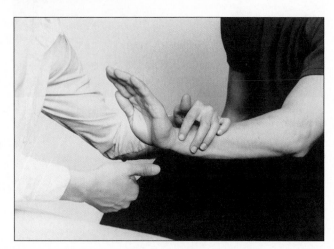

Figure 5-114 Screen position: extensor carpi ulnaris.

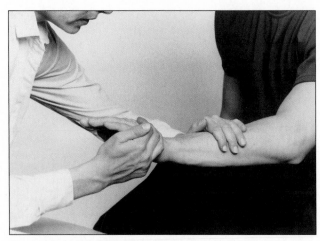

Figure 5-115 Resistance: extensor carpi ulnaris.

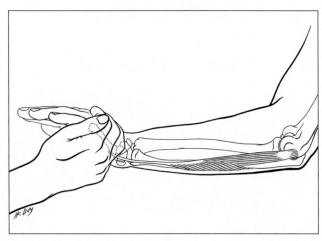

Figure 5-116 Extensor carpi ulnaris.

Gravity Eliminated: Extensor Carpi Ulnaris

Start Position. The patient is sitting or supine. The forearm is in slight pronation and supported on a table or powder board. The wrist is flexed in radial deviation. The fingers and thumb are flexed (Fig. 5-117).

Stabilization. The therapist stabilizes the forearm proximal to the wrist.

End Position. The patient extends the wrist with simultaneous ulnar deviation through full ROM (Fig. 5-118).

Substitute Movement. The long finger extensors (extensor digitorum communis, extensor indicis, extensor digiti minimi). Extensor carpi radialis longus and brevis.

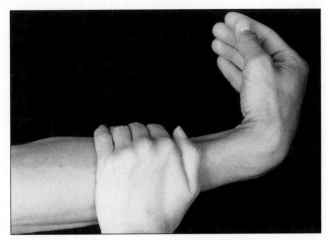

Figure 5-117 Start position: extensor carpi ulnaris.

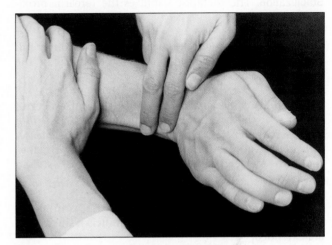

Figure 5-118 End position: extensor carpi ulnaris.

Wrist Extension (Not Shown)

Against Gravity: Extensor Carpi Radialis Longus, Extensor Carpi Radialis Brevis, and Extensor Carpi Ulnaris

Form 5-27

Start Position. The patient is sitting or supine. If sitting, the forearm is pronated and supported on a table. The wrist is flexed and the fingers and thumb are relaxed.

Stabilization. The therapist stabilizes the forearm proximal to the wrist.

Movement. The patient extends the wrist through full ROM. The patient should be instructed to keep the thumb and fingers relaxed.

Palpation. *Extensor carpi radialis longus:* dorsal aspect of the wrist at the base of the second metacarpal. *Extensor carpi radialis brevis:* base of the third metacarpal. *Extensor carpi ulnaris:* on the dorsal aspect of the wrist proximal to the fifth metacarpal and distal to the ulnar styloid process.

Substitute Movement. Extensor digitorum communis, extensor digiti minimi, and extensor indicis if the fingers are extended.

Resistance Location. Applied on the dorsal aspect of the hand over the metacarpals.

Resistance Direction. Wrist flexion.

Gravity Eliminated: Extensor Carpi Radialis Longus, Extensor Carpi Radialis Brevis, and Extensor Carpi Ulnaris

Start Position. The patient is sitting or supine. The forearm is in midposition and supported on a table or powder board. The wrist is flexed, and the fingers and thumb are relaxed.

Stabilization. The therapist stabilizes the forearm proximal to the wrist.

End Position. The patient extends the wrist through full ROM.

Substitute Movement. Extensor digitorum, extensor digiti minimi, extensor indicis.

Finger and Thumb Muscles

Gravity is not considered to be a factor in manual muscle testing of the fingers and thumb because the weight of the part is small in comparison to the strength of the muscle.[21] The muscles of the fingers and toes may be tested in either a gravity eliminated or an against gravity position for all grades. Table 5-6 gives a description of the grading for the fingers and toes.

TABLE 5-6	Grading for the Fingers and Toes
Numeral	**Description**
	The patient is able to actively move through:
5	The full available ROM against maximal resistance, gravity eliminated or against gravity
4	The full available ROM against moderate resistance, gravity eliminated or against gravity
3	The full available ROM, gravity eliminated or against gravity
2	Part of the available ROM, gravity eliminated or against gravity
1	None of the available ROM, but there is a palpable or observable flicker of a muscle contraction, gravity eliminated or against gravity
0	None of the available ROM, and there is no palpable or observable muscle contraction, gravity eliminated or against gravity

Finger Metacarpophalangeal Extension

Extensor Digitorum Communis, Extensor Indicis Proprius, and Extensor Digiti Minimi

Form 5-28

Start Position. The patient is sitting or supine. The forearm is pronated, the wrist is in a neutral position, and the fingers are flexed (Fig. 5-119).

Stabilization. The therapist stabilizes the metacarpals.

Movement. The patient extends all four MCP joints while maintaining flexion at the IP joints (Fig. 5-120).

Palpation (Fig. 5-121). *Extensor digitorum:* the tendons to each finger can be palpated on the dorsum of the hand proximal to each metacarpal head. *Extensor indicis:* medial to the extensor digitorum tendon to the index finger. *Extensor digiti minimi:* lateral to the extensor digitorum tendon to the little finger.

Substitute Movement. Stabilization of the wrist prevents the tenodesis effect of wrist flexion and subsequent MCP extension.[14,19]

Resistance Location. Dorsal aspect of the proximal phalanx of each finger (Figs. 5-122 and 5-123).

Resistance Direction. MCP flexion.

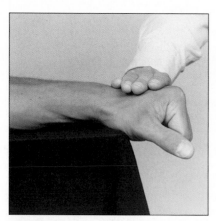

Figure 5-119 Start position: extensor digitorum, extensor indicis proprius, and extensor digiti minimi.

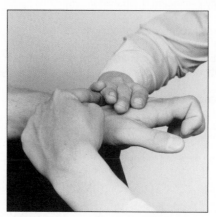

Figure 5-120 Screen position: extensor digitorum, extensor indicis, and extensor digiti minimi.

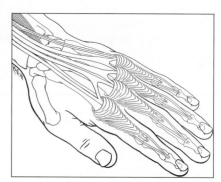

Figure 5-121 Extensor expansion.

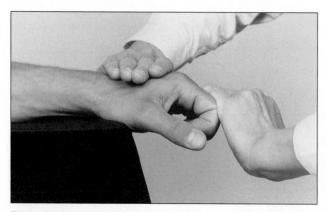

Figure 5-122 Resistance: extensor digitorum, extensor indicis, and extensor digiti minimi.

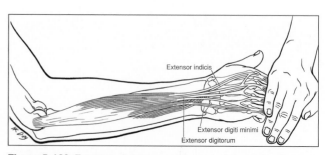

Figure 5-123 Extensor digitorum, extensor indicis, and extensor digiti minimi.

Metacarpophalangeal Abduction

Dorsal Interossei and Abductor Digiti Minimi

Start Position. The patient is sitting or supine. Dorsal interossei (Fig. 5-124): the forearm is pronated and supported on a table, the wrist is in neutral, and the fingers are extended and adducted. Abductor digiti minimi (Fig. 5-125): the forearm is supinated.

Forms 5-29, 5-30

Stabilization. Dorsal interossei: the therapist stabilizes the dorsum of the hand over the metacarpal bones and wrist. Abductor digiti minimi: the therapist stabilizes the wrist and lateral three metacarpals. The adjacent finger away from which the finger is moving may also be stabilized.

Movement. Dorsal interossei (Fig. 5-126): the patient abducts the index finger toward the thumb, the middle finger toward the index finger and then ring finger, and the ring finger toward the little finger. To prevent assistance from an adjacent finger, the nontest digits may require stabilization. Abductor digiti minimi (Fig. 5-127): the patient abducts the little finger.

Palpation. The *first dorsal interosseous* is palpated on the radial aspect of the second metacarpal (see Fig. 5-126). The remaining interossei cannot be palpated. *Abductor digiti minimi* is palpated on the ulnar aspect of the fifth metacarpal (see Fig. 5-127).

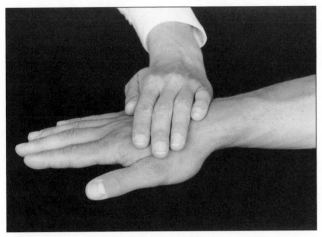

Figure 5-124 Start position: dorsal interossei.

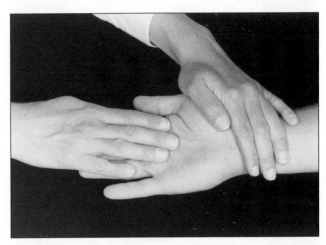

Figure 5-125 Start position: abductor digiti minimi.

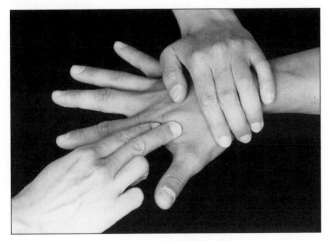

Figure 5-126 Screen position: dorsal interossei.

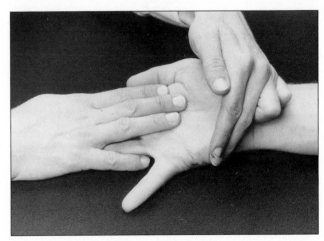

Figure 5-127 Screen position: abductor digiti minimi.

Substitute Movement. Maintain the MCP joints in neutral position to avoid finger abduction through contraction of the extensor digitorum communis.

Resistance Location. Against the proximal phalanx of the digit being tested. The therapist resists on the radial side of the index and middle fingers and the ulnar side of the middle, ring (Figs. 5-128 and 5-129), and little fingers (Figs. 5-130 and 5-131).

Resistance Direction. Adduction.

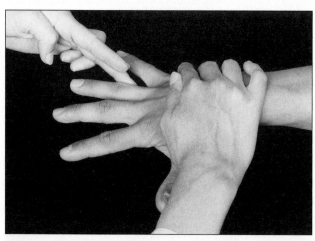

Figure 5-128 Resistance: fourth dorsal interosseous.

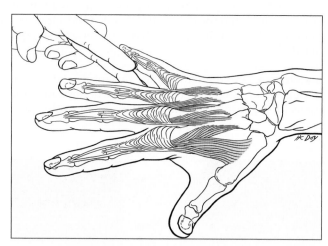

Figure 5-129 Dorsal interossei.

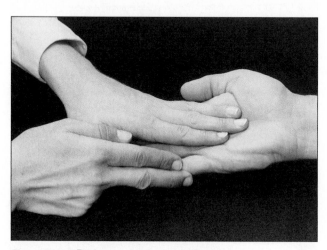

Figure 5-130 Resistance: abductor digiti minimi.

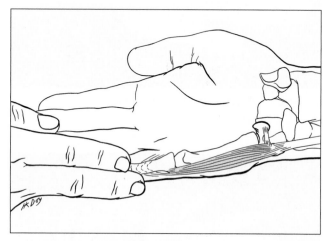

Figure 5-131 Abductor digiti minimi.

Metacarpophalangeal Adduction

Palmar Interossei

Form 5-31

Start Position. The patient is sitting or supine. If sitting, the forearm is supinated and supported on a table, the wrist is in neutral, and the fingers are abducted (Fig. 5-132).

Stabilization. The therapist stabilizes the metacarpal bones and wrist. The adjacent finger toward which the finger is moving may also be stabilized (not shown).

Movement. The patient adducts the index, ring, and little finger toward the middle finger (Fig. 5-133).

Palpation. These muscles cannot be palpated.

Substitute Movement. None.

Resistance Location. Against the proximal phalanx of the digit being tested (Figs. 5-134 and 5-135). The therapist resists on the ulnar aspect of the index finger and on the radial aspect of the ring and fifth fingers.

Resistance Direction. Abduction.

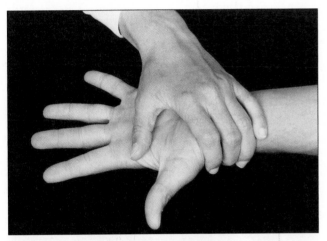

Figure 5-132 Start position: palmar interossei.

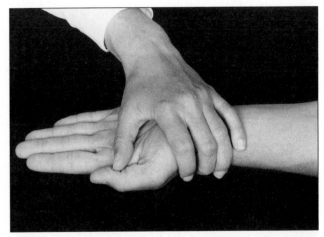

Figure 5-133 Screen position: palmar interossei.

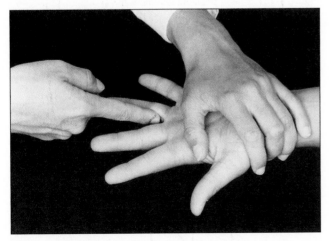

Figure 5-134 Resistance: third palmar interosseous.

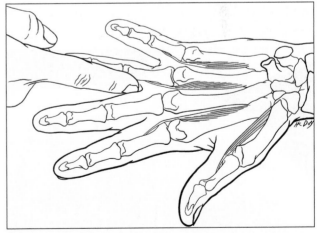

Figure 5-135 Palmar interossei.

Finger Metacarpophalangeal Flexion and Interphalangeal Extension

Lumbricales

The interossei muscles also flex the MCP joints and simultaneously extend the IP joints. The interossei have been isolated for testing as abductors and adductors. Should the interossei be strong, weakness elicited in this muscle test may be attributed to lumbricales. Accessory muscle: flexor digiti minimi (MCP joint flexion).

Form 5-32

Start Position. The patient is sitting or supine. The forearm is pronated or in midposition, supported on a table. The wrist is in a neutral position, the MCP joints are extended and adducted, and the IP joints are slightly flexed (Fig. 5-136).

Stabilization. The therapist stabilizes the metacarpals.

Movement. The patient flexes the MCP joints while simultaneously extending the IP joints (Fig. 5-137). The fingers are allowed to abduct to prevent assistance from adjacent fingers in static adduction.

Palpation. The lumbricales cannot be palpated.

Substitute Movement. Extensor digitorum communis.

Resistance Location. Applied on the volar surface of the proximal phalanx and the dorsal surface of the middle phalanx (Figs. 5-138 and 5-139).

Resistance Direction. MCP extension and IP flexion.

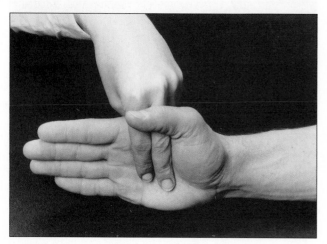

Figure 5-136 Start position: lumbricales.

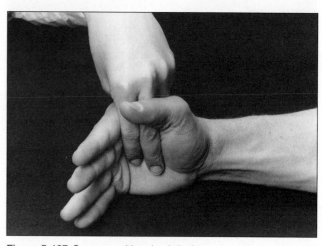

Figure 5-137 Screen position: lumbricales.

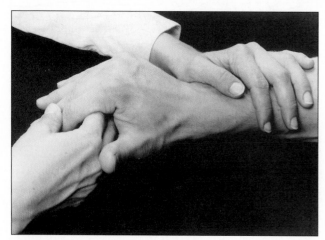

Figure 5-138 Resistance: first lumbricalis.

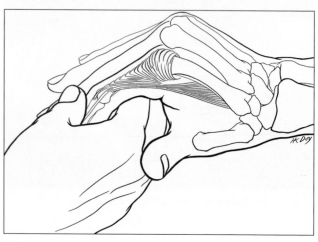

Figure 5-139 First lumbricalis.

Fifth Finger Metacarpophalangeal Flexion

Flexor Digiti Minimi

Form 5-33 Accessory muscles: fourth lumbricalis, fourth palmar interosseous, and abductor digiti minimi.

Start Position. The patient is sitting or supine. If sitting, the forearm is supinated and supported on a table. The wrist is in a neutral position and the fingers are extended (Fig. 5-140).

Stabilization. The therapist stabilizes the metacarpals.

Movement. The patient flexes the MCP joint of the little finger while maintaining IP joint extension (Fig. 5-141).

Palpation. On the hypothenar eminence medial to abductor digiti minimi.

Substitute Movement. The patient may attempt to use flexor digitorum superficialis and profundus. Ensure that no flexion of the IP joints occurs. If flexion cannot be initiated, the patient may abduct the little finger through the action of abductor digiti minimi.

Resistance Location. Applied on the volar aspect of the proximal phalanx of the little finger (Figs. 5-142 and 5-143).

Resistance Direction. Extension.

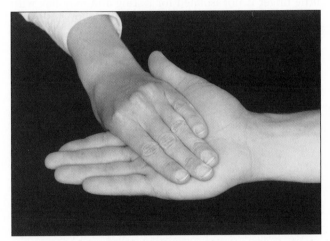

Figure 5-140 Start position: flexor digiti minimi.

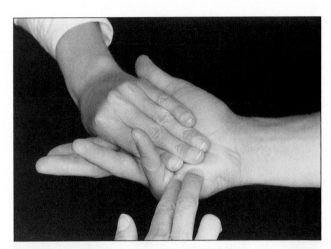

Figure 5-141 Screen position: flexor digiti minimi.

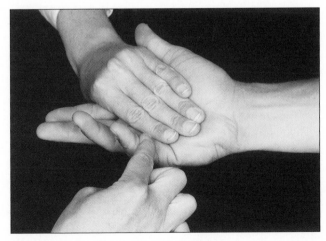

Figure 5-142 Resistance: flexor digiti minimi.

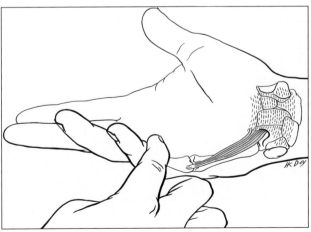

Figure 5-143 Flexor digiti minimi.

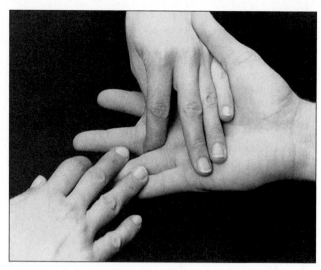

Figure 5-144 Start position: flexor digitorum superficialis.

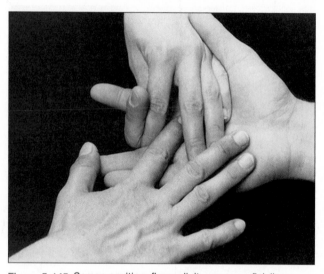

Figure 5-145 Screen position: flexor digitorum superficialis.

Finger Proximal Interphalangeal Flexion

Flexor Digitorum Superficialis

 Accessory muscle: flexor digitorum profundus.

Form 5-34

Start Position. The patient is sitting or supine. In sitting, the forearm is supinated and supported on a table. The wrist is in a neutral position or slight extension and the fingers are extended. To rule out the contribution of flexor digitorum profundus, the fingers not being tested may be held in extension[24] (Fig. 5-144).

Stabilization. The therapist stabilizes the metacarpals and the proximal phalanx of the finger being tested.

Movement. The patient flexes the PIP joint of each finger while maintaining DIP joint extension (Fig. 5-145). The little finger is not isolated for testing and may flex with the ring finger. Isolated action of the little finger superficialis is not always possible.[25]

Palpation. On the volar surface of the wrist between the palmaris longus and flexor carpi ulnaris tendons or on the proximal phalanx.

Substitute Movement. Flexor digitorum profundus. The flexor digitorum profundus tendons to the ulnar three fingers often originate from a common muscle belly; thus, the action of the profundus is interdependent in these fingers.[26] Therefore, holding the nontest fingers in extension eliminates normal function of the profundus tendon of the test finger.

Resistance Location. Applied on the volar surface of the middle phalanx (Figs. 5-146 and 5-147).

Resistance Direction. Extension.

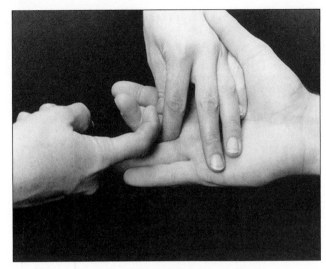

Figure 5-146 Resistance: flexor digitorum superficialis.

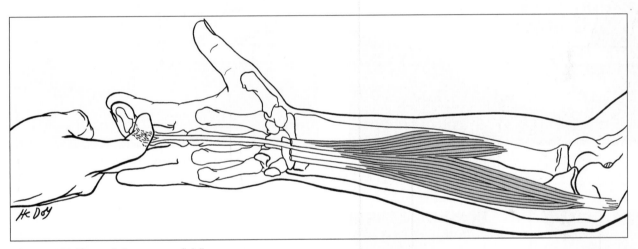

Figure 5-147 Flexor digitorum superficialis.

Finger Distal Interphalangeal Flexion

Flexor Digitorum Profundus

Start Position. The patient is sitting or supine. If sitting, the forearm is supinated and supported on a table. The wrist is in a neutral position or slight extension and the test finger is in extension (Fig. 5-148).

Form 5-35

Stabilization. The therapist stabilizes the proximal and middle phalanges of the test finger.

Movement. The patient flexes the DIP joint through full ROM (Fig. 5-149).

The flexor digitorum profundus tendons to the ulnar three fingers often originate from a common muscle belly; thus, the action of the profundus is interdependent in these fingers and the nontest fingers should be held in slight flexion during testing.[26]

Palpation. On the volar surface of the middle phalanx.

Resistance Location. Applied on the volar aspect of the distal phalanx (Figs. 5-150 and 5-151).

Resistance Direction. Extension.

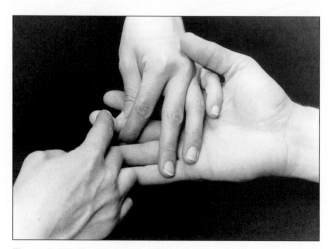

Figure 5-148 Start position: flexor digitorum profundus.

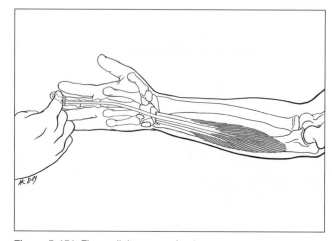

Figure 5-149 Screen position: flexor digitorum profundus.

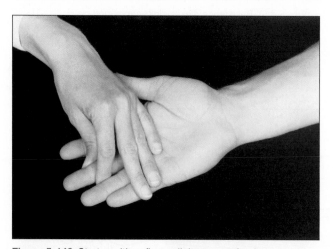

Figure 5-150 Resistance: flexor digitorum profundus.

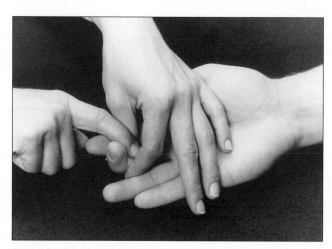

Figure 5-151 Flexor digitorum profundus.

Thumb Interphalangeal Flexion

Flexor Pollicis Longus

Form 5-36

Start Position. The patient is sitting or supine. The forearm is supinated, the wrist is in a neutral position, and the thumb is extended (Fig. 5-152).

Stabilization. The therapist stabilizes the wrist, the thumb metacarpal, and proximal phalanx.

Movement. The patient flexes the IP joint through full ROM (Fig. 5-153).

Palpation. Volar aspect of the proximal phalanx.

Substitute Movement. The relaxation of the thumb following extension of the IP joint may give the appearance of contraction of flexor pollicis longus.

Resistance Location. Applied on the volar surface of the distal phalanx (Figs. 5-154 and 5-155).

Resistance Direction. Extension.

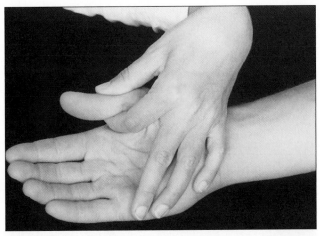

Figure 5-152 Start position: flexor pollicis longus.

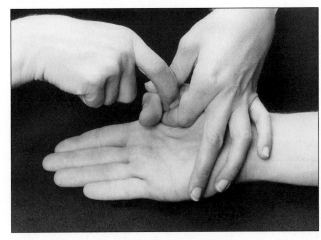

Figure 5-153 Screen position: flexor pollicis longus.

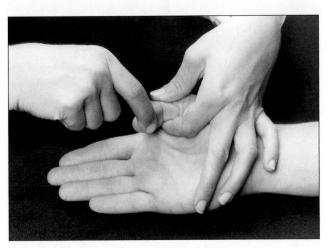

Figure 5-154 Resistance: flexor pollicis longus.

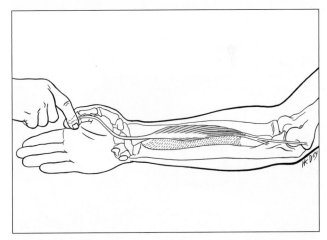

Figure 5-155 Flexor pollicis longus.

Thumb Metacarpophalangeal Flexion

Flexor Pollicis Brevis

Accessory muscle: flexor pollicis longus.

Form 5-37

Start Position. The patient is sitting or supine. The forearm is supinated, the wrist is in a neutral position, and the thumb is extended and adducted (Fig. 5-156).

Stabilization. The therapist stabilizes the wrist and thumb metacarpal.

Movement. The patient flexes the MCP joint while maintaining extension of the IP joint to minimize the action of flexor pollicis longus (Fig. 5-157).

Palpation. Proximal to the MCP joint on the middle of the thenar eminence, medial to abductor pollicis brevis.

Substitute Movement. Flexor pollicis longus.

Resistance Location. Applied on the volar aspect of the proximal phalanx (Figs. 5-158 and 5-159).

Resistance Direction. Extension.

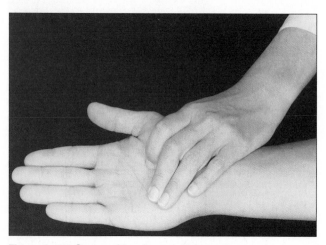

Figure 5-156 Start position: flexor pollicis brevis.

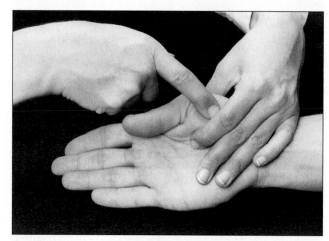

Figure 5-157 Screen position: flexor pollicis brevis.

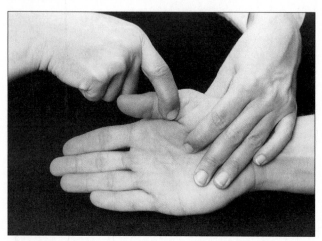

Figure 5-158 Resistance: flexor pollicis brevis.

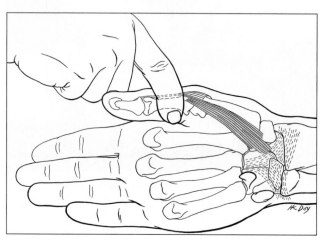

Figure 5-159 Flexor pollicis brevis.

Thumb Interphalangeal Extension

Extensor Pollicis Longus

Start Position. The patient is sitting or supine. The forearm is in midposition or slight pronation and the wrist is in a neutral position. The thumb is adducted with the MCP joint extended and the IP joint flexed (Fig. 5-160).

Form 5-38

Stabilization. The therapist stabilizes the thumb metacarpal and proximal phalanx.

Movement. The patient extends the IP joint through full ROM (Fig. 5-161A).

Palpation. On the dorsal surface of the proximal phalanx or on the ulnar border of the anatomical snuff box (see Fig. 5-161B).

Substitute Movement. Positioning of the thumb in adduction limits the extensor action of abductor pollicis brevis and flexor pollicis brevis.[24] Rebound of contraction of flexor pollicis longus.

Resistance Location. Applied on the dorsal aspect of the distal phalanx (Figs. 5-162 and 5-163).

Resistance Direction. Flexion.

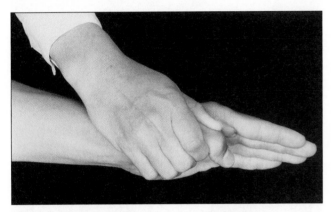

Figure 5-160 Start position: extensor pollicis longus.

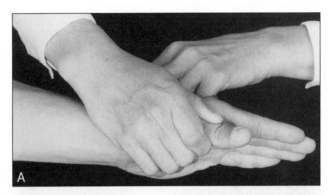

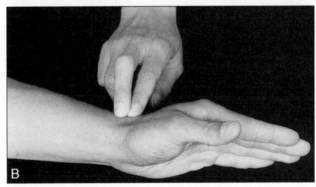

Figure 5-161 **A.** Screen position: extensor pollicis longus.
B. Palpation: extensor pollicis longus.

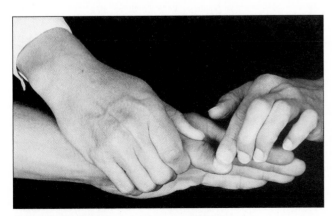

Figure 5-162 Resistance: extensor pollicis longus.

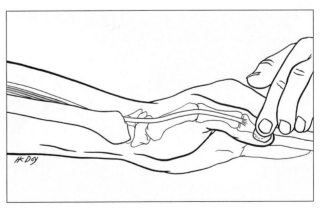

Figure 5-163 Extensor pollicis longus.

Thumb Metacarpophalangeal Extension

Extensor Pollicis Brevis

Accessory muscle: extensor pollicis longus.

Form 5-39   **Start Position.** The patient is sitting or supine. The forearm is in midposition or slightly pronated and the wrist is in a neutral position. The thumb MCP and IP joints are flexed (Fig. 5-164).

Stabilization. The therapist stabilizes the first metacarpal.

Movement. The patient extends the MCP joint of the thumb while maintaining slight flexion of the IP joint (Fig. 5-165A).

Palpation. On the dorsoradial aspect of the wrist at the base of the shaft of the thumb metacarpal. It forms the radial border of the anatomical snuff box and is medial to the tendon of abductor pollicis longus (see Fig. 5-165B).

Substitute Movement. Extensor pollicis longus.

Resistance Location. Applied on the dorsal surface of the proximal phalanx (Figs. 5-166 and 5-167).

Resistance Direction. Flexion.

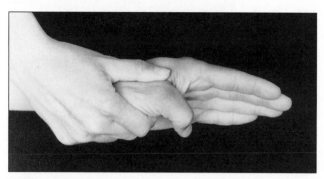

Figure 5-164 Start position: extensor pollicis brevis.

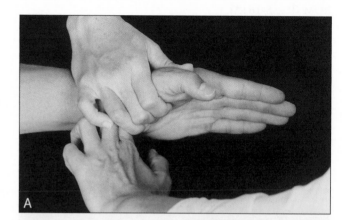

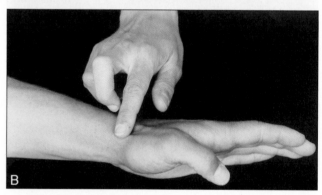

Figure 5-165 **A.** Screen position: extensor pollicis brevis. **B.** Palpation: extensor pollicis brevis.

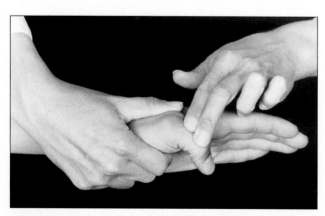

Figure 5-166 Resistance: extensor pollicis brevis.

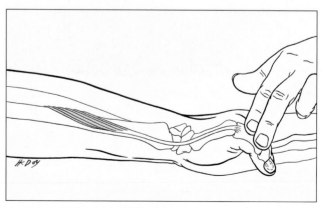

Figure 5-167 Extensor pollicis brevis.

Thumb Radial Abduction

Abductor Pollicis Longus

 Start Position. The patient is sitting or supine. The forearm is in supination and the wrist is in neutral. The thumb is adducted against the volar aspect of the index finger (Fig. 5-168).

Form 5-40

Stabilization. The therapist stabilizes the wrist and second metacarpal.

Movement. The patient abducts the thumb in a radial direction through full ROM (Fig. 5-169). The thumb is taken away from the index finger at an angle of 45°[24] toward extension.

Palpation. On the lateral aspect of the wrist at the base of the thumb metacarpal, and on the radial side of extensor pollicis brevis.

Substitute Movement. Palmar abduction may be attempted through the action of abductor pollicis brevis.[27]

Resistance Location. Applied on the lateral aspect of the thumb metacarpal (Figs. 5-170 and 5-171).

Resistance Direction. Adduction and flexion.

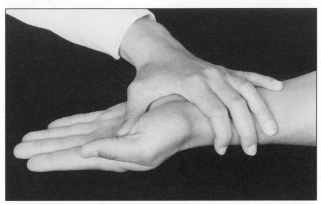

Figure 5-168 Start position: abductor pollicis longus.

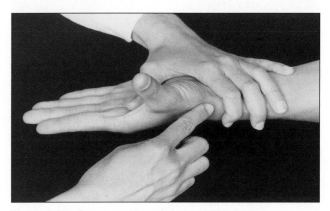

Figure 5-169 Screen position: abductor pollicis longus.

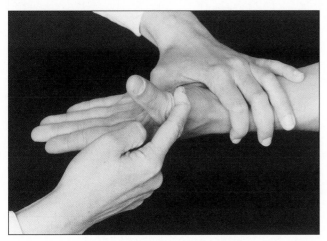

Figure 5-170 Resistance: abductor pollicis longus.

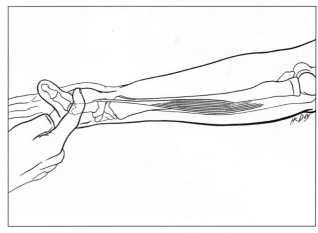

Figure 5-171 Abductor pollicis longus.

Thumb Palmar Abduction

Abductor Pollicis Brevis

Form 5-41

Start Position. The patient is sitting or supine. The forearm is in supination and the wrist is in a neutral position. The thumb is adducted against the volar aspect of the index finger (Fig. 5-172).

Stabilization. The therapist stabilizes the wrist and the second metacarpal.

Movement. The patient abducts the thumb through full ROM (Fig. 5-173). The thumb is taken away at a right angle to the index finger.[24]

Palpation. On the lateral aspect of the thumb metacarpal.

Substitute Movement. Radial abduction may be attempted through the action of abductor pollicis longus.[27]

Resistance Location. Applied on the lateral aspect of the proximal phalanx (Figs. 5-174 and 5-175).

Resistance Direction. Adduction.

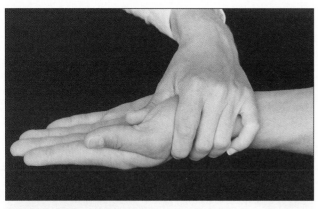

Figure 5-172 Start position: abductor pollicis brevis.

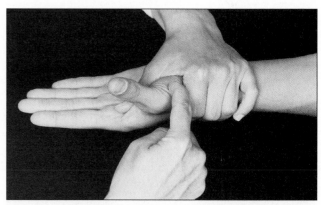

Figure 5-173 Screen position: abductor pollicis brevis.

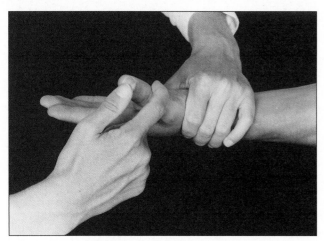

Figure 5-174 Resistance: abductor pollicis brevis.

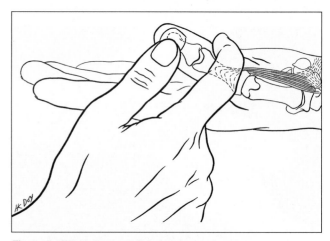

Figure 5-175 Abductor pollicis brevis.

Thumb Adduction

Adductor Pollicis

Accessory muscle: flexor pollicis brevis.

Form 5-42

Start Position. The patient is sitting or supine. The forearm is supinated. The wrist is in a neutral position and the fingers are extended. The MCP and IP joints of the thumb are flexed and the thumb is in palmar abduction (Fig. 5-176).

Stabilization. The therapist stabilizes the wrist and the second through fifth metacarpals.

Movement. The patient adducts the thumb while maintaining flexion of the MCP and IP joints (Fig. 5-177). If the patient has difficulty maintaining flexion, the MCP and IP joints may be held in extension.

Palpation. On the palmar surface of the hand between the first and second metacarpals.

Substitute Movement. Flexor pollicis longus and extensor pollicis longus.[19,24]

Resistance Location. Applied on the medial aspect of the proximal phalanx (Figs. 5-178 and 5-179).

Resistance Direction. Palmar abduction.

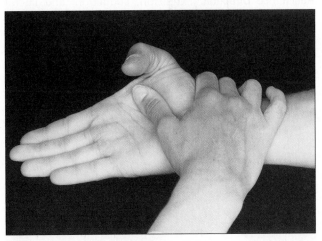

Figure 5-176 Start position: adductor pollicis.

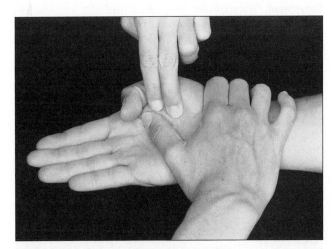

Figure 5-177 Screen position: adductor pollicis.

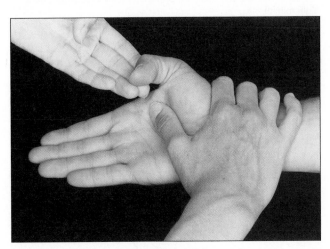

Figure 5-178 Resistance: adductor pollicis.

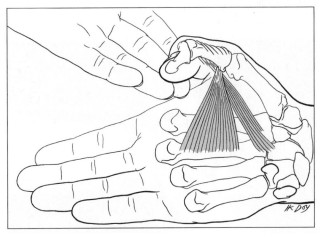

Figure 5-179 Adductor pollicis.

Opposition of the Thumb and Fifth Finger

Opponens Pollicis and Opponens Digiti Minimi)

 Accessory muscles: abductor pollicis brevis, adductor pollicis brevis, and flexor pollicis brevis.

Form 5-43

Start Position. The patient is sitting or supine. The forearm is supinated and the wrist is in a neutral position (Fig. 5-180). The fingers are extended and the MCP and IP joints of the thumb are extended. The thumb is in palmar abduction because the opponens pollicis cannot oppose effectively until the thumb is abducted.[24]

Stabilization. The therapist stabilizes the distal forearm. The thumb may be supported in abduction if the abductor pollicis brevis is weak.

Movement. The patient flexes and medially rotates the thumb metacarpal toward the little finger, and the little finger flexes and rotates toward the thumb so that the pads of the finger and thumb touch (Fig. 5-181). The distal phalanges remain in extension throughout movement.

Palpation. *Opponens pollicis:* lateral to abductor pollicis brevis on the radial aspect of the shaft of the thumb metacarpal. *Opponens digiti minimi:* on the volar surface of the shaft of the fifth metacarpal (see Fig. 5-181).

Substitute Movement. Toward the end of range, the patient may flex the distal joints of the thumb and finger to give the appearance of full opposition. This substitution is absent if, in full opposition, the thumbnail is observed to lie in a plane parallel to the plane of the palm.

Resistance Location. Both movements are resisted simultaneously and resistance is applied on the volar surfaces of the thumb metacarpal and fifth metacarpal (Figs. 5-182 and 5-183).

Resistance Direction. Extension, adduction, and lateral rotation.

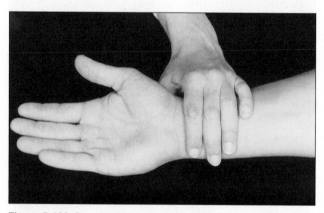

Figure 5-180 Start position: opponens pollicis and opponens digiti minimi.

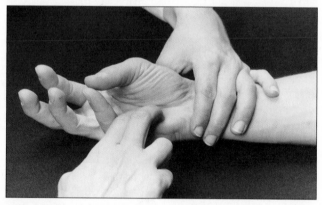

Figure 5-181 Screen position: opponens pollicis and opponens digiti minimi.

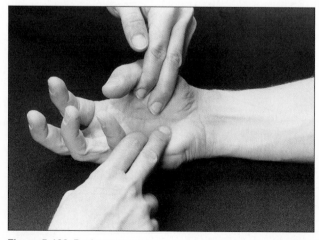

Figure 5-182 Resistance: opponens pollicis and opponens digiti minimi.

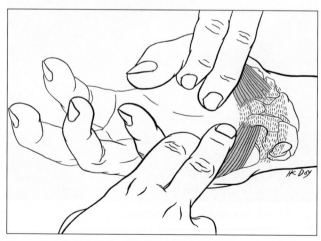

Figure 5-183 Opponens pollicis and opponens digiti minimi.

FUNCTIONAL APPLICATION

Joint Function: Wrist

The wrist optimizes the function of the hand to touch, grasp, or manipulate objects. Wrist motion positions the hand in space relative to the forearm and serves to transmit load between the hand and forearm.[28] Because of wrist motion and static positioning, the wrist serves to control the length–tension relations of the extrinsic muscles of the hand.

Wrist position effects finger ROM. Moving the wrist from a flexed position into extension causes synergistic finger flexion at the MCP, PIP, and DIP joints of the fingers due to passive tension in the long finger flexors.[29] As the wrist moves from an extended position into flexion, the fingers extend due to passive tension in the long finger extensors and the hand opens.

Functional Range of Motion: Wrist

Wrist extension and ulnar deviation are the most important positions or movements[30] for activities of daily living

(ADL). In most daily activities, the wrist assumes a position of extension for the purpose of stabilization of the hand and flexion of the distal joints (Fig. 5-184). However, in the performance of perineal hygiene activities and dressing activities at the back (Fig. 5-185), the wrist assumes a flexed posture.

Two approaches have been used to determine the wrist ROM required to successfully perform ADL:

In *one approach,* the wrist ROM was assessed as normal subjects performed ADL. Brumfield and Champoux[31] evaluated 15 ADL and found the normal functional range of wrist motion for most activities was between 10° flexion and 35° extension. Palmer and coworkers,[32] evaluating 52

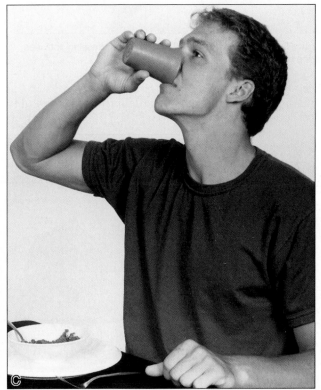

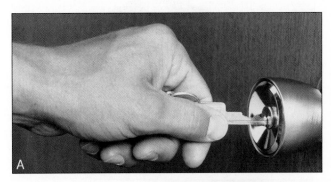

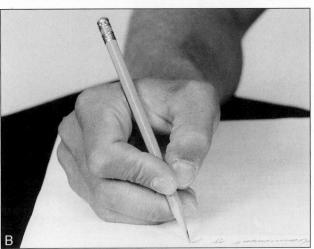

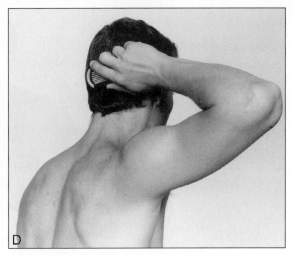

Figure 5-184 In most ADL the wrist assumes a position of extension. **A.** Unlocking a door with a key. **B.** Writing. **C.** Drinking from a cup. **D.** Brushing one's hair.

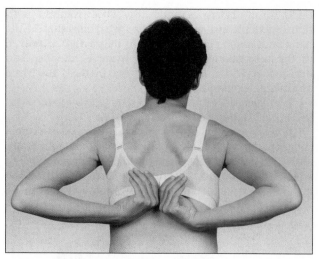

Figure 5-185 The wrist is flexed in performing dressing activities at the back.

standardized tasks, found comparable required ranges of 5° flexion and 30° extension. Normal functional range for ulnar deviation was 15° and radial deviation 10°.[32]

Higher values (54° flexion, 60° extension, 40° ulnar deviation, and 17° radial deviation) for the maximum wrist motion required for ADL were reported by Ryu and colleagues[30] in evaluating 31 activities. The authors suggested differing methods of data analysis and the design and application of the goniometer as possible reasons for these values being higher compared to other studies.

More specific ROM requirements for feeding activities (Fig. 5-186) (i.e., drinking from a cup or glass, eating using a fork or spoon, and cutting using a knife) are from approximately 3° wrist flexion to 35° wrist extension[31,33] and from 20° ulnar deviation to 5° radial deviation.[33]

Using *another approach*, wrist ROM was artificially restricted and the ability to complete ADL was assessed. Nelson[34] evaluated the ability to perform 125 ADL (activities of work or recreation were not included) with the

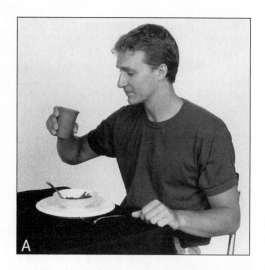

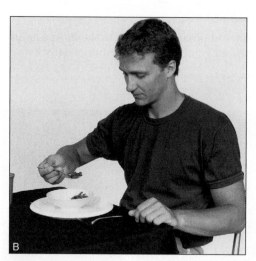

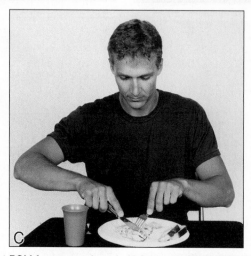

Figure 5-186 Wrist ROM from approximately 3° flexion to 35° extension (31, 33) and from 20° ulnar deviation and 5° radial deviation (33) are required for feeding activities.
A. Drinking from a cup. **B.** Eating using a spoon. **C.** Eating using a knife and fork.

wrist splinted to allow for only 5° flexion, 6° extension, 7° radial deviation, and 6° ulnar deviation. With the wrist splinted in this manner, 123 ADL could be completed. Therefore, marked loss of wrist ROM may not significantly hinder a patient's ability to carry out ADL.

Franko and colleagues[35] used objective ROM parameters, an objective timed test, and subjective surveys to evaluate functional differences between unrestricted (100%), partially (42%), and highly (15%) restricted normal wrist ROM conditions. The objective timed test included contemporary ADL not studied previously, such as, the use of a computer mouse, cell phone, and typing on a computer keyboard and handheld device. The researchers concluded that as wrist ROM decreased objective and subjective functional limitation increased; however, "all subjects in both highly and partially restricted motion conditions had a surprisingly high degree of functional motion, suggesting that a direct correlation does not exist between loss of motion and loss of function."[35(p495.e6)]

Coupled Wrist Motion[11,36]

Wrist movements are coupled during dynamic tasks. Wrist radial deviation occurs with maximal wrist extension, and ulnar deviation occurs with maximal wrist flexion.

Finger Position Effects Wrist ROM

Gehrmann and coworkers[12] assessed wrist ROM with the fingers unconstrained and held in three different flexed positions. With increased finger flexion angles, wrist flexion and ulnar deviation ROM significantly decreased. Flexed finger positions occur when gripping a handle or tool and in these situations wrist ROM may be reduced.

Joint Function: Hand

The hand has multiple functions associated with ADL. The primary functions are to grasp, manipulate objects, communicate, and receive sensory information from the environment. The grasping function is isolated for presentation in this section.

Functional Range of Motion: Hand

Full opening of the hand is not required for grasping tasks in daily self-care activities but may be required for grasp in leisure or occupational tasks. When grasping an object, the shape, size, and weight of the object influence the degree of finger flexion, the area of palmar contact, and thumb position (Fig. 5-187). The thumb may or may not be included in the grip[10] (see Fig. 5-187A). When grasping different-sized cylinders, the DIP joint angle remains constant and the fingers adjust to the new cylinder size through changes in the joint angles at the MCP and PIP joints.[37]

Pieniazek and colleagues[38] evaluated the flexion and extension ROM at the MCP, PIP, and DIP joints of the hand during three ADL, combing the hair, closing a zip fastener, and answering a telephone call. The ROM values were about midrange and never reach maximal flexion/extension values. The pattern of relative mobility was similar in all fingers, being greatest at the MCP joints and decreasing from the PIP to the DIP joints, except for the index finger where PIP joint motion was greater than that at the MCP joint.

Hume and coworkers[39] reported the MCP and IP joint ROM needed to perform many ADL. No significant differences in the functional positions of the individual fingers were found; therefore, the finger positions were reported as one. The ROM at the MCP joints of the fingers and thumb were 33°–73° flexion and 10°–32° flexion, respectively. The PIP and DIP joint ROM of the fingers was 36°–86° flexion and 20°–61° flexion, respectively. The ROM of the IP joint of the thumb was 2°–43° flexion.

Arches of the Hand

The arches of the hand are described in Table 5-7. The arches are observed with the forearm supinated and the hand resting on a table (Fig. 5-188).

The carpal arch, a relatively fixed segment, is covered by the flexor retinaculum. This arrangement functions to maintain the long finger flexors close to the wrist joint, thus reducing the ability of these muscles to produce wrist flexion and enhancing the synergistic action of the wrist flexors and extensors in power grip.[19]

In the relaxed position of the hand, a gently cupped concavity is normally observed. When gripping or manipulating objects, the palmar concavity becomes deeper and more gutter-shaped. When the hand is opened fully, the palm flattens. The guttering and flattening of the palm results from the mobility available at the rays of the ring and little fingers and thumb. Each ray consists of the metacarpal and phalanges of a finger or the thumb. These rays flex, rotate, and move toward the center of the palm so the pads of the fingers and thumb are positioned to meet. This motion occurs at the CM joints. The mobile peripheral rays move around the fixed metacarpals of the index and middle fingers.

The Grasping Function of the Wrist and Hand

The two terms that relate to the grasping function of the hand are prehension and grip. Tubiana and colleagues[19] point out that there is a fundamental difference in the meaning of the two terms. They define prehension as "… all the functions that are put into play when an object is grasped by the hands-intent, permanent sensory control, and a mechanism of grip".[19(p161)] Grip is defined as "the manual mechanical component of prehension".[19(p161)]

Napier[40] categorizes grip into two main gripping postures: power grip and precision grip. He emphasizes that these two postures provide the anatomical basis for all skilled or unskilled activities of the hand and that power

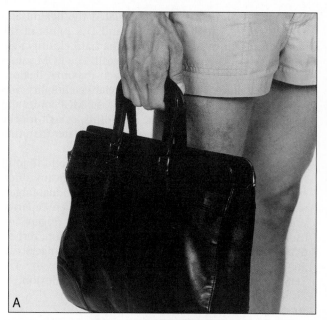

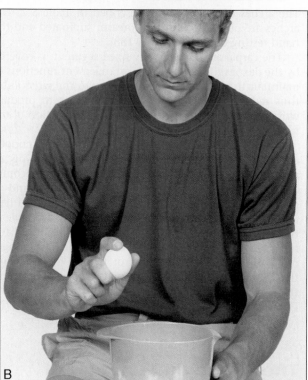

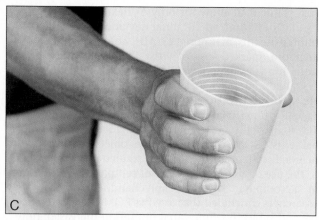

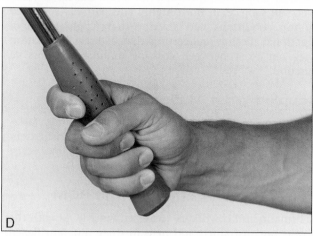

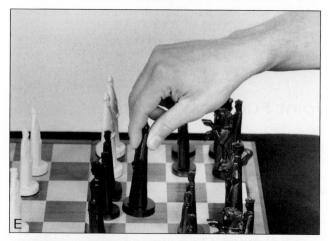

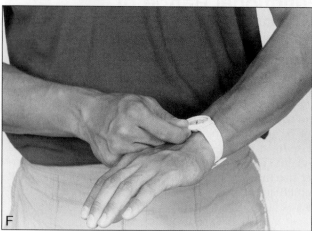

Figure 5-187 When grasping an object, the shape, size, and/or weight of the object influence the degree of finger flexion, the area of palmar contact, and thumb position, as observed when **(A)** carrying a briefcase, **(B)** cracking an egg, **(C)** holding a large cup, **(D)** gripping the handle of a hammer, **(E)** moving a chess piece, and **(F)** winding a watch.

TABLE 5-7 Arches of the Hand[19]

Arch	Location	Keystone	Mobility
Carpal arch	Distal row of carpal bones	Capitate	Fixed
	Proximal row of carpal bones	–	Mobile
Metacarpal arch	Level of metacarpal heads	Third metacarpal head	Mobile
Longitudinal arches	Carpals and each of the five rays*	MCP joints	Mobile; fixed (index and middle metacarpal)

*Ray: the metacarpal and phalanges of one finger or the thumb.

and precision are the dominant characteristics in all prehensile activities. Power grips are used when power or force is required in a grasping activity (Fig. 5-189). The object is held in a clamp, formed by the flexed fingers and the palm, with optional counterpressure on the object being applied by the thumb.

When precision is required in an activity, the hand assumes a precision grip posture (Fig. 5-190). The object is pinched between the volar aspects of the fingers and the opposed thumb. Precision grip[40] involves stabilization of an object between the finger(s) and thumb. The function of precision grip is to secure the object so that the more proximal limb segments can move the object. An object may also be manipulated in the hand. Landsmeer[41] refers to this manipulation function as "precision handling."[41(p. 165)] The first phase is positioning the fingers and thumb to hold the object and the second phase is the actual manipulation or handling of the object.

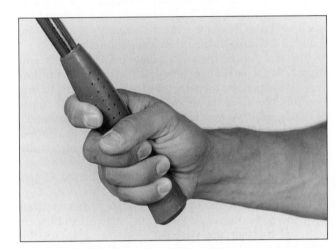

Figure 5-189 Power grip.

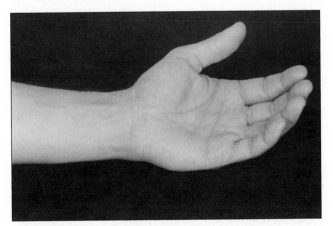

Figure 5-188 Palmar arches. Observe the transverse palmar concavities at the levels of the distal row of carpal bones and the metacarpal bones and the longitudinal concavities along the rays of each finger.

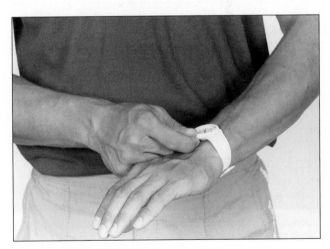

Figure 5-190 Precision grip.

The following description of wrist and hand function is limited to an analysis of power grip, precision grip, and precision handling. Emphasis is placed on the phases of the gripping process, movement patterns, static positioning, and muscle activity of the respective grip.

Power Grip

There are four phases of power grip: opening the hand, positioning the fingers, approaching the fingers or fingers and thumb to the object, and the actual grip.[41] Each phase is a prerequisite of effective grip.

Opening Phase (Fig. 5-191)

Opening is an intuitive action and the amount is predetermined by intent to grasp a specific object.[42] The hand assumes a posture that will accommodate the physical structure of the object. Full opening is not required for grasping tasks in daily self-care activities but may be required for grasp in leisure or occupational tasks.

The position of the wrist influences the fingers and thumb. Wrist flexion permits full extension of the fingers[19,43] to open the hand for grasp of large objects. In this position, the tip of the thumb is level with the PIP joints of the fingers.[44] As the distance between the open hand's fingers and thumb encompasses excess space in relation to the object, the MCP joints of the fingers are often fully extended, whereas the IP joints are always flexed to a certain degree so that the gripping surfaces of the fingers face the object.[42]

The opening phase is a dynamic phase,[41] characterized by concentric muscle contraction. Active opening is achieved through the synergistic muscle action of the wrist flexors and the finger extensors.[43-45] The long extensors of the fingers extend the MCP joints and have a secondary wrist extensor action. To prevent the extensor action from occurring at the wrist, the wrist flexors function as counteracting synergists, keeping the wrist in a neutral position or flexion.[43] The integrity of extensor digitorum is essential for creating active finger opening.[42] The larger the object to be grasped, the more the fingers abduct and the thumb radially abducts and/or extends.

Finger and Thumb (Optional) Positioning Phase (see Fig. 5-191)

The choice of finger position occurs in conjunction with the opening phase and adjustment to the desired position occurs at the MCP and IP joints.[41] The integrity of the activity of extensor digitorum in extending the MCP joints and lumbricales in creating a grip position is essential in this phase of grip.[42] When ulnar deviation of one or more MCP joints is a component of the intended grip, the interossei replace the lumbricales.[42]

Approach Phase (Fig. 5-192)

The movement pattern identified for this phase is wrist extension, finger and thumb flexion, and adduction. As in the opening phase, the position of the wrist influences the fingers and thumb. Wrist extension permits full flexion of the fingers[19,43] as one grasps an object. As the object is approached, the fingers usually flex simultaneously and close around the object[43] so the palm of the hand contacts the object. Flexor digitorum profundus is the critical muscle used in free closing of the hand.[46] The wrist extensors function to stabilize the wrist and prevent wrist flexion by profundus and superficialis.[43] The thenar muscles, when the thumb is involved, are active as the thumb approaches the object for its final position of adduction and/or opposition. Both the position and muscle activity are influenced by the shape of the object to be grasped.

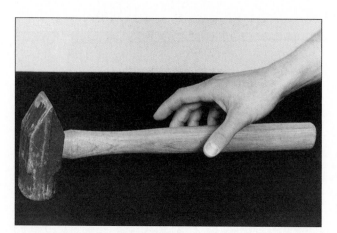

Figure 5-191 Power grip: opening phase and finger/optional thumb positioning phase.

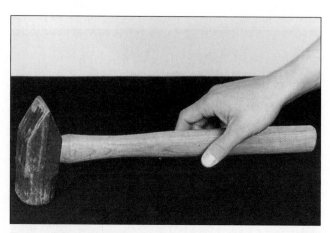

Figure 5-192 Power grip: approach phase.

Static Grip Phase (Fig. 5-193)

This phase is a power or stabilization phase and is characterized by isometric muscle contraction. The function of the hand complex is to stabilize an object so that it can be moved by the proximal limb segments[41] and contributes to the aggregate power of the arm.

The power grip has three significant characteristics: 1. the wrist is held in neutral or extension, 2. the fingers are maintained in flexion and abduction or adduction, and 3. the volar surfaces of the fingers and portions of the palm make forceful contact with the object. The thumb may or may not be included in the grip.[10] For example, in grasping a briefcase (Fig. 5-194), the thumb does not contribute to the grip and this grip is referred to as a hook grasp. In grasping a cylindrical object, such as a hammer or a cup (Fig. 5-195), the thumb does contribute to the grip. When included for force, the thumb may be flexed and adducted. When included for an element of precision, it is usually abducted and flexed.

The shape, size, and/or weight of the object influence the degree of finger flexion, the area of palmar contact, and thumb position. When grasping different sized cylinders, the DIP joint angle remains constant and the fingers adjust to the new cylinder size through changes in the joint angles at the MCP and PIP joints.[37] It should also be noted that as the diameter of a cylindrical object increases, the total grip strength has been shown to decrease.[47]

The ability of the two ulnar fingers to flex and rotate at the CM joints and flex beyond 90° at the MCP joints contributes to digitopalmar contact on the ulnar side of the hand. Research by Bendz[48] shows the hypothenar muscles, notably the flexor digiti minimi and the abductor digiti minimi, contract to flex the fifth metacarpal and proximal phalanx of the fifth digit. The abductor digiti minimi also rotates the fifth metacarpal. These muscles contract to provide strength to the grip, but for full strength the flexor carpi ulnaris is subsequently recruited to augment the contractions of the flexor and abductor digiti minimi via the common attachment of these muscles to the pisiform bone.[48] However, the ring and little finger can generate only about 70% of the force of the index and middle fingers, so that power require-

ments fall to the radial fingers.[49,50] As increased force is required in the grasp, the wrist ulnarly deviates. The greatest force generated at the phalanges is obtained when the wrist is in ulnar deviation.[49] Within the general classification of Napier's[40] descriptors of power grip, various subgroups of postures can be identified. Kamakura and associates[51] identify five patterns of power grip. These patterns have the three general characteristics previously specified. Specific patterns may be differentiated according to the involvement of the thumb, degree of range of movement, finger position, and/or the amount of digitopalmar contact area. Sollerman and Sperling[52] developed a code system that classifies hand grips according to the participation of the various parts of the hand, the positioning of the fingers and the joints, the contact surfaces, and the relationship between the longitudinal axis of the object and the hand. The postural details described in both studies illustrate the immense variety of ways that one can grasp an object and the concomitant muscle activity that may exist in these postures.

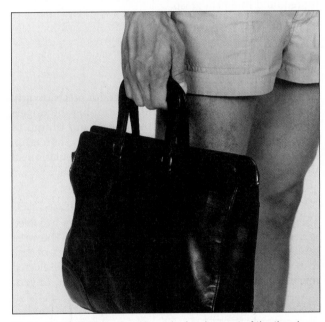

Figure 5-194 Power grip without the involvement of the thumb.

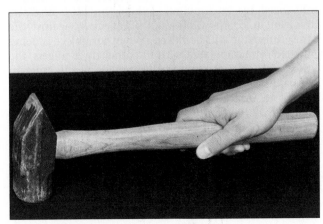

Figure 5-193 Power grip: static grip phase.

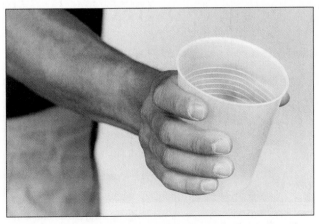

Figure 5-195 Power grip with the thumb contributing to the grip.

Long and associates[46] present electromyographic data of intrinsic-extrinsic muscle activity involved in five classifications of power grip: simple squeeze, hammer squeeze, screwdriver squeeze, disc grip, and spherical grip. The following summary of their findings provides insight into the muscle activity patterns involved in the static grip phase of hand posture.

The extrinsic finger flexors provide the major gripping force. Flexor digitorum profundus and superficialis both contribute to power grip with superficialis increasing its participation as force requirements increase. The major intrinsic participation is provided through the interossei. They abduct or adduct the proximal phalanx to align the fingers with the object so that the extrinsic flexors can provide the gripping power. The interossei also provide gripping power as they flex the metacarpophalangeal joints.

When the thumb is adducted and flexed in power grip, the muscle power is provided through the isometric contraction of adductor pollicis[44–46,53] and flexor pollicis longus.[44,45] Flexor pollicis brevis contributes to the stability required in a firm grasp.[44,53]

Precision Grip and Precision Handling

Three common phases can be identified for precision grip and handling: opening the hand, positioning the fingers and thumb, and approaching the fingers and thumb to the object. The last phase in precision grip is static grip. The last phase in precision handling is manipulation of the object.

Opening Phase (Fig. 5-196)

The amount of opening and number of fingers involved varies with the shape and purpose of the object. The wrist position also varies with the purpose of the object or task to be performed and location of the object. The elected opening posture is that which positions the wrist, fingers,

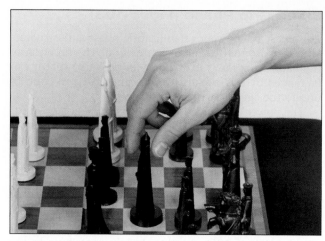

Figure 5-197 Precision grip or handling: approach phase.

and thumb for the subsequent function of stabilization or manipulation. Because of the infinite number of ways that an object can be stabilized or manipulated, the range of movement and muscle activity is more variable than power grip. The same pattern of movement is evident but as more precision is demanded, finer motor control is required.

Finger and Thumb Positioning Phase (see Fig. 5-196)

As indicated in power grip, adjustment of the fingers and thumb to the object occurs concurrently with the opening phase with many positions possible through the positioning of the MCP and IP joints. However, in precision grip or handling the thumb is always involved and is positioned to achieve opposition to bring it into pad-to-pad contact with the finger or fingers.

Approach Phase (Fig. 5-197)

The movement pattern and muscular requirements of the wrist are similar to power grip. The wrist can either move into extension while the MCP joints flex or remain in flexion with the MCP joints flexing. The MCP joints of the index, middle, and ring fingers usually flex in precision grip and precision handling. The MCP joint of the little finger may be flexed or extended. The position is influenced by its function. When the little finger is involved in compression on the object or against the other fingers, it will be flexed. When an object is being pinched or manipulated with the other three fingers, the little finger may be extended to provide tactile input to the hand or to contribute to stabilization of the hand on a working surface. There is no deviation at the wrist.[40] In addition to finger MCP flexion, there is abduction or adduction of one or more fingers. The PIP joint(s) of the finger(s) flex or extend.[54] Although IP flexion is required for subsequent manipulation, flexion or extension may be required in precision grip. The DIP joints may be flexed or extended. As in power grip, the integrity of the flexor digitorum profundus is critical to approaching an object in a flexion pattern. Lumbrical activity is a prerequisite to the initiation of an extension approach.[55]

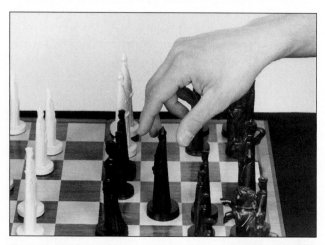

Figure 5-196 Precision grip or handling: opening phase and finger and thumb positioning phase.

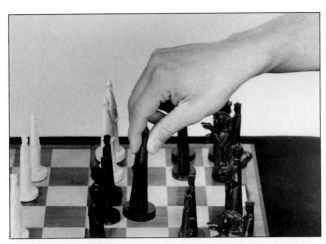

Figure 5-198 Precision grip: static grip phase.

The approach of the thumb incorporates the movement of opposition as the function of the thumb is to oppose the fingers. Opposition is a sequential movement incorporating abduction, flexion, and adduction of the first metacarpal, with simultaneous rotation.[10] Thenar muscle control occurs through opponens pollicis, flexor pollicis brevis, abductor pollicis brevis, and adductor pollicis.

Precision Grip (Fig. 5-198)

When the fingers and thumb contact the object, the hand grips the object. Precision grip[40] involves stabilization of an object between the finger(s) and thumb. The function of precision grip is to secure an object so that the more proximal limb segments can move the object.

There are five hand postures that illustrate the characteristics of precision grip and are used frequently in ADL: pulp pinch (Fig. 5-199), tripod pinch (Fig. 5-200), five-pulp pinch (Fig. 5-201), lateral pinch (Fig. 5-202), and tip pinch (Fig. 5-203). They share the common characteristic of pinch between the thumb and one or more fingers. Sollerman and Sperling[56] report that of the hand postures used in ADL, the first four pinch postures are used 65% of the time. The specific posture assumed when pinching an object is influenced by the purpose of the object.[40,57] Pulp pinch and lateral pinch are isolated for analysis of posture and muscular activity.

Pulp Pinch (see Figs. 5-199, 5-200, and 5-201)

The object is pinched between the pulp of the thumb and the pulp of one or more fingers. The thumb and finger(s) are opposed to each other. The most commonly used fingers are the index finger and/or middle finger. The index finger is of significant value in activities. It is strong, can abduct, has relative independence of its musculature, and has proximity to the thumb.[19] The middle finger adds an element of strength to precision grip (tripod pinch). The ring and little fingers contribute to five-pulp pinch.

The thumb assumes a position of CM flexion, abduction, and rotation. The MCP joints and IP joints can be

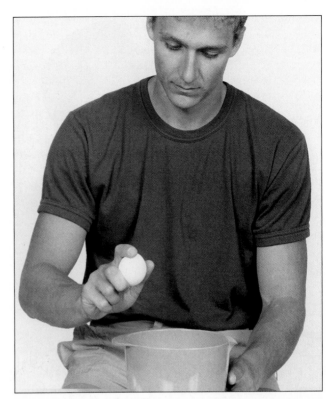

Figure 5-199 Pulp pinch.

flexed or fully extended. The compression force for stabilization of the object is achieved through the muscular contraction of opponens pollicis, adductor pollicis, and flexor pollicis brevis.[46] The adductor pollicis increases its contribution as increased pressure is required. The flexor pollicis longus contributes to distal phalanx compression when the distal phalanx is flexed.[45,53]

The radial three fingers are normally flexed at the MCP joint. The little finger may be flexed or extended. The DIP joints of the fingers may be flexed or extended. When flexed, the flexor digitorum profundus plays a key role in the compression. When the distal joint is extended, flexor digitorum superficialis is the muscle recruited for mainte-

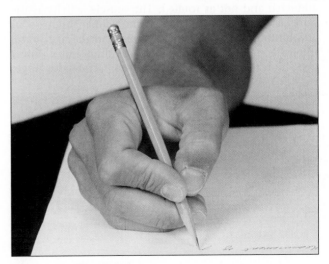

Figure 5-200 Tripod pinch.

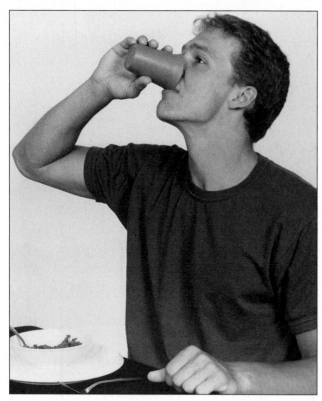

Figure 5-201 Five-pulp pinch.

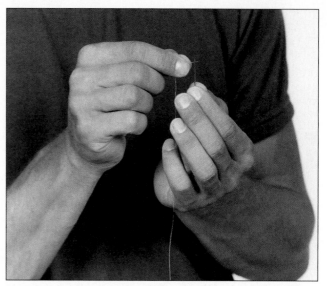

Figure 5-203 Tip pinch of a needle with precision handling of the thread.

nance of position. These extrinsic muscles contribute to the power in pinch with assistance being provided by the first palmar and dorsal interosseous and first lumbricalis.[46] It has been suggested by Maier and colleagues[58] that the intrinsic muscles may even play a primary role in production of low isometric forces in precision grip.

Lateral Pinch (see Fig. 5-202)

The difference between this form of pinch and pulp pinch is that the thumb pulp stabilizes an object against the side of the index finger with counterpressure being provided by the index finger. The thumb is more adducted and not as rotated. The muscle activity is the same as pulp pinch except that the palmar interosseous and lumbricalis reduce their activity and the first dorsal interosseous is very active in providing index finger abduction force to stabilize the object.[46] The index finger

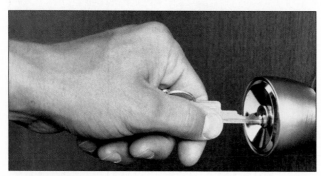

Figure 5-202 Lateral pinch.

is flexed at the MCP joint and may be flexed or extended at the PIP and DIP joints.[54] Although flexion of the proximal phalanx is the most commonly used posture, extension may be the desired posture in precision grip of objects with flat surfaces such as a plate, book, or magazine. The lumbricales and dorsal interosseous muscles are active in the extension posture.[54]

Precision Handling (see Fig. 5-203)

This term refers to manipulation of an object using the fingers and thumb.[41] The dominant characteristic in precision handling is manipulation through concentric muscle contraction. The static phase is very brief and pressure applied to the object is light. In most daily activities, the wrist usually assumes a position of extension for the purposes of stabilization of the hand and flexion of the distal joints. However, in the performance of perineal hygiene activities and dressing activities at the back, the wrist assumes a flexed posture. The finger and thumb position is partly determined by the size and shape of the object but the major determinant is that the object requires a change in position.[46]

Long and associates[46] describe two types of manipulation that characterize precision handling with involvement of the thumb and radial two fingers: translation and rotation. In translation, the object is pushed away from or returned to the palm by the fingertips. There is a handling phase and return phase for each motion sequence. Translation toward the palm involves the motion sequences of flexion at the MCP and IP joints (handling phase) and extension of the IP joints (return phase). Translation toward the palm is under the control of the extrinsic flexors and interossei in the handling phase and lumbricales in the return phase. Translation away from the palm involves the motion sequences of flexion at the MCP joints with extension of the IP joints (handling phase) and flexion at the MCP and IP joints (return phase). The interossei and lumbrical muscles are dominant in translation away from the palm.

In rotation, the object is rotated in a clockwise or counter-clockwise direction. The rotation of the object is accomplished through the interossei muscles as they abduct and adduct. The lumbrical muscles function to extend the IP joints and are active in both rotations.

During precision handling, the thenar triad of flexor pollicis brevis, opponens pollicis, and abductor pollicis brevis are active. Adductor pollicis only becomes active when force is required against the index finger.

Precision handling usually involves the radial two fingers and thumb. However, the remaining two fingers may be involved in manipulation or stabilization. The hypothenar muscles are active when the little finger is flexed and abducted through the activity of abductor digiti minimi, opponens digiti minimi, and flexor digiti minimi.[53]

References

1. Kapandji AI. *The Physiology of the Joints. Vol 1. The Upper Limb*, 6th ed. New York, NY: Churchill Livingstone Elsevier; 2007.
2. Standring S, ed. *Gray's Anatomy: The Anatomical Basis of Clinical Practice*. 39th ed. London: Elsevier Churchill Livingstone; 2005.
3. Norkin CC, White DJ. *Measurement of Joint Motion: A Guide to Goniometry*. 4th ed. Philadelphia, PA: FA Davis; 2009.
4. Daniels L, Worthingham C. *Muscle Testing: Techniques of Manual Examination*. 5th ed. Philadelphia, PA: WB Saunders; 1986.
5. Magee DJ. *Orthopedic Physical Assessment*. 5th ed. Philadelphia, PA: Saunders Elsevier; 2008.
6. American Academy of Orthopaedic Surgeons. *Joint Motion: Method of Measuring and Recording*. Chicago, IL: AAOS; 1965.
7. Berryman Reese N, Bandy WD. *Joint Range of Motion and Muscle Length Testing*. 2nd ed. Philadelphia, PA: Saunders Elsevier; 2010.
8. Cyriax J. *Textbook of Orthopaedic Medicine, Vol 1. Diagnosis of Soft Tissue Lesions*. 8th ed. London: Bailliere Tindall; 1982.
9. Knutson JS, Kilgore KL, Mansour JM, Crago PE. Intrinsic and extrinsic contributions to the passive movement at the metacarpophalangeal joint. *J Biomech*. 2000; 33:1675–1681.
10. Li Z-M, Kuxhaus L, Fisk JA, Christophel TH. Coupling between wrist flexion–extension and radial-ulnar deviation. *Clin Biomech*. 2005;20:177–183.
11. Levangie PK, Norkin CC. *Joint Structure and Function: A Comprehensive Analysis*. 4th ed. Philadelphia, PA: FA Davis; 2005.
12. Gehrmann SV, Kaufmann RA, Li Z-M. Wrist circumduction reduced by finger constraints. *J Hand Surg*. 2008;33A:1287–1292.
13. Neumann DA. *Kinesiology of the Musculoskeletal System: Foundations for Physical Rehabilitation*. 2nd ed. St Louis, MO: Mosby Elsevier; 2010.
14. Scott AD, Trombly CA. Evaluation. In: Trombly CA. *Occupational Therapy for Physical Dysfunction*. 2nd ed. Baltimore, MD: Williams & Wilkins; 1983.
15. Kato M, Echigo A, Ohta H, Ishiai S, Aoki M, Tsubota S, Uchiyama E. The accuracy of goniometric measurements of proximal interphalangeal joints in fresh cadavers: Comparison between methods of measurement, types of goniometers, and fingers. *J Hand Ther*. 2007;20(1):12–18.
16. Swanson AB, Goran-Hagert C, DeGroot Swanson G. Evaluation of impairment of hand function. In: Hunter JM,
17. Steginck Jansen CW, Patterson R, Viegas SF. Effects of fingernail length on finger and hand performance. *J Hand Ther*. 2000;13:211–217.
18. deKraker M, Selles RW, Schreuders TAR, Stam HJ, Hovius SER. Palmar abduction: reliability of 6 measurment methods in healthy adults. *J Hand Surg*. 2009;34A:523–530.
19. Tubiana R, Thomine JM, Macklin E. *Examination of the Hand and Wrist*. 2nd ed. St. Louis, MO: Mosby; 1996.
20. Soames RW, ed. Skeletal system. Salmons S, ed. Muscle. *Gray's Anatomy*. 38th ed. New York, NY: Churchill Livingstone; 1995.
21. Kendall FP, McCreary EK, Provance PG, Rodgers MM, Romani WA. *Muscles Testing and Function*. 5th ed. Baltimore, MD: Williams & Wilkins; 2005.
22. Woodburne RT. *Essentials of Human Anatomy*. 5th ed. London: Oxford University Press; 1973.
23. Sebastin SJ, Lim AYT, Bee WH, Wong TCM, Methil BV. Does the absence of the palmaris longus affect grip and pinch strength?. *J Hand Surg*. 2005;30B(4):406–408.
24. Wynn Parry CB. *Rehabilitation of the Hand*. 4th ed. London: Butterworths; 1981.
25. Baker DS, Gaul JS, Williams VK, Graves M. The little finger superficialis—clinical investigation of its anatomic and functional shortcomings. *J Hand Surg*. 1981;6:374–378.
26. Aulincino PL. Clinical examination of the hand. In: Hunter JM, Macklin EJ, Callahan AD. *Rehabilitation of the Hand: Surgery and Therapy*. 4th ed. St. Louis, MO: Mosby; 1995.
27. Pedretti LW. Evaluation of muscle strength. In: Pedretti LW. *Occupational Therapy Practice Skills for Physical Dysfunction*. 2nd ed. St. Louis, MO: CV Mosby; 1985.
28. Nordin M, Frankel VH. *Basic Biomechanics of the Musculoskeletal System*. 3rd ed. Philadelphia, PA: Lippincott Williams & Wilkins; 2001.
29. Su F-C, Chou YL, Yang CS, Lin GT, An KN. Movement of finger joints induced by synergistic wrist motion. *Clin Biomech*. 2005;20:491–497.
30. Ryu J, Cooney WP, Askew LJ, et al. Functional ranges of motion of the wrist joint. *J Hand Surg [Am]*. 1991;16:409–419.
31. Brumfield RH, Champoux JA. A biomechanical study of normal functional wrist motion. *Clin Orthop Relat Res*. 1984; 187:23–25.
32. Palmer AK, Werner FW, Murphy DM, Glisson R. Functional wrist motion: a biomechanical study. *J Hand Surg [Am]*. 1985;10:39–46.
33. Safaee-Rad R, Shwedyk E, Quanbury AO, Cooper JE. Normal functional range of motion of upper limb joints during performance of three feeding activities. *Arch Phys Med Rehabil*. 1990;71:505–509.
34. Nelson DL. Functional wrist motion. *Hand Clin*. 1997;13: 83–92.
35. Franko OI, Zurakowski D, Day CS. Functional disability of the wrist: Direct correlation with decreased wrist motion. *J Hand Surg*. 2008;33A:485.e1–485.e9.
36. Wigderowitz CA, Scott I, Jariwala A, Arnold GP, Abboud RJ. Adapting the Fastrak® System for three-dimensional measurement of the motion of the wrist. *J Hand Surg Eur Vol*. 2007;32E(6):700–704.
37. Lee JW, Rim K. Measurement of finger joint angles and maximum finger forces during cylinder grip activity. *J Biomed Eng*. 1991;13:152–162.
38. Pieniazek M, Chwala W, Szczechowicz J, Pelczar-Pieniazek M. Upper limb joint mobility ranges during activities of daily living determined by three-dimensional motion analysis—preliminary report. *Ortop Traumatol Rehabil*. 2007;9(4): 413–422.

Schneider LH, Mackin EJ, Bell JA. *Rehabilitation of the Hand*. St. Louis, MO: CV Mosby; 1978.

39. Hume MC, Gellman H, McKellop H, Brumfield RH. Functional range of motion of the joints of the hand. *J Hand Surg [Am].* 1990;15:240–243.

40. Napier JR. The prehensile movements of the human hand. *J Bone Joint Surg [Br].* 1956;38:902–913.

41. Landsmeer JMF. Power grip and precision handling. *Ann Rheum Dis.* 1962;21:164–169.

42. Benz P. The motor balance of the fingers of the open hand. *Scand J Rehabil Med.* 1980;12:115–121.

43. Smith LK, Weiss EL, Lehmkuhl LD. *Brunnstrom's Clinical Kinesiology.* 5th ed. Philadelphia, PA: FA Davis; 1996.

44. Tubiana R. Architecture and functions of the hand. In: Tubiana R, Thomine JM, Mackin E, eds. *Examination of the Hand & Upper Limb.* Philadelphia, PA: WB Saunders; 1984.

45. Norkin CC, Levangie PK. *Joint Structure & Function: A Comprehensive Analysis.* 2nd ed. Philadelphia, PA: FA Davis; 1992.

46. Long C, Conrad PW, Hall EA, Furler SL. Intrinsic-extrinsic muscle control of the hand in power grip and precision handling. *J Bone Joint Surg [Am].* 1970;52:853–867.

47. Radhakrishnan S, Nagaravindra M. Analysis of hand forces in health and disease during maximum isometric grasping of cylinders. *Med Biol Eng Comput.* 1993;31:372–376.

48. Bendz P. The functional significance of the fifth metacarpus and hypothenar in two useful grips of the hand. *Am J Phys Med Rehabil.* 1993;72:210–213.

49. Hazelton FT, Smidt GL, Flatt AE, Stephens RI. The influence of wrist position on the force produced by the finger flexors. *J Biomech.* 1975;8:301–306.

50. MacDermid JC, Lee A, Richards RS, Roth JH. Individual finger strength: Are the ulnar digits "powerful"?. *J Hand Ther.* 2004;17:364–367.

51. Kamakura N, Matsuo M, Ishii H, Mitsuboshi F, Miura Y. Patterns of static prehension in normal hands. *Am J Occup Ther.* 1980;34:437–445.

52. Sollerman C, Sperling L. Evaluation of ADL function-especially hand function. *Scand J Rehabil Med.* 1978;10:139–143.

53. Basmajian JV, DeLuca CJ. *Muscles Alive: Their Function Revealed by Electromyography.* 5th ed. Baltimore, MD: Williams & Wilkins; 1985.

54. Benz P. Systemization of the grip of the hand in relation to finger motor systems. *Scand J Rehabil Med.* 1974;6:158–165.

55. Benz P. Motor balance in formation and release of the extension grip. *Scand J Rehabil Med.* 1980;12:155–160.

56. Sollerman C, Sperling L. Classification of the hand grip: a preliminary study. *Am J Occup Med.* 1976;18:395–398.

57. Sperling L, Jacobson-Sollerman C. The grip pattern of the healthy hand during eating. *Scand J Rehabil Med.* 1977;9:115–121.

58. Maier MA, Hepp-Reymond M-C. EMG activation patterns during force production in precision grip. *Exp Brain Res.* 1995;103:108–122.

Chapter 6

Hip

ARTICULATIONS AND MOVEMENTS

The hip joint is a ball-and-socket joint (Fig. 6-1) formed proximally by the cup-shaped, concave surface of the pelvic acetabulum and distally by the ball-shaped, convex head of the femur. Movements at the hip joint include flexion, extension, abduction, adduction, and internal and external rotation.

From the anatomical position, the hip joint may be flexed and extended in the sagittal plane, with movement occurring around a frontal axis, and abducted and adducted in the frontal plane about a sagittal axis (Fig. 6-2). With the hip positioned in 90° of flexion, hip internal and external rotation occurs in the frontal plane about a sagittal axis (Fig. 6-3). Hip rotation can also be

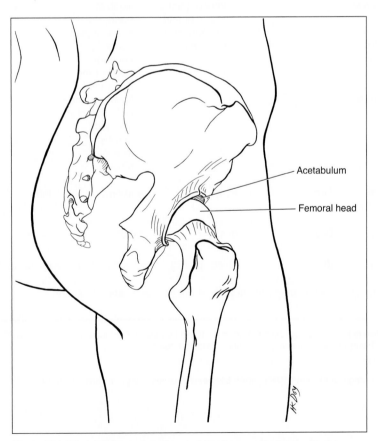

Figure 6-1 Hip joint: the convex head of the femur articulates with the concave surface of the acetabulum.

performed in the anatomical position, with movement occurring in the transverse plane about a longitudinal (vertical) axis.

Movements at the hip joint can result from movement of the femur on the pelvis, pelvis on the femur, or movement of the femur and pelvis. Hip joint range of motion (ROM) and muscle strength assessment techniques are performed by moving the femur on the fixed pelvis. Motions occurring at the more central joints can augment movement at the hip joint. Therefore, when assessing hip ROM and muscle strength, the pelvis is stabilized to avoid lumbo-pelvic movement that would augment hip movement and give the appearance of greater hip ROM than is actually present. The movements of the hip joint are described in Table 6-1.

TABLE 6-1   Joint Structure: Hip Movements

	Flexion	Extension	Abduction	Adduction	Internal Rotation	External Rotation
Articulation[1,2]	Hip	Hip	Hip	Hip	Hip	Hip
Plane	Sagittal	Sagittal	Frontal	Frontal	Horizontal	Horizontal
Axis	Frontal	Frontal	Sagittal	Sagittal	Longitudinal	Longitudinal
Normal limiting factors[1,3–6]* (see Fig. 6-4A and B)	Soft tissue apposition of the anterior thigh and the abdomen (knee is flexed); tension in the posterior hip joint capsule and gluteus maximus	Tension in the anterior joint capsule, the iliofemoral, ischiofemoral, and pubofemoral ligaments and iliopsoas	Tension in the pubofemoral and ischiofemoral ligaments, the inferior band of the iliofemoral ligament, the inferior joint capsule, and hip adductor muscles	Soft tissue apposition of the thighs With the contralateral leg in abduction or flexion; tension in the iliotibial band, the superior joint capsule, superior band of the iliofemoral ligament, the ischiofemoral ligament, and hip abductor muscles	Tension in the ischiofemoral ligament, the posterior joint capsule, and the external rotator muscles	Tension in the iliofemoral and pubofemoral ligaments, the anterior joint capsule, and the medial rotator muscles
Normal end feel[3,7]	Soft/firm	Firm	Firm	Soft/firm	Firm	Firm
Normal AROM[8]†	0–120°	0–30°	0–45°	0–30°	0–45°	0–45°
(AROM[9])	(0–120°)	(0–20°)	(0–40° to 45°)	(0–25° to 30°)	(0–35° to 40°)	(0–35° to 40°)
Capsular pattern[7,10]	The order of restriction may vary: flexion, abduction, and internal rotation					

*There is a paucity of definitive research that identifies the normal limiting factors (NLF) of joint range of motion. The NLF and end feels listed here are based on a knowledge of anatomy, clinical experience, and available references.

†AROM, active range of motion.

Note: Normal hip extension range of motion (ROM) varies between sources, ranging from 10° to 30°.[4,8,9,11–13]

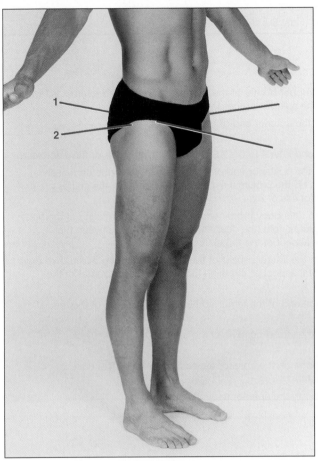

Figure 6-2 Hip joint axes: *(1)* abduction–adduction and *(2)* flexion-extension.

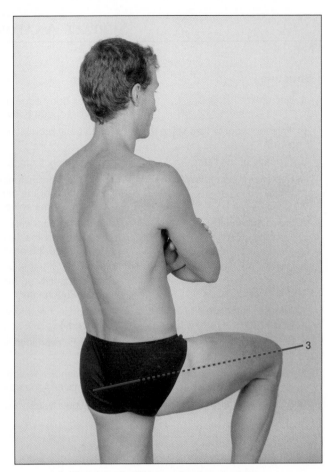

Figure 6-3 Hip joint axis: *(3)* internal–external rotation.

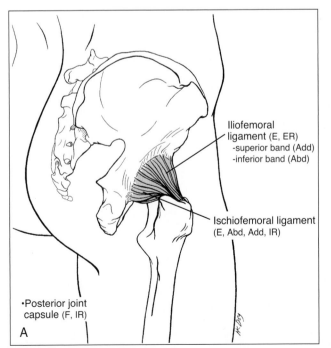

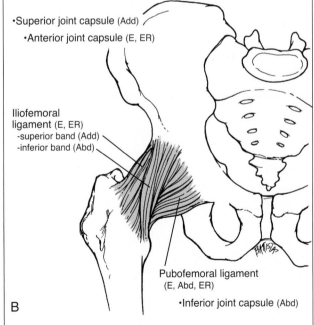

Iliofemoral ligament (E, ER)
-superior band (Add)
-inferior band (Abd)

Ischiofemoral ligament (E, Abd, Add, IR)

•Posterior joint capsule (F, IR)

A

•Superior joint capsule (Add)
•Anterior joint capsule (E, ER)

Iliofemoral ligament (E, ER)
-superior band (Add)
-inferior band (Abd)

Pubofemoral ligament (E, Abd, ER)

•Inferior joint capsule (Abd)

B

Figure 6-4 **Normal Limiting Factors. A.** Posterolateral view of the hip joint showing noncontractile structures that normally limit motion. **B.** Anterolateral view of the hip joint showing noncontractile structures that normally limit motion. *Motion limited by structure is identified in brackets, using the following abbreviations: *F*, flexion; *E*, extension; *Abd*, abduction; *Add*, adduction; *ER*, external rotation; *IR*, internal rotation. Muscles normally limiting motion are not illustrated.

SURFACE ANATOMY (Figs. 6-5 through 6-9)

Structure	Location
1. Iliac crest	A convex bony ridge on the upper border of the ilium; the top of the iliac crest is level with the space between the spinous processes of L4 and L5.
2. Anterior superior iliac spine (ASIS)	Round bony prominence at the anterior end of the iliac crest.
3. Tubercle of the ilium	Approximately 5 cm above and lateral to the ASIS along the lateral lip of the iliac crest.
4. Posterior superior iliac spine (PSIS)	Round bony prominence at the posterior end of the iliac crest, felt subcutaneously at the bottom of the dimples on the proximal aspect of the buttocks; the spines are at the level of the spinous process of S2.
5. Ischial tuberosity	With the hip passively flexed, this bony prominence is lateral to the midline of the body and just proximal to the gluteal fold (the deep transverse groove between the buttock and the posterior aspect of the thigh).
6. Greater trochanter	With the tip of the thumb on the lateral aspect of the iliac crest, the tip of the third digit placed distally on the lateral aspect of the thigh locates the upper border of the greater trochanter.
7. Adductor tubercle	Medial projection at the distal end of the femur at the proximal aspect of the medial epicondyle.
8. Lateral epicondyle of the femur	Small bony prominence on the lateral condyle of the femur.
9. Patella	Large triangular sesamoid bone on the anterior aspect of the knee. The base is proximal and the apex distal.
10. Anterior border of the tibia	Subcutaneous bony ridge along the anterior aspect of the leg.

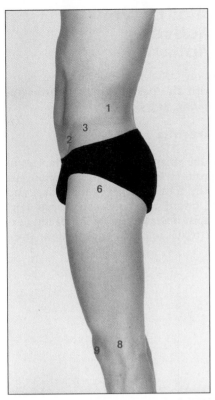

Figure 6-5 Lateral aspect of the trunk and thigh.

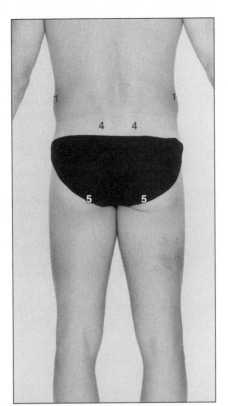

Figure 6-6 Posterior aspect of the trunk and thigh.

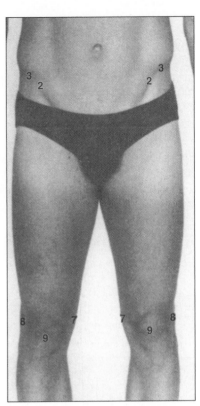

Figure 6-7 Anterior aspect of the trunk and thigh.

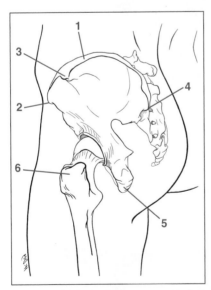

Figure 6-8 Bony anatomy, posterolateral aspect of the pelvis and thigh.

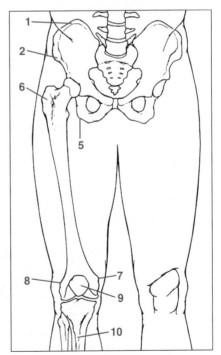

Figure 6-9 Bony anatomy, anterior aspect of the pelvis, thigh, and knee.

RANGE OF MOTION ASSESSMENT AND MEASUREMENT

 Practice Makes Perfect

To aid you in practicing the skills covered in this section, or for a handy review, use the practical testing forms found at http://thepoint.lww.com/Clarkson3e.

General Scan: Lower Extremity Active Range of Motion

Active range of motion (AROM) of the lower extremity joints is scanned with the patient either non-weight-bearing or weight-bearing, as follows:

Non-Weight-Bearing

1. The patient is in the supine position with the legs in the anatomical position. In supine-lying position, the patient extends the toes, dorsiflexes the ankle, and brings the heel toward the contralateral hip (Fig. 6-10A). The therapist observes the AROM of hip flexion, abduction, external rotation, knee flexion, ankle

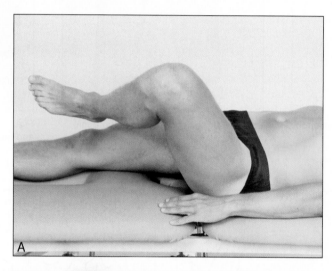

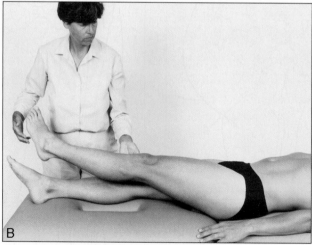

Figure 6-10 **A.** Non-weight-bearing scan: AROM of lower extremity. **B.** Non–weight-bearing scan: AROM of lower extremity.

dorsiflexion, and toe extension. As the patient attempts to touch the contralateral hip, the level reached by the heel may be used as a guide of AROM of the hip and knee joints.

2. The patient flexes the toes, plantarflexes the ankle, extends the knee, and adducts, internally rotates, and extends the hip to move the great toe toward the corner on the other side of the plinth (Fig. 6-10B). The therapist observes the AROM of hip adduction, internal rotation, knee extension, ankle plantarflexion, and toe flexion.

Weight-Bearing

1. The patient squats (Fig. 6-11A). The therapist observes bilateral hip flexion, knee flexion, ankle dorsiflexion, and toe extension ROM.

2. Standing, the patient rises onto the toes (Fig. 6-11B). The therapist observes hip extension, knee extension, ankle plantarflexion, and toe extension ROM bilaterally.

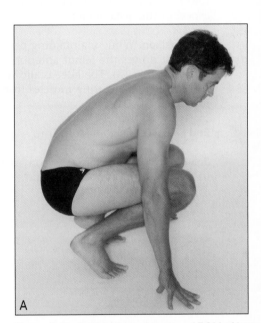
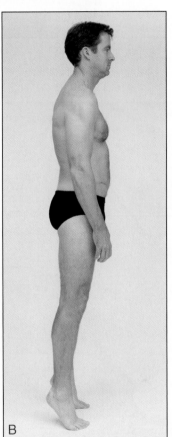

Figure 6-11 A. Weight-bearing scan: AROM of lower extremity. **B.** Weight-bearing scan: AROM of lower extremity.

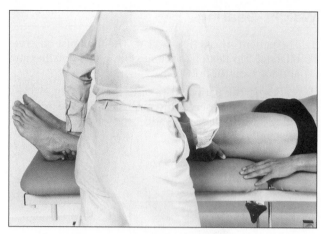

Figure 6-12 Start position: hip flexion.

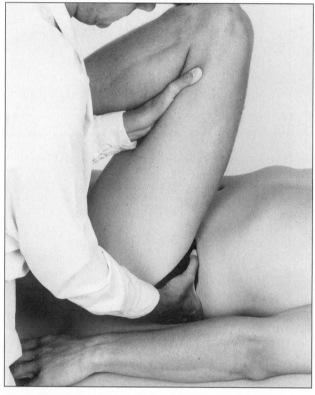

Figure 6-13 Soft or firm end feel at limit of hip flexion.

Hip Flexion

AROM Assessment

Substitute Movement. Posterior pelvic tilt and flexion of the lumbar spine.

PROM Assessment

Start Position. The patient is supine. The hip and knee on the test side are in the anatomical position (Fig. 6-12). The pelvis is in the neutral position; that is, the ASISs and the symphysis pubis are in the same frontal plane and the right and left ASISs are in the same transverse plane.[11,14]

Form 6-1

Stabilization. The therapist stabilizes the ipsilateral pelvis at the ASIS and iliac crest to maintain a neutral position. The trunk is stabilized through body positioning.

Therapist's Distal Hand Placement. The therapist raises the lower extremity off the plinth and grasps the posterior aspect of the distal femur.

End Position. While maintaining pelvic stabilization, the therapist moves the femur anteriorly to the limit of hip flexion (Fig. 6-13). The knee is allowed to flex to prevent the two-joint hamstring muscles from limiting hip flexion ROM.

End Feel. Hip flexion—soft/firm.

Joint Spin.[6] Hip flexion—the convex femoral head spins in the fixed concave acetabulum.

Measurement: Universal Goniometer

Start Position. The patient is supine. The hip and knee on the test side are in the anatomical position (Fig. 6-14). The pelvis is in the neutral position.

Stabilization. The trunk is stabilized through body positioning and the therapist stabilizes the ipsilateral pelvis.

Goniometer Axis. The axis is placed over the greater trochanter of the femur (Fig. 6-15).

Stationary Arm. Parallel to the midaxillary line of the trunk.

Movable Arm. Parallel to the longitudinal axis of the femur, pointing toward the lateral epicondyle.

End Position. The hip is moved to the limit of hip flexion (120°) (Fig. 6-16). The knee is allowed to flex to prevent hamstring muscles from limiting hip flexion ROM.

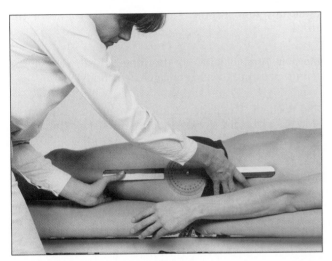

Figure 6-14 Start position: hip flexion.

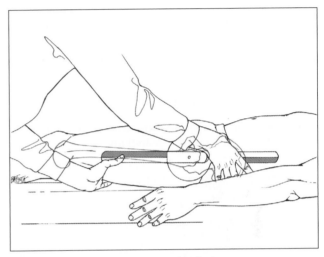

Figure 6-15 Goniometer alignment: hip flexion.

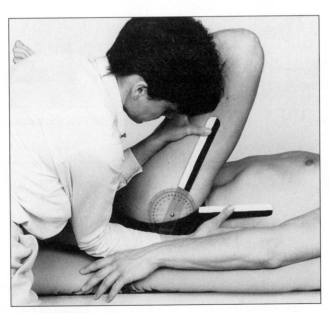

Figure 6-16 End position: hip flexion.

Hip Extension

AROM Assessment

Substitute Movement. Anterior pelvic tilt and extension of the lumbar spine.

PROM Assessment

Form 6-2

Start Position. The patient is prone. Both hips and knees are in the anatomical position. The feet are over the end of the plinth (Fig. 6-17).

Stabilization. The therapist stabilizes the pelvis.

Therapist's Distal Hand Placement. The therapist grasps the anterior aspect of the distal femur.

End Position. The therapist moves the femur posteriorly to the limit of hip extension (Fig. 6-18).

End Feel. Hip extension—firm.

Joint Spin.[6] Hip extension—the convex femoral head spins in the fixed concave acetabulum.

Measurement: Universal Goniometer

Start Position. The patient is prone. The hips and knees are in the anatomical position. The feet are over the end of the plinth (Fig. 6-19).

Stabilization. The pelvis is stabilized through strapping. Alternatively, a second therapist may assist to manually stabilize the pelvis.

Goniometer Axis. The axis is placed over the greater trochanter of the femur.

Stationary Arm. Parallel to the midaxillary line of the trunk.

Movable Arm. Parallel to the longitudinal axis of the femur, pointing toward the lateral epicondyle.

End Position. The patient's knee is maintained in extension to place the rectus femoris on slack. The hip is moved to the limit of hip extension (30°) (Fig. 6-20).

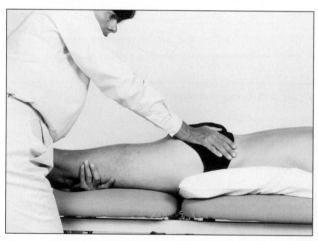

Figure 6-17 Start position: hip extension.

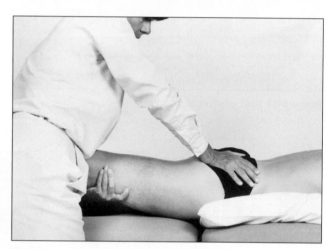

Figure 6-18 Firm end feel at limit of hip extension.

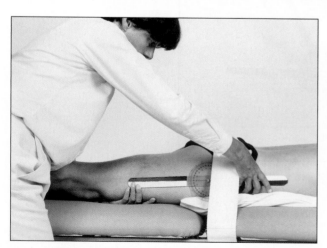

Figure 6-19 Start position: hip extension.

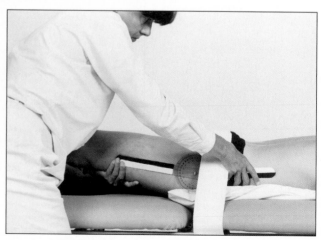

Figure 6-20 End position: hip extension.

Hip Abduction

AROM Assessment

Substitute Movement. External rotation and flexion of the hip, hiking of the ipsilateral pelvis.

PROM Assessment

Form 6-3

Start Position. The patient is supine; the pelvis is level and the lower extremities are in the anatomical position (Fig. 6-21).

Stabilization. The therapist stabilizes the ipsilateral pelvis. If additional stabilization of the trunk and pelvis is required, the contralateral lower extremity may be positioned in hip abduction with the knee flexed over the edge of the plinth and the foot supported on a stool (see Fig. 6-26).

Therapist's Distal Hand Placement. The therapist grasps the medial aspect of the distal femur.

End Position. The therapist moves the femur to the limit of hip abduction motion (Fig. 6-22).

End Feel. Hip abduction—firm.

Joint Glide. Hip abduction—the convex femoral head glides inferiorly on the fixed concave acetabulum.

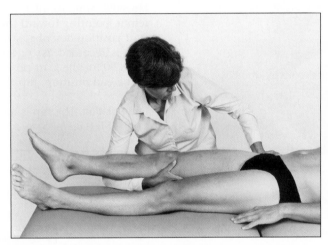

Figure 6-21 Start position for hip abduction.

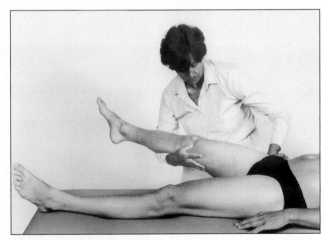

Figure 6-22 Firm end feel at the limit of hip abduction.

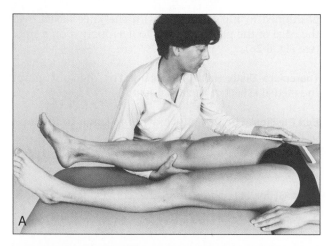

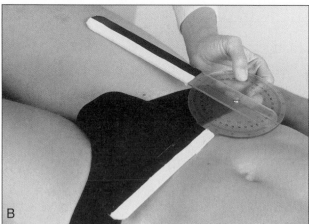

Figure 6-23 **A.** Start position: hip abduction. **B.** Goniometer alignment.

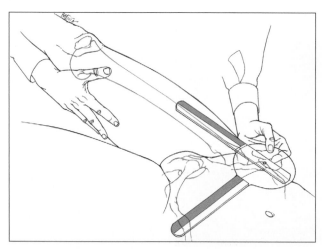

Figure 6-24 Goniometer alignment: hip abduction and adduction.

Measurement: Universal Goniometer

Start Position. The patient is supine with the lower extremities in the anatomical position (Fig. 6-23A). Ensure the pelvis is level.

Stabilization. The therapist stabilizes the ipsilateral pelvis. If additional stabilization of the trunk and pelvis is required, the contralateral lower extremity may be positioned in hip abduction with the knee flexed over the edge of the plinth and the foot supported on a stool (see Fig. 6-26).

Goniometer Axis. The axis is placed over the ASIS on the side being measured (Figs. 6-23B and 6-24).

Stationary Arm. Along a line that joins the two ASISs.

Movable Arm. Parallel to the longitudinal axis of the femur, pointing toward the midline of the patella. In the start position described, the goniometer will indicate 90°. This is recorded as 0°. For example, if the goniometer reads 90° at the start position for hip abduction and 60° at the end position, hip abduction PROM would be 30°.

End Position. The hip is moved to the limit of hip abduction (45°) (Fig. 6-25).

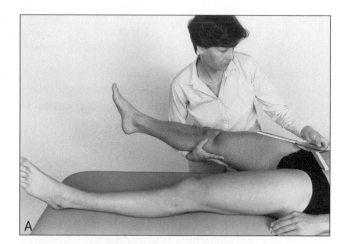

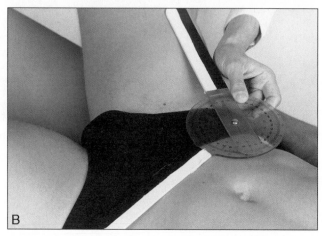

Figure 6-25 **A.** End position: hip abduction. **B.** Goniometer alignment.

Hip Adduction

AROM Assessment

Substitute Movement. Hip internal rotation, hiking of the contralateral pelvis.

PROM Assessment

Start Position. The patient is supine, the pelvis is level, and the lower extremity is in the anatomical position. The hip on the nontest side is abducted to allow full ROM in adduction on the test side. The abducted nontest limb may remain on the plinth or the knee may be flexed over the edge of the plinth with the foot supported on a stool (Fig. 6-26).

Form 6-4

Stabilization. The therapist stabilizes the ipsilateral pelvis.

Therapist's Distal Hand Placement. The therapist grasps the distal femur.

End Position. The therapist moves the femur to the limit of hip adduction ROM (Fig. 6-27).

End Feel. Hip adduction—soft/firm.

Joint Glide. Hip adduction—the convex femoral head glides superiorly on the fixed concave acetabulum.

Measurement: Universal Goniometer

Start Position. The patient is supine with the lower extremity in the anatomical position. The hip on the nontest side is abducted to allow full range of hip adduction on the test side. The pelvis is level.

Stabilization. The therapist stabilizes the ipsilateral pelvis.

Goniometer Axis. The axis is placed over the ASIS on the side being measured. The goniometer is aligned the same as for hip abduction ROM measurement (see Fig. 6-24).

Stationary Arm. Along a line that joins the two ASISs.

Movable Arm. Parallel to the longitudinal axis of the femur, pointing toward the midline of the patella. In the start position described, the goniometer will indicate 90°. This is recorded as 0°. For example, if the goniometer reads 90° at the start position for hip adduction and 105° at the end position, hip adduction PROM would be 15°.

End Position. The hip is moved to the limit of hip adduction (30°) (Fig. 6-28).

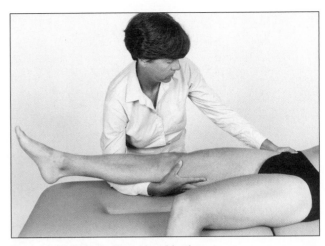

Figure 6-26 Start position: hip adduction.

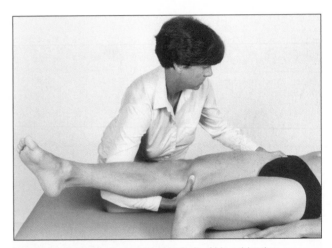

Figure 6-27 Soft or firm end feel at limit of hip adduction.

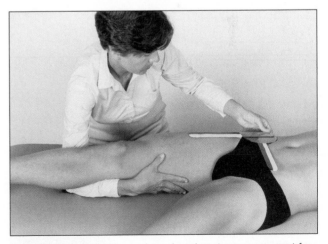

Figure 6-28 End position: universal goniometer measurement for hip adduction.

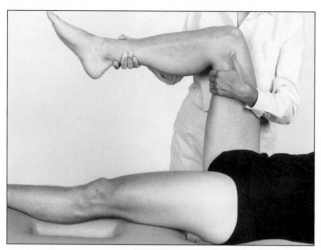

Figure 6-29 Start position: hip internal and external rotation.

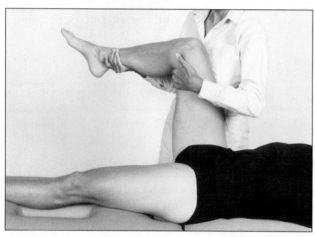

Figure 6-30 Firm end feel at the limit of hip internal rotation.

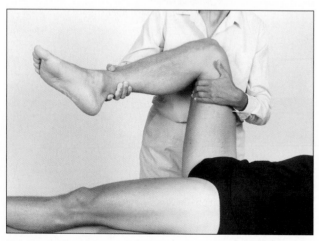

Figure 6-31 Firm end feel at the limit of hip external rotation.

Hip Internal and External Rotation

AROM Assessment

Substitute Movement. Lateral tilting of the pelvis. In sitting, the patient shifts body weight to raise the pelvis and lift the buttocks off the sitting surface.

PROM Assessment

Start Position. The patient is sitting or supine with the hip and knee flexed to 90° (Fig. 6-29).

Form 6-5, 6-6 **Stabilization.** The pelvis is stabilized through body positioning. The therapist maintains the position of the femur, without restricting movement.

Therapist's Distal Hand Placement. The therapist grasps the distal tibia and fibula.

End Position. The therapist moves the tibia and fibula in a lateral direction to the limit of hip internal rotation (Fig. 6-30) and in a medial direction to the limit of hip external rotation (Fig. 6-31). The stresses on the knee joint should be considered and caution exercised.

End Feels. *Hip internal rotation—firm; hip external rotation—firm.*

Joint Glides. *Hip internal rotation*—the convex femoral head glides on the fixed concave acetabulum in a posterior direction with the hip in anatomical position, and in an inferior direction with the hip in a position of 90° flexion.

Hip external rotation—the convex femoral head glides on the fixed concave acetabulum in an anterior direction with the hip in anatomical position, and in a superior direction with the hip in a position of 90° flexion.

Measurement: Universal Goniometer

Start Position. The patient is sitting. In sitting, the hip being measured is in 90° of flexion and neutral rotation with the knee flexed to 90°. A pad is placed under the distal thigh to keep the thigh in a horizontal position. The contralateral hip is abducted and the foot is supported on a stool (Fig. 6-32).

Alternate Starting Positions

- Supine with the lower extremities in anatomical position,
- Supine with the hip and knee flexed to 90° (see Fig. 6-29),
- Sit-lying (i.e., supine with the knees flexed 90° over the end of the plinth), and
- Prone with the knee flexed 90° (see Fig. 6-37).

Hip rotation PROM is greater when measured with the patient prone than sitting.[15] To accurately evaluate patient progress, the position used to measure hip rotation PROM should be charted,[15] and the same position used on subsequent measurement.

Stabilization. The pelvis is stabilized through body positioning. The therapist maintains the position of the femur without restricting movement. In sitting, the patient grasps the edge of the plinth. In prone, the pelvis is stabilized through strapping (Fig. 6-37).

Goniometer Axis. The axis is placed over the midpoint of the patella (Figs. 6-33 and 6-34).

Stationary Arm. Perpendicular to the floor.

Movable Arm. Parallel to the anterior midline of the tibia.

End Positions. Internal rotation (Figs. 6-34 and 6-35): The hip is moved to the limit of hip internal rotation (45°) as the leg and foot move in a lateral direction.

External rotation (Figs. 6-36 and 6-37): The hip is moved to the limit of hip external rotation (45°) as the leg and foot move in a medial direction.

Hip rotation PROM measurements may not accurately reflect hip rotation ROM if the measurement technique is influenced by mobility at the knee joint. Harris-Hayes and colleagues[16] measured hip rotation PROM in prone with the knee flexed 90°, with and without the tibiofemoral joint stabilized. The researchers found a clinically relevant increase in hip rotation PROM in women (not men), attributed to motion at the knee joint.

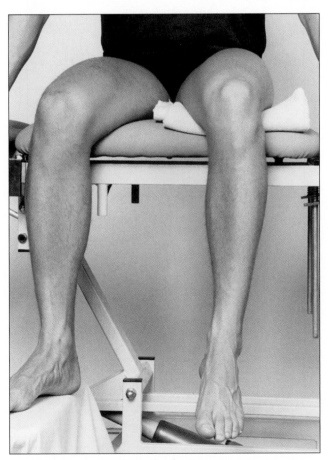

Figure 6-32 Start position: hip internal and external rotation.

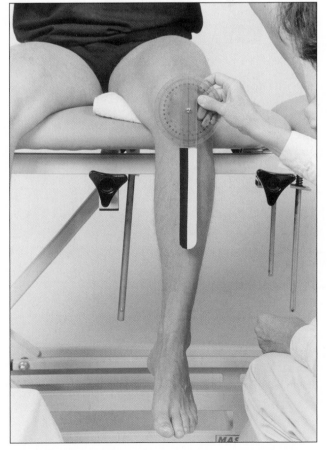

Figure 6-33 Start position: goniometer placement for hip internal and external rotation.

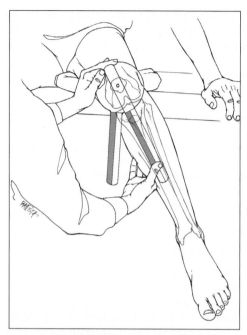

Figure 6-34 Goniometer alignment: hip internal rotation and external rotation. Illustrated with the hip in internal rotation.

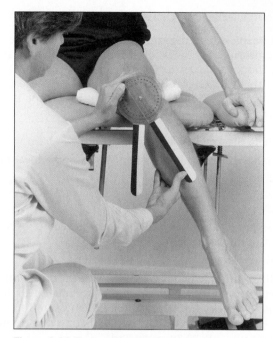

Figure 6-35 End position: internal rotation.

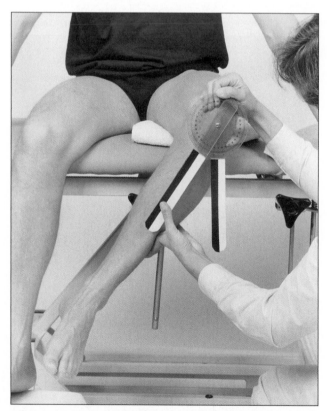

Figure 6-36 End position: external rotation.

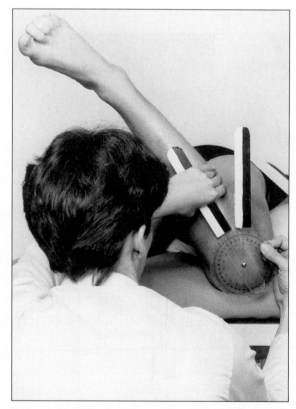

Figure 6-37 Alternate test position: prone with the knee flexed 90° and the hip in external rotation.

Measurement: OB Goniometer

The procedure for measurement of hip internal and external rotation PROM is the same as described for Measurement: Universal Goniometer, except for the placement and use of the OB Goniometer.

OB Goniometer Placement. The strap is placed around the lower leg proximal to the ankle. The dial is placed on the anterior aspect of the lower leg (Figs. 6-38, 6-39, and 6-40).

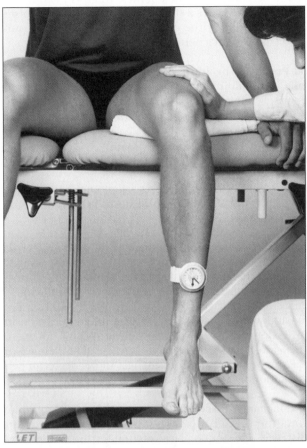

Figure 6-38 Start position: OB goniometer measurement hip rotation.

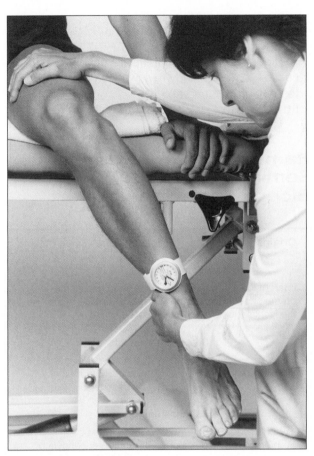

Figure 6-39 Internal rotation.

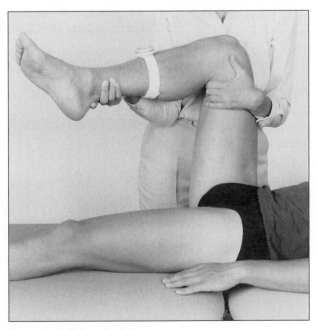

Figure 6-40 External rotation.

MUSCLE LENGTH ASSESSMENT AND MEASUREMENT

Practice Makes Perfect

To aid you in practicing the skills covered in this section, or for a handy review, use the practical testing forms found at http://thepoint.lww.com/Clarkson3e.

Hamstrings (Semitendinosus, Semimembranous, Biceps Femoris)

Origins[2]	Insertions[2]
Semitendinosus	
Inferomedial impression on the superior aspect of the ischial tuberosity	Proximal part of the medial surface of the tibia.
Semimembranosus	
Superolateral aspect of the ischial tuberosity	Tubercle on the posterior aspect of the medial tibial condyle.
Biceps Femoris	
a. Long head: inferomedial impression of the superior aspect of the ischial tuberosity; lower portion of the sacrotuberous ligament	Head of the fibula; slip to the lateral condyle of the tibia; slip to the lateral collateral ligament.
b. Short head: lateral lip of the linea aspera and lateral supracondylar line	

Passive Straight Leg Raise (PSLR)

Start Position. The patient is supine with the lower extremities in the anatomical position (Fig. 6-41). The low back and sacrum should be flat on the plinth.[11] Ankle dorsiflexion limits the ROM of SLR,[17] therefore the test is performed with the ankle relaxed in plantarflexion.

Form 6-7

Stabilization. It is difficult to stabilize the pelvis when performing PSLR, and pelvic rotation is not eliminated from the movement.[18] However, the therapist must ensure that excessive anterior or posterior pelvic tilt is avoided through use of a precise start position, adequate stabilization, and observation of pelvic motion. To stabilize the pelvis, the patient's nontest thigh is held on the plinth with the use of a strap (Fig. 6-41), or the therapist's knee is placed over the distal aspect of the anterior surface of the patient's nontest thigh (not shown).

End Position. The hip is flexed to the limit of motion while maintaining knee extension so that the biceps femoris, semitendinosus, and semimembranosus are put on full stretch (Figs. 6-42 and 6-43). The ankle is relaxed in plantarflexion during the test.

End Feel. Hamstrings on stretch—firm.

Measurement. The therapist uses a goniometer to measure and record the available hip flexion PROM (Figs. 6-42, 6-43, and 6-44).

Universal Goniometer Placement. The goniometer is placed the same as for hip flexion. A second therapist may assist to align and read the goniometer. Normal ROM and hamstring length is about 80° hip flexion.[11] Youdas and colleagues[19] assessed the PSLR ROM of 214 men and women, aged 20 to 79 years, and reported mean hip flexion PROM of 76° for women and 69° for men. When interpreting test results, consider that changes in PSLR might also result from changes in the degree of pelvic rotation.[20]

OB Goniometer Placement. This measurement procedure allows the therapist to easily assess PSLR ROM without assistance. The strap is placed around the distal thigh and the dial is placed on the lateral aspect of the thigh (Fig. 6-45).

Alternate Positions—Passive Knee Extension (PKE) and Sitting

These alternate techniques used to evaluate hamstring muscle length are described in Chapter 7.

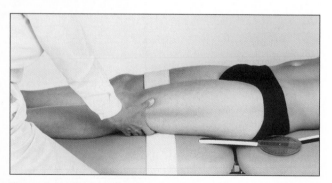

Figure 6-41 Start position: length of hamstrings.

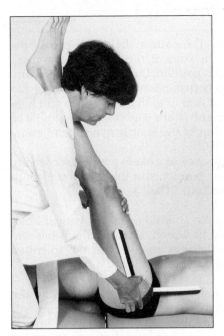

Figure 6-42 End position: universal goniometer measurement of hamstrings length.

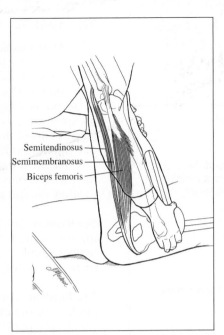

Figure 6-43 Hamstring muscles on stretch.

Semitendinosus
Semimembranosus
Biceps femoris

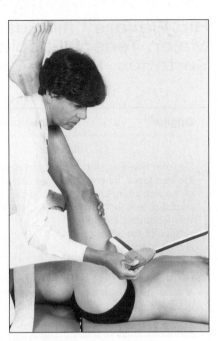

Figure 6-44 Reading goniometer: hamstrings length.

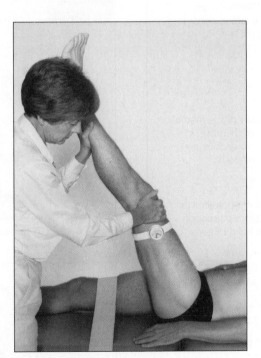

Figure 6-45 End position: OB goniometer measurement of hamstrings length.

Hip Flexors[11] (Iliacus, Psoas Major, Tensor Fascia Latae, Sartorius, Rectus Femoris)

Origins[2]	Insertions[2]
Iliacus	
Superior two-thirds of the iliac fossa, inner lip of the iliac crest; ventral sacroiliac and iliolumbar ligaments; and the upper surface of the lateral aspect of the sacrum.	Lateral side of the tendon of psoas major; and into the lesser trochanter.
Psoas Major	
Anterior aspects of the transverse processes of all of the lumbar vertebrae; sides of the bodies and intervertebral discs of T12 and all the lumbar vertebrae.	Lesser trochanter of the femur.
Tensor Fascia Latae	
Anterior aspect of the outer lip of the iliac crest; outer surface and notch below the ASIS; and the deep surface of the fascia latae.	Via the iliotibial tract onto the lateral condyle of the tibia.
Sartorius	
ASIS and the upper half of the notch below it.	Upper part of the medial surface of the tibia (anterior to gracilis and semitendinosus).
Rectus Femoris	
a. Straight head: anterior aspect of the anterior inferior iliac spine.	Base of the patella, via the quadriceps tendon into the tibial tuberosity.
b. Reflected head: groove above the acetabulum and the capsule of the hip joint.	

Thomas Test

Start Position. The patient sits at the end of the plinth with the edge of the plinth at mid-thigh level. From this position, the patient is assisted into supine. Using both hands, the patient holds the hip of the nontest leg in flexion so that the sacrum and lumbar spine are flat on the plinth (Fig. 6-46). Care should be taken to avoid flexion of the lumbar spine due to excessive hip flexion ROM.

Form 6-8

(*Note:* In the presence of excessive hip flexor length, the patient's hips are positioned at the edge of the plinth to allow the full available ROM.[11])

Stabilization. The supine position, and the patient holding the nontest hip in flexion, stabilizes the pelvis and lumbar spine. The therapist observes the ASIS to ensure there is no pelvic tilting during the test.

End Position. The test leg is allowed to fall toward the plinth into hip extension (Fig. 6-47). As the test leg falls toward the plinth, the therapist ensures: (1) the knee is free to move into extension to avoid placing the rectus femoris on stretch, and (2) the thigh remains in neutral adduction/abduction and rotation.

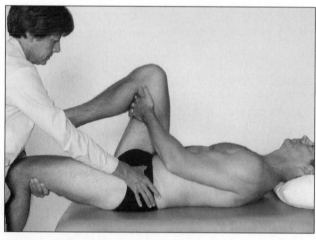

Figure 6-46 Start position: length of hip flexors.

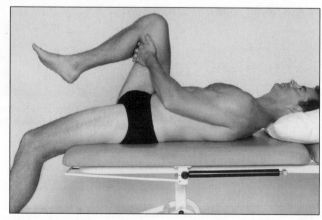

Figure 6-47 End position: thigh touching plinth indicates normal length of hip flexors.

If the thigh touches the plinth (Fig. 6-47), the hip flexors, that is, iliopsoas, is considered to be of normal length.[11]

If the thigh does not touch the plinth (Fig. 6-48), the therapist passively extends the knee and if:

1. The thigh touches the plinth (Fig. 6-49), shortness of rectus femoris restricted the hip extension ROM.

2. There is no change in the position of the thigh; the therapist applies slight overpressure on the anterior aspect of the thigh to passively move the femur posteriorly to the limit of movement (Figs. 6-50 and 6-51). The end feel is evaluated to determine if iliopsoas shortness is the cause of the hip extension ROM restriction. Note that a flexion deformity at the hip can be obscured by an increased lumbar lordosis.[21]

End Feel. Iliacus and psoas major on stretch—firm.

Measurement. With shortness of the hip flexors, that is, iliopsoas, the angle between the midaxillary line of the trunk and the longitudinal axis of the femur represents the degree of hip flexion contracture (Figs. 6-50 and 6-51).

Universal Goniometer Placement. The same as for hip flexion-extension with the axis over the greater trochanter of the femur (Figs. 6-50 and 6-51).

Additional Considerations. If a restriction of hip joint extension is present (i.e., the thigh does not rest on the plinth) with the knee joint in extension, shortness of the iliopsoas, sartorius, or tensor fascia latae muscles may contribute to the limited ROM. The muscle shortness causing the restriction can be determined using the following criteria[11]:

A. Shortness of the *sartorius* should be suspected if the hip joint assumes a position of external rotation and abduction and/or the knee flexes at the restricted limit of hip extension.

B. Shortness of the *tensor fascia latae* may be suspected if the thigh is observed to abduct as the hip joint extends. If during testing the thigh is abducted as the hip is extended, and this results in increased hip extension, there is shortness of the tensor fascia latae. Specific length testing of tensor fascia latae should be performed to confirm this finding. Van Dillen and colleagues[22] suggest that abducting the hip may place the anterior fibers of the gluteus medius and minimus on slack and thus also contribute to the increase in hip extension. If hip abduction makes no difference to the restricted hip extension ROM, the *iliopsoas* muscle is shortened and preventing the full movement.

If the thigh is prevented from abducting during testing, a shortened tensor fascia latae may also produce hip internal rotation, lateral deviation of the patella, external rotation of the tibia, or knee extension.

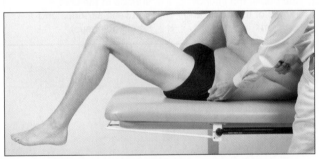

Figure 6-48 End position: thigh does not touch plinth.

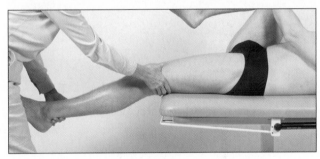

Figure 6-49 Thigh touches plinth with knee extended.

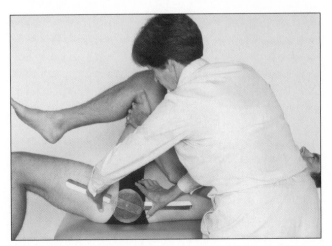

Figure 6-50 Goniometer measurement: length of shortened hip flexors.

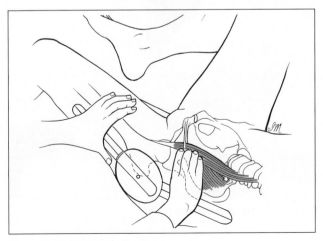

Figure 6-51 Hip flexors on stretch.

Hip Adductors (Adductor Longus, Adductor Brevis, Adductor Magnus, Pectineus, and Gracilis)

Start Position. The patient is supine with the lower extremity in the anatomical position. On the non-test side, the hip is abducted, the knee is flexed, and the foot rests on a stool beside the plinth (Fig. 6-52).

Form 6-9

Stabilization. The therapist stabilizes the ipsilateral pelvis.

End Position. The hip is abducted to the limit of motion so that the hip adductor muscles are put on full stretch (Fig. 6-53).

End Feel. Hip adductors on stretch—firm.

Origins[2]	Insertions[2]
Adductor Longus	
Front of the pubis in the angle between the crest and the symphysis.	Middle third of the linea aspera of the femur.
Adductor Brevis	
External surface of the inferior pubic ramus between gracilis and obturator externus.	Line between lesser trochanter and linea aspera; upper part of the linea aspera.
Adductor Magnus	
External surface of the inferior ramus of the pubis adjacent to the ischium; the external surface of the inferior ramus of the ischium; and the inferolateral aspect of the ischial tuberosity.	Medial margin of the gluteal tuberosity of the femur; medial lip of the linea aspera; medial supracondylar line; adductor tubercle.
Pectineus	
Pecten pubis between the iliopectineal eminence and the pubic tubercle.	Line between the lesser trochanter and the linea aspera.
Gracilis	
Lower half of the body of the pubis; the inferior ramus of the pubis and ischium.	Upper part of the medial surface of the tibia (between sartorius and semitendinosus).

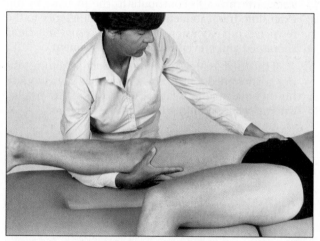

Figure 6-52 Start position: length of hip adductors.

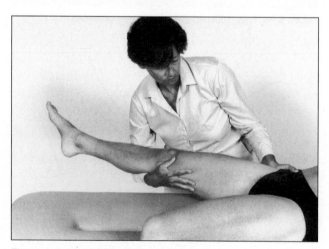

Figure 6-53 Hip adductors on stretch.

Measurement. If the hip adductors are shortened, hip abduction PROM will be restricted proportional to the decrease in muscle length. The therapist uses a goniometer to measure and record the available hip abduction PROM (Figs. 6-54 and 6-55).

Universal Goniometer Placement. The goniometer is placed the same as for hip abduction (Fig. 6-55).

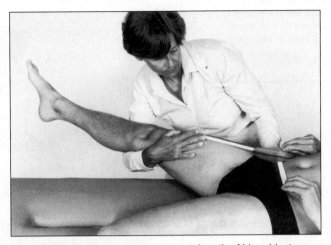

Figure 6-54 Goniometer measurement: length of hip adductors.

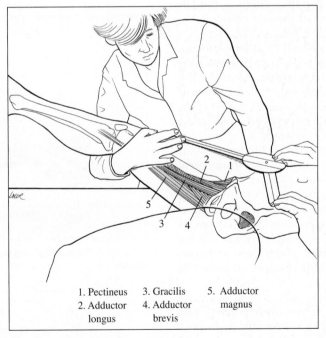

1. Pectineus
2. Adductor longus
3. Gracilis
4. Adductor brevis
5. Adductor magnus

Figure 6-55 Hip adductors on stretch.

Tensor Fascia Latae (Iliotibial Band)—Ober's Test[23]

Origin[2]	Insertion[2]
Tensor Fascia Latae	
Anterior aspect of the outer lip of the iliac crest; the outer surface and notch below the ASIS; and the deep surface of the fascia latae.	Via the iliotibial tract onto the anterolateral aspect of the lateral condyle of the tibia.

Start Position. The patient is in the side-lying position on the nontest side and holds the nontest leg in hip and knee flexion to flatten the lumbar spine. The therapist stands behind and against the patient's pelvis to maintain the side-lying position. The hip is positioned in abduction and then extension to stretch the iliotibial band over the greater trochanter. The hip is in neutral rotation and the knee is positioned in 90° flexion (Fig. 6-56).

Form 6-10

Stabilization. The position of the nontest leg stabilizes the pelvis and lumbar spine; the therapist stabilizes the lateral pelvis at the superior aspect of the iliac crest.

End Position. The test leg is allowed to fall toward the plinth. The therapist may apply slight overpressure on the lateral aspect of the thigh to passively adduct the hip to the limit of movement (not shown). With shortness of the tensor fascia latae, the hip remains abducted (Figs. 6-57 and 6-58). If the leg cannot be passively adducted to the horizontal, there is maximal tightness; if the horizontal position is reached, there is moderate tightness; and if the leg falls below horizontal but does not completely reach the plinth, there is minimal tightness.[24]

Note that tightness of the tensor fascia latae at the hip can be obscured by a downward lateral tilt of the pelvis on the test side that may be accompanied by trunk lateral flexion on the opposite side. The position of the test leg must be carefully maintained in hip extension and neutral or slight external rotation to perform an accurate test of tensor fascia latae tightness.

If the rectus femoris muscle is tight or there is a need to decrease stress in the region of the knee, the Ober's Test may be modified (Modified Ober's Test) and performed with the knee in extension[11] (not shown). Note that the degree of hip adduction ROM used to indicate the length of tensor fascia latae will be more restricted with the knee in flexion (Ober's Test) than with the knee in extension (Modified Ober's Test).[25,26] Therefore, these tests should not be used interchangeably[26] when assessing tensor fascia latae muscle length.

End Feel. Tensor fascia latae (iliotibial band) on stretch—firm.

Measurement. If the tensor fascia latae is shortened, hip adduction PROM will be restricted proportional to the decrease in muscle length.

Universal Goniometer Placement. The goniometer is placed the same as for hip abduction/adduction. A second therapist is required to assist with the alignment and reading of the goniometer.

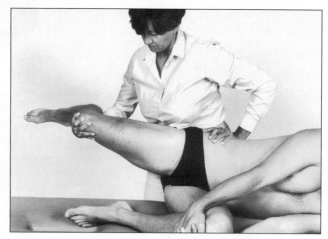

Figure 6-56 Ober's Test start position: length of tensor fascia latae.

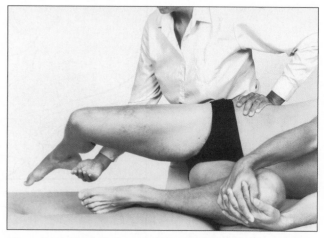

Figure 6-57 Ober's Test end position: tensor fascia latae on stretch.

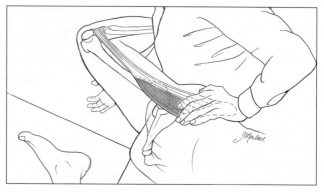

Figure 6-58 Ober's Test: tensor fascia latae on stretch.

Alternate Measurement: Ober's Test: Trunk Prone

Form 6-11

Kendall and colleagues[11] describe the "Modified Ober Test: Trunk Prone" to assess tensor fascia latae muscle length. This test provides better stabilization than the Ober's Test.

Start Position. The patient is standing at the end of the plinth and flexes the hips so the trunk is resting on the plinth (Fig. 6-59). The nontest leg is placed under the plinth with the hip and knee flexed. The patient positions the arms overhead and grasps the sides of the plinth. The therapist supports the test leg and, while maintaining the knee in 90° flexion and the hip in neutral rotation, moves the hip into full abduction, followed by full extension to stretch the iliotibial band over the greater trochanter.

Stabilization. The therapist stabilizes the posterior aspect of the ipsilateral pelvis to prevent anterior pelvic tilt. It is also important the therapist stabilize the lateral aspect of the pelvis to prevent elevation of the contralateral pelvis, and downward lateral tilt of the ipsilateral pelvis. The patient's arm position aids in preventing lateral pelvic tilt. The weight of the trunk offers stabilization.

End Position. With the hip maintained in full extension and neutral rotation, the hip is adducted to the limit of motion to place the tensor fascia latae on full stretch (Fig. 6-60). If the tensor fascia latae is shortened, hip adduction PROM with the hip in extension, will be restricted proportional to the decrease in muscle length.

End Feel. Tensor fascia latae on stretch—firm.

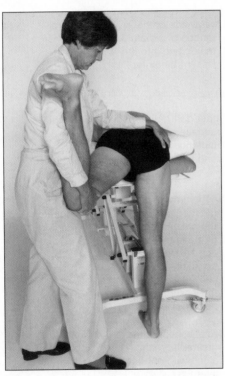

Figure 6-59 Start position: Ober's Test: Trunk Prone.

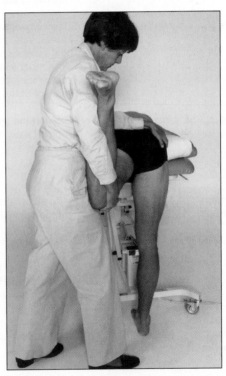

Figure 6-60 End position: tensor fascia latae on stretch.

MUSCLE STRENGTH ASSESSMENT (TABLE 6-2)

 Practice Makes Perfect

To aid you in practicing the skills covered in this section, or for a handy review, use the practical testing forms found at http://thepoint.lww.com/Clarkson3e.

TABLE 6-2   Muscle Actions, Attachments, and Nerve Supply: the Hip[27]

Muscle	Primary Muscle Action	Muscle Origin	Muscle Insertion	Peripheral Nerve	Nerve Root
Psoas major	Hip flexion	Anterior aspects of the transverse processes of all of the lumbar vertebrae; sides of the bodies and intervertebral discs of T12 and all of the lumbar vertebrae	Lesser trochanter of the femur	Ventral rami of the lumbar	L123
Iliacus	Hip flexion	Superior two-thirds of the iliac fossa, inner lip of the iliac crest; the ventral sacroiliac and iliolumbar ligaments; and the upper surface of the lateral aspect of the sacrum	Lateral side of the tendon of psoas major; and into the lesser trochanter	Femoral	L23
Sartorius	Hip flexion, abduction, and external rotation Knee flexion	ASIS and the upper one half of the notch below it	Upper part of the medial surface of the tibia (anterior to gracilis and semitendinosus)	Femoral	L23
Obturator internus	Hip external rotation	Pelvic surface of the inferior ramus of the pubis and ischium and the superior ramus of the pubis; the pelvic surface of the obturator membrane; above and behind the obturator foramen, as far as the upper part of the greater sciatic foramen	Anterior impression on the medial aspect of the greater trochanter of the femur, superior and anterior to the trochanteric fossa (after passing through the lesser sciatic notch)	Nerve to obturator internus	L5S1
Gemellus superior	Hip external rotation	Dorsal aspect of the spine of the ischium	Medial aspect of the greater trochanter along with obturator internus	Nerve to obturator internus	L5S1
Gemellus inferior	Hip external rotation	Superior aspect of the tuberosity of the ischium	Medial aspect of the greater trochanter along with obturator internus	Nerve to quadratus femoris	L5S1
Obturator externus	Hip external rotation	Superior and inferior pubic ramus and the inferior ramus of the ischium; medial two-thirds of the outer surface of the obturator membrane; medial side of the obturator foramen	Trochanteric fossa of the greater trochanter of the femur	Obturator	L34
Quadratus femoris	Hip external rotation	Upper portion of the external aspect of the ischial tuberosity	Quadrate tubercle and area of bone just below it on the femur	Nerve to quadratus femoris	L5S1

(continued)

TABLE 6-2 *Continued*

Muscle	Primary Muscle Action	Muscle Origin	Muscle Insertion	Peripheral Nerve	Nerve Root
Pectineus	Hip adduction	Pecten pubis between the iliopectineal eminence and the pubic tubercle	Line between the lesser trochanter and the linea aspera	Femoral	L23
Adductor longus	Hip adduction	Front of the pubis in the angle between the crest and the symphysis	Middle third of the linea aspera of the femur	Obturator	L234
Adductor brevis	Hip adduction	External surface of the inferior pubic ramus between gracilis and obturator externus	Line between lesser trochanter and linea aspera; upper part of linea aspera	Obturator	L23
Gracilis	Hip adduction	Lower half of the body of the pubis; the inferior ramus of the pubis and ischium	Upper part of the medial surface of the tibia (between sartorius and semitendinosus)	Obturator	L23
Adductor magnus	Hip adduction	External surface of the inferior ramus of the pubis adjacent to the ischium; the external surface of the inferior ramus of the ischium; and the inferolateral aspect of the ischial tuberosity	Medial margin of the gluteal tuberosity of the femur; medial lip of the linea aspera; and the medial supracondylar line; adductor tubercle	Obturator, Sciatic (tibial division)	L234
Piriformis	Hip external rotation	Pelvic surface of the sacrum between the second to fourth sacral foramina, and gluteal surface of the ilium adjacent to the posterior inferior iliac spine	Medial aspect of the upper border of the greater trochanter of the femur (after passing through the greater sciatic foramina)	Branches from	L5S12
Gluteus maximus	Hip extension	Posterior gluteal line of the ilium and the iliac crest above and behind the line; aponeurosis of the erector spinae; dorsal surface of the lower part of the sacrum and the side of the coccyx; and sacrotuberous ligament	Iliotibial tract and gluteal tuberosity	Inferior gluteal	L5S12
Tensor fascia latae	Hip flexion, abduction, and internal rotation (through the iliotibial tract—knee extension)	Anterior aspect of the outer lip of the iliac crest; the outer surface and notch below the ASIS; and the deep surface of the fascia lata	Iliotibial tract	Superior gluteal	L45S1
Gluteus medius	Hip abduction and internal rotation	Outer surface of the ilium between the iliac crest and posterior gluteal line above and the anterior gluteal line below	Oblique ridge, downwards and forwards, on the lateral surface of the greater trochanter	Superior gluteal	L45S1
Gluteus minimus	Hip abduction and internal rotation	Outer surface of the ilium between the anterior and inferior gluteal lines and the margin of the greater sciatic notch	Anterolateral aspect of the greater trochanter	Superior gluteal	L45S1

Hip Flexion

Against Gravity: Iliopsoas

Accessory muscles: rectus femoris, sartorius, tensor fascia latae, and pectineus.

Form
6-12   **Start Position.** The patient is sitting with the knee flexed and foot unsupported. The contralateral foot is supported on a stool (Fig. 6-61).

Alternate Start Position. The patient is supine. The hip and knee are in the anatomical position. The leg not being tested is flexed at the hip and knee (Fig. 6-62). In this position, gravity assists hip flexion beyond 90°. Resistance is added equal to the weight of the limb to compensate when assessing a grade 3 (not shown).

Stabilization. The therapist stabilizes the pelvis by placing the hand over the ipsilateral iliac crest. If sitting, the patient also grasps the edge of the plinth to stabilize the proximal body segments.

Movement. The patient flexes the hip through full ROM. The knee is allowed to flex (Fig. 6-63). In the supine position, the hip and knee are flexed (Fig. 6-64). Beyond 90°, gravity assists motion and the therapist can add resistance.

Palpation. Iliacus and psoas major are not easily palpated.

Substitute Movement. Substitution by the accessory muscles can be observed through additional movement patterns: abduction and external rotation via sartorius; abduction and internal rotation via tensor fascia latae.[4]

Resistance Location. Applied over the anterior aspect of the thigh proximal to the knee joint (Figs. 6-65, 6-66, and 6-67).

Resistance Direction. Hip extension.

Figure 6-61 Start position: iliopsoas.

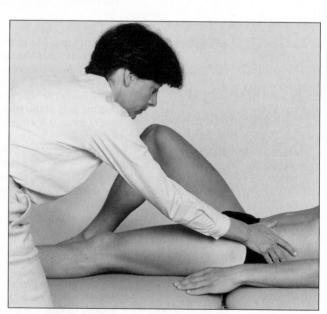

Figure 6-62 Alternate start position: iliopsoas.

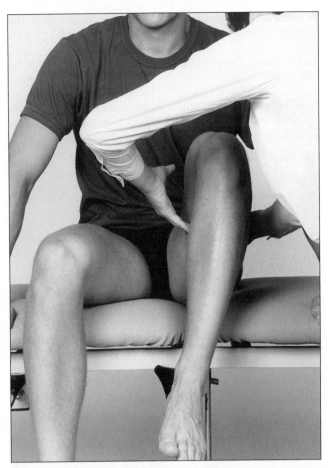

Figure 6-63 Screen position: iliopsoas.

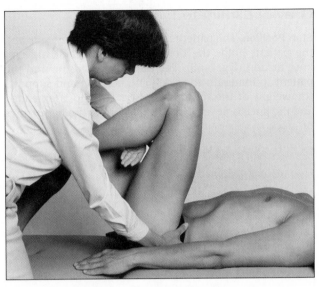

Figure 6-64 Alternate screen position: iliopsoas.

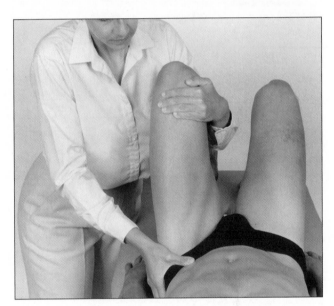

Figure 6-66 Resistance in alternate test position: iliopsoas.

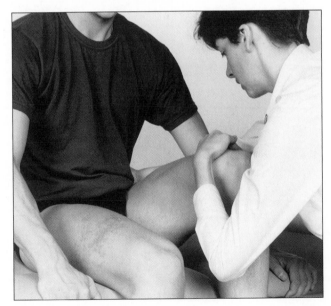

Figure 6-65 Resistance: iliopsoas.

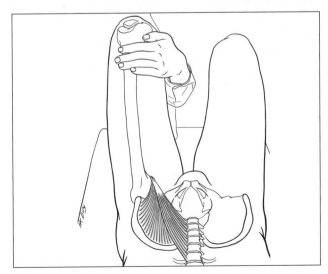

Figure 6-67 Iliopsoas.

Gravity Eliminated: Iliopsoas

Start Position. The patient is lying on the nontest side and the patient holds the nontest leg in maximal hip and knee flexion (Fig. 6-68). The therapist stands behind the patient to maintain the side-lying position and supports the weight of the lower extremity. The hip is extended and the knee is flexed. Knee flexion places the hamstrings on slack.

Stabilization. The position of the nontest leg stabilizes the lumbar spine; the therapist stabilizes the pelvis.

End Position. The patient flexes the hip through full ROM (Fig. 6-69).

Substitute Movement. Hip abduction with hip external or internal rotation[4] and posterior pelvic tilt through the abdominal muscles.[28]

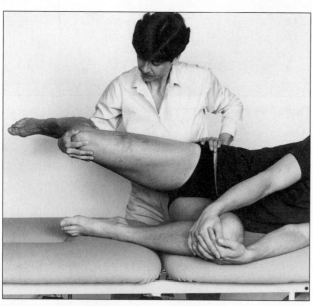

Figure 6-68 Start position: iliopsoas.

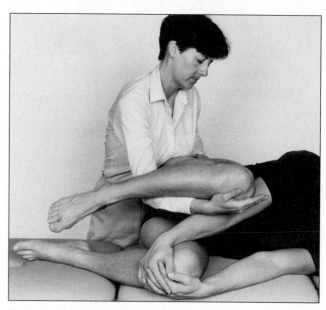

Figure 6-69 End position: iliopsoas.

Hip Flexion, Abduction, and External Rotation with Knee Flexion

Against Gravity: Sartorius

Accessory muscles: iliopsoas, rectus femoris, and tensor fascia latae.

Form 6-13

Start Position. The patient is supine with both legs in the anatomical position (Fig. 6-70).

Alternate Start Position. The patient is sitting with the knee flexed and the foot unsupported. The contralateral foot is supported on a stool (Fig. 6-71).

Stabilization. The weight of the trunk in supine. In sitting, the therapist stabilizes the pelvis at the ipsilateral iliac crest, and the patient grasps the edge of the plinth.

Movement. The patient flexes, abducts, and externally rotates the hip and flexes the knee (Figs. 6-72 and 6-73).

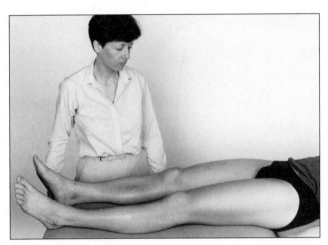

Figure 6-70 Start position: sartorius.

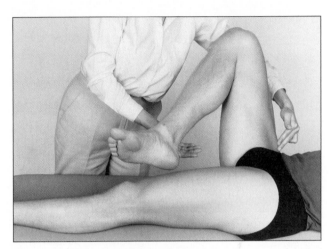

Figure 6-72 Screen position: sartorius.

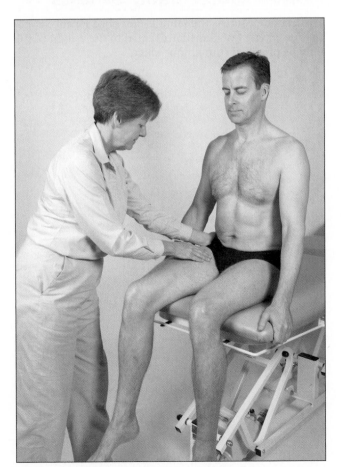

Figure 6-71 Alternate start position: sartorius.

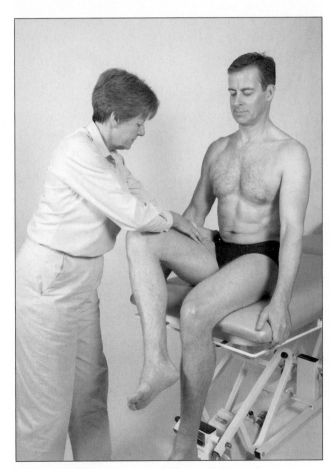

Figure 6-73 Alternate screen position: sartorius.

Palpation. On the anterior aspect of the thigh medial to tensor fascia latae.

Substitute Movement. Iliopsoas and rectus femoris. To ensure the correct movement, the heel of the test leg should pass just above and parallel to the shin of the contralateral leg. The activity in tensor fascia latae decreases when hip flexion is combined with external rotation.[29]

Resistance Locations. Applied at the same time: (1) at the anterolateral aspect of the thigh proximal to the knee joint, and (2) at the posterior aspect of the lower leg proximal to the ankle joint (Figs. 6-74, 6-75 and 6-76).

Resistance Direction. (1) Hip extension, adduction, and internal rotation; (2) knee extension.

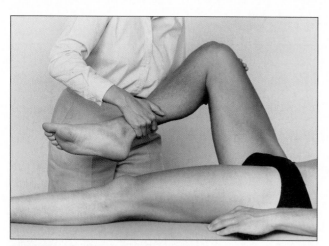

Figure 6-74 Resistance: sartorius.

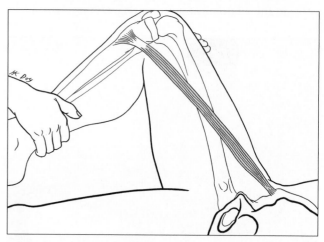

Figure 6-75 Sartorius.

Assisted Against Gravity: Sartorius

The test procedure is the same as described for the supine against gravity test. Assistance, equal to the weight of the limb, is provided throughout range.

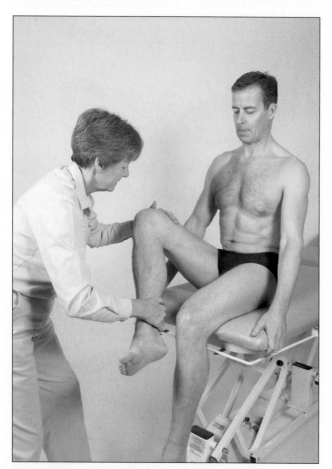

Figure 6-76 Resistance: sartorius alternate position.

Hip Extension

Against Gravity: Gluteus Maximus, Biceps Femoris, Semitendinosus, and Semimembranosus

 Accessory muscles: adductor magnus, piriformis, and gluteus medius.

Form
6-14   **Start Position.** This position is indicated for testing patients with tight hip flexors (Fig. 6-77).

The patient is standing with the trunk flexed and thorax resting on the plinth. The leg not being tested is placed under the table so that the hip and knee are flexed. The test leg hip is flexed and the knee is extended.

Alternate Start Position. The patient is prone with the legs in the anatomical position and two pillows are placed under the pelvis to flex the hips (Fig. 6-78).

Stabilization. The therapist or a pelvic strap is used to stabilize the pelvis. The patient grasps the edges of the plinth; the weight of the trunk offers stabilization.

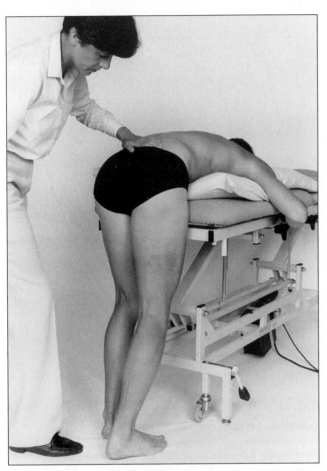

Figure 6-77 Start position: hip extensors.

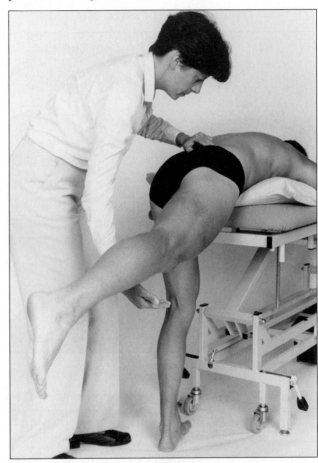

Figure 6-79 Screen position: hip extensors.

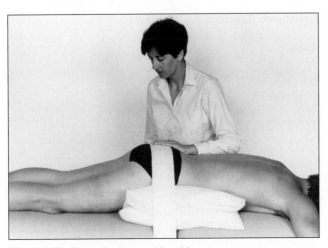

Figure 6-78 Alternate start position: hip extensors.

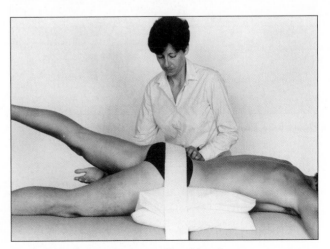

Figure 6-80 Alternate screen position: hip extensors.

Movement. The patient extends the hip with the knee held in extension (Figs. 6-79 and 6-80). The patient is instructed to maintain external rotation to gain maximum contraction of the gluteus maximus. Extending the hip with the knee actively flexed places the hamstrings in a shortened position and this test position has been advocated for isolation of gluteus maximus.[4] Although some of the efficiency of hamstrings may be decreased when the knee is actively maintained in flexion,[5,30] the hamstrings are active in maintaining knee flexion and cannot be eliminated.[30,31] The therapist can passively hold the knee in flexion to isolate the gluteus maximus, but it is difficult to maintain the knee position while applying pressure to the thigh.[31]

The knee must be held in extension in the presence of rectus femoris tightness.

Palpation. Gluteus maximus: medial to its insertion on the gluteal tuberosity or adjacent to its origin from the posterior aspect of the ilium (see Fig. 6-85B).

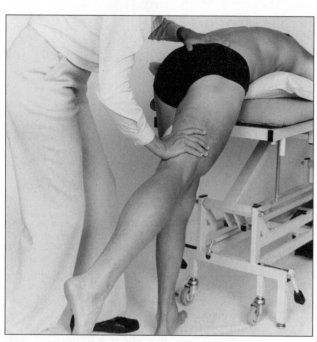

Figure 6-81 Resistance: hip extensors.

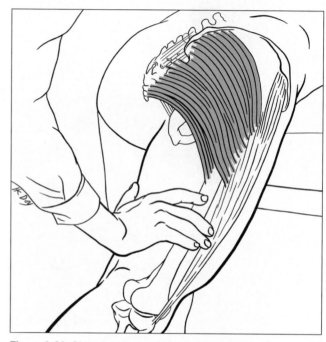

Figure 6-82 Gluteus maximus.

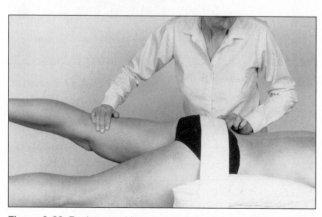

Figure 6-83 Resistance: hip extensors alternate position.

Substitute Movement. Lumbar spine extension.

Resistance Location. Applied on the posterior aspect of the thigh proximal to the knee joint (Figs. 6-81, 6-82, and 6-83).

Resistance Direction. Hip flexion.

Gravity Eliminated: Gluteus Maximus, Biceps Femoris, Semitendinosus, and Semimembranosus

Start Position. The patient is lying on the nontest side with the hip and the knee flexed (Fig. 6-84).

Stabilization. The patient holds the nontest leg in maximal hip and knee flexion to stabilize the trunk and pelvis and prevent lumbar spine extension.

End Position. The patient extends the hip through full ROM (Fig. 6-85A). The knee is allowed to extend if tightness is present in rectus femoris.

Substitute Movement. Hip abduction or adduction.

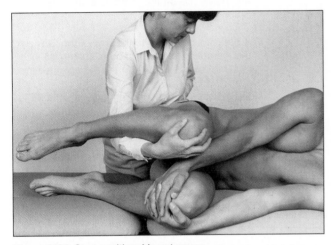

Figure 6-84 Start position: hip extensors.

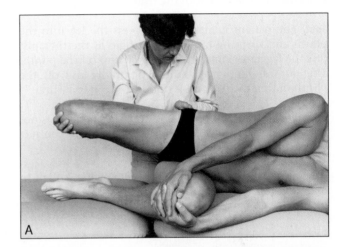

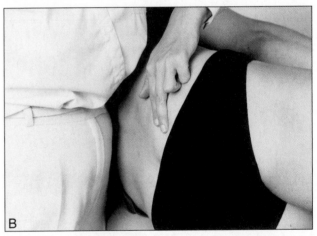

Figure 6-85 A. End position: hip extensors. **B.** The therapist is palpating the gluteus maximus.

Supine Hip Extensor Test[32]

The supine hip extensor test is a reliable and valid method to assess hip extensor muscle strength grades 2 through 5[32] for patients who cannot lie prone.

Start Position. The patient is supine with heels off the end of the plinth and the arms held off the plinth and folded across the chest (Fig. 6-86). The therapist cups both hands under the heel of the test leg.

Stabilization. The weight of the trunk.

Test. The patient is instructed to press the leg into the plinth and keep the hip and body rigid as the therapist lifts the leg approximately 35 in. (~90 cm) off the plinth. The nontest limb may also involuntarily rise off the plinth during the test and is not of concern in testing.

Palpation. In the supine test position, the therapist is not able to palpate or observe hip extensor muscle contraction to assess grades of 1 or 0.

Grading. Grading is based on the ability of the patient to maintain full hip extension, and the resistance to movement felt by the therapist as the hip flexes.

Grade	Description
	As the therapist lifts the leg off the plinth, the patient's:
5	Hip position remains in the start position (i.e., hip extension)*, and the pelvis and leg rise off the plinth as a unit (Fig. 6-87).
4	Hip flexes up to about 30° before the patient is able to resist further hip flexion and the leg and pelvis rise off the plinth as a unit (Fig. 6-88).
	The patient's hip flexes to the limit of the SLR as the therapist lifts the leg approximately 35 in. (~90 cm) off the plinth and the therapist feels:
3	Good resistance to the movement with little or no pelvic rise off the plinth (Fig. 6-89).
2	Minimal resistance (i.e., greater than the weight of the leg) to the movement with no pelvic rise off the plinth (Fig. 6-89).

*In the presence of a hip flexion contracture the start position of hip extension cannot be assumed and therefore grade 5 cannot be assessed using the supine hip extension test.

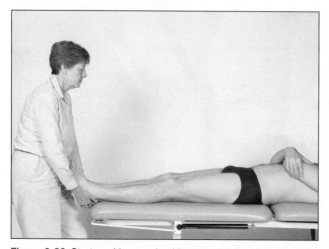

Figure 6-86 Start position: supine hip extension test.

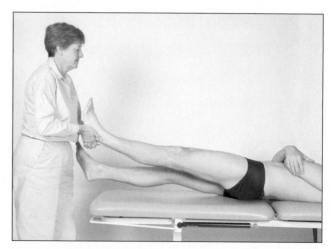

Figure 6-87 Grade 5: hip extended, leg and pelvis rise off plinth.

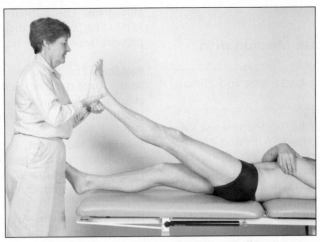

Figure 6-88 Grade 4: hip flexes ~30°, leg and pelvis rise off plinth.

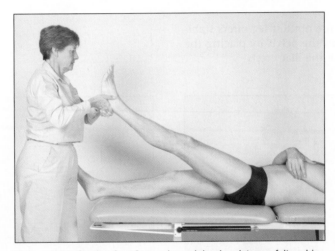

Figure 6-89 Grades 3 or 2: good or minimal resistance felt as hip flexes.

Hip Abduction

Against Gravity: Gluteus Medius and Gluteus Minimus

 Accessory muscles: tensor fascia latae and gluteus maximus (upper fibers).

Form
6-15 **Start Position.** The patient lies on the nontest side with the hip and knee maintained in flexion by the patient to stabilize the trunk and pelvis (Fig. 6-90). The therapist stands behind and against the patient's buttocks to maintain the side-lying position. The hip of the leg to be tested is slightly extended and in neutral rotation.

Widler and colleagues[33] assessed the validity and reliability of assessing unilateral hip abductor muscle strength in the side-lying, supine, and standing positions. These researchers[33] found the side-lying position to be the most valid and reliable position for assessing hip abductor muscle strength.

Stabilization. The position of the nontest leg offers stabilization; the therapist stabilizes the pelvis by placing the hand on the superior aspect of the iliac crest.

Movement. The patient abducts the hip through full ROM. The patient is instructed to lead with the heel to prevent flexion of the hip (Fig. 6-91).

Palpation. The *gluteus medius* is palpated just distal to the lateral lip of the iliac crest or proximal to the greater trochanter of the femur. *Gluteus minimus* lies deep to gluteus medius and is not palpable.

Substitute Movement. Hip flexion through iliacus and psoas major, pelvic elevation through quadratus lumborum. The patient may abduct the leg with hip flexion and internal rotation through the action of tensor fascia latae.

Resistance Location. Applied on the lateral aspect of the thigh proximal to the knee (Figs. 6-92, 6-93, and 6-94).

Resistance Direction. Hip adduction.

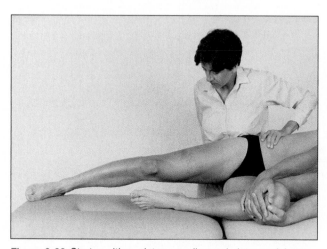

Figure 6-90 Start position: gluteus medius and gluteus minimus.

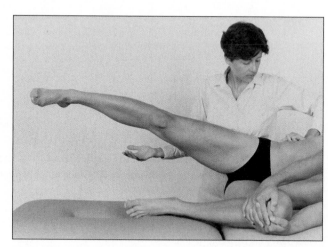

Figure 6-91 Screen position: gluteus medius and gluteus minimus.

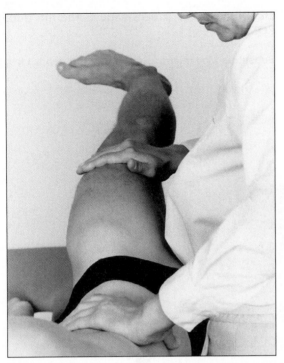

Figure 6-92 Resistance: gluteus medius and gluteus minimus.

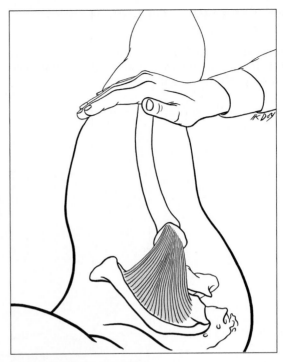

Figure 6-93 Gluteus medius.

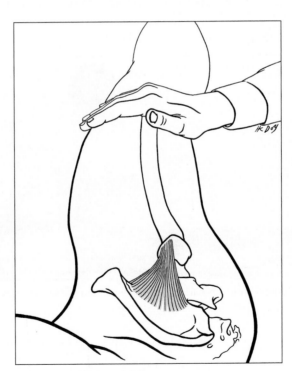

Figure 6-94 Gluteus minimus.

Gravity Eliminated: Gluteus Medius and Gluteus Minimus

Start Position. The patient is supine with the lower extremity in the anatomical position (Fig. 6-95). The therapist supports the weight of the limb.

Stabilization. The therapist stabilizes the pelvis.

End Position. The patient abducts the hip through full ROM (Fig. 6-96).

Substitute Movement. Hip flexion and pelvic elevation.

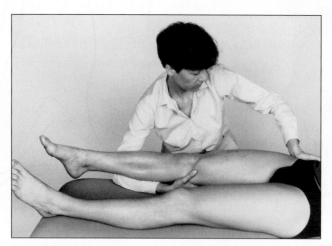

Figure 6-95 Start position: gluteus medius and gluteus minimus.

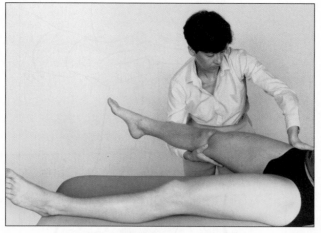

Figure 6-96 End position: gluteus medius and gluteus minimus.

Hip Abduction and Hip Flexion

Against Gravity: Tensor Fascia Latae

 Accessory muscles: gluteus medius and gluteus minimus.

Form 6-16 **Start Position.** The patient is lying on the side not being tested and supports the nontest leg in maximal hip and knee flexion (Fig. 6-97). The leg on the test side is placed in 10° to 20° of hip flexion and in internal rotation. The pelvis is rolled backward and the therapist stands behind and against the patient's buttocks to maintain this position in side-lying. The knee is in extension.

Stabilization. The position of the nontest leg offers stabilization; the therapist stabilizes the pelvis by placing a hand on the superior aspect of the iliac crest.

Movement. The patient abducts the hip through full ROM and slightly flexes the hip (Fig. 6-98).

Palpation. Lateral to the upper portion of sartorius or distal to the greater trochanter on the iliotibial band.

Substitute Movement. Quadratus lumborum (pelvic elevation), iliacus and psoas major (hip flexion), and gluteus medius and minimus (hip abduction).

Resistance Location. Applied on the anterolateral aspect of the thigh proximal to the knee joint (Figs. 6-99 and 6-100).

Resistance Direction. Hip adduction and extension.

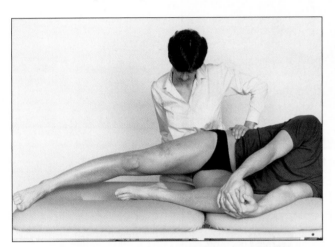

Figure 6-97 Start position: tensor fascia latae.

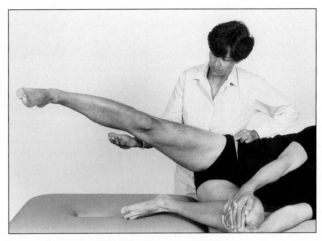

Figure 6-98 Screen position: tensor fascia latae.

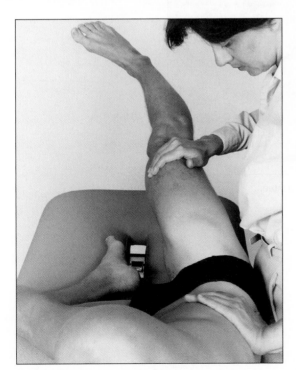

Figure 6-99 Resistance: tensor fascia latae.

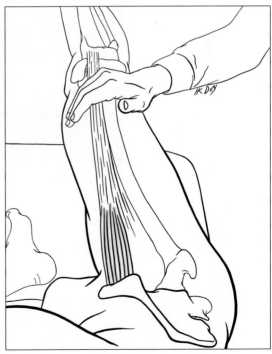

Figure 6-100 Tensor fascia latae.

Gravity Eliminated: Tensor Fascia Latae

Start Position. The patient is supine. The therapist supports the weight of the lower extremity in 10° to 20° of hip flexion, internal rotation, and knee extension, and maintains the support throughout movement (Fig. 6-101).

Stabilization. The weight of the patient's trunk offers stabilization.

End Position. The patient abducts the hip through full ROM and slightly flexes the hip (Fig. 6-102).

Substitute Movement. Quadratus lumborum, iliacus, psoas major, and gluteus medius and minimus.

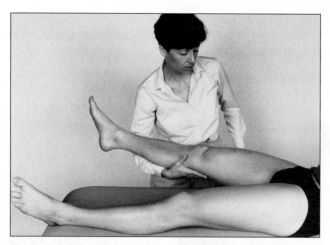

Figure 6-101 Start position: tensor fascia latae.

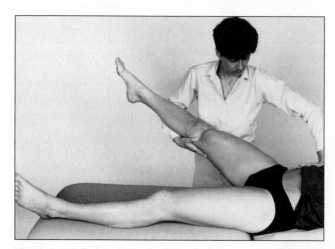

Figure 6-102 End position: tensor fascia latae.

Clinical Test: Weakness of Hip Abductor Mechanism

The hip abductor muscles primarily function to maintain a level pelvis during unilateral stance.[30] Assumption of a unilateral stance occurs in walking when one leg is swinging forward and the other foot maintains contact with the ground. In standing with one foot off the ground, the weight of the head, arms, trunk, and ipsilateral limb acts to rotate the pelvis in a downward direction on the unsupported side.[30] This downward rotation must be balanced around the femoral head by contraction of the contralateral hip abductors.[30] In the presence of weakness or paralysis of the abductors of the stance leg, the pelvis on the contralateral unsupported side will drop. Weakness or paralysis may be clinically detected through the Trendelenburg test.[5,21,34]

Trendelenburg Test. The patient is standing on the leg to be tested and places the hands lightly on a table to maintain balance (not shown). The contralateral hip and knee are flexed so that the foot clears the floor. The therapist stands behind the patient and observes the posture of the pelvis and trunk. A negative Trendelenburg sign (Fig. 6-103) indicates no abductor weakness. The PSISs are level or slightly inclined toward the unsupported side. A positive Trendelenburg sign (Fig. 6-104) indicates abductor weakness. The PSISs are not level and the pelvis drops on the unsupported side. As a compensatory balance mechanism for hip abductor weakness, the patient will shift the trunk over the involved side stance leg (i.e., the side of the weak hip abductors).

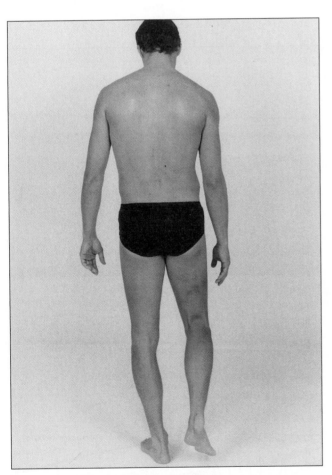

Figure 6-103 Negative Trendelenburg sign.

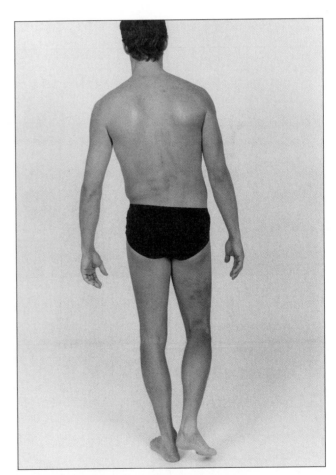

Figure 6-104 Positive Trendelenburg sign.

Hip Adduction

Against Gravity: Adductor Longus, Adductor Brevis, Adductor Magnus, Pectineus, and Gracilis

Start Position. The patient lies on the test side. The therapist stands behind and against the patient's buttocks to maintain the side-lying position. The hip of the nontest leg is abducted about 25° to 30° and held in position by the therapist providing support under the medial aspect of the thigh and knee (Fig. 6-105). Alternatively, the hip adductors may be tested with the patient supine, and the therapist offers resistance to hip adduction equal to the weight of the limb to resemble the against gravity situation.

Form 6-17

Stabilization. The patient grasps the edge of the plinth.

Movement. The hip is adducted until the test limb contacts the uppermost limb (Fig. 6-106). The patient is instructed not to rotate the limb during the test.

Palpation. The adductors are palpated as a group on the medial and distal aspect of the thigh.

Resistance Location. Applied on the medial aspect of the thigh proximal to the knee joint (Figs. 6-107 and 6-108).

Resistance Direction. Hip abduction.

Substitute Movement. Rolling posteriorly out of the side-lying position and internally rotating the hip to use the hip flexors. Rolling anteriorly out of the side-lying position and externally rotating the hip to use the hip extensors.

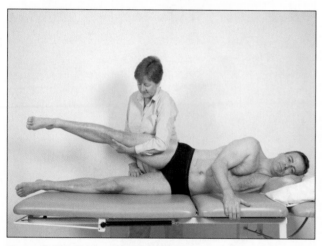

Figure 6-105 Start position: hip adductors.

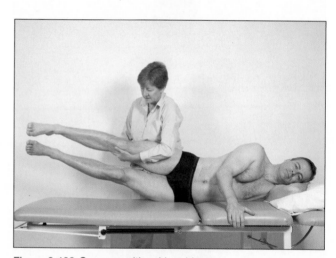

Figure 6-106 Screen position: hip adductors.

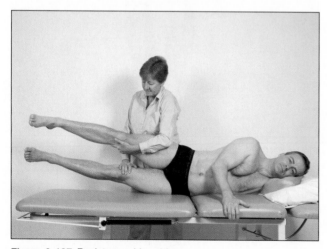

Figure 6-107 Resistance: hip adductors.

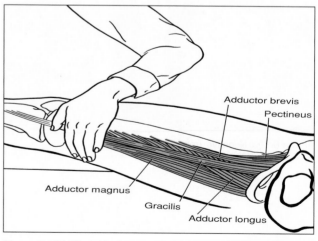

Figure 6-108 Hip adductors.

Gravity Eliminated: Adductor Longus, Adductor Brevis, Adductor Magnus, Pectineus, and Gracilis

Start Position. The patient is supine. The hip to be tested is in about 25° to 30° abduction, neutral rotation, and extension (Fig. 6-109). The therapist supports the weight of the limb.

Stabilization. The weight of the body with the patient in supine and the therapist stabilizes the pelvis.

End Position. The patient adducts the hip through full ROM (Fig. 6-110).

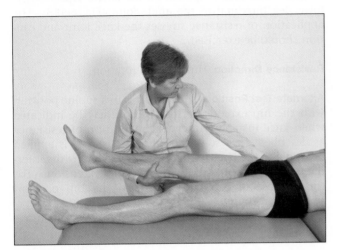

Figure 6-109 Start position: hip adductors.

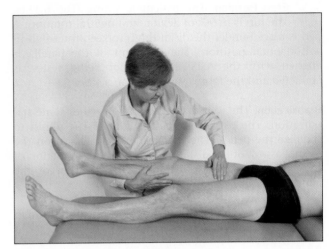

Figure 6-110 End position: hip adductors.

Hip Internal Rotation

Against Gravity: Gluteus Medius, Gluteus Minimus, and Tensor Fascia Latae

 Accessory muscle: adductor longus.

Form 6-18 **Start Position.** The patient is sitting (Fig. 6-111). The hip is in 90° of flexion and neutral rotation. A pad is placed under the distal thigh to keep the thigh in a horizontal position. The midpoint of the patella is aligned with the ASIS. The leg not being tested is abducted and the foot is supported on a stool.

Stabilization. The weight of the trunk provides some stabilization. The patient grasps the edge of the plinth to stabilize the pelvis. The therapist places a hand on the medial aspect of the distal thigh to prevent adduction of the hip. The therapist maintains the position of the femur, without restricting movement.

Movement. The patient internally rotates the hip through full ROM (Fig. 6-112).

Palpation. Refer to previous test descriptions for palpation of gluteus medius, gluteus minimus, and tensor fascia latae.

Substitute Movement. Pelvic elevation, contralateral trunk side flexion, and hip adduction.

Resistance Location. Applied on the lateral aspect of the lower leg proximal to the ankle joint (Fig. 6-113). The application of resistance stresses the knee joint and caution should be exercised.

Resistance Direction. Hip external rotation.

Alternate Test Position. The patient is in a supine position with the hip extended. This position may be indicated when knee instability prevents application of resistance as described. In a supine position, resistance is applied proximal to the knee joint. The force exerted by the internal rotators is greater in hip flexion than extension.[35] For the purpose of interrater reliability, the hip position should be recorded.

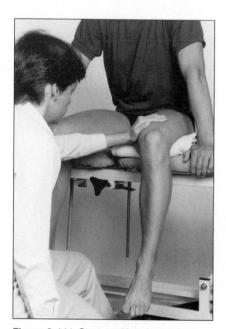

Figure 6-111 Start position: internal rotators.

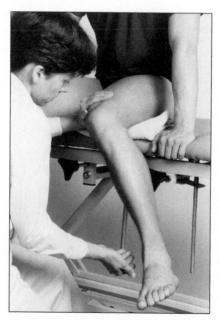

Figure 6-112 Screen position: hip internal rotators.

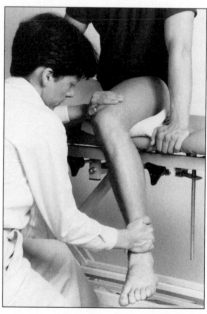

Figure 6-113 Resistance: internal rotators.

Gravity Eliminated: Gluteus Medius, Gluteus Minimus, and Tensor Fascia Latae

Start Position. The patient is supine. The therapist supports the leg in a position of 90° of hip flexion, neutral rotation, and knee flexion (Fig. 6-114).

Stabilization. The patient grasps the edge of the plinth for stabilization of the pelvis.

End Position. The patient internally rotates the hip through full ROM (Fig. 6-115). The therapist's supporting hand on the medial aspect of the thigh should allow full rotation and prevent hip adduction. The movement is repeated and the therapist palpates the muscles.

Substitute Movement. Hip adduction and knee flexion.

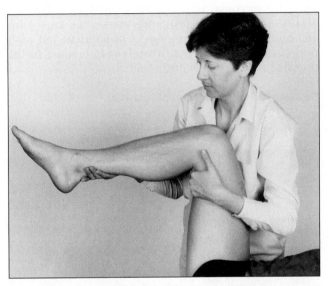

Figure 6-114 Start position: internal rotators.

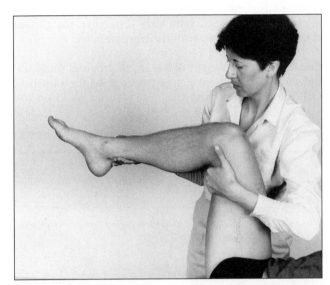

Figure 6-115 End position: internal rotators.

Hip External Rotation

Against Gravity: Piriformis, Obturator Externus, Gemellus Superior, Quadratus Femoris, Gemellus Inferior, and Obturator Internus

 Accessory muscle: gluteus maximus in hip extension.

Form 6-19 **Start Position.** The patient is sitting (Fig. 6-116). The hip is in 90° of flexion and neutral rotation. A pad is placed under the distal thigh to keep the thigh in a horizontal position. The midpoint of the patella is aligned with the ASIS. With knee instability, the patient is in a supine position with the hip extended.

Stabilization. The weight of the trunk provides some stabilization. The patient grasps the edge of the plinth to stabilize the pelvis. The therapist places a hand on the anterolateral aspect of the distal thigh to prevent hip abduction and flexion. The therapist maintains the position of the femur, without restricting movement.

Movement. The patient externally rotates the hip through full ROM (Fig. 6-117).

Palpation. The external rotators are too deep to palpate.

Substitute Movement. Hip flexion and abduction; ipsilateral trunk side flexion.

Resistance Location. Applied on the medial aspect of the lower leg proximal to the ankle joint (Figs. 6-118 and 6-119). Application of resistance stresses the knee joint and caution should be exercised. The alternate test position described for internal rotators may be used in the presence of knee instability.

Resistance Direction. Internal rotation.

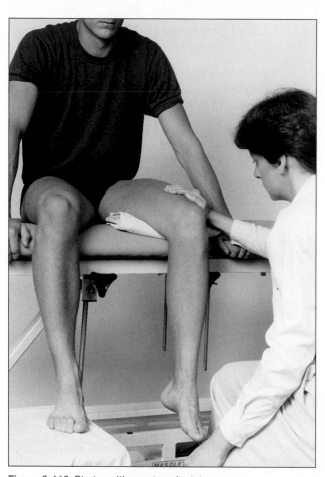

Figure 6-116 Start position: external rotators.

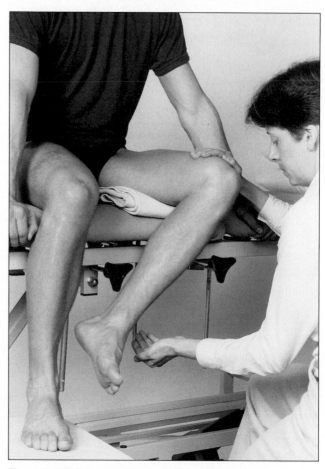

Figure 6-117 Screen position: external rotators.

Gravity Eliminated: Piriformis, Obturator Externus, Gemellus Superior, Quadratus Femoris, Gemellus Inferior, and Obturator Internus

Start Position. The position is the same as described for internal rotation.

End Position. The patient externally rotates the hip through full ROM (Fig. 6-120).

Substitute Movement. Hip flexion and abduction and knee flexion.

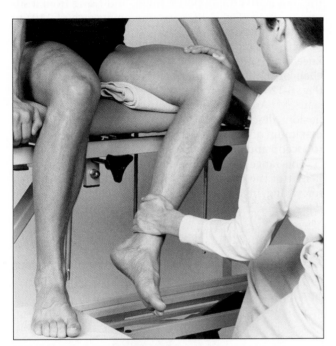

Figure 6-118 Resistance: external rotators.

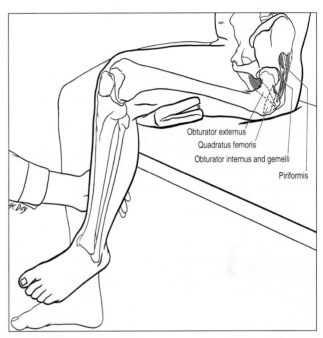

Figure 6-119 External rotators.

Obturator externus
Quadratus femoris
Obturator internus and gemelli
Piriformis

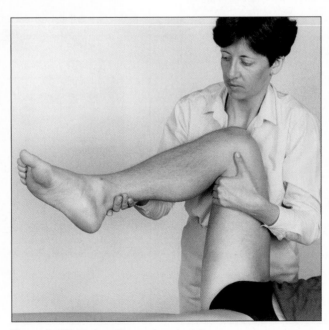

Figure 6-120 End position: external rotators.

FUNCTIONAL APPLICATION

Joint Function[30]

The hip joint transmits forces between the ground and the pelvis to support the body weight and acts as a fulcrum during single-leg stance. With the foot fixed on the ground, hip movement enables the body to be moved closer to or farther away from the ground. Hip motion brings the foot closer to the trunk and positions the lower limb in space.

Functional Range of Motion

Common activities of daily living (ADL) can be accomplished in a normal manner with hip ROM of at least 120° flexion, 20° abduction, and 20° external rotation.[36] In performing functional activities, hip movements are accompanied at various points in the ROM by lumbar-pelvic motions.[37] These motions extend the functional range capabilities of the hip joint.

Hip Flexion and Extension

The normal AROM for hip flexion is 0° to 120° and extension is 0° to 30°.[8] Full hip flexion and extension ranges of motion are required for many ADL. Standing requires 0° or slight hip extension.[38] Using electrogoniometric measures, it has been found that without using compensatory movement patterns at other joints, activities such as squatting to pick up an object from the ground, tying a shoe lace with the foot on the ground (Fig. 6-121) or with the foot across the opposite thigh, and rising from a sitting position (Fig. 6-122) require an average of 110° to 120° of hip flexion.[36]

Activities requiring less than 90° of hip flexion include kneeling,[39] sitting on the floor cross-legged,[39] sitting in a chair of standard height,[36] putting on a pair of trousers (Fig. 6-123), and ascending (Fig. 6-124) and descending stairs.[36,40] Ascending stairs requires an average of 67° hip flexion, descending an average of 36° hip flexion.[36] A maximum of about 1° to 2° hip extension may be required to ascend and descend stairs.[40]

The range required for sitting is determined by the height of the chair. About 84° of hip flexion is required for sitting in a standard chair.[36] To sit from standing

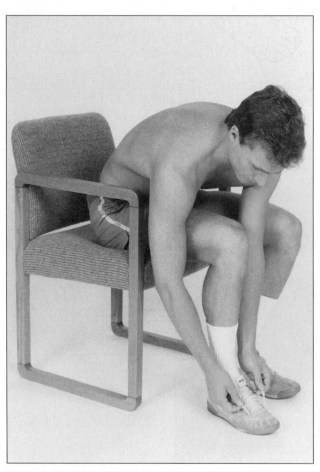

Figure 6-121 Tying a shoelace with the foot flat on the floor requires approximately 120° of hip flexion.[36]

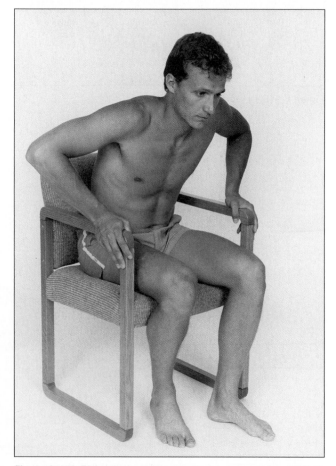

Figure 6-122 Rising from a sitting position requires at least 90° of hip flexion.[36]

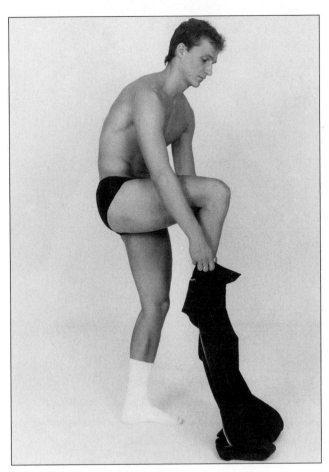

Figure 6-123 Donning a pair of trousers.

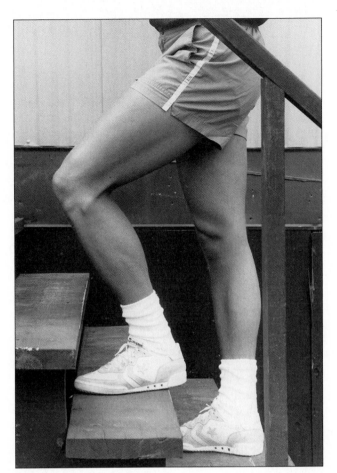

Figure 6-124 Ascending stairs.

requires an average of 104° hip flexion;[36] to rise from sitting requires an average of 98° to 101° hip flexion ROM.[41] These ranges increase with decreased chair height and decrease with increased chair height.

Hip Abduction and Adduction

The normal AROM at the hip for abduction is 0° to 45°; for adduction, it is 0° to 30°.[8] Most daily functions do not require the full ranges of hip abduction and adduction.

Many ADL can be performed within an arc of 0° to 20° of hip abduction.[36] Squatting to pick up an object, and sitting with the foot across the opposite thigh (Fig. 6-125) are examples of activities performed within this ROM. Mounting a men's bicycle (Fig. 6-126) may require the full range of hip abduction bilaterally. Positions essential in ADL used by Asian and Eastern cultures such as squatting, cross-legged sitting, and kneeling require about 30° to 40° hip abduction ROM.[39,42]

Hip adduction in ADL is illustrated when sitting with the thighs crossed (Fig. 6-127) and when standing on one leg; the leg one stands on adducts as a result of the pelvis dropping on the contralateral side.

Hip Internal and External Rotation

The AROM of hip internal and external rotation is 0° to 45° in both directions.[8] The extremes of these rotational motions are seldom used in ADL. Ranges of 0° to 20° external rotation are required for most ADL.[36] Mounting a bicycle (Fig. 6-126), sitting on a chair with the foot across the opposite thigh (Fig. 6-125) to tie a shoelace, or visually observing the skin on the sole of the foot when performing foot hygiene activities illustrate the use of hip external rotation. Positions essential in ADL used by Asian and Eastern cultures require full hip external rotation ROM for cross-legged sitting on the floor[39,42] and lesser average hip external rotation ROM for kneeling (25°) and squatting (19°).[39]

Walking and pivoting on one leg to turn are examples of functional activities that utilize hip internal rotation.

Gait

A normal walking pattern requires hip motion in the sagittal, frontal, and horizontal planes. In the sagittal plane, about 10° to 20° of hip extension is required at terminal stance, and 30° of hip flexion is required at the end of swing phase and the beginning of stance phase as the limb is advanced forward to take the next step (from the Rancho Los Amigos gait analysis forms as cited in Levangie and Norkin[38]).

With the feet fixed on the ground, the femoral heads can act as fulcrums for the pelvis as it tilts anteriorly and posteriorly. The pelvis can also tilt laterally, causing the

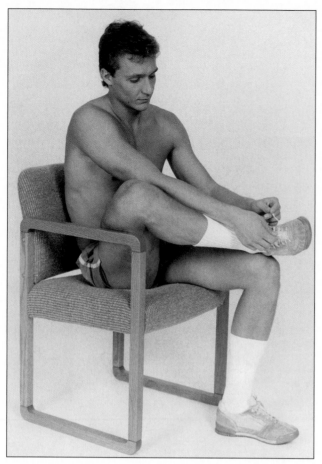

Figure 6-125 Sitting with the foot across the opposite thigh requires hip flexion, abduction, and external rotation: external rotators and sartorius muscle function.

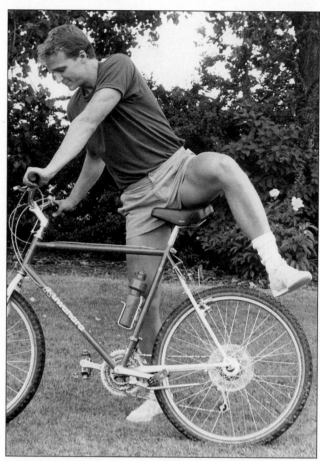

Figure 6-126 Mounting a bicycle requires hip flexion, abduction, and external rotation.

iliac crests to move either superiorly or inferiorly. Lateral tilting of the pelvis occurs when one leg is off the ground, the hip joint of the supporting leg acts as a fulcrum, and the tilting results in relative abduction and adduction at the hip joints.[38] When walking, there is a lateral tilt of the pelvis inferiorly on the unsupported side during the swing phase of the gait cycle. This dropping of the pelvis on the unsupported side results in ipsilateral hip abduction. As the pelvis drops, the inferior aspect of the pelvis moves toward the femur of the stance leg, producing hip adduction on this side. About 7° of hip abduction is required at initial swing, and 5° of hip adduction is required at the end of the stance phase of the gait cycle.[43]

Pelvic rotation occurs in the horizontal plane about a vertical axis. Rotations of the thigh occur relative to the pelvis. As the swinging leg advances during locomotion, the pelvis rotates forward on the same side. The fulcrum for this forward rotation of the pelvis is the head of the femur on the supporting leg. As the supporting or stance leg is fixed on the ground, the pelvis rotates around the femoral head, resulting in internal rotation at the hip joint. As the pelvis moves forward on the swing side, the swinging leg moves forward in the sagittal plane in the line of progression, resulting in external rotation of the hip during the swing phase of the gait cycle. During

the normal gait cycle, about 5° of internal rotation and 9° of external rotation are required at the hip joint.[43] External rotation occurs at the end of the stance phase and through most of the swing phase, and internal rotation occurs at terminal swing before initial contact to the end of the stance phase.[43] Refer to Appendix D for further description and illustrations of the positions and motions at the hip joint during gait.

Hip flexion and extension ROM requirements for running are greater than for walking and vary depending on the speed of running. When running average peak hip flexion ROM is 65° and hip extension ROM is 20°.[38]

Muscle Function

Hip Flexion

Iliacus and psoas major (often referred to as iliopsoas) are the primary flexors of the hip joint. Tensor fascia latae (anteromedial fibers),[44] rectus femoris, sartorius, gracilis, and the hip adductors assist the iliopsoas. The hip adductors assist in flexion when the hip is in an extended position.[30] Gracilis flexes the hip primarily in the initial stages of the motion[45] and with the knee in extension but not

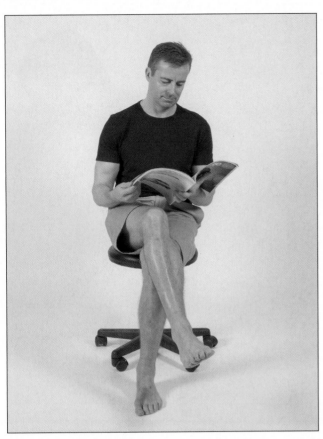

Figure 6-127 Hip adduction.

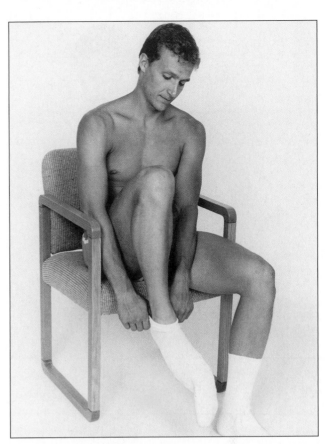

Figure 6-128 Iliopsoas muscle function.

with the knee flexed.[46] The action of the adductors and gracilis in hip flexion is illustrated in the action of kicking a ball and swimming using the flutter kick. The action of sartorius as a hip flexor, abductor, external rotator, and knee flexor[47] is illustrated when positioning the foot across the thigh in sitting (Fig. 6-125).

The iliopsoas is the only flexor effective in flexing the hip beyond 90° in the sitting position[32] in activities such as raising the lower limb to sit with the thighs crossed (Fig. 6-127) and pulling on a sock (Fig. 6-128). The hip flexor muscles contract with the abdominals to raise the trunk when moving in bed from supine to sitting. The iliopsoas controls the movement of the trunk and pelvis as one leans backward in sitting[32] to look overhead or lowers the trunk to lie down in bed from a sitting position. Other activities that require contraction of the hip flexors include donning a pair of trousers (Fig. 6-123), climbing a ladder, ascending stairs (Fig. 6-124), and stepping in and out of the bathtub.

Hip Extension

The hip extensor muscles are the gluteus maximus, semimembranosus, semitendinosus, biceps femoris, and adductor magnus.[48] The contribution of the five hip extensors in functional activities is partly determined by the position of the hip joint and the magnitude of the

force required to perform hip extension. The hamstrings usually initiate the movement of hip extension[49] and the gluteus maximus contracts when the thigh moves beyond the anatomical position, into hyperextension, or when extension occurs against resistance.[46,49] The hamstrings produce motion at the hip and knee joints. According to Németh and colleagues[50], the position of the knee has no effect on the strength of hip extension with the knee flexed between 0° and 90°. The adductor magnus acts as a hip extensor from 90° to 0° of hip flexion; its effect as a hip extensor is somewhat less in men in the final 30° of the extension motion as the anterior portion of the muscle becomes ineffective as an extensor.[48]

The action of the hip extensors is illustrated in activities where the body is raised,[51,52] such as getting up from sitting[53] (Fig. 6-129), climbing stairs (Fig. 6-124), and jumping. The hip extensors contract in lifting activities performed with the knees and hips flexed[49,54,55] (Fig. 6-130). The extensors control the forward movement of the pelvis when leaning forward in the sitting or standing positions and initiate and perform the posterior motion of the pelvis to sit or stand upright again.[30,54,56] The gluteus maximus contracts when one holds a crouch position[52] to change a car tire or look into a low cupboard.

In the standing position, thigh extension is performed by the hamstrings and when resistance is added to the movement the gluteus maximus assists to extend the hip.[46] Thus, the extensors contract to propel one forward

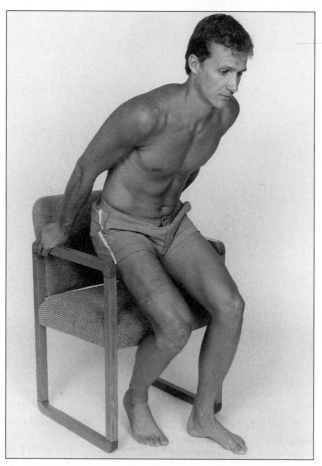

Figure 6-129 The hip extensors function when the body is raised when getting up from a chair.

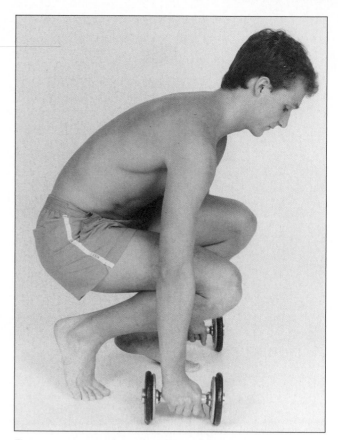

Figure 6-130 Hip extensor muscle function.

when skating. The gluteus maximus contracts strongly to extend the thigh at the extreme of movement, as the hip is hyperextended.[49,52]

Hip Abduction

The muscles responsible for hip abduction are the gluteus medius, gluteus minimus, and tensor fascia latae. The upper fibers of the gluteus maximus assist with abduction when force is required.[57] The main function of the hip abductor muscles is to keep the pelvis level when one foot is off the ground. When standing on one leg, the hip joint of the supporting leg and the pelvis act as a first-class lever. The head of the femur represents the fulcrum and the pelvis, the lever arm. With one foot off the ground, the pelvis is unsupported and will drop down on the same side due to the torque created by the weight of the head, arms, trunk, and leg causing the pelvis to rotate around the head of the femur of the stance leg. The hip abductor muscles on the stance side contract with a reversed origin and insertion to pull the iliac crest (pelvis) down on the same side, causing the pelvis to rotate around the head of the femur and rise on the unsupported side. The pelvic leveling action of the hip abductors in single leg stance is illustrated in walking, running, and kicking a ball.

In single leg stance, the hip abductors may not be required to contract to keep the pelvis level if the trunk is shifted over the supporting leg so that the line of gravity of the head, arms, and trunk falls through the hip joint.

If the pelvis is allowed to drop on the non-weight-bearing side when standing on one leg, the fascia latae and the iliotibial tract become taut on the weight-bearing side to maintain the posture of the pelvis and the hip abductors do not contract.[58]

The hip abductors may contract bilaterally in activities that require abduction of the non-weight-bearing extremity such as standing when mounting a bicycle (Fig. 6-126) and performing karate (Fig. 6-131).

Hip Adduction

Activities such as climbing a rope,[30] kicking a ball across the front of the body, and horseback riding require contraction of the hip adductors that includes the adductor magnus, adductor longus, adductor brevis, gracilis, and pectineus. Janda and Stara (cited in Basmajian and DeLuca[57]) suggest that the hip adductors function primarily as postural muscles in various activities rather than prime movers for hip adduction.

Hip Internal Rotation

The primary internal rotators of the hip include the tensor fascia latae, anterior fibers of the gluteus medius and

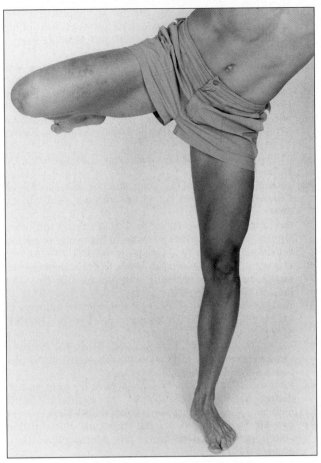

Figure 6-131 Hip abductor muscle function.

of the exact location of the line of gravity, there is little muscular activity at the hip in symmetrical standing. Electromyography has shown no activity in the gluteus maximus, medius, and minimus in easy standing.[56] There appears to be variable activity in the iliopsoas muscles because Basmajian[62] recorded slight to moderate activity and Joseph and Williams[56] detected no activity in standing using electromyography.

Gait[63]

The hamstrings and gluteus maximus contract at the end of the swing phase and the beginning of the stance phase to decelerate the forward swinging extremity and to extend the hip at initial contact and loading response. The gluteus maximus inserts into the iliotibial band and as the muscle contracts, it pulls the band posteriorly. The tensor fascia latae contracts at the beginning of the stance phase to prevent the posterior displacement of the iliotibial band. The hip abductors, gluteus medius and minimus, contract on the side of the weight-bearing extremity when the pelvis is unsupported on the contralateral side during the swing phase of the gait cycle. The contraction of the gluteus medius and minimus prevents the pelvis from dropping on the unsupported side during the swing phase. The hip flexors, iliopsoas and rectus femoris,[64] and tensor fascia latae contract at the end of the stance phase and early swing phase to initiate hip flexion. The activity of the hip adductors is variable, but these muscles are active during the swing phase of the gait cycle. The hip adductors contract to keep the extremity in the midline and may assist in maintaining hip flexion at the end of swing phase.[65]

Montgomery and colleagues[66] provide a description of the hip muscle activity during running.

minimus,[14] and the hip adductor muscles.[59,60] The semimembranosus and semitendinosus internally rotate the hip when the hip is in extension.[46] The internal rotators are active in walking or when pivoting on one foot in the standing position.[30]

Hip External Rotation

The piriformis, obturator internus, obturator externus, quadratus femoris, and gemellus superior and inferior, and sartorius externally rotate the hip joint. The piriformis and obturator internus function most effectively as external rotators when the thigh is extended and become less effective as the thigh is flexed.[14] The gluteus maximus and biceps femoris also rotate the hip externally when the hip is in extension.[46] Mounting a bicycle (Fig. 6-126), performing karate (Fig. 6-131), and positioning the foot across the opposite thigh to tie a shoelace (Fig. 6-125) require contraction of the external rotators of the hip.

Standing Posture

The line of gravity shifts in relation to the hip joint and may pass either slightly anterior to, slightly posterior to, or through the hip joint in the sagittal plane.[61] Regardless

References

1. Kapandji AI. *The Physiology of the Joints. Vol 2. The Lower Limb.* 6th ed. New York, NY: Churchill Livingstone Elsevier; 2011.
2. Standring S, ed. *Gray's Anatomy: The Anatomical Basis of Clinical Practice.* 39th ed. London: Elsevier Churchill Livingstone; 2005.
3. Norkin CC, White DJ. *Measurement of Joint Motion: A Guide to Goniometry.* 4th ed. Philadelphia, PA: FA Davis; 2009.
4. Daniels L, Worthingham C. *Muscle Testing: Techniques of Manual Examination.* 5th ed. Philadelphia, PA: WB Saunders; 1986.
5. Norkin CC, Levangie PK. *Joint Structure and Function: A Comprehensive Analysis.* Philadelphia, PA: FA Davis; 1983.
6. Neumann DA. *Kinesiology of the Musculoskeletal System: Foundations for Rehabilitation.* 2nd ed. St. Louis, MO: Mosby Elsevier; 2010.
7. Magee DJ. *Orthopedic Physical Assessment.* 5th ed. St. Louis, MO: Saunders Elsevier; 2008.
8. American Academy of Orthopaedic Surgeons. *Joint Motion: Method of Measuring and Recording.* Chicago, IL: AAOS; 1965.
9. Berryman Reese N, Bandy WD. *Joint Range of Motion and Muscle Length Testing.* 2nd ed. St. Louis, MO: Saunders Elsevier; 2010.
10. Cyriax J. *Textbook of Orthopaedic Medicine. Vol 1. Diagnosis of Soft Tissue Lesions.* 8th ed. London: Bailliere Tindall; 1982.

11. Kendall FP, McCreary EK, Provance PG, Rogers MM, Romani WA. *Muscles Testing and Function with Posture and Pain.* 5th ed. Baltimore, MD: Lippincott Williams & Wilkins; 2005.

12. Cailliet R. *Soft Tissue Pain and Disability.* Philadelphia, PA: FA Davis; 1977.

13. Boone DC, Azen SP. Normal range of motion of joints in male subjects. *J Bone Joint Surg.* 1979;61:756–759.

14. Steindler A. *Kinesiology of the Human Body Under Normal and Pathological Conditions.* Springfield, IL: Charles C Thomas; 1955.

15. Hollman JH, Burgess B, Bokermann JC. Passive hip rotation range of motion: effects of testing position and age in runners and non-runners. *Physiother Theor Pract.* 2003;19:77–86.

16. Harris-Hayes M, Wendl PM, Sahrmann SA, Van Dillen LR. Does stabilization of the tibiofemoral joint affect passive prone hip rotation range of motion measures in unimpaired individuals? A preliminary report. *Physiother Theor Pract.* 2007;23:315–323.

17. Gajdosik RL, LeVeau BF, Bohannon RW. Effects of ankle dorsiflexion on active and passive unilateral straight leg raising. *Phys Ther.* 1985;65:1478–1482.

18. Bohannon RW. Cinematographic analysis of the passive straight-leg-raising test for hamstring muscle length. *Phys Ther.* 1982;62:1269–1274.

19. Youdas JW, Krause DA, Hollman JH, Harmsen WS, Laskowski E. The influence of gender and age on hamstring muscle length in healthy adults. *J Orthop Sports Phys Ther.* 2005;35:246–252.

20. Bohannon R, Gajdosik R, LeVeau BF. Contribution of pelvic and lower limb motion to increases in the angle of passive straight leg raising. *Phys Ther.* 1985;65:474–476.

21. Salter RB. *Textbook of Disorders and Injuries of the Musculoskeletal System.* 2nd ed. Baltimore, MD: Williams & Wilkins; 1983.

22. Van Dillen LR, McDonnell MK, Fleming DA, Sahrmann SA. Effect of knee and hip position on hip extension range of motion in individuals with and without low back pain. *J Orthop Sports Phys Ther.* 2000;30:307–316.

23. Ober FR. Back strain and sciatica. *JAMA.* 1935;104:1580–1583.

24. Gose JC, Schweizer P. Iliotibial band tightness. *J Orthop Sports Phys Ther.* 1989;10:399–407.

25. Gajdosik RL, Sandler MM, Marr HL. Influence of knee positions and gender on the Ober test for length of the iliotibial band. *Clin Biomech.* 2003;18:77–79.

26. Berryman Reese N, Bandy WD. Use of an inclinometer to measure flexibility of the iliotibial band using the Ober test and the modified Ober test: differences in magnitude and reliability of measurements. *J Orthop Sports Phys Ther.* 2003;33:326–330.

27. Soames RW, ed. Skeletal system. Salmons S, ed. Muscle. *Gray's Anatomy.* 38th ed. New York, NY: Churchill Livingstone; 1995.

28. Trombly CA. Evaluation of biomechanical and physiological aspects of motor performance. In: Trombly CA, ed. *Occupational Therapy for Physical Dysfunction.* 4th ed. Baltimore, MD: Williams & Wilkins; 1995.

29. Carlsoo S, Fohlin L. The mechanics of the two-joint muscles rectus femoris, sartorius and tensor fascia latae in relation to their activity. *Scand J Rehabil Med.* 1969;1:107–111.

30. Smith LK, Weiss EL, Lehmkuhl LD. *Brunnstrom's Clinical Kinesiology.* 5th ed. Philadelphia, PA: FA Davis; 1996.

31. Kendall FP, McCreary EK, Provance PG. *Muscles Testing and Function.* 4th ed. Baltimore, MD: Williams & Wilkins; 1993.

32. Perry J, Weiss WB, Burnfield JM, Gronley JK. The supine hip extensor manual muscle test: A reliability and validity study. *Arch Phys Med Rehabil.* 2004;85:1345–1350.

33. Widler KS, Glatthorn JF, Bizzini M, Impellizzeri FM, Munzinger U, Leunig M, Maffiuletti NA. Assessment of hip abductor muscle strength. A validity and reliability study. *J Bone Joint Surg [Am].* 2009;91:2666–2672.

34. Hoppenfeld S. *Physical Examination of the Spine and Extremities.* New York, NY: Appleton-Century-Crofts; 1976.

35. Jarvis DK. Relative strength of the hip rotator muscle groups. *Phys Ther Rev.* 1952;32:500–503.

36. Johnston RC, Smidt GL. Hip motion measurements for selected activities of daily living. *Clin Orthop Relat Res.* 1970; 72:205–215.

37. Cailliet R. *Low Back Pain Syndrome.* 2nd ed. Philadelphia, PA: FA Davis; 1968.

38. Levangie PK, Norkin CC. *Joint Structure and Function. A Comprehensive Analysis.* 3rd ed. Philadelphia, PA: FA Davis; 2001.

39. Hemmerich A, Brown H, Smith S, Marthandam SSK, Wyss UP. Hip, knee, and ankle kinematics of high range of motion activities of daily living. *J Orthop Res.* 2006;24:770–781.

40. Livingston LA, Stevenson JM, Olney SJ. Stairclimbing kinematics on stairs of differing dimensions. *Arch Phys Med Rehabil.* 1991;72:398–402.

41. Ikeda ER, Schenkman ML, Riley PO, Hodge WA. Influence of age on dynamics of rising from a chair. *Phys Ther.* 1991;71: 473–481.

42. Kapoor A, Mishra SK, Kewangan SK, Mody BS. Range of movements of lower limb joints in cross-legged sitting posture. *J Arthroplasty.* 2008;23:451–453.

43. Johnston RC, Smidt GL. Measurement of hip-joint motion during walking. Evaluation of an electrogoniometric method. *J Bone Joint Surg [Am].* 1969;51:1083–1094.

44. Paré EB, Stern JT, Schwartz JM. Functional differentiation within the tensor fasciae latae. *J Bone Joint Surg [Am].* 1981; 63:1457–1471.

45. Jonsson B, Steen B. Function of the gracilis muscle. An electromyographic study. *Acta Morphol Neerl Scand.* 1964;6:325–341.

46. Wheatley MD, Jahnke WD. Electromyographic study of the superficial thigh and hip muscles in normal individuals. *Arch Phys Med.* 1951;32:508–515.

47. Johnson CE, Basmajian JV, Dasher W. Electromyography of sartorius muscle. *Anat Rec.* 1972;173:127–130.

48. Németh G, Ohlsén H. In vivo moment arm lengths for hip extensor muscles at different angles of hip flexion. *J Biomech.* 1985;18:129–140.

49. Fischer FJ, Houtz SJ. Evaluation of the function of the gluteus maximus muscle. *Am J Phys Med.* 1968;47:182–191.

50. Németh G, Ekholm J, Arborelius UP, Harms-Ringdahl K, Schüldt K. Influence of knee flexion on isometric hip extensor strength. *Scand J Rehabil Med.* 1983;15:97–101.

51. Németh G, Ekholm J, Arborelius UP. Hip joint load and muscular activation during rising exercises. *Scand J Rehabil Med.* 1984;16:93–102.

52. Karlsson E, Jonsson B. Function of the gluteus maximus muscle. *Acta Morphol Neerl Scand.* 1965;6:161–169.

53. Wretenberg P, Arborelius UP. Power and work produced in different leg muscle groups when rising from a chair. *Eur J Appl Physiol.* 1994;68:413–417.

54. Németh G, Ekholm J, Arborelius UP. Hip load moments and muscular activity during lifting. *Scand J Rehabil Med.* 1984;16:103–111.

55. Vakos JP, Nitz AJ, Threlkeld AJ, Shapiro R, Horn T. Electromyographic activity of selected trunk and hip muscles during a squat lift. *Spine.* 1994;19:687–695.

56. Joseph J, Williams PL. Electromyography of certain hip muscles. *J Anat.* 1957;91:286–294.

57. Basmajian JV, DeLuca CJ. *Muscles Alive: Their Functions Revealed by Electromyography.* 5th ed. Baltimore, MD: Williams & Wilkins; 1985.

58. Inman VT. Functional aspects of the abductor muscles of the hip. *J Bone Joint Surg [Am].* 1947;29:607–619.

59. Williams M, Wesley W. Hip rotator action of the adductor longus muscle. *Phys Ther Rev.* 1951;31:90–92.

60. Basmajian JV. *Muscles Alive: Their Functions Revealed by Electromyography.* 4th ed. Baltimore, MD: Williams & Wilkins; 1978.

61. Soderberg GL. *Kinesiology: Application to Pathological Motion.* 2nd ed. Baltimore, MD: Williams & Wilkins; 1997.

62. Basmajian JV. Electromyography of iliopsoas. *Anat Rec.* 1958;132:127–132.

63. Inman VT, Ralston HJ, Todd F. *Human Walking.* Baltimore, MD: Williams & Wilkins; 1981.

64. Rab GT. Muscle. In: Rose J, Gamble JG, eds. *Human Walking.* 2nd ed. Baltimore, MD: Williams & Wilkins; 1994.

65. Norkin CC, Levangie PK. *Joint Structure and Function: A Comprehensive Analysis.* 2nd ed. Philadelphia, PA: FA Davis; 1992.

66. Montgomery WH, Pink M, Perry J. Electromyographic analysis of hip and knee musculature during running. *Am J Sports Med.* 1994;22:272–278.

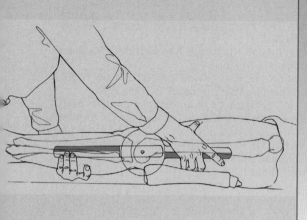

Chapter

7

Knee

ARTICULATIONS AND MOVEMENTS

The knee is made up of the tibiofemoral and patellofemoral articulations (Fig. 7-1). The tibiofemoral articulation is a bicondylar joint formed proximally by the convex condyles of the femur and distally by the concave surfaces of the tibial condyles. The congruency of these surfaces is enhanced by the menisci located between the articulating surfaces.[1] From the anatomical position, the tibiofemoral joint may be flexed and extended in the sagittal plane, with movement occurring around a frontal axis (Fig. 7-2). Rotation also occurs at the tibiofemoral joint and is an essential component of normal range of motion (ROM) at the knee. Rotation occurs in the horizontal plane around a longitudinal axis (Fig. 7-2). At the beginning of knee flexion from full extension, the tibia automatically rotates internally on the femur, and at the end of knee extension, the tibia automatically rotates externally. The external rotation at the end of knee extension locks the knee in full extension and is referred to as the "screw home mechanism." The greatest range of tibial rotation is available when the knee is flexed 90°.[2] Knee movements are described in Table 7-1.

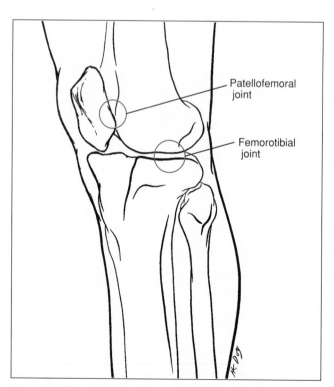

Figure 7-1 Knee joint articulations, anterolateral view.

Patellofemoral joint

Femorotibial joint

The patellofemoral articulation (Fig. 7-1), an incongruous joint, is also contained within the capsule of the knee joint. The patellar articular surface, divided by a vertical ridge, is flat or slightly convex mediolaterally and superoinferiorly,[13] and articulates with the anterior surface of the femur, a surface that is divided by the intercondylar groove and is concave mediolaterally and convex superoinferiorly.[1] The "motion of the patella relative to the femur or femoral groove in knee flexion and extension" is referred to as patellar tracking.[14(p. 241)] The gliding of the patella on the femur during knee flexion and extension is essential for normal motion at the knee. In full knee flexion, the patella slides distally and lies in the intercondylar notch.[13] In full knee extension, the patella slides proximally and the lower portion of the patellar surface articulates with the anterior surface of the femur.[1] In addition to proximal-distal glide, the patella glides medial-laterally during knee joint movement.[15] At the beginning of knee flexion, the patella shifts slightly medial, and as knee flexion increases, the patella gradually shifts laterally.[14]

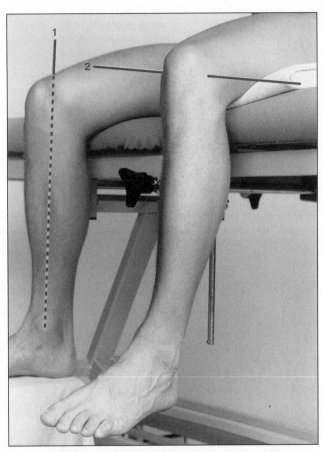

Figure 7-2 Knee joint axes: *(1)* tibial internal-external rotation; *(2)* flexion-extension.

TABLE 7-1   Joint Structure: Knee Movements

	Flexion	Extension	Internal Rotation	External Rotation
Articulation[1,3]	Femorotibial Patellofemoral	Femorotibial Patellofemoral	Femorotibial	Femorotibial
Plane	Sagittal	Sagittal	Horizontal	Horizontal
Axis	Frontal	Frontal	Longitudinal	Longitudinal
Normal limiting factors[2–6]★ (see Fig. 7-3A and B)	Tension in the rectus femoris (with the hip in extension); tension in the vasti muscles; soft tissue apposition of the posterior aspects of the calf and thigh or the heel and buttock	Tension in parts of both cruciate ligaments, the medial and lateral collateral ligaments, the posterior aspect of the capsule, and the oblique popliteal ligament	Tension in the cruciate ligaments	Tension in the collateral ligaments
Normal end feel[4,7]	Firm/soft	Firm	Firm	Firm
Normal AROM[8]† (AROM[9])	0–135° (0–140° to 145°)	135–0° (0°)	40°[11] to 58°[12] total active range at 90° knee flexion	
Capsular pattern[7,10]	Tibiofemoral joint: flexion, extension			

*Note: There is a paucity of definitive research that identifies the normal limiting factors (NLF) of joint motion. The NLF and end feels listed here are based on knowledge of anatomy, clinical experience, and available references.

†AROM, active range of motion.

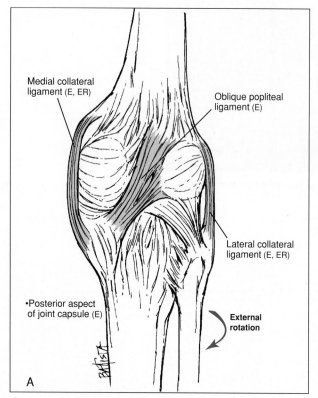

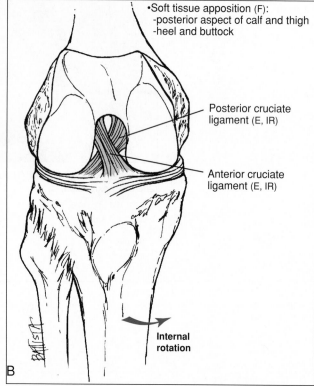

Figure 7-3 **Normal Limiting Factors. A.** Posterior view of the knee showing noncontractile structures that normally limit motion. **B.** Anterior view of the knee showing noncontractile structures that normally limit motion. Motion limited by structure is identified in brackets, using the following abbreviations: E, extension; ER, external rotation; IR, internal rotation. Muscles normally limiting motion are not illustrated.

SURFACE ANATOMY (Figs. 7-4 and 7-5)

Structure	Location
1. Greater trochanter	The superior border of the greater trochanter can be found with the tip of the thumb placed on the iliac crest at the midline and the tip of the third finger placed distally on the lateral aspect of the thigh.
2. Patella	Large triangular sesamoid bone on the anterior aspect of the knee. The base is proximal and the apex distal.
3. Ligamentum patellae tendon	Extends from the apex of the patella to the tibial tuberosity (patellar ligament or patellar tendon). As the patient attempts to extend the knee, the edges of the tendon are palpable.
4. Tibial tuberosity	Bony prominence at the proximal end of the anterior border of the tibia and the insertion of the ligamentum patellae.
5. Tibial plateaus	The upper edges of the medial and lateral tibial plateaus are located in the soft tissue depressions on either side of the ligamentum patellae. Follow the plateaus medially and laterally to ascertain the knee joint line.
6. Head of the fibula	A round bony prominence on the lateral aspect of the leg on a level with the tibial tuberosity.
7. Lateral malleolus	The prominent distal end of the fibula on the lateral aspect of the ankle.
8. Lateral epicondyle of the femur	Small bony prominence on the lateral condyle of the femur.

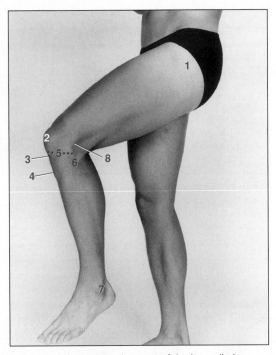

Figure 7-4 Anterolateral aspect of the lower limb.

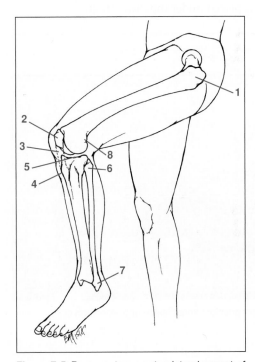

Figure 7-5 Bony anatomy, anterolateral aspect of the lower limb.

RANGE OF MOTION ASSESSMENT AND MEASUREMENT

 Practice Makes Perfect

To aid you in practicing the skills covered in this section, or for a handy review, use the practical testing forms found at http://thepoint.lww.com/Clarkson3e.

Knee Flexion-Extension

AROM Assessment

Substitute Movement. Hip flexion.

PROM Assessment

Forms
7-1, 7-2

Start Position. The patient is supine with the hip and knee in the anatomical position (Fig. 7-6). A towel is placed under the distal thigh.

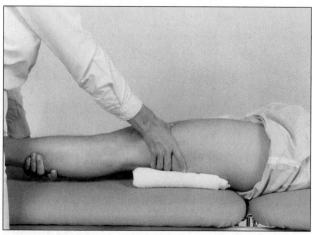

Figure 7-6 Start position: knee flexion and extension or hyperextension.

Stabilization. The pelvis is stabilized by the weight of the patient's body. The therapist stabilizes the femur.

Therapist's Distal Hand Placement. The therapist grasps the distal tibia and fibula.

End Positions. The therapist moves the lower leg to flex the hip and knee to the limit of knee flexion (Fig. 7-7).

The therapist extends the knee to the limit of knee extension/hyperextension (Fig. 7-8).

End Feels. *Flexion*—firm/soft; *extension/hyperextension*—firm.

Joint Glides. *Flexion*—the concave tibial condyles glide posteriorly on the fixed convex femoral condyles. *Extension*—the concave tibial condyles glide anteriorly on the fixed convex femoral condyles.

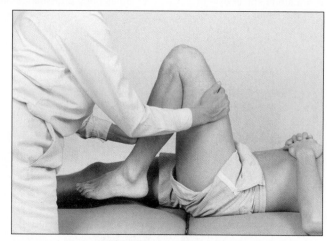

Figure 7-7 Firm or soft end feel at the limit of knee flexion.

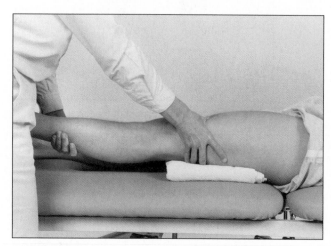

Figure 7-8 Firm end feel at the limit of knee extension or hyperextension.

Measurement: Universal Goniometer

Start Position. The patient is supine. The hip is in the anatomical position and the knee is in extension (0°) (Fig. 7-9). A towel is placed under the distal thigh.

Stabilization. The pelvis is stabilized by the weight of the patient's body. The therapist stabilizes the femur.

Goniometer Axis. The axis is placed over the lateral epicondyle of the femur (Fig. 7-10).

Stationary Arm. Parallel to the longitudinal axis of the femur, pointing toward the greater trochanter.

Movable Arm. Parallel to the longitudinal axis of the fibula, pointing toward the lateral malleolus.

End Position. From the start position of knee extension, the hip and knee are flexed (Fig. 7-11). The heel is moved toward the buttock to the limit of knee flexion (135°).

Hyperextension. The femur is stabilized, and the lower leg is moved in an anterior direction beyond 0° of extension (Fig. 7-12). Knee hyperextension from 0° to 10° may be present.

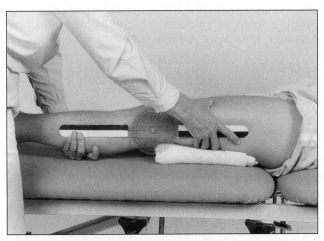

Figure 7-9 Start position: goniometer placement for knee flexion and extension/hyperextension.

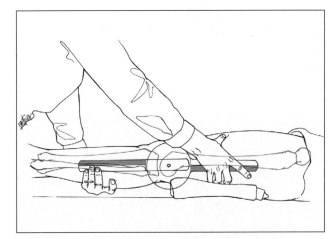

Figure 7-10 Goniometer placement for knee flexion and extension.

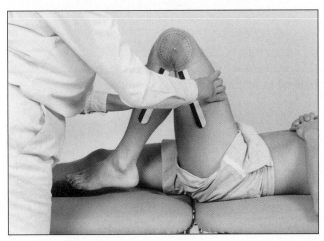

Figure 7-11 Knee flexion.

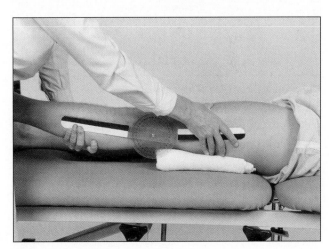

Figure 7-12 Knee hyperextension.

Patellar Mobility— Distal Glide

PROM Assessment

Form 7-3

Start Position. The patient is supine; a roll supports the knee joint in slight flexion (Fig. 7-13).

Stabilization. The femur rests on the plinth.

Procedure[16]. The heel of one hand is against the base of the patella, with the forearm lying along the thigh. The other hand is placed on top, and both hands move the patella in a distal direction to the end of the movement. Movement of the patella in a posterior direction compresses the patella against the femur and should be avoided. The therapist records whether the movement is full or restricted. The patella moves vertically a total of 8 cm from full flexion to full extension of the knee.[17]

End Feel. Firm.

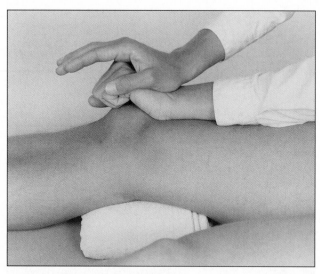

Figure 7-13 Distal glide of the patella.

Patellar Mobility— Medial-Lateral Glide

PROM Assessment

Form 7-4

Start Position. The patient is supine; a roll supports the knee joint in slight flexion (Fig. 7-14).

Stabilization. The therapist stabilizes the femur and tibia.

Procedure. The palmar aspects of the thumbs are placed on the lateral border of the patella. The pads of the index fingers are placed on the medial border of the patella. The thumbs move the patella medially, and the index fingers move the patella laterally in a side-to-side motion. With the knee in extension, passive movement of the patella should average 9.6 mm medially and 5.4 mm laterally.[18] Excessive, normal, or restricted ROM is recorded.

End Feel. Firm.

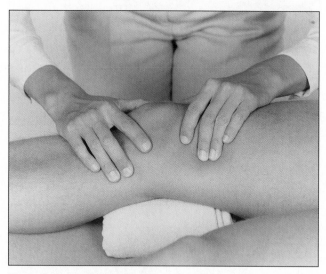

Figure 7-14 Medial-lateral glide of the patella.

Tibial Rotation

Tibial rotation is an essential component of normal ROM at the knee. Assessment of total rotation ROM is more reliable than assessment of internal and external tibial rotation because of the difficulty of defining the zero start position for the individual movements.[19] The greatest range of tibial rotation is available when the knee is flexed 90°.[13]

AROM Assessment

Substitute Movement. Tibial internal rotation—hip internal rotation, ankle dorsiflexion/plantarflexion, subtalar joint inversion, forefoot adduction. Tibial external rotation—hip external rotation, ankle dorsiflexion/plantarflexion, subtalar joint eversion, forefoot abduction.

PROM Assessment

Form 7-5

Start Position. The patient is sitting with the knee in 90° flexion and the tibia in full internal rotation (Fig. 7-15A). A pad is placed under the distal thigh to maintain the thigh in a horizontal position.

Stabilization. The therapist stabilizes the femur.

Procedure. From full internal rotation, the therapist rotates the tibia externally through the full available ROM (Fig. 7-16A). The total range of tibial rotation is observed (average total active range, about 40° in women[11] and 58° in men[12]) and recorded as excessive, normal, or restricted.

End Feels. *Internal rotation*—firm; *external rotation*—firm.

Joint Spin. The proximal concave surface of the tibia spins on the convex condyles of the fixed femur. This spin occurs in conjunction with roll and glide of the articular surface during flexion and extension at the knee joint.

Measurement: OB Goniometer

Start Position. The patient is sitting with the knee in 90° flexion and the tibia in full internal rotation (Fig. 7-15A). A pad is placed under the distal thigh to maintain the thigh in a horizontal position. In the start position, the fluid-filled container of the goniometer is rotated until the 0° arrow lines up directly underneath the compass needle (Fig. 7-15B).

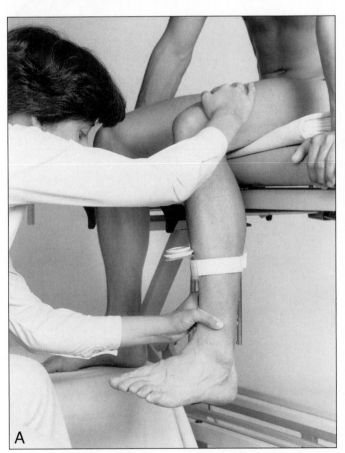

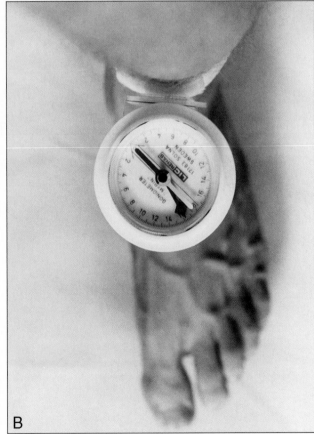

Figure 7-15 A. and B. Start position for total tibial rotation: tibial internal rotation.

Goniometer Placement. The strap is placed around the leg distal to the gastrocnemius muscle, and the dial is placed on the right-angle extension plate on the anterior aspect of the leg.

Stabilization. The therapist stabilizes the femur.

End Position. From full internal rotation, the therapist rotates the tibia externally through the full available PROM (see Fig. 7-16A). The number of degrees the compass needle moves away from the 0° arrow on the compass dial is recorded as the total range of tibial rotation (see Fig. 7-16B) (average total active range, about 40° in women[11] and 58° in men[12]).

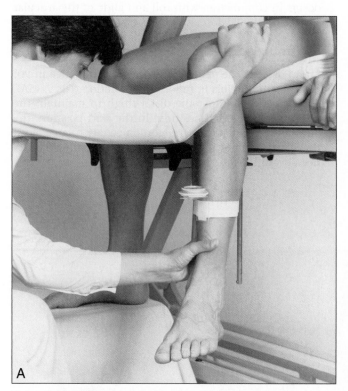
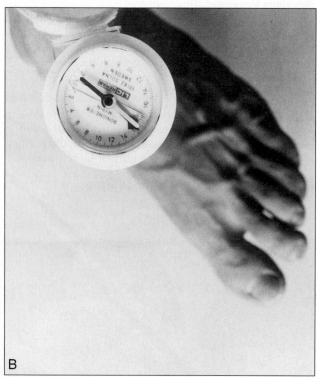

Figure 7-16 A and B. End position for total tibial rotation: tibial external rotation.

MUSCLE LENGTH ASSESSMENT AND MEASUREMENT

Practice Makes Perfect

To aid you in practicing the skills covered in this section, or for a handy review, use the practical testing forms found at http://thepoint.lww.com/Clarkson3e.

Hamstrings (Semitendinosus, Semimembranosus, Biceps Femoris)

Origins[1]	Insertions[1]
Semitendinosus	
Inferomedial impression on the superior aspect of the ischial tuberosity	Proximal part of the medial surface of the tibia.
Semimembranosus	
Superolateral aspect of the ischial tuberosity	Tubercle on the posterior aspect of the medial tibial condyle.
Biceps Femoris	
a. Long head: inferomedial impression of the superior aspect of the ischial tuberosity; lower portion of the sacrotuberous ligament	Head of the fibula; slip to the lateral condyle of the tibia; slip to the lateral collateral ligament.
b. Short head: lateral lip of the linea aspera and lateral supracondylar line	

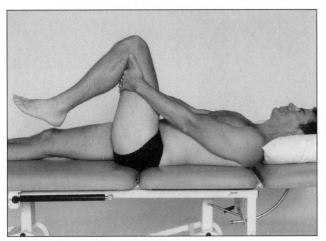

Figure 7-17 PKE: hamstrings length.

Passive Knee Extension (PKE) Supine[20]

 Start Position. The patient is supine (Fig. 7-17). The hip is flexed to 90°. The patient supports the thigh in this position by placing both hands around the distal thigh. If the patient cannot hold this position, the therapist stabilizes the thigh. The knee is flexed, and the ankle is relaxed in plantarflexion.

Form 7-6

Stabilization. The patient or the therapist stabilizes the femur to maintain the hip in 90° flexion. Posterior tilt of the pelvis is avoided through use of a precise start position, observation of pelvic motion, and if necessary use of a strap placed over the anterior aspect of the distal thigh on the nontest side (see Fig. 6-41).

Goniometer Placement. The goniometer is placed the same as for knee flexion (Fig. 7-18). Should the therapist stabilize the thigh, a second therapist may be required to assist with the alignment and reading of the universal goniometer.

End Position. While maintaining the hip in 90° flexion, the knee is extended to the limit of motion so that the hamstring muscles are put on full stretch (Fig. 7-18). The ankle is relaxed in plantarflexion during the test.

The angle of knee flexion is used to indicate the hamstring muscle length. If the knee cannot be extended beyond 20° knee flexion, according to some sources[21,22] this indicates hamstring tightness. However, Youdas and colleagues[23] performed the PKE test with 214 men and women, aged 20–79 years, and reported mean knee flexion PROM of 28° for women and 39° for men.

End Feel. Hamstrings on stretch—firm.

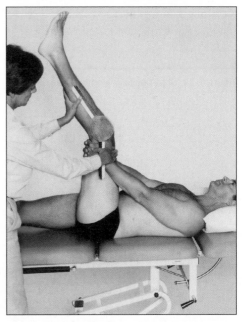

Figure 7-18 End position: universal goniometer measurement of knee flexion for hamstrings length.

Alternate Position—Sitting

Start Position. The patient is sitting, grasps the edge of the plinth, and has the nontest foot supported on a stool (Fig. 7-19). A pad is placed under the distal thigh to maintain the thigh in a horizontal position. The ankle on the test side is relaxed in plantarflexion.

Form 7-7

Stabilization. The therapist stabilizes the femur. The patient grasps the edge of the plinth and is instructed to maintain the upright sitting position.

Goniometer Placement. The goniometer is placed the same as for knee flexion-extension (Fig. 7-20).

End Position. The therapist extends the knee to the limit of motion so that hamstrings are put on full stretch (Fig. 7-20). The ankle is relaxed in plantarflexion throughout the test movement to prevent gastrocnemius muscle tightness from limiting knee ROM.

End Feel. Hamstrings on stretch—firm.

Substitute Movement. The patient leans back to posteriorly tilt the pelvis, extending the hip joint to place the hamstrings on slack, and thus allow increased knee extension (Fig. 7-21).

Alternate Position—Passive Straight Leg Raise (PSLR)

The PSLR technique used to evaluate hamstring muscle length is described in Chapter 6. Note: the PKE and PSLR tests should not be used interchangeably when assessing hamstring muscle length.[22]

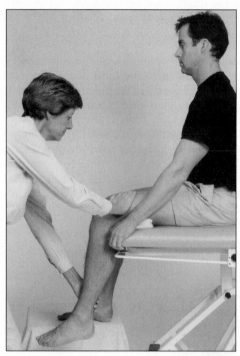

Figure 7-19 Start position: length of hamstrings.

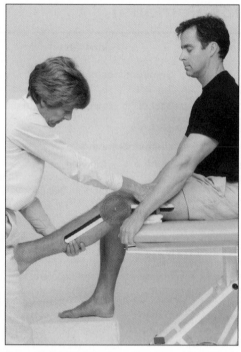

Figure 7-20 Goniometer measurement: length of hamstrings.

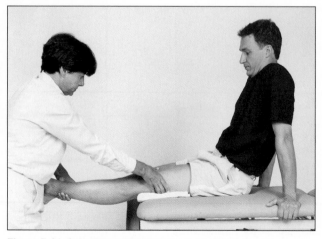

Figure 7-21 Substitute movement: backward lean during hamstrings length test.

Rectus Femoris

Origins[1]	Insertion[1]
Rectus Femoris	
a. Straight head: anterior inferior iliac spine.	Base of the patella, via the quadriceps tendon into the tibial tuberosity.
b. Reflected head: groove above the acetabulum and the capsule of the hip joint.	

Start Position. The patient is prone. To position the pelvis in a posterior tilt, the nontest leg is over the side of the plinth with the hip flexed and the foot on the floor (Fig. 7-22). This positioning of the nontest leg has been shown to effectively tilt the pelvis posteriorly, and thus increase hip extension of the test leg to better ensure maximum stretch of the rectus femoris muscle.[24] The test leg is in the anatomical position with the knee in extension (0°). A towel may be placed under the thigh to eliminate pressure on the patella.

Form 7-8

Stabilization. The patient's prone position with the nontest leg over the side of the plinth with the hip flexed and the foot on the floor stabilizes the pelvis. A strap may also be placed over the buttocks to stabilize the pelvis. The therapist stabilizes the femur.

Goniometer Placement. The goniometer is placed the same as for knee flexion-extension.

End Position. The lower leg is moved in a posterior direction so that the heel approximates the buttock to the limit of knee flexion. Decreased length of the rectus femoris restricts the range of knee flexion when the patient is prone (Fig. 7-23).

End Feel. Rectus femoris on stretch—firm.

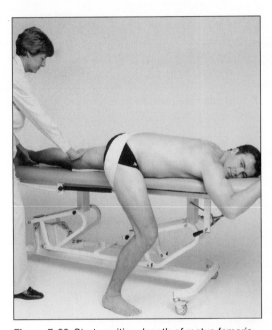

Figure 7-22 Start position: length of rectus femoris.

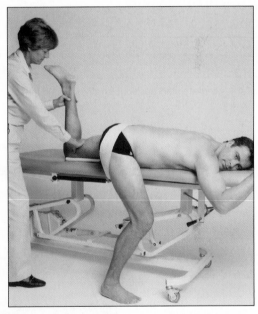

Figure 7-23 End position: length of rectus femoris.

Alternate Position—Ely's Test

 Start Position. The patient is prone. A towel may be placed under the thigh to eliminate pressure on the patella. The leg is in the anatomical position with the knee in extension (0°) (Fig. 7-24).

Form 7-9

Stabilization. The patient's prone position stabilizes the pelvis. A strap may also be placed over the buttocks to stabilize the pelvis. The therapist observes the pelvis to ensure there is no tilting. The therapist stabilizes the femur.

Goniometer Placement. The goniometer is placed the same as for knee flexion-extension.

End Position. The lower leg is moved in a posterior direction so the heel approximates the buttock to the limit of knee flexion. Decreased length of the rectus femoris restricts the range of knee flexion when the patient is prone (Fig. 7-25).

End Feel. Rectus femoris on stretch—firm.

Substitute Movement. The patient anteriorly tilts the pelvis and flexes the hip to place the rectus femoris on slack, and thus allows increased knee flexion (Fig. 7-26).

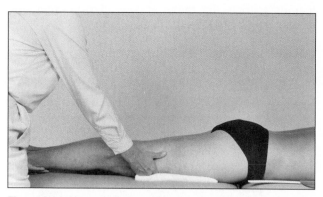

Figure 7-24 Alternate start position: length of rectus femoris.

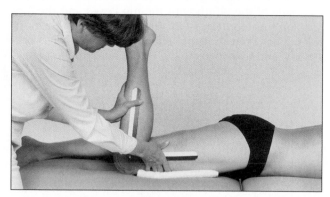

Figure 7-25 Goniometer measurement: length of rectus femoris.

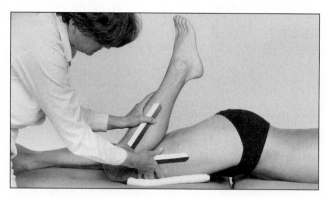

Figure 7-26 Substitute movement: anterior pelvic tilt and hip flexion placing rectus femoris on slack.

Alternate Position—Thomas Test Position

Start Position. The patient sits at the end of the plinth with the edge of the plinth at midthigh level. From this position, the patient is assisted into supine. Using both hands, the patient holds the hip of the nontest leg in flexion so that the sacrum and lumbar spine are flat on the plinth. Care should be taken to avoid flexion of the lumbar spine due to excessive hip flexion ROM. With the hip abducted, the hip is extended to the limit of motion[25] (Fig. 7-27).

Stabilization. The patient's supine position and holding of the nontest hip in flexion stabilizes the pelvis and lumbar spine. The therapist observes the anterior superior iliac spine (ASIS) to ensure there is no pelvic tilting. The therapist stabilizes the femur.

Goniometer Placement. The goniometer is placed the same as for knee flexion-extension.

End Position. The knee is flexed to the limit of motion to assess shortness of the rectus femoris (Figs. 7-28 and 7-29). If the rectus femoris is shortened, knee flexion PROM will be restricted proportional to the decrease in muscle length. Knee flexion of less than 80° indicates the degree of muscle shortening.[26]

End Feel. Rectus femoris on stretch—firm.

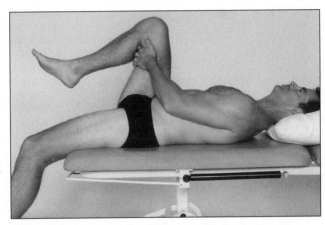

Figure 7-27 Alternate start position: length of rectus femoris.

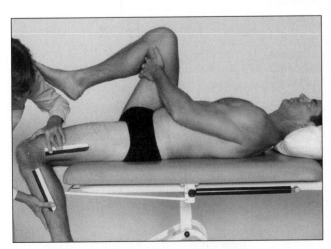

Figure 7-28 End position: length of rectus femoris.

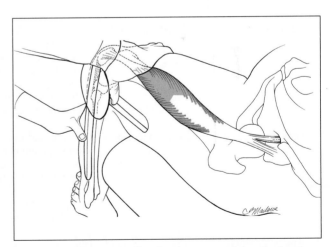

Figure 7-29 Alternate goniometer measurement: length of rectus femoris.

MUSCLE STRENGTH ASSESSMENT (TABLE 7-2)

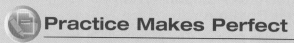

Practice Makes Perfect

To aid you in practicing the skills covered in this section, or for a handy review, use the practical testing forms found at http://thepoint.lww.com/Clarkson3e.

TABLE 7-2 **Muscle Actions, Attachments, and Nerve Supply: the Knee[27]**

Muscle	Primary Muscle Action	Muscle Origin	Muscle Insertion	Peripheral Nerve	Nerve Root
		Hamstrings			
Semimembranosus	Knee flexion Internal rotation of the flexed knee	Superolateral aspect of the ischial tuberosity	Tubercle on the posterior aspect of the medial tibial condyle	Sciatic (tibial portion)	L5S12
Semitendinosus	Knee flexion Internal rotation of the flexed knee	Inferomedial impression on the superior aspect of the ischial tuberosity	Proximal part of the medial surface of the tibia	Sciatic (tibial portion)	L5S12
Biceps femoris	Knee flexion External rotation of the flexed knee	a. Long head: inferomedial impression of the superior aspect of the ischial tuberosity; lower portion of the sacrotuberous ligament b. Short head: lateral lip of the linea aspera and lateral supracondylar line	Head of the fibula; slip to the lateral condyle of the tibia; slip to the lateral collateral ligament	Sciatic (tibial and common peroneal portions)	L5S12
		Quadriceps			
Vastus medialis	Knee extension	Lower part of the intertrochanteric line and the spiral line, medial lip of the linea aspera, proximal part of the supracondylar line, the adductor tendons of longus and magnus, and the intermuscular septum	Medial border of the patella, via the quadriceps tendon into the tibial tuberosity	Femoral	L234
Vastus lateralis	Knee extension	Superior part of the intertrochanteric line, anterior and inferior borders of the greater trochanter, lateral lip of the gluteal tuberosity, and the upper half of the lateral lip of the linea aspera	Lateral border and base of the patella, via the quadriceps tendon into the tibial tuberosity	Femoral	L234
Vastus intermedius	Knee extension	Upper two-thirds of the anterior and lateral surfaces of the femoral shaft	Base of the patella, via the quadriceps tendon into the tibial tuberosity	Femoral	L234
Rectus femoris	Hip flexion Knee extension	a. Straight head: anterior aspect of the anterior inferior iliac spine b. Reflected head: groove above the acetabulum and the capsule of the hip joint	Base of the patella, via the quadriceps tendon into the tibial tuberosity	Femoral	L234

Knee Flexion

Against Gravity: Biceps Femoris, Semitendinosus, and Semimembranosus

Accessory muscles: gastrocnemius, popliteus, gracilis, and sartorius.

Form 7-11

Research[28,29] appears to support the practice of testing the hamstrings as a group with the tibia positioned in neutral rotation, and isolating the medial and lateral hamstrings by positioning the tibia in either internal or external rotation, respectively.

Start Position. The patient is in the prone-lying position with a pillow under the abdomen (Fig. 7-30). The knee is in extension, the tibia is in neutral rotation, and the foot is over the end of the plinth. The rectus femoris may limit the range of knee flexion in the prone position.

Stabilization. A pelvic strap stabilizes the pelvis. The therapist stabilizes the thigh.

Movement. The patient flexes the knee through full ROM (Fig. 7-31).

Palpation. *Biceps femoris:* proximal to the knee joint on the lateral margin of the popliteal fossa. *Semitendinosus:* proximal to the knee joint on the medial margin of the popliteal fossa. *Semimembranosus:* proximal to the knee joint on either side of the semitendinosus tendon.[30]

Substitute Movement. Sartorius (producing hip flexion and external rotation) and gracilis (producing hip adduction).[5]

Resistance Location. Applied proximal to the ankle joint on the posterior aspect of the leg (Fig. 7-32). Walmsley and Yang[31] found that with the hip at or near 0°, a strong knee flexion contraction could not be performed beyond 90° because of discomfort. It is not uncommon to experience cramping of the hamstring muscles if too much resistance is applied as the knee moves into greater degrees of flexion.[26]

Resistance Direction. Knee extension.

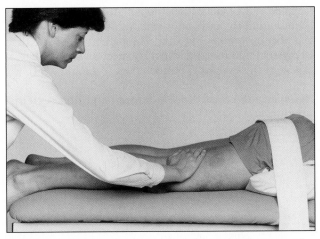

Figure 7-30 Start position: biceps femoris, semitendinosus, and semimembranosus.

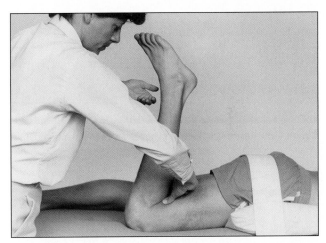

Figure 7-31 Screen position: biceps femoris, semitendinosus, and semimembranosus.

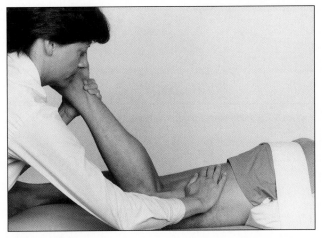

Figure 7-32 Resistance: biceps femoris, semitendinosus, and semimembranosus.

Isolation of the Medial Hamstrings. The medial hamstrings (semitendinosus and semimembranosus) internally rotate the tibia during knee flexion. The patient holds the tibia in internal rotation and brings the heel toward the lateral aspect of the ipsilateral buttock (Figs. 7-33 and 7-34).

Resistance Direction. Knee extension and tibial external rotation.

Isolation of the Lateral Hamstring. The lateral hamstring (biceps femoris) externally rotates the tibia during knee flexion. The patient holds the tibia in external rotation and brings the heel toward the contralateral buttock (Figs. 7-35 and 7-36).

Resistance Direction. Knee extension and tibial internal rotation.

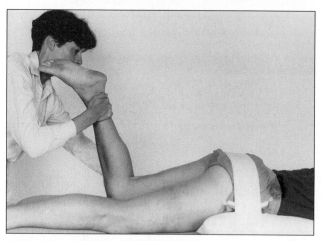

Figure 7-33 Resistance: semitendinosus and semimembranosus.

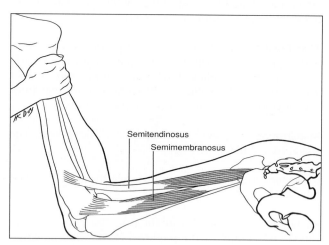

Figure 7-34 Semitendinosus and semimembranosus.

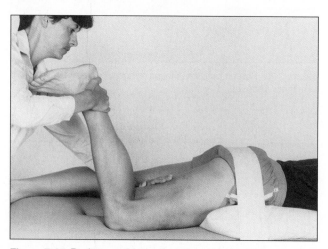

Figure 7-35 Resistance: biceps femoris.

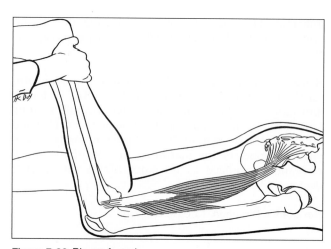

Figure 7-36 Biceps femoris.

Gravity Eliminated: Biceps Femoris, Semitendinosus, and Semimembranosus

Start Position. The patient is side-lying on the nontest side (Fig. 7-37). The therapist supports the weight of the lower extremity. The hip is in anatomical position with the knee extended.

Stabilization. The therapist stabilizes the thigh.

End Position. The patient flexes the knee through full ROM (Fig. 7-38).

Substitute Movement. Hip flexion resulting in passive knee flexion.

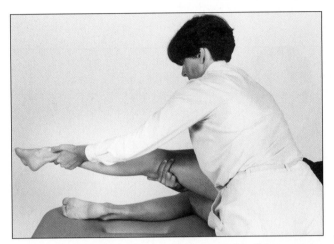

Figure 7-37 Start position: biceps femoris, semitendinosus, and semimembranosus.

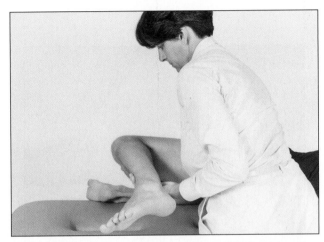

Figure 7-38 End position: biceps femoris, semitendinosus, and semimembranosus.

Knee Extension

Against Gravity: Rectus Femoris, Vastus Intermedius, Vastus Lateralis, and Vastus Medialis

Start Position. The patient is sitting (Fig. 7-39). The knee is flexed and a pad is placed under the distal thigh to maintain the thigh in a horizontal position.

Form 7-12

Stabilization. The therapist stabilizes the thigh and the patient grasps the edge of the plinth.

Movement. The patient extends the knee through full ROM (Fig. 7-40). If the hamstrings are tight, the patient may lean back to relieve the tension on the hamstrings during the movement. The patient may attempt to lean back during the test to place the rectus femoris muscle on stretch and increase the contribution from this muscle to produce knee extension.[30]

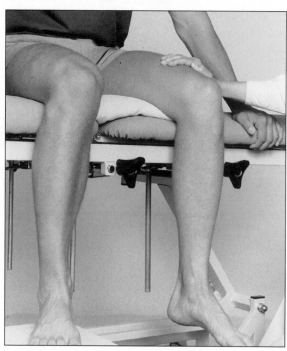

Figure 7-39 Start position: rectus femoris, vastus intermedius, vastus lateralis, and vastus medialis.

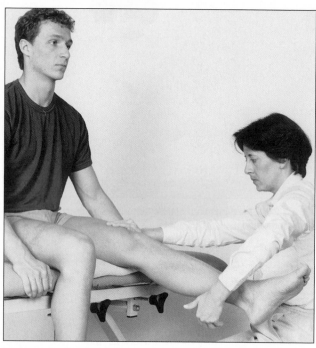

Figure 7-40 Screen position: rectus femoris, vastus intermedius, vastus lateralis, and vastus medialis.

Palpation. *Rectus femoris:* on the anterior midthigh. *Vastus intermedius:* too deep to palpate. *Vastus lateralis:* lateral aspect midthigh. *Vastus medialis:* medial aspect distal thigh. The *quadriceps muscle group* may be palpated proximal to the tibial tuberosity at the patellar tendon.

Substitute Movement. Tensor fascia latae (observe internal rotation of the hip).[26]

Resistance Location. Applied on the anterior surface of the distal end of the leg (Figs. 7-41 and 7-42). Ensure the patient does not lock the knee in full extension (close-packed position).

Resistance Direction. Knee flexion.

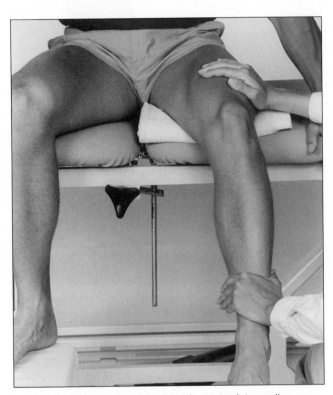

Figure 7-41 Resistance: rectus femoris, vastus intermedius, vastus lateralis, and vastus medialis.

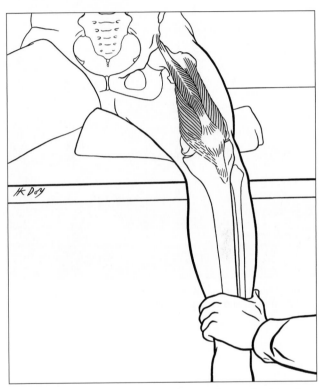

Figure 7-42 Rectus femoris, vastus intermedius, vastus lateralis, and vastus medialis.

Gravity Eliminated: Rectus Femoris, Vastus Intermedius, Vastus Lateralis, and Vastus Medialis

Start Position. The patient is side-lying on the nontest side (Fig. 7-43). The therapist supports the weight of the lower extremity. The hip is in anatomical position with the knee flexed.

Stabilization. The therapist stabilizes the thigh.

End Position. The patient extends the knee through full ROM (Fig. 7-44).

Substitute Movement. Hip extension from a flexed position can result in passive knee extension.[5]

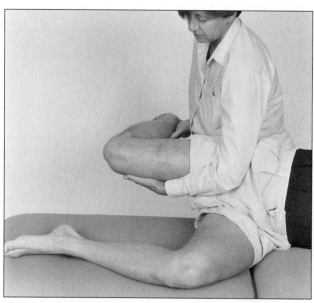

Figure 7-43 Start position: rectus femoris, vastus intermedius, vastus lateralis, and vastus medialis.

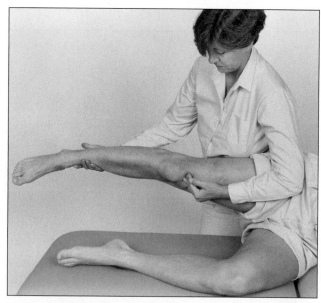

Figure 7-44 End position: rectus femoris, vastus intermedius, vastus lateralis, and vastus medialis.

FUNCTIONAL APPLICATION

Joint Function

The knee joint functions to support the body weight and to shorten or lengthen the lower limb.[2] Knee flexion with the foot planted lowers the body closer to the ground, while knee extension raises the body.[30] With the foot off the ground, foot orientation in space is provided[2] by flexing or extending the knee or rotating the tibia. The rotational mobility of the knee joint makes twisting movements of the body possible when the foot is planted on the ground.[30] In walking, the knee joint acts as a shock absorber, decreases the vertical displacement of the body, and through knee flexion shortens the lower limb to allow the toes to clear the ground during the swing phase of the gait cycle.[32,33]

Functional Range of Motion

The normal AROM at the knee is from 0° of extension to 135° of flexion. Full extension is required for normal function, but many daily activities require less than 135° of knee flexion. Rowe and colleagues[34] suggest 0° to at least 110° of knee flexion would be an appropriate target for rehabilitation. A target of 110° knee flexion would enable one to walk, sit in and stand up from a chair, and negotiate stairs. Using the bath would require greater ROM of approximately 135° flexion to be performed in a normal manner.

The knee must be fully extended to stand erect (Fig. 7-45). Full or near-full knee extension is required to reach a height (Fig. 7-46) or to contact a distant object or surface with the foot, such as depressing the brake pedal of a car or going downstairs (Fig. 7-47). When dressing, the knee is extended to put on a pair of trousers (Fig. 7-48) or shorts. The fully extended position of the knee usually occurs in asymmetrical postures; for example, prolonged standing when one leg is used to support most of the body weight or when powerful thrusting motions[1] such as jumping are performed.

Daily activities involving ranges of knee motion up to an average of 117° of flexion include lifting an object off the floor (Fig. 7-49), sitting down in a chair (Fig. 7-50), descending and ascending stairs (Figs. 7-47 and 7-51), and tying a shoelace [36] or pulling on a sock (Fig. 7-52). Many of the daily functions previously mentioned require on average less than 25° of tibial rotation.[36] The knee flexion ROM required for selected activities of daily living (ADL) is shown in Table 7-3.

Far greater knee flexion ROM is utilized by non-Western cultures accustomed to performing ADL such as squatting, cross-legged sitting, and kneeling[38,39] (Table 7-4). A range with a mean minimum of 135° knee flexion when sitting cross-legged[39] to a mean maximum of about 157° flexion when squatting with the heels up,[38] is required for these ADL. Positions (i.e., squatting, cross-legged sitting, and kneeling) essential for ADL in Asian and Eastern cultures all require high knee flexion ROM accompanied by tibial internal rotation ROM up to an average maximum of 33° for cross-legged sitting.[38] To achieve the knee flexion ROM required to squat and kneel, the hip is flexed placing

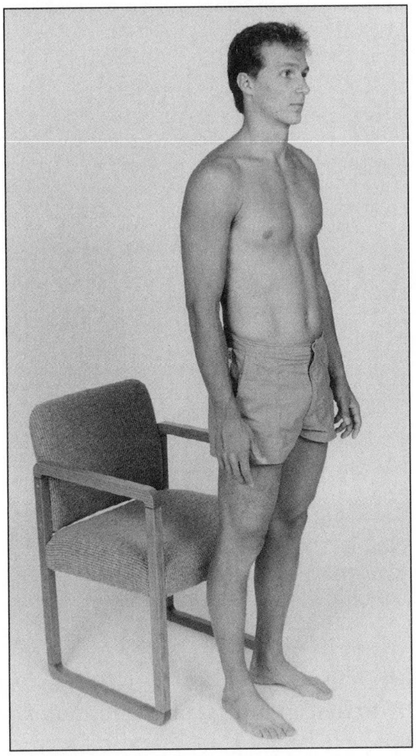

Figure 7-45 Full knee extension is required to stand erect.

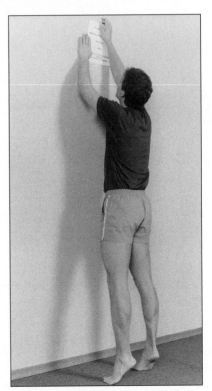

Figure 7-46 To reach a height, full or near-full knee extension is required.

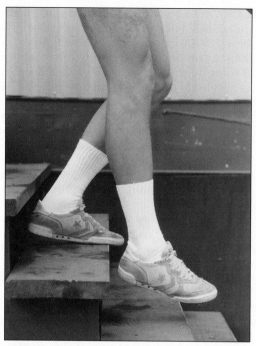

Figure 7-47 Going down stairs requires: an average of 86° to 107° of knee flexion, full or near-full knee extension,[35] and eccentric quadriceps contraction.

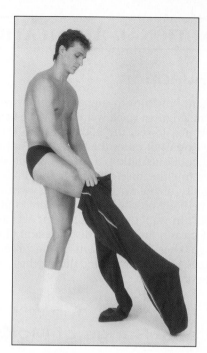

Figure 7-48 The knee is in extension to put on a pair of trousers.

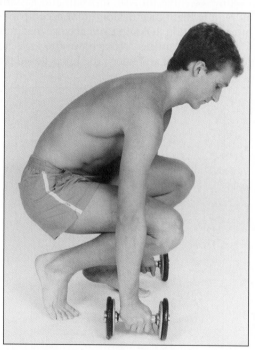

Figure 7-49 Lifting an object off the floor requires an average of 117° of knee flexion.[36]

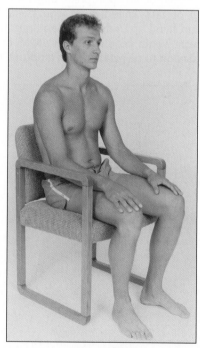

Figure 7-50 To sit down in a chair requires an average of 93° of knee flexion.[36]

rectus femoris on slack, and body weight assists in passively flexing the knee joint.

Livingston and coworkers[35] evaluated the knee flexion ROM required to ascend and descend three stairs of different dimensions. Depending on the stair dimensions and subject height, the maximum knee flexion ROM required ranged between averages of 83° and 105° to ascend, and 86° and 107° to descend the stairs. Minimum knee flexion ROM averages of between 1° or 2° and 15° were required to ascend or descend stairs. It appears that changes of ROM at the knee joint, rather than the hip and ankle, are used to adjust to different stair dimensions.[35]

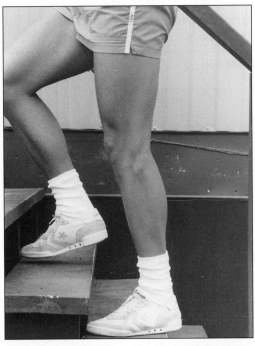

Figure 7-51 Climbing stairs requires an average of 83° to 105° of knee flexion and full or near-full knee extension.[35]

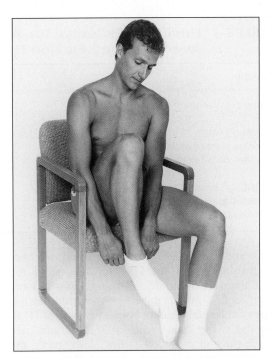

Figure 7-52 Knee range within the arc of 0° to 117° of flexion.

Gait

Walking requires a ROM from about 0° of knee extension as the leg advances forward to make initial contact with the ground (Fig. 7-53), to a maximum of about 60° of knee flexion at initial swing so that the foot clears the ground as the extremity is advanced forward (from the Rancho Los Amigos gait analysis forms, as cited in the work of Levangie and Norkin[2]). The tibia rotates internally on the femur at the end of the swing phase and maintains the position of internal rotation through the stance phase until preswing, when the tibia externally rotates through to midswing.[40] An average of about 13° of tibial rotation is required for normal gait.[41] For further description and illustrations of the positions and motions at the knee joint during gait, see Appendix D.

TABLE 7-3 Knee Flexion ROM Average Values Required for ADL

Activity	Knee Flexion
Taking a bath[34]	135°
Tying shoe: sitting and bringing the foot up from the floor*	106°
Sitting: without touching the chair with the hands*	93°
Lifting object from floor*	
Bending at hips to reach down	71°
Back straight, bending knees	117°
Stairs[†]	
Ascending	83–105°
Descending	86–107°
Walking[‡]	60°
Fast-paced running[37] (faster than 7.5-minute mile)	103°

*Knee flexion ROM for 30 subjects were measured from the subject's normal stance position and not anatomical zero position.[36]

[†]Knee flexion ROM for 15 subjects during ascent and descent of three stairs of different dimensions. Maximum knee flexion ROM requirements varied depending on the stair dimensions and subject height.[35]

[‡]Data from the Rancho Los Amigos gait analysis forms as cited in Levangie and Norkin.[2]

TABLE 7-4 **Positions Essential for ADL in Asian and Eastern Cultures: Average Knee Flexion ROM Values Required**

Activity	Knee Flexion
Sitting cross-legged	135°[39]–150°[38]
Kneeling[38] with:	
ankles plantarflexed	144°
ankles dorsiflexed	155°
Squatting[38] with:	
heels down	154°
heels up	157°

Pink and colleagues[37] investigated and described the ROM requirement at the knee for slow-paced running (slower than an 8-minute mile) and fast-paced running (faster than a 7.5-minute mile). Fast-paced running required a range of knee joint motion from an average of 11° flexion at terminal swing to an average 103° maximum knee flexion near the end of middle swing. Slower-paced running required less flexion throughout most of the swing phase compared to fast-paced running.

Muscle Function

Knee Flexors

The knee flexors include the biceps femoris, semitendinosus, semimembranosus, sartorius, gracilis, popliteus, and

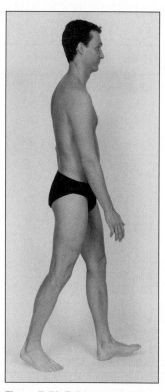

Figure 7-53 Full knee extension is required for normal gait.

gastrocnemius. The majority of the knee flexors are biarticular muscles and also produce movement at either the hip or ankle joints. The popliteus and short head of biceps femoris are the only monoarticular knee flexors.

The gracilis muscle contributes to the knee flexor moment at all knee joint angles.[42] The gastrocnemius also flexes the knee joint at all knee joint angles, and controls knee hyperextension.[17] The contribution of gastrocnemius to knee flexion is greatest with the knee joint in full extension and decreases as the knee is flexed regardless of ankle joint position.[43] Gastrocnemius knee flexion torque is greater when the ankle is dorsiflexed than when the ankle is positioned in plantarflexion.[43]

With the exception of gastrocnemius, the knee flexors rotate the tibia. Biceps femoris contracts to externally rotate and flex the tibia on the femur. The other knee flexors internally rotate the tibia on the femur.

The action of popliteus is negligible as a knee flexor, but the muscle functions to internally rotate the tibia on the femur,[44] contracting at the initiation of knee flexion to unlock the knee joint.[45] When loads are carried while walking downhill, popliteus activity is increased to stabilize the knee at midstance, from that of level or downhill walking.[46] When a crouch position is assumed, the popliteus contracts to prevent the forward displacement of the femur on the tibia,[45] in activities such as squatting to pick up an object (Fig. 7-49).

The action of the knee flexors is illustrated in sitting when the ankle is placed across the opposite thigh (Fig. 7-54) or when the legs are crossed at the ankles with the feet positioned under the chair. In standing, the knee flexors contract to allow one to inspect the sole of the foot. The flexors contract when knee flexion is forced at the end of the ROM, for example, when pulling on a sock (Fig. 7-52). When walking or running, the knee flexors contract eccentrically to decelerate the leg as the knee extends to take a step forward. Activities such as ascending stairs do not require contraction of the knee flexors because the knee is flexed passively[17] due to active hip flexion.

The knee flexors that function as rotators initiate and control knee rotation in activities such as running and turning.[30] These muscles are also active in squatting and kneeling when the trunk and upper extremities produce knee motions on the fixed tibia.[30]

a chair, jumping, ascending stairs (Fig. 7-51), and rising to get out of the bathtub.

When the foot is not fixed on the ground, the knee extensors contract when the knee is extended against resistance, including the weight of the leg. Kicking a ball, pulling on a pair of trousers, and swimming using the frog kick require contraction of the knee extensors.

Standing Posture

There is no contraction of the quadriceps in the standing position because the line of gravity tends to fall anterior to the knee joint. Using electromyography, Portnoy and Morin[53] found that the hamstrings and gastrocnemius muscles contract in standing. These muscles may function to prevent the knee from extending or hyperextending.[30]

Gait

The knee extensors and flexors contract simultaneously to stabilize the knee in the extended position to prepare for initial contact.[54] During the first part of the stance phase, the quadriceps contract eccentrically to prevent knee flexion from occurring at initial contact and loading response as the weight is transferred to the limb. The quadriceps may or may not contract from loading response to midstance to extend the knee. At higher walking speeds, the quadriceps may contract to prevent excessive knee flexion and initiate knee extension at initial swing.[33] The hamstrings contract eccentrically at terminal swing to decelerate the forward-swinging limb.[54] The sartorius is active throughout the swing phase of the gait cycle, assisting with hip flexion required for toe clearance and external rotation of the hip as the pelvis rotates forward on the same side.[55] The gracilis contracts at the end of the stance phase and the beginning of the swing phase of the gait cycle.[56] The popliteus internally rotates the tibia on the femur and maintains this position from midswing through to preswing.[40]

Montgomery and colleagues[57] provide a description of the knee muscle activity during running.

References

1. Standring S, ed. *Gray's Anatomy: The Anatomical Basis of Clinical Practice*. 39th ed. London: Elsevier Churchill Livingstone; 2001.
2. Levangie PK, Norkin CC. *Joint Structure and Function. A Comprehensive Analysis*. 3rd ed. Philadelphia: FA Davis; 2001.
3. Kapandji IA. *The Physiology of the Joints. Vol. 2. The Lower Limb*. 6th ed. New York: Churchill Livingstone Elsevier; 2011.
4. Norkin CC, White DJ. *Measurement of Joint Motion: A Guide to Goniometry*. 4th ed. Philadelphia: FA Davis Company; 2009.
5. Daniels L, Worthingham C. *Muscle Testing: Techniques of Manual Examination*. 5th ed. Philadelphia: WB Saunders; 1986.
6. Woodburne RT. *Essentials of Human Anatomy*. 5th ed. London: Oxford University Press; 1973.
7. Magee DJ. *Orthopedic Physical Assessment*. 5th ed. St. Louis: Saunders Elsevier; 2008.
8. American Academy of Orthopaedic Surgeons. *Joint Motion: Method of Measuring and Recording*. Chicago: AAOS; 1965.
9. Berryman Reese N, Bandy WD. *Joint Range of Motion and Muscle Length Testing*. 2nd ed. St. Louis: Saunders Elsevier; 2010.

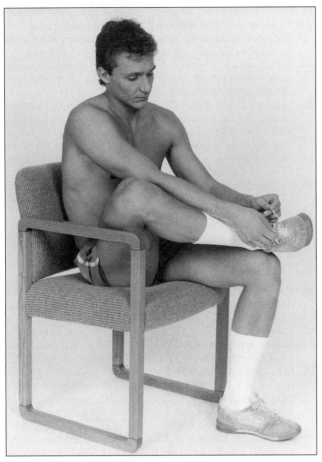

Figure 7-54 The knee flexors contract to position the foot across the opposite thigh.

Knee Extensors

The extensors of the knee are the rectus femoris, vastus medialis, vastus lateralis, and vastus intermedius. The rectus femoris acts at the hip and knee joints and is more effective as a knee extensor if the hip is extended and the muscle is placed on stretch.[47] Okamoto found that the hip must be stabilized for the rectus femoris to act fully as a knee extensor (cited in Basmajian and DeLuca[48]). The vastus medialis contracts with the other vasti muscles through the full ROM to perform knee extension.[49-52] The inferior oblique fibers of vastus medialis are thought to function at terminal extension to prevent the lateral displacement of the patella by drawing the patella medially.[48]

Two main patterns of movement occur in the lower limb during ADL. One pattern includes hip flexion, knee flexion, and ankle dorsiflexion.[47] In this pattern, the knee extensors usually contract eccentrically to control knee flexion. This is illustrated in activities when the foot is fixed on the ground and the body is moved closer to the ground, such as squatting to lift an object off the floor, sitting down in a chair, and descending stairs (Fig. 7-47). The other common movement pattern of the lower limb consists of hip extension, knee extension, and ankle plantarflexion.[47] In this pattern, the knee extensors normally contract concentrically to extend the knee joint. This synergy is illustrated when rising out of

10. Cyriax J. *Textbook of Orthopaedic Medicine. Vol. 1. Diagnosis of Soft Tissue Lesions.* 8th ed. London: Bailliere Tindall; 1982.
11. Mossberg KA, Smith LK. Axial rotation of the knee in women. *J Orthop Sports Phys Ther.* 1983;4(4):236–240.
12. Osternig LR, Bates BT, James SL. Patterns of tibial rotary torque in knees of healthy subjects. *Med Sci Sports Exerc.* 1980;12:195–199.
13. Levangie PK, Norkin CC. *Joint Structure and Function. A Comprehensive Analysis.* 4th ed. Philadelphia: FA Davis, 2005.
14. Katchburian MV, Bull AMJ, Shih Y-F, Heatley FW, Amis AA. Measurement of patellar tracking: assessment and analysis of the literature. *Clin Orthop Relat Res.* 2003;412:241–259.
15. Heegaard J, Leyvraz P-F, Van Kampen A, Rakotomanana L, Rubin PJ, Blankevoort L. Influence of soft structures on patellar three-dimensional tracking. *Clin Orthop Relat Res.* 1994;299:235–243.
16. Kaltenborn FM. *Mobilization of the Extremity Joints: Examination and Basic Treatment Techniques.* 3rd ed. Oslo: Olaf Norlis Bokhandel; 1985.
17. Soderberg GL. *Kinesiology: Application to Pathological Motion.* 2nd ed. Baltimore: Williams & Wilkins; 1997.
18. Skalley TC, Terry GC, Teitge RA. The quantitative measurement of normal passive medial and lateral patellar motion limits. *Am J Sports Med.* 1993;21:728–732.
19. Zarins B, Rowe CR, Harris BA, Watkins MP. Rotational motion of the knee. *Am J Sports Med.* 1983;11:152–156.
20. Holt KS. *Assessment of Cerebral Palsy. I. Muscle Function, Locomotion and Hand Function.* London: Lloyd-Luke Medical Books; 1965.
21. Palmer ML, Epler ME. *Clinical Assessment Procedures in Physical Therapy.* Philadelphia: JB Lippincott; 1990.
22. Davis DS, Quinn RO, Whiteman CT, Williams JD, Young CR. Concurrent validity of four clinical tests used to measure hamstring flexibility. *J Strength Cond Res.* 2008;22(2):583–588.
23. Youdas JW, Krause DA, Hollman JH, Harmsen WS, Laskowski E. The influence of gender and age on hamstring muscle length in healthy adults. *J Orthop Sports Phys Ther.* 2005;35:246–252.
24. Hamberg J, Bjorklund M, Nordgren B, Sahistedt B. Stretchability of the rectus femoris muscle: investigation of validity and intratester reliability of two methods including x-ray analysis of pelvic tilt. *Arch Phys Med Rehab.* 1993;74:263–270.
25. Van Dillen LR, McDonnell MK, Fleming DA, Sahrmann SA. Effect of knee and hip position on hip extension range of motion in individuals with and without low back pain. *Orthop Sports Phys Ther.* 2000;30:307–316.
26. Kendall FP, McCreary EK, Provance PG, Rodgers MM, Romani WA. *Muscles Testing and Function.* 5th ed. Baltimore: Williams & Wilkins; 2005.
27. Soames RW, ed. Skeletal system. Salmons S, ed. Muscle. In: *Gray's Anatomy.* 38th ed. New York: Churchill Livingstone; 1995.
28. Fiebert IM, Haas JM, Dworkin KJ, LeBlanc WG. A comparison of medial versus lateral hamstring electromyographic activity and force output during isometric contractions. *Isokinetics and Exercise Science.* 1992;2:47–55.
29. Fiebert IM, Pahl CH, Applegate EB, Spielholz NI, Beernik K. Medial-lateral hamstring electromyographic activity during maximum isometric knee flexion at different angles. *Isokinetics and Exercise Science.* 1996;6:157–162.
30. Smith LK, Weiss EL, Lehmkuhl LD. *Brunnstrom's Clinical Kinesiology.* 5th ed. Philadelphia: FA Davis; 1996.
31. Walmsley RP, Yang JF. Measurement of maximum isometric knee flexor movement. *Physiother Can.* 1980;32:83–86.
32. Edelstein JE. Biomechanics of normal ambulation. *J Can Physiother Assoc.* 1965;17:174–185.
33. Inman VT, Ralston HJ, Todd F. *Human Walking.* Baltimore: Williams & Wilkins; 1981.
34. Rowe PJ, Myles CM, Walker C, Nutton R. Knee joint kinematics in gait and other functional activities measured using flexible electrogoniometry: how much knee motion is sufficient for normal daily life? *Gait and Posture.* 2000;12:143–155.
35. Livingston LA, Stevenson JM, Olney SJ. Stairclimbing kinematics on stairs of differing dimensions. *Arch Phys Med Rehab.* 1991;72:398–402.
36. Laubenthal KN, Smidt GL, Kettelkamp DB. A quantitative analysis of knee motion during activities of daily living. *Phys Ther.* 1972;52:34–42.
37. Pink M, Perry J, Houglum PA, Devine DJ. Lower extremity range of motion in the recreational sport runner. *Am J Sports Med.* 1994;22:541–549.
38. Hemmerich A, Brown H, Smith S, Marthandam SSK, Wyss UP. Hip, knee, and ankle kinematics of high range of motion activities of daily living. *J Orthop Res.* 2006;24:770–781.
39. Kapoor A, Mishra SK, Kewangan SK, Mody BS. Range of movements of lower limb joints in cross-legged sitting posture. *J Arthroplasty.* 2008;23:451–453.
40. Mann RA, Hagy JL. The popliteus muscle. *J Bone Joint Surg [Am].* 1977;59:924–927.
41. Kettelkamp DB, Johnson RJ, Smidt GL, Chao EYS, Walker M. An electrogoniometric study of knee motion in normal gait. *J Bone Joint Surg [Am].* 1970;52:775–790.
42. Yucesoy CA, Ates F, Akgün U, Karahan M. Measurement of human gracilis muscle isometric force as a function of knee angle, intraoperatively. *J Biomech.* 2010;43:2665–2671.
43. Li L, Landin D, Grodesky J, Myers J. The function of gastrocnemius as a knee flexor at selected knee and ankle angles. *J Electromyogr Kinesiol.* 2002;12:385–390.
44. Basmajian JV, Lovejoy JF. Functions of the popliteus muscle in man. *J Bone Joint Surg [Am].* 1971;53:557–562.
45. Barnett CH, Richardson AT. The postural function of the popliteus muscle. *Ann Phys Med.* 1953;1:177–179.
46. Davis M, Newsam CJ, Perry J. Electromyograph analysis of the popliteus muscle in level and downhill walking. *Clin Orthop.* 1995;310:211–217.
47. Norkin CC, Levangie PK. *Joint Structure & Function: A Comprehensive Analysis.* Philadelphia: FA Davis; 1983.
48. Basmajian JV, DeLuca CJ. *Muscles Alive: Their Functions Revealed by Electromyography.* 5th ed. Baltimore: Williams & Wilkins; 1985.
49. Duarte Cintra AI, Furlani J. Electromyographic study of quadriceps femoris in man. *Electromyogr Clin Neurophysiol.* 1981;21:539–554.
50. Lieb FJ, Perry J. Quadriceps function. *J Bone Joint Surg [Am].* 1971;53:749–758.
51. Signorile JF, Kacsik D, Perry A, Robertson B, Williams R, Lowensteyn I, Digel S, Caruso J, LeBlanc WG. The effect of knee and foot position on the electromyographical activity of the superficial quadriceps. *J Orthop Sports Phys Ther.* 1995;22:2–9.
52. Salzman A, Torburn L, Perry J. Contribution of rectus femoris and vasti to knee extension. *Clin Orthop.* 1993;290:236–243.
53. Portnoy H, Morin F. Electromyographic study of postural muscles in various positions and movements. *Am J Physiol.* 1956;186:122–126.
54. Rab GT. Muscle. In: Rose J, Gamble JG, eds. *Human Walking.* 2nd ed. Baltimore: Williams & Wilkins; 1994.
55. Johnson CE, Basmajian JV, Dasher W. Electromyography of sartorius muscle. *Anat Rec.* 1972;173:127–130.
56. Jonsson B, Steen B. Function of the gracilis muscle: An electromyographic study. *Acta Morphol Neerl-Scand.* 1964;6:325–341.
57. Montgomery WH, Pink M, Perry J. Electromyographic analysis of hip and knee musculature during running. *Am J Sports Med.* 1994;22:272–278.

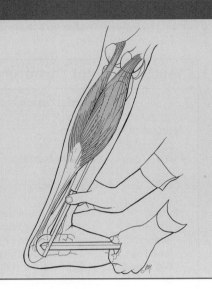

Ankle and Foot

ARTICULATIONS AND MOVEMENTS

Articulations of the ankle and foot are illustrated in Figure 8-1. The articulations at which range of motion (ROM) is commonly measured are the talocrural (ankle) joint, the subtalar joint, and the metatarsophalangeal (MTP) and interphalangeal (IP) joints of the great toe. The movements of these joints are described in Tables 8-1 and 8-2.

The ankle joint is classified as a hinge joint. The proximal concave articulating surface of the joint, commonly referred to as the ankle mortise, is formed by the medial aspect of the lateral malleolus, the distal tibia, and the lateral aspect of the medial malleolus. This concave surface is mated with the convex surface of the body of the talus. The primary movements at the ankle, dorsiflexion, and plantarflexion, occur around an oblique frontal axis in an oblique sagittal plane (Fig. 8-2). With the ankle in plantarflexion, the narrower posterior aspect of the body of the talus lies within the mortise and allows additional motion to occur at the joint. This movement is slight and includes side-to-side gliding, rotation, and abduction and adduction.[2]

The subtalar joint consists of two separate articulations between the talus and calcaneus that are separated by the tarsal canal. Posterior to the tarsal canal, the concave surface on the inferior aspect of the talus articulates with the convex posterior facet on the superior surface of

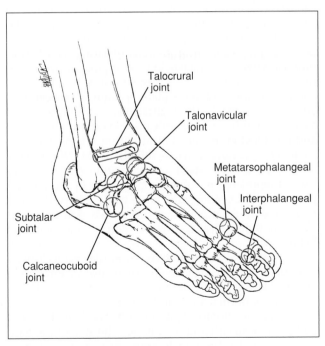

Figure 8-1 Ankle and foot articulations.

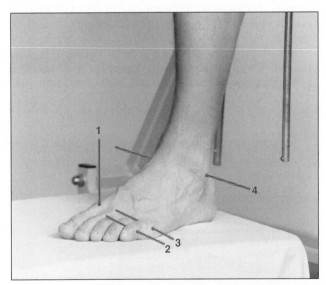

Figure 8-2 Ankle and foot axes: (1) metatarsophalangeal (MTP) joint abduction–adduction; (2) interphalangeal (IP) joint flexion–extension; (3) MTP joint flexion–extension; (4) talocrural joint dorsiflexion–plantarflexion.

TABLE 8-1 Joint Structure: Ankle and Foot Movements

	Plantarflexion	Dorsiflexion	Inversion	Eversion
Articulation[1,2]	Talocrural	Talocrural	Subtalar	Subtalar
Plane	Oblique sagittal	Oblique sagittal	Oblique frontal	Oblique frontal
Axis	Oblique frontal	Oblique frontal	Oblique sagittal	Oblique sagittal
Normal limiting factors[1–6]* (see Fig. 8-4 A and B)	Tension in the anterior joint capsule, anterior portion of the deltoid, anterior talofibular ligaments, and the ankle dorsiflexors; contact between the talus and the tibia	Tension in the posterior joint capsule, the deltoid, calcaneofibular and posterior talofibular ligaments, and the soleus; contact between the talus and the tibia	Tension in the lateral collateral ligament, ankle evertors, lateral talocalcaneal ligaments, cervical ligament, and the lateral joint capsule	Contact between the talus and calcaneus; tension in the medial joint capsule, medial collateral ligaments, medial talocalcaneal ligament, tibialis posterior, flexor hallucis longus and flexor digitorum longus
Normal end feel[3,7]	Firm/hard	Firm/hard	Firm	Hard/firm
Normal AROM[8]† (AROM[9])	0–50° (0–40° to 50°)	0–20° (0–15° to 20°)	0–5°: forefoot 0–35° (0–30° to 35°)	0–5°: forefoot 0–15° (0–20°)
Capsular pattern[7,10]	Talocrural joint: plantarflexion, dorsiflexion Subtalar joint: varus (i.e., inversion), valgus (i.e., eversion)			

*There is a paucity of definitive research that identifies the normal limiting factors (NLF) of joint motion. The NLF and end feels listed here are based on knowledge of anatomy, clinical experience, and available references.

†AROM, active range of motion.

the calcaneus. Anterior to the canal, the convex head of the talus articulates with the concave middle and anterior facets on the superior surface of the calcaneus. The subtalar joint axis runs posteroanteriorly, obliquely upward from the transverse plane and medial to the sagittal plane (Fig. 8-3). Owing to the obliqueness of the joint axis and the opposite shapes of the surfaces of the two joints (i.e.,

talar surfaces: posteriorly concave, anteriorly convex; calcaneal surfaces: posteriorly convex, anteriorly concave) that make up the subtalar joint, movement at the subtalar joint occurs in three planes and is identified as supination and pronation. In non–weight-bearing (NWB) conditions, when the subtalar joint is supinated, the calcaneus inverts in the frontal plane around a sagittal axis, adducts in the transverse plane around a vertical axis, and plantarflexes in the sagittal plane around a frontal axis.[5] Pronation includes calcaneal eversion, abduction, and dorsiflexion. In the clinical setting it is not possible to directly measure triplanar subtalar ROM. "By convention, single-axis calcaneal inversion and eversion is considered representative of triplanar motion of the subtalar joint."[11(p. 430)] Therefore, the more easily observed movements of inversion and eversion[5] are assessed and measured in the clinical setting to indicate subtalar joint ROM.

Movement at the transverse tarsal (i.e., talocalcaneonavicular and calcaneocuboid articulations), intertarsal, tarsometatarsal, and intermetatarsal joints (Fig. 8-1) is essential for normal ankle and foot function. These joints function to accommodate motions between the hindfoot and forefoot to either raise or flatten the arch of the foot, and thus enable the foot to conform to the supporting surface. In the clinical setting, it is not possible to directly measure movements at these joints.

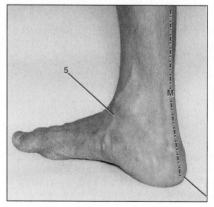

Figure 8-3 Subtalar joint axis:
(5) inversion–eversion (M, midline of leg and heel).

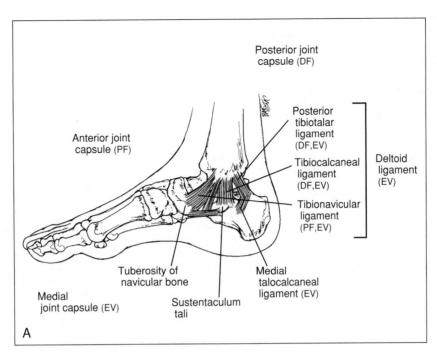

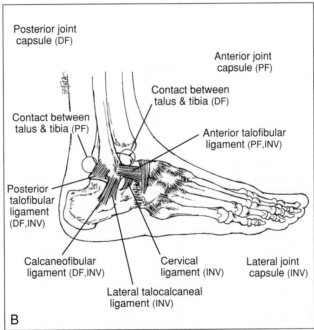

Figure 8-4 Normal Limiting Factors. A. Medial view of the ankle and foot showing noncontractile structures that normally limit motion at the ankle and subtalar joints. **B.** Lateral view of the ankle and foot showing noncontractile structures that normally limit motion at the ankle and subtalar joints. Motion limited by structures is identified in brackets, using the following abbreviations: *F,* flexion; *E,* extension; *Abd,* abduction; *Add,* adduction. Muscles normally limiting motion are not illustrated.

The MTP and IP joints of the toes make up the distal articulations of the foot (Fig. 8-1). The MTP joints are ellipsoidal joints,[2] each formed proximally by the convex head of the metatarsal articulating with the concave base of the adjacent proximal phalanx. The movements at the MTP articulations include flexion, extension, abduction, and adduction. Flexion and extension movements occur in the sagittal plane around a frontal axis, and the movements of abduction/adduction occur in the transverse plane around a vertical axis (Fig. 8-2). The IP joints are classified as hinge joints, formed by the convex head of the proximal phalanx articulating with the concave base of the adjacent distal phalanx. The IP joints allow flexion and extension movements of the toes.

TABLE 8-2   Joint Structure: Toe Movements

	Flexion	Extension	Abduction	Adduction
Articulation[1,2]	Metatarsophalangeal (MTP), proximal interphalangeal (PIP), distal interphalangeal (DIP) (second to fifth toes)	MTP PIP DIP	MTP	MTP
Plane	Sagittal	Sagittal	Transverse	Transverse
Axis	Frontal	Frontal	Vertical	Vertical
Normal limiting factors[3,4,6]* (see Fig. 8-5)	MTP: tension in the dorsal joint capsule, extensor muscles, collateral ligaments PIP: soft tissue apposition between the plantar aspects of the phalanges; tension in the dorsal joint capsule, collateral ligaments DIP: tension in the dorsal joint capsule, collateral ligaments, and oblique retinacular ligaments	MTP: tension in the plantar joint capsule, plantar ligament, flexor muscles PIP: tension in the plantar joint capsule, plantar ligament DIP: tension in the plantar joint capsule, plantar ligament	MTP: tension in the medial joint capsule, collateral ligaments, adductor muscles, fascia and skin of the web spaces, and the plantar interosseous muscles	MTP: contact between the toes
Normal end feel[3,7]	MTP firm PIP soft/firm DIP firm	MTP firm PIP firm DIP firm	Firm	Soft
Normal AROM[8]	Great toe MTP 0–45° IP 0–90° Toes 2–5 MTP 0–40° PIP 0–35° DIP 0–60°	Great toe MTP 0–70° IP 0° Toes 2–5 MTP 0–40° IP 0°		
Capsular pattern[7,10]	First MTP joint: extension, flexion Second to fifth MTP joints: variable, tend to fix in extension with the IP joints in flexion			

*There is a paucity of definitive research that identifies the normal limiting factors (NLF) of joint motion. The NLF and end feels listed here are based on knowledge of anatomy, clinical experience, and available references.

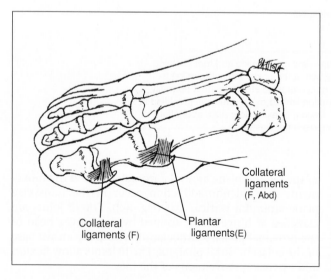

Collateral ligaments (F, Abd)

Collateral ligaments (F)

Plantar ligaments (E)

Figure 8-5 **Normal Limiting Factors.** Anteromedial view of the foot showing noncontractile structures that normally limit motion at the MTP and IP joints (medial collateral ligaments not shown). Motion limited by structures is identified in brackets, using the following abbreviations: *F,* flexion; *E,* extension; *Abd,* abduction; *Add,* adduction. Muscles normally limiting motion are not illustrated.

SURFACE ANATOMY (Figs. 8-6 through 8-8)

Structure	Location
1. Head of the fibula	Round bony prominence on the lateral aspect of the leg level with the tibial tuberosity.
2. Anterior border of the tibia	Subcutaneous bony ridge along the anterior aspect of the leg.
3. Achilles tendon	Prominent ridge on the posterior aspect of the ankle; tendon edges are palpable proximal to the posterior aspect of the calcaneus.
4. Medial malleolus	Prominent distal end of the tibia on the medial aspect of the ankle.
5. Lateral malleolus	Prominent distal end of the fibula on the lateral aspect of the ankle.
6. Tuberosity of the navicular bone	About 2.5 cm inferior and anterior to the medial malleolus.
7. Base of the fifth metatarsal bone	Small bony prominence at the midpoint of the lateral border of the foot.
8. Head of the first metatarsal	Round bony prominence at the medial aspect of the ball of the foot, at the base of the great toe.
9. Calcaneus	Posterior aspect of the heel.

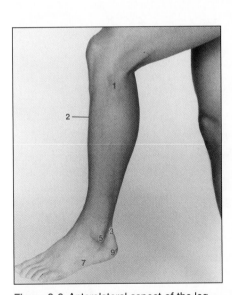

Figure 8-6 Anterolateral aspect of the leg and foot.

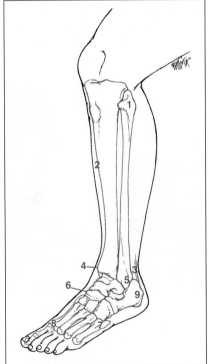

Figure 8-7 Bony anatomy, anterolateral aspect of the leg and foot.

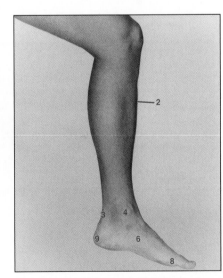

Figure 8-8 Medial aspect of the leg and foot.

RANGE OF MOTION ASSESSMENT AND MEASUREMENT

Practice Makes Perfect

To aid you in practicing the skills covered in this section, or for a handy review, use the practical testing forms found at http://thepoint.lww.com/Clarkson3e.

Ankle Dorsiflexion and Plantarflexion

AROM Assessment

Substitute Movement. Dorsiflexion—knee extension, toe extension. Plantarflexion—knee flexion, toe flexion.

PROM Assessment

Ankle Dorsiflexion

Form 8-1

Start Position. The patient is supine. A roll is placed under the knee to position the knee in about 20° to 30° flexion and place the gastrocnemius on slack (Fig. 8-9A). The ankle is in the anatomical or neutral position with the foot perpendicular to the lower leg (see Fig. 8-9B).

Stabilization. The therapist stabilizes the tibia and fibula.

Therapist's Distal Hand Placement. The therapist grasps the posterior aspect of the calcaneus and places the forearm against the plantar aspect of the forefoot (Fig. 8-10).

End Position. The therapist applies traction to the calcaneus and using the forearm moves the dorsal aspect of the foot toward the anterior aspect of the lower leg to the limit of ankle dorsiflexion (Fig. 8-10).

End Feel. Dorsiflexion—firm/hard.

Joint Glide. Dorsiflexion—convex body of the talus glides posteriorly on the fixed concave ankle mortise.

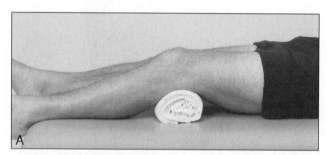
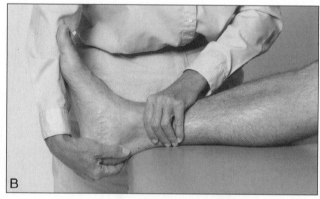

Figure 8-9 **A.** Position of knee in 20° to 30° flexion for assessment of ankle dorsiflexion. **B.** Start position: ankle dorsiflexion.

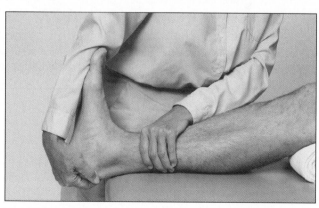

Figure 8-10 Firm or hard end feel at the limit of ankle dorsiflexion.

Ankle Plantarflexion

Form
8-2

Start Position. The patient is supine. A roll is placed under the knee to maintain about 20° to 30° knee flexion, and the ankle is in the neutral position (Fig. 8-11).

Stabilization. The therapist stabilizes the tibia and fibula.

Therapist's Distal Hand Placement. The therapist grasps the dorsum of the foot with the radial border of the index finger over the anterior aspects of the talus and calcaneus.

End Position. The therapist moves the talus and calcaneus in a downward direction to the limit of ankle plantarflexion (Fig. 8-12).

End Feel. Plantarflexion—firm/hard.

Joint Glide. Plantarflexion—convex body of the talus glides anteriorly on the fixed concave ankle mortise.

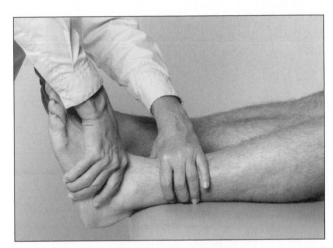

Figure 8-11 Start position for ankle plantarflexion.

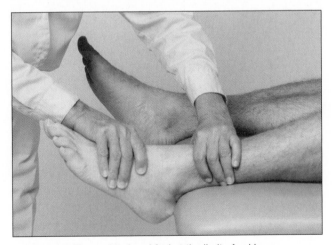

Figure 8-12 Firm or hard end feel at the limit of ankle plantarflexion.

Measurement: Universal Goniometer

Ankle Dorsiflexion and Plantarflexion

Start Position. The patient is supine with a roll placed under the knee to maintain about 20° to 30° knee flexion and place the gastrocnemius on slack (see Fig. 8-9A). The ankle is in the anatomical position 0° (Fig. 8-13). Alternatively, the patient may be sitting with the knee flexed to 90° and the ankle in anatomical position (Fig. 8-14).

Stabilization. The therapist stabilizes the tibia and fibula.

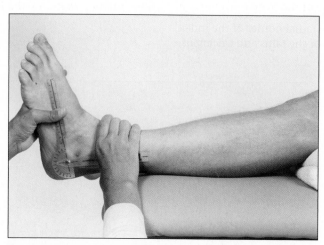

Figure 8-13 Start position for ankle dorsiflexion and plantarflexion.

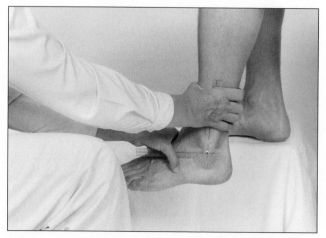

Figure 8-14 Alternate start position for ankle dorsiflexion and plantarflexion.

Goniometer Axis. The axis is placed inferior to the lateral malleolus (Fig. 8-15). This measurement may also be obtained by placing the axis inferior to the medial malleolus (not shown).

Stationary Arm. Parallel to the longitudinal axis of the fibula, pointing toward the head of the fibula.

Movable Arm. Parallel to the sole of the heel (see reference line Fig. 8-15), to eliminate forefoot movement from the

measurement. In the start position described, the goniometer will indicate 90°. This is recorded as 0°. For example, if the goniometer reads 90° at the start position for ankle dorsiflexion and 80° at the end position, the ankle dorsiflexion PROM would be 10°.

End Positions. Dorsiflexion (20°) (Fig. 8-16): The ankle is flexed with the dorsal aspect of the foot approximating the anterior aspect of the lower leg. Plantarflexion (50°) (Fig. 8-17): The ankle is extended to the limit of motion.

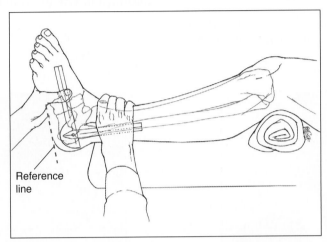

Reference line

Figure 8-15 Goniometer alignment for ankle dorsiflexion and plantarflexion.

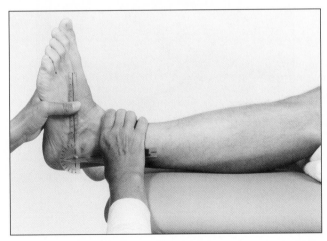

Figure 8-16 Dorsiflexion.

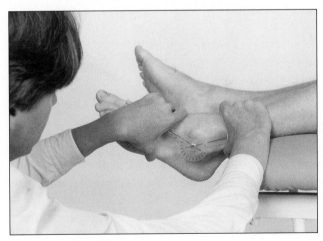

Figure 8-17 Plantarflexion.

Alternate Measurement

This test may be contraindicated for patients with poor standing balance or generalized or specific lower extremity weakness.

Start Position. The patient is standing erect (Fig. 8-18). The nontest foot is off the ground or only lightly touching the ground to assist with balance (Fig. 8-19).

Stabilization. The patient uses the parallel bars or other stable structure for balance. The foot on the test side is stabilized by the patient's body weight.

End Position. The patient is instructed to maintain the foot on the test side flat on the floor, with the toes pointing forward, and to flex the knee as far as possible (Fig. 8-19). *Note:* If the soleus muscle is shortened, the patient will feel a muscle stretch over the posterior aspect of the calf and ankle dorsiflexion ROM will be restricted proportional to the decrease in muscle length.

Measurement: Universal Goniometer

The therapist measures and records the available ankle dorsiflexion PROM. The goniometer is placed as described for measuring ankle dorsiflexion ROM (see Fig. 8-15). Ankle dorsiflexion PROM measured in weight-bearing (WB) is greater than in NWB positions. If dorsiflexion is measured in WB, this is noted when recording the ROM.

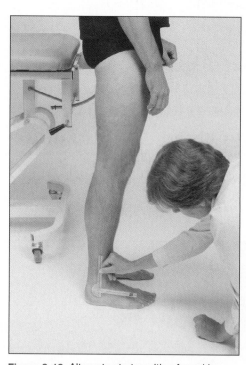

Figure 8-18 Alternate start position for ankle dorsiflexion.

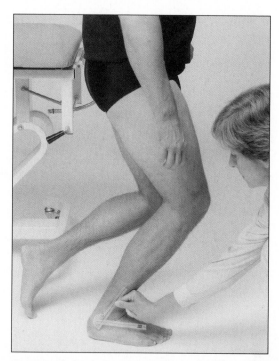

Figure 8-19 Goniometer measurement for ankle dorsiflexion.

Measurement: OB Goniometer

Goniometer Placement. The strap is placed around the lower leg proximal to the ankle. The dial is placed on the lateral aspect of the lower leg (Fig. 8-20). With the patient in the start position, the inclination needle is aligned with the 0° arrow of the fluid-filled container. At the end position, the number of degrees the inclination needle moves away from the 0° arrow on the inclinometer dial is recorded as the ankle dorsiflexion PROM (Fig. 8-21). (Alternatively, a standard inclinometer can be placed on the anterior border of the tibia to measure ankle dorsiflexion in standing [not shown].)

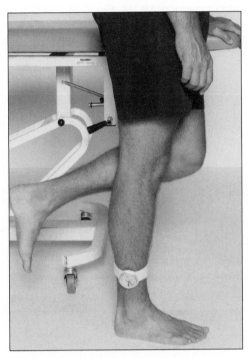

Figure 8-20 Start position for OB goniometer measurement of ankle dorsiflexion.

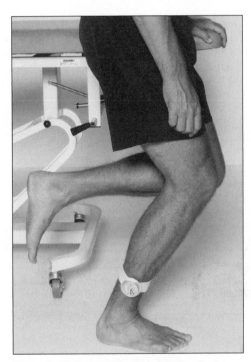

Figure 8-21 End position for ankle dorsiflexion.

Subtalar Inversion and Eversion

AROM Assessment

Substitute Movement. Inversion—hip external rotation. Eversion—hip internal rotation.

Measurement: Universal Goniometer

Form 8-3

Start Position. The patient is supine (Fig. 8-22). A roll is placed under the knee to maintain slight flexion. The ankle is in the neutral position. A piece of paper, adhered to a flat surface, is placed under the heel. A flat-surfaced object (Plexiglass or book) is placed against the full sole of the foot. A line is drawn along the Plexiglass or book as shown in Figure 8-22.

Stabilization. The therapist stabilizes the tibia and fibula.

End Positions. The foot is placed in inversion to the limit of motion (Fig. 8-23). The Plexiglass is again positioned against the full sole of the foot in this position and a line is again drawn along the Plexiglass (Fig. 8-24). The process is repeated at the limit of eversion AROM (Figs. 8-25 and 8-26).

Goniometer Axis and Arms. The goniometer is placed on the line graphics to obtain a measure of the arc of movement (Figs. 8-27 and 8-28).

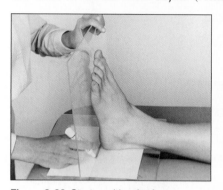

Figure 8-22 Start position for foot inversion and eversion AROM.

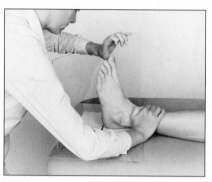

Figure 8-23 Placement of the foot in inversion.

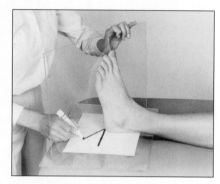

Figure 8-24 Inversion.

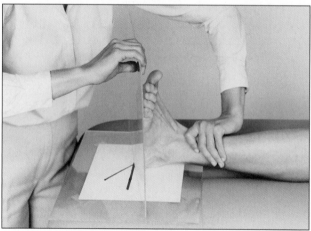

Figure 8-25 Placement of the foot in eversion.

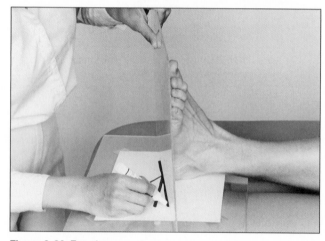

Figure 8-26 Eversion.

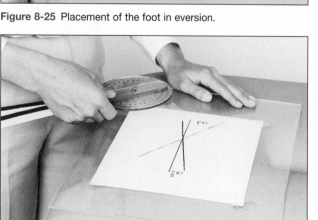

Figure 8-27 Completed measurements of inversion and eversion AROM.

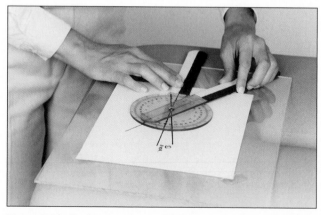

Figure 8-28 Goniometer placement for measurement of inversion AROM.

PROM Assessment

Start Position. The patient is supine. The ankle is in the neutral position (Fig. 8-29).

Forms
8-4, 8-5 **Stabilization.** The therapist stabilizes the talus immediately anterior and inferior to the medial and lateral malleoli. Current research[11] appears to support positioning the ankle in dorsiflexion to assist in stabilizing the talus, as the wider anterior aspect of the body of the talus is wedged within the mortise.

Therapist's Distal Hand Placement. The therapist grasps the posterior aspect and sides of the calcaneus.

End Positions. The therapist moves the calcaneus inward to the limit of inversion (Fig. 8-30) and outward to the limit of eversion (Fig. 8-31).

End Feels. *Inversion*—firm; *eversion*—hard/firm.

Joint Glides. *Inversion*—(1) posterior subtalar joint surfaces: the convex surface of the calcaneus glides laterally on the fixed concave surface of the talus; (2) anterior subtalar joint surfaces: the concave surfaces of the middle and anterior facets of the calcaneus glide medially on the fixed convex surface of the head of the talus. *Eversion*—(1) posterior subtalar joint surfaces: the convex surface of the calcaneus glides medially on the fixed concave surface of the talus; (2) anterior subtalar joint surfaces: the concave surfaces of the middle and anterior facets of the calcaneus glide laterally on the fixed convex surface of the head of the talus.

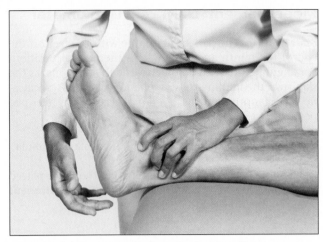

Figure 8-29 Start position for inversion and eversion.

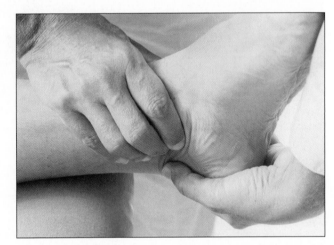

Figure 8-30 Firm end feel at the limit of inversion.

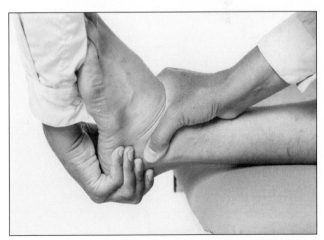

Figure 8-31 Hard or firm end feel at the limit of eversion.

Measurement: Universal Goniometer

Start Position. The patient lies prone with the feet off the end of the plinth and the ankle in the neutral position. For alignment of the goniometer, the therapist marks the skin over the midlines of the superior aspect of the calcaneus posteriorly and the inferior aspect of the heel pad posteriorly (Fig. 8-32A).

Stabilization. The therapist stabilizes the tibia and fibula.

Goniometer Axis. The axis is placed over the mark placed at the midline of the superior aspect of the calcaneus (Figs. 8-32B and 8-33).

Stationary Arm. Parallel to the longitudinal axis of the lower leg.

Movable Arm. Lies along the midline of the posterior aspect of the calcaneus. Use the mark on the heel pad posteriorly to assist in maintaining alignment of the movable arm.

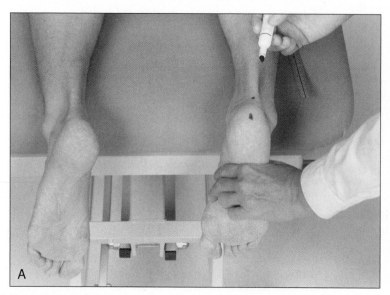
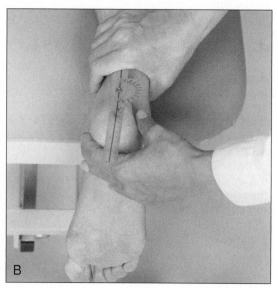

Figure 8-32 A. Subtalar inversion and eversion. Points marked for alignment of goniometer. **B.** Goniometer alignment for subtalar joint inversion and eversion.

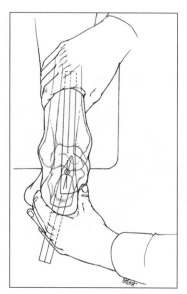

Figure 8-33 Goniometer placement for inversion and eversion. Shown with the subtalar joint of the left foot in eversion.

End Positions. The calcaneus is passively inverted (Fig. 8-34) and then passively everted (Fig. 8-35) to the limit of inversion (5°) and to the limit of eversion (5°), respectively.

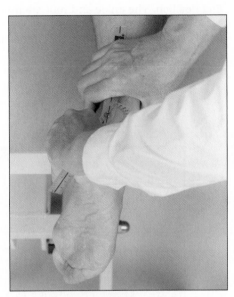

Figure 8-34 End position for measurement of right subtalar joint inversion.

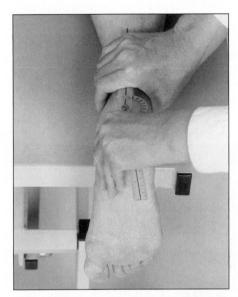

Figure 8-35 End position for measurement of right subtalar joint eversion.

Ankle and Foot Supination/ Pronation: Inversion/Eversion Components

The inversion and eversion components of ankle and foot supination and pronation occur mainly at the subtalar and transverse tarsal (i.e., talocalcaneonavicular and calcaneocuboid) joints.

Ankle and Foot Supination: Inversion Component

AROM Assessment

Substitute Movement. Tibial internal rotation, knee flexion, hip external rotation, hip abduction.

PROM Assessment

Start Position. The patient is sitting with the ankle and foot in anatomical position (Fig. 8-36).

Form 8-6 **Stabilization.** The therapist stabilizes the tibia and fibula.

Therapist's Distal Hand Placement. The therapist grasps the lateral aspect of the forefoot.

End Position. The ankle and foot are inverted (Fig. 8-37).

End Feel. Ankle and foot are inverted—firm.

Figure 8-36 Start position: ankle and foot supination: inversion component.

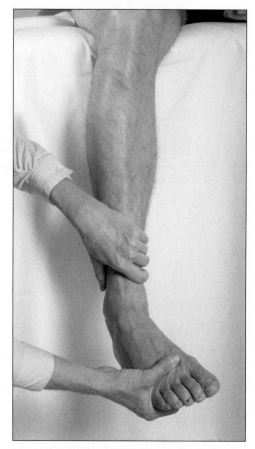

Figure 8-37 Firm end feel at the limit of ankle and foot supination: inversion component.

Measurement: Universal Goniometer

Start Position. The patient is sitting with the ankle and foot in anatomical position.

Stabilization. The therapist stabilizes the tibia and fibula.

Goniometer Axis. The axis is placed anterior to the talocrural (ankle) joint midway between the medial and lateral malleoli (Fig. 8-38).

Stationary Arm. Parallel to the midline of the tibia, pointing toward the tibial tuberosity.

Movable Arm. Parallel to the midline of the second metatarsal.

End Position. Ankle and foot supination: inversion component (Fig. 8-39).

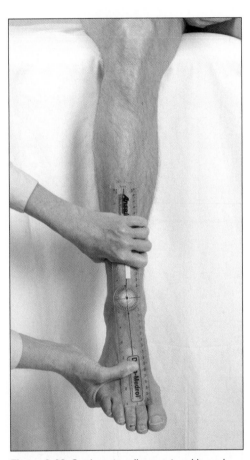

Figure 8-38 Goniometer alignment: ankle and foot supination: inversion component.

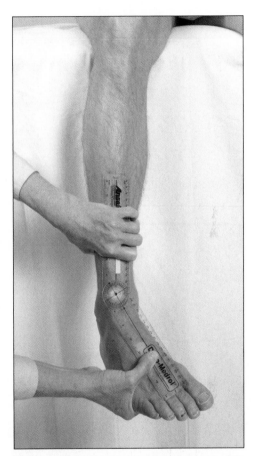

Figure 8-39 End position for measurement: ankle and foot supination: inversion component.

Ankle and Foot Pronation: Eversion Component

AROM Assessment

Substitute Movement. Tibial external rotation, knee extension, hip internal rotation, hip adduction.

PROM Assessment

Form 8-7

Start Position. The patient is sitting with the ankle and foot in anatomical position (Fig. 8-40).

Stabilization. The therapist stabilizes the tibia and fibula.

Therapist's Distal Hand Placement. The therapist grasps the medial aspect of the forefoot.

End Position. The ankle and foot are everted (Fig. 8-41).

End Feel. Ankle and foot eversion—firm/hard.

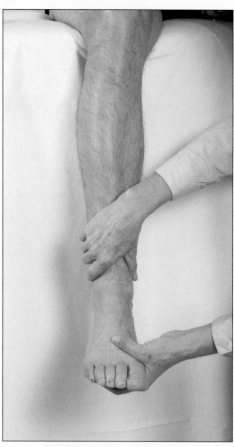

Figure 8-40 Start position: ankle and foot pronation: eversion component.

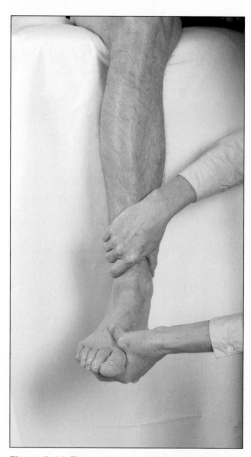

Figure 8-41 Firm or hard end feel at the limit of ankle and foot pronation: eversion component.

Measurement: Universal Goniometer

Start Position. The patient is sitting with the ankle and foot in anatomical position.

Stabilization. The therapist stabilizes the tibia and fibula.

Goniometer Axis. The axis is placed anterior to the talocrural (ankle) joint midway between the medial and lateral malleoli (Fig. 8-42).

Stationary Arm. Parallel to the midline of the tibia, pointing toward the tibial tuberosity.

Movable Arm. Parallel to the midline of the second metatarsal.

End Position. Ankle and foot pronation: eversion component (Fig. 8-43).

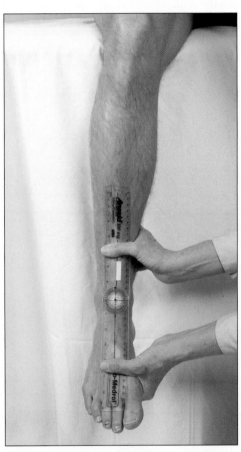

Figure 8-42 Goniometer alignment: ankle and foot pronation: eversion component.

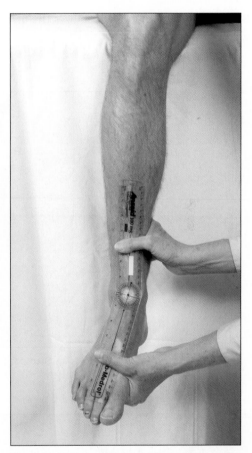

Figure 8-43 End position for measurement: ankle and foot pronation: eversion component.

MTP Joint Flexion and Extension of the Great Toe

AROM Assessment

Substitute Movement. *MTP flexion:* Ankle plantar flexion, *MTP extension:* Ankle dorsiflexion.

PROM Assessment

Forms
8-8, 8-9

Start Position. The patient is supine. The ankle and toes are in the neutral position (Fig. 8-44).

Stabilization. The therapist stabilizes the first metatarsal.

Therapist's Distal Hand Placement. The therapist grasps the proximal phalanx.

End Positions. The therapist moves the proximal phalanx of the great toe to the limit of MTP joint flexion (Fig. 8-45) and MTP joint extension (Fig. 8-46).

End Feels. *MTP joint flexion*—firm; *MTP joint extension*—firm.

Joint Glides. *MTP joint flexion*—the concave base of the proximal phalanx glides in a plantar direction on the fixed convex head of the adjacent metatarsal. *MTP joint extension*—the concave base of the proximal phalanx glides in a dorsal direction on the fixed convex head of the adjacent metatarsal.

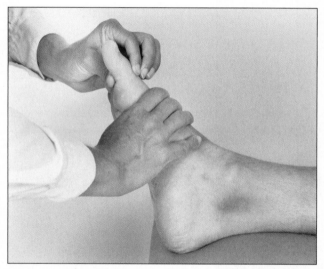

Figure 8-44 Start position for MTP joint flexion and extension.

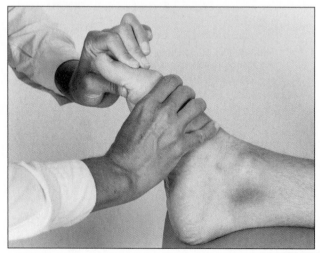

Figure 8-45 Firm end feel at limit of MTP joint flexion of the great toe.

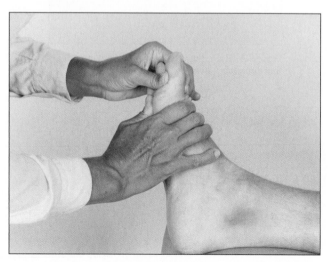

Figure 8-46 Firm end feel at limit of MTP joint extension of the great toe.

Measurement: Universal Goniometer

Start Position. The patient is supine or sitting. The ankle and toes are in the neutral position (Fig. 8-47).

Stabilization. The therapist stabilizes the first metatarsal.

Goniometer Axis. For MTP joint flexion, the axis is placed over the dorsum of the MTP joint (Fig. 8-47). For MTP joint extension, the goniometer axis is placed over the plantar aspect of the MTP joint (not shown). Alternatively, the axis can be placed over the MTP joint axis on the medial aspect of the great toe (Figs. 8-49 and 8-50).

Stationary Arm. Parallel to the longitudinal axis of the first metatarsal.

Movable Arm. Parallel to the longitudinal axis of the proximal phalanx of the great toe.

End Positions. The MTP joint is flexed to the limit of MTP joint flexion (45° for the great toe) (Fig. 8-48). The MTP joint of the toe being measured is extended to the limit of MTP joint extension (70° for the great toe) (Figs. 8-49 and 8-50).

MTP Joint Flexion/Extension of the Lesser Four Toes

Flexion and extension at the MTP joints of the lesser four toes is normally not measured using a universal goniometer. The MTP joints of the lesser four toes are flexed to the limit of MTP joint flexion (40°) and extended to the limit of MTP joint extension (40°). The ROM is observed and recorded as either full or decreased.

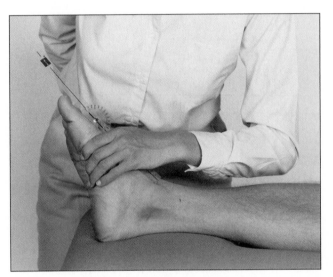

Figure 8-47 Start position for MTP joint flexion.

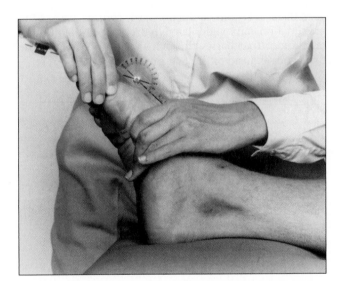

Figure 8-48 MTP joint flexion of the great toe.

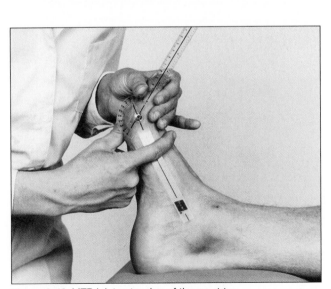

Figure 8-49 MTP joint extension of the great toe.

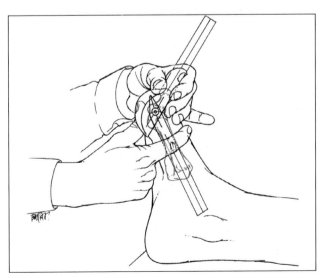

Figure 8-50 Goniometer alignment for MTP joint flexion and extension.

MTP Joint Abduction and Adduction of the Great Toe

PROM Assessment (MTP Joint Abduction)

Start Position. The patient is supine. The ankle and great toe are in the neutral position.

Forms 8-10, 8-11 **Stabilization.** The therapist stabilizes the first metatarsal.

Therapist's Distal Hand Placement. The therapist grasps the proximal phalanx of the great toe.

End Position. The therapist moves the proximal phalanx to the limit of MTP joint abduction (Fig. 8-51).

End Feel. MTP joint abduction—firm.

Joint Glide. MTP joint abduction—the concave base of the proximal phalanx glides laterally (relative to the midline of the foot that passes through the second toe) on the fixed convex head of the first metatarsal.

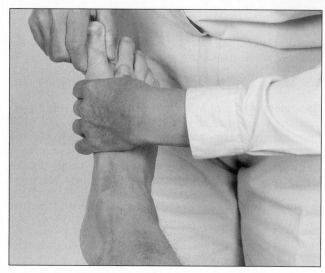

Figure 8-51 Firm end feel at limit of MTP joint abduction.

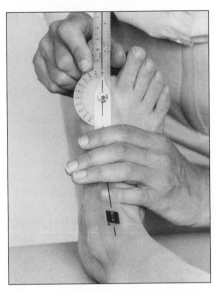

Figure 8-52 Start position for MTP joint abduction and adduction.

Measurement: Universal Goniometer

Start Position. The patient is supine or sitting. The ankle and toes are in the neutral position (Fig. 8-52).

Stabilization. The therapist stabilizes the first metatarsal and the foot proximal to the MTP joint.

Goniometer Axis. The axis is placed on the dorsum of the first MTP joint (Figs. 8-52 and 8-53).

Stationary Arm. Parallel to the longitudinal axis of the first metatarsal.

Movable Arm. Parallel to the longitudinal axis of the proximal phalanx of the great toe.

End Positions. The MTP joint is abducted to the limit of motion (Fig. 8-54) and adducted to the limit of motion (Fig. 8-55).

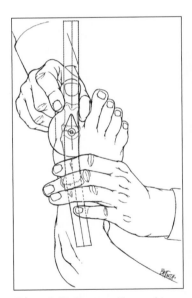

Figure 8-53 Start position and goniometer alignment for MTP joint abduction and adduction.

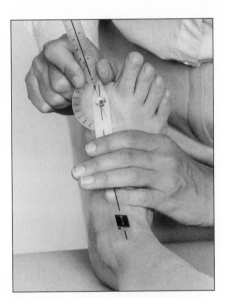

Figure 8-54 MTP joint abduction.

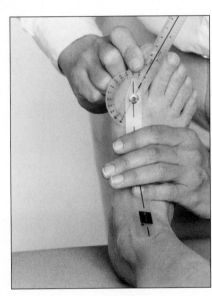

Figure 8-55 MTP joint adduction.

IP Joint Flexion/Extension of the Great Toe

AROM Assessment

Substitute Movement. *IP joint flexion:* MTP joint flexion, ankle plantarflexion. *IP joint extension:* MTP joint extension, ankle dorsiflexion.

PROM Assessment

Start Position. The patient is supine. The ankle and great toe are in the neutral position.

Forms 8-12, 8-13

Stabilization. The therapist stabilizes the proximal phalanx of the great toe.

Therapist's Distal Hand Placement. The therapist grasps the distal phalanx of the great toe.

End Positions. The therapist moves the distal phalanx to the limit of IP joint flexion (Fig. 8-56) and IP joint extension (Fig. 8-57).

End Feels. *IP joint flexion*—soft/firm; *IP joint extension*—firm.

Joint Glides. *IP joint flexion*—the concave base of the distal phalanx of the great toe glides in a plantar direction on the fixed convex head of the proximal phalanx of the great toe. *IP joint extension*—the concave base of the distal phalanx of the great toe glides in a dorsal direction on the fixed convex head of the proximal phalanx of the great toe.

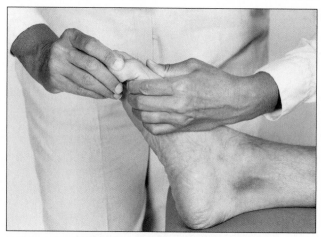

Figure 8-56 Soft or firm end feel at limit of IP joint flexion.

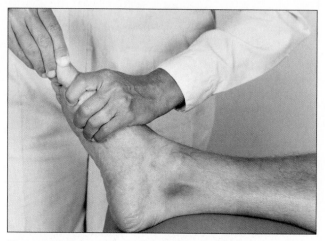

Figure 8-57 Firm end feel at limit of IP joint extension.

Measurement: Universal Goniometer

Start Position. The patient is supine or sitting. The ankle and toes are in the neutral position (Fig. 8-58).

Stabilization. The therapist stabilizes the proximal phalanx.

Goniometer Axis. The axis is placed over the dorsal aspect of the IP joint for flexion (Fig. 8-58) and the plantar aspect of the IP joint for extension (not shown).

Stationary Arm. Parallel to the longitudinal axis of the proximal phalanx.

Movable Arm. Parallel to the longitudinal axis of the distal phalanx.

End Positions. The IP joint is flexed to the limit of IP joint flexion (90° for the great toe) (Fig. 8-59). The IP joint is extended to the limit of IP joint extension (0° for the great toe; not shown).

MTP and IP Joint Flexion/Extension of the Lesser Four Toes

The lesser four toes are flexed and extended as a group, and the ROM is observed and recorded as either full or decreased.

Flexion and extension at the MTP and IP joints of the lesser four toes are normally not measured using a universal goniometer. However if used, the goniometer is placed according to the same principles used for measuring finger MTP and IP joint flexion and extension ROM.

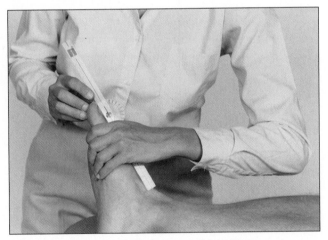

Figure 8-58 Start position for great toe IP joint flexion.

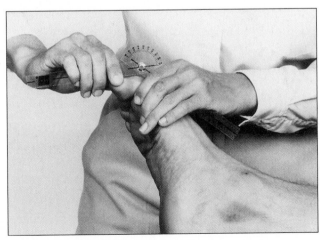

Figure 8-59 IP joint flexion of the great toe.

Muscle Length Assessment and Measurement

Practice Makes Perfect

To aid you in practicing the skills covered in this section, or for a handy review, use the practical testing forms found at http://thepoint.lww.com/Clarkson3e.

Gastrocnemius

Origins[2]	Insertion[2]
Gastrocnemius	
a. Medial head: proximal and posterior aspect of the medial condyle of the femur posterior to the adductor tubercle.	Via the Achilles tendon into the calcaneus.
b. Lateral head: lateral and posterior aspect of the lateral condyle of the femur; lower part of the supracondylar line.	

Form 8-14

Start Position. The patient is standing erect with the lower extremity in the anatomical position. The patient is positioned facing a stable plinth or wall.

End Position. The patient places the nontest leg ahead of the test leg and leans forward to place the hands on the plinth or wall (Fig. 8-60). The patient is instructed to maintain the foot on the test side flat on the floor, with the toes pointing forward, and to keep the knee in full extension as the leg moves over the foot. As the patient leans closer toward the supporting surface the leg moves over the foot to the limit of ankle dorsiflexion and the gastrocnemius is placed on full stretch. Research[12] supports the use of ankle dorsiflexion PROM as an indicator of Achilles tendon length.

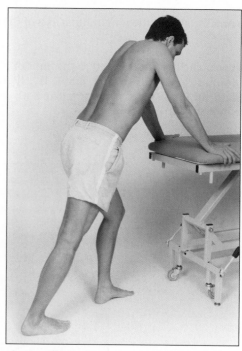

Figure 8-60 End position for measurement of the length of gastrocnemius.

Measurement. If the gastrocnemius is shortened, ankle dorsiflexion ROM will be restricted proportional to the decrease in muscle length. The therapist measures and records the available ankle dorsiflexion PROM.

Universal Goniometer Placement. The goniometer is placed as described for measuring ankle dorsiflexion ROM (Figs. 8-61 and 8-62).

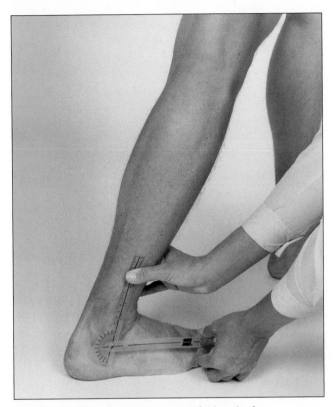

Figure 8-61 Goniometer measurement for length of gastrocnemius.

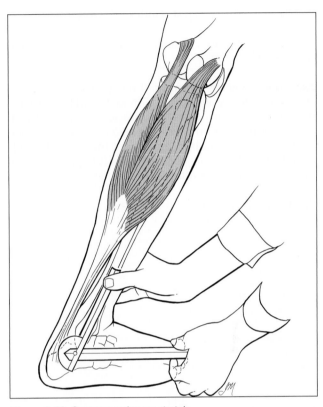

Figure 8-62 Gastrocnemius on stretch.

OB Goniometer Placement. The strap is placed around the lower leg proximal to the ankle (Fig. 8-63). The dial is placed on the lateral aspect of the lower leg. With the patient in the start position, the inclination needle is aligned with the 0° arrow of the fluid-filled container. At the end position, the number of degrees the inclination needle moves away from the 0° arrow on the inclinometer dial is recorded to represent the length of the gastrocnemius muscle.

Note: If the contralateral (i.e., nontest) leg is not placed ahead of the test leg, ensure the heel of the nontest leg is raised slightly off the floor. This position ensures a true test for gastrocnemius tightness on the test side because the amount of forward lean the patient achieves will not be limited by contralateral gastrocnemius tightness, if present.

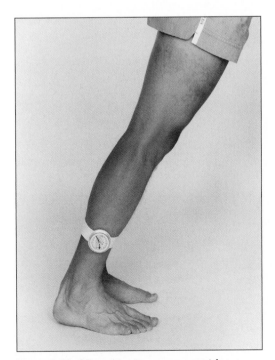

Figure 8-63 OB goniometer measurement for gastrocnemius muscle length.

Alternate Test

Start Position. The patient is supine. The leg is in the anatomical position with the knee in extension (0°) (Fig. 8-64).

Stabilization. The therapist stabilizes the lower leg.

End Position. The foot is moved to the limit of ankle dorsiflexion (Fig. 8-65).

Assessment and Measurement. If the gastrocnemius muscle is shortened, ankle dorsiflexion ROM will be restricted proportional to the decrease in muscle length. The therapist either observes the available PROM or uses a universal goniometer to measure and record the available ankle dorsiflexion PROM. A second therapist is required to measure the PROM when using a goniometer.

End Feel. Gastrocnemius on stretch—firm.

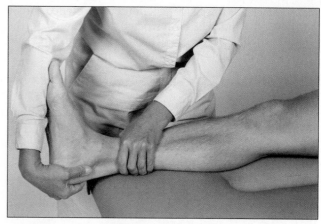

Figure 8-64 Alternate start position for gastrocnemius length.

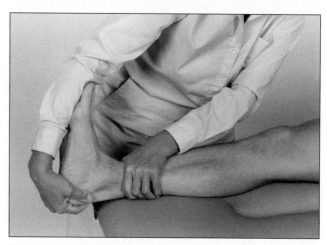

Figure 8-65 Gastrocnemius on stretch.

MUSCLE STRENGTH ASSESSMENT (TABLE 8-3)

Practice Makes Perfect

To aid you in practicing the skills covered in this section, or for a handy review, use the practical testing forms found at http://thepoint.lww.com/Clarkson3e.

TABLE 8-3   Muscle Actions, Attachments, and Nerve Supply: The Ankle and Foot[2]

Muscle	Primary Muscle Action	Muscle Origin	Muscle Insertion	Peripheral Nerve	Nerve Root
Tibialis anterior	Ankle dorsiflexion Foot inversion	Lateral condyle of the tibia; proximal half to two thirds of the lateral surface of the shaft of the tibia; anterior aspect of the interosseous membrane	Medial and inferior surfaces of the medial cunieform bone; medial aspect of the base of the first metatarsal bone	Deep peroneal	L45
Gastrocnemius	Ankle plantarflexion Knee flexion	a. Medial head: proximal and posterior aspect of the medial condyle of the femur posterior to the adductor tubercle b. Lateral head: lateral and posterior aspect of the lateral condyle of the femur; lower part of the supracondylar line	Via the Achilles tendon into the calcaneum	Tibial	S12
Soleus	Ankle plantarflexion	Posterior aspect of the head and proximal one fourth of the shaft of the fibula; soleal line and middle third of the medial border of the tibia	Via the Achilles tendon into the calcaneum	Tibial	S12
Tibialis posterior	Foot inversion	Upper two thirds of the posterolateral surface of the tibia below the soleal line; posterior surface of the interosseous membrane; medial aspect of the proximal two thirds of the fibula	Tuberosity of the navicular bone; expansions to the medial, intermediate, and lateral cuneiforms, the cuboid and the bases of the second, third and fourth metatarsals; tendinous band passes to the tip and distal margin of the sustentaculum tali	Tibial	L45
Peroneus longus	Foot eversion Ankle plantarflexion	Head and upper two thirds of the lateral surface of the fibula; a few fibers from the lateral condyle of the tibia	Lateral side of the base of the first metatarsal and medial cuneiform bones	Superficial peroneal	L5S1
Peroneus brevis	Foot eversion	Lower two thirds of the lateral surface of the fibula	Tubercle on the lateral aspect of the base of the fifth metatarsal bone	Superficial peroneal	L5S1

TABLE 8-3   Continued

Muscle	Primary Muscle Action	Muscle Origin	Muscle Insertion	Peripheral Nerve	Nerve Root
Flexor hallucis brevis	Flexion of the MTP joint of the great toe	Medial part of the plantar surface of the cuboid bone and adjacent part of the lateral cuneiform bone	Medial and lateral aspects of the base of the proximal phalanx of the great toe	Medial plantar	S12
Flexor hallucis longus	Flexion of the IP joint of the great toe	Distal two thirds of the posterior surface of the fibula; posterior surface of the interosseous membrane	Plantar aspect of the base of the distal phalanx of the great toe	Tibial	L5S12
Flexor digitorum longus	Flexion of the DIP joints of the lateral four toes	Posterior surface of the middle three fifths of the tibia below the soleal line	Plantar aspects of the bases of the distal phalanges of the lateral four toes	Tibial	L5S12
Flexor digitorum brevis	Flexion of the PIP joints of the lateral four toes	Medial process of the calcaneal tuberosity; plantar fascia	Medial and lateral aspects of the middle phalanges of the lateral four toes	Medial plantar	S12
Flexor digiti minimi brevis	Flexion of the MTP joint of the fifth toe	Medial plantar aspect of the base of the fifth metatarsal; sheath of peroneus longus	Lateral side of the base of the proximal phalanx of the fifth toe	Lateral plantar	S23
Lumbricales	Flexion of the MTP joints Extension of the IP joints of the toes	First lumbricalis: medial aspect of flexor digitorum longus tendon; Second to fourth lumbricales: adjacent sides of the flexor digitorum longus tendons	Medial aspects of the dorsal digital expansions on the proximal phalanges of the lateral four toes	First lumbricalis: medial plantar Second to fourth lumbricales: lateral plantar	S23
Abductor hallucis	Abduction of the great toe	Medial process of the calcaneal tuberosity; flexor retinaculum and plantar aponeurosis	Medial aspect of the base of the proximal phalanx of the great toe	Medial plantar	S12
Abductor digiti minimi	Abduction and flexion of the fifth toe	Medial and lateral processes of the calcaneal tuberosity; the bone between the tuberosities; plantar fascia	Lateral aspect of the base of the proximal phalanx of the fifth toe	Lateral plantar	S123
Dorsal interossei	Abduction of the second, third, and fourth toes Flexion of the MTP joints	Adjacent sides of metatarsal bones	First interosseous: medial aspect of the base of the proximal phalanx of the second toe; second to fourth interossei: lateral aspects of the bases of the proximal phalanges of the second, third, and fourth toes; dorsal digital expansions	Lateral plantar	S23

(continued)

TABLE 8-3 *Continued*

Muscle	Primary Muscle Action	Muscle Origin	Muscle Insertion	Peripheral Nerve	Nerve Root
Plantar interossei	Adduction of the third, fourth, and fifth toes Flexion of the MTP joints	Bases and medial aspects of the third, fourth, and fifth metatarsal bones	Medial aspects of the bases of the proximal phalanges of the third, fourth, and fifth toes; dorsal digital expansions	Lateral plantar	S23
Adductor hallucis	Adduction of the great toe	a. Oblique head: bases of the second, third, and fourth metatarsal bones; sheath of peroneus longus b. Transverse head: plantar MTP ligaments of the third, fourth, and fifth toes and the deep transverse metatarsal ligaments between them	Lateral sesamoid bone and the base of the first phalanx of the great toe	Lateral plantar	S23
Extensor hallucis longus	Extension of the IP joint of the great toe	Middle half of the medial surface of the fibula; anterior aspect of the interosseous membrane	Dorsal surface of the base of the distal phalanx of the great toe	Deep peroneal	L5
Extensor digitorum longus	Extension of the MTP and IP joints of the lesser four toes	Lateral condyle of the tibia; proximal three fourths of the medial surface of the fibula; anterior surface of the interosseous membrane	Dorsal aspect of the base of the middle phalanx of the lesser four toes; dorsal aspect of the base of the distal phalanx of the lesser four toes	Deep peroneal	L5S1
Extensor digitorum brevis	Extension of the first MTP joint Extension of the phalanges of the middle three toes	Anterior superolateral surface of the calcaneum	Medial part of the muscle (extensor hallucis brevis): dorsal aspect of the base of the proximal phalanx of the great toe tendons to the second, third, and fourth toes: into the lateral aspect of the corresponding extensor digitorum longus tendons	Deep peroneal	L5S1

Ankle Dorsiflexion and Foot Inversion

Against Gravity: Tibialis Anterior

Form 8-15

Start Position. The patient is sitting. The ankle is in plantarflexion and the foot is in slight eversion (Fig. 8-66).

Stabilization. The lower leg is supported against the therapist's thigh and the therapist stabilizes the lower leg proximal to the ankle.

Movement. The patient dorsiflexes the ankle and inverts the foot through full ROM (Fig. 8-67). The patient is instructed to keep the toes relaxed.

Palpation. The tibialis anterior is the most medial tendon on the anteromedial aspect of the ankle joint or medial to the anterior border of the tibia.

Resistance Location. Applied on the dorsomedial aspect of the forefoot (Figs. 8-68 and 8-69).

Resistance Direction. Ankle plantarflexion and foot eversion.

Substitute Movement. Extensor digitorum longus and extensor hallucis longus (toe extension); these muscles extend the toes before acting to dorsiflex the ankle.[13]

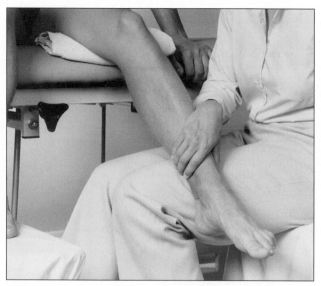

Figure 8-66 Start position: tibialis anterior.

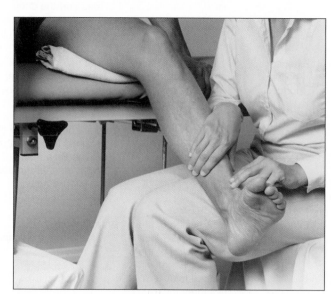

Figure 8-67 Screen position: tibialis anterior.

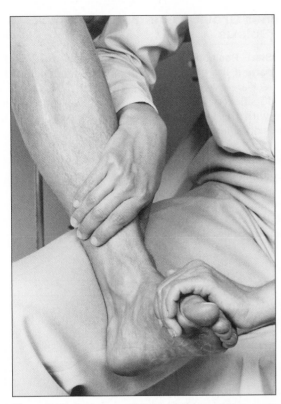

Figure 8-68 Resistance: tibialis anterior.

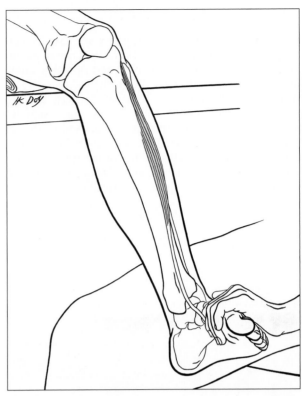

Figure 8-69 Tibialis anterior.

Gravity Eliminated: Tibialis Anterior

Start Position. The patient is in a side-lying position on the test side. The knee is flexed to place the gastrocnemius on slack, the ankle is in plantarflexion, and the foot is in slight eversion (Fig. 8-70).

Stabilization. The therapist stabilizes the lower leg proximal to the ankle. By placing the hand underneath the leg the friction of the table is eliminated.

End Position. The patient dorsiflexes the ankle and inverts the foot through full ROM (Fig. 8-71).

Substitute Movement. Extensor hallucis longus and extensor digitorum longus (toe extension).

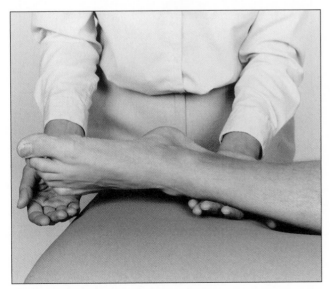

Figure 8-70 Start position: tibialis anterior.

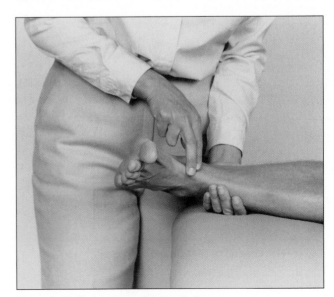

Figure 8-71 End position: tibialis anterior.

Ankle Plantarflexion

The gastrocnemius and soleus muscles are tested when ankle plantarflexion is performed with the knee in extension. Gastrocnemius muscle activity and isometric ankle plantarflexion strength have been shown to decrease with increasing knee flexion, most significantly at knee flexion angles greater than 45°.[14] Soleus muscle activity (evaluated at 90°, 45°, and 0° knee flexion) was greatest at 90° knee flexion and least at full knee extension.[15] Therefore, the more specific testing of the soleus muscle strength is performed with the knee flexed to at least 45° when the gastrocnemius muscle is placed on slack.

Against Gravity: Gastrocnemius and Soleus

Start Positions. Gastrocnemius (Fig. 8-72): The patient lies prone with the knee extended and the feet are over the edge of the plinth. The ankle is dorsiflexed. Soleus (Fig. 8-73): The patient lies prone with the knee on the test side flexed to 90°. The ankle is dorsiflexed.

Form 8-16

Stabilization. The therapist stabilizes the lower leg proximal to the ankle.

Movement. The patient plantarflexes the ankle through full ROM (Figs. 8-74 and 8-75). The patient is instructed to keep the toes relaxed.

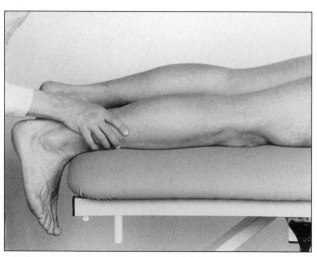

Figure 8-72 Start position: gastrocnemius.

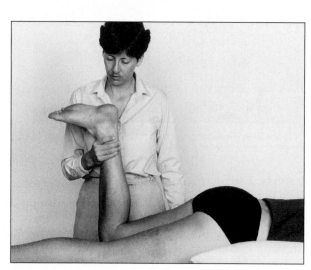

Figure 8-73 Start position: soleus.

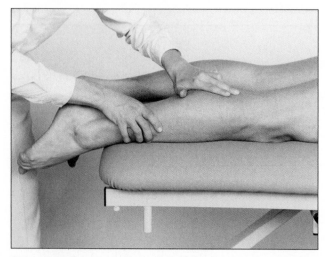

Figure 8-74 Screen position: gastrocnemius.

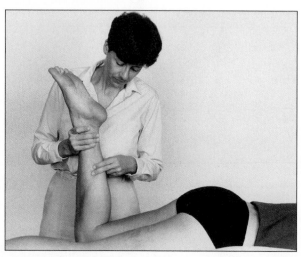

Figure 8-75 Screen position: soleus.

Palpation. *Gastrocnemius:* medial and lateral margin of the popliteal fossa distal to the knee joint. *Soleus:* on either side of gastrocnemius midway down the calf.

Resistance Location. Applied on the posterior aspect of the calcaneum (Figs. 8-76 through 8-79).

Resistance Direction. In a downward and anterior direction to dorsiflex the ankle.

Recording. Record the grade and indicate this is an NWB test.

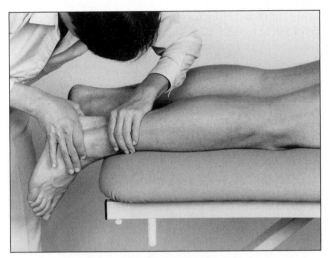

Figure 8-76 Resistance: gastrocnemius.

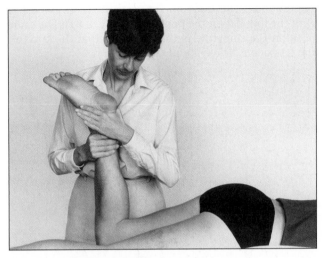

Figure 8-78 Resistance: soleus.

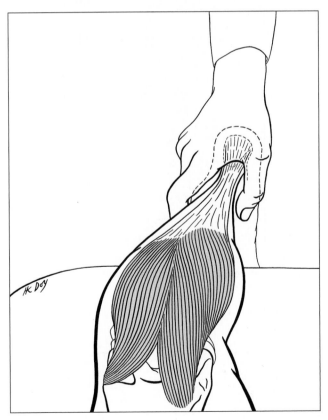

Figure 8-77 Gastrocnemius.

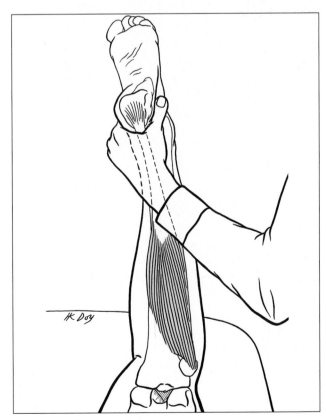

Figure 8-79 Soleus.

Alternate Against Gravity: Gastrocnemius and Soleus

Form 8-17

This test may be contraindicated for patients with poor standing balance or generalized or specific lower extremity weakness.

Start Positions. Gastrocnemius (Fig. 8-80): The patient is standing. The patient raises the foot off the floor on the nontest side. The knee on the test side is in extension with the foot flat on the floor. Soleus (Fig. 8-81): The same position is assumed with the exception that the knee on the test side is flexed about 45°.

Although knee joint test angles are on average, well maintained during gastrocnemius and soleus muscle testing in young subjects,[16] this may vary between individuals based on age, ability to understand instructions, and other factors. Knee joint position should be monitored during each test condition to ensure knee angles are maintained during the WB tests.

Stabilization. The patient may use the parallel bars or other stable structure for balance but should be instructed not to bear weight through their hands. Alternatively, the therapist may provide this support.

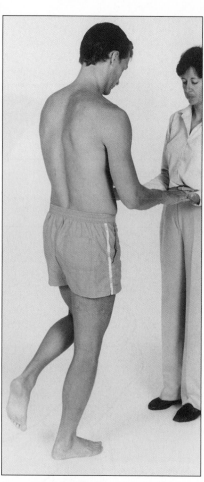

Figure 8-80 Alternate start position: gastrocnemius.

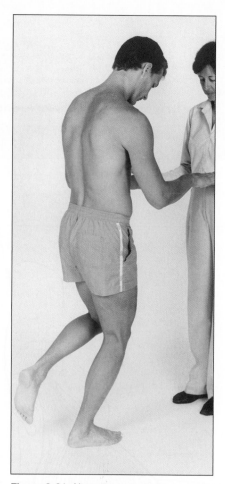

Figure 8-81 Alternate start position: soleus.

Movement. The patient plantarflexes the ankle to go up on the toes (Figs. 8-82 and 8-83) and repeats the movement until fatigued or instructed to stop.

Resistance. Body weight resists the movement.

Grading.
5 = Maintaining the heel fully off the floor through more than six repetitions;
4 = Maintaining the heel fully off the floor through three to five repetitions with subsequent attempts resulting in decreased range; and
3 = Maintaining the heel off the floor through one to two repetitions only with subsequent attempts resulting in decreased range.

Lunsford and Perry[17] studied 203 normal subjects between 20 and 59 years of age and recommended 25 standing heel-rise repetitions be required for a grade of 5. Parameters for other grades were not studied. However, Jan and colleagues[18] studied the heel-rise capabilities of 180 healthy sedentary subjects between 21 and 80 years of age and found few could perform the 20 repetitions for "normal" plantarflexor muscle strength. Significant differences were found in number of repetitions possible based on age and sex, with heel-rise repetitions decreasing with increased age, and women performing fewer repetitions than men.

Following a recent systematic review of the literature,[19] no general consensus and description of definitive standardized testing parameters or normal values of the heel-rise test could be established. Therefore, it is important to record the grading standard used to assess ankle plantarflexion strength.

Recording. Record the grade, grading standard used, and indicate this is a WB test.

Substitute Movement. (1) Soleus: flexion of the knee joint when testing gastrocnemius; (2) gastrocnemius: extension of the knee joint when testing soleus; (3) pushing down on parallel bars or other support (alternate test only); (4) leaning body forward (alternate test only); and (5) when testing NWB: downward movement of the forefoot or toe flexion (through the action of tibialis posterior, peroneus longus, peroneus brevis, flexor hallucis longus, and flexor digitorum longus) giving the appearance of ankle plantarflexion. Ensure upward movement of the heel.

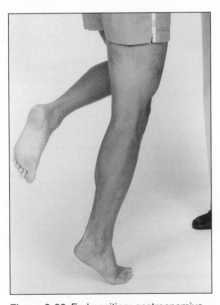

Figure 8-82 End position: gastrocnemius.

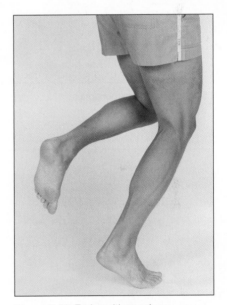

Figure 8-83 End position: soleus.

Gravity Eliminated: Gastrocnemius and Soleus

Start Positions. For both muscle tests, the patient is in a side-lying position with the nontest side lower extremity flexed. Gastrocnemius (Fig. 8-84): the knee is extended and the ankle is dorsiflexed. Soleus (Fig. 8-85): the knee is flexed to 90° and the ankle is dorsiflexed.

Stabilization. The lower leg is stabilized and supported proximal to the ankle joint.

End Position. The patient plantarflexes the ankle through full ROM for gastrocnemius (Fig. 8-86) and for soleus (Fig. 8-87).

Substitute Movement. Forefoot movement or toe flexion as described in the against gravity test.

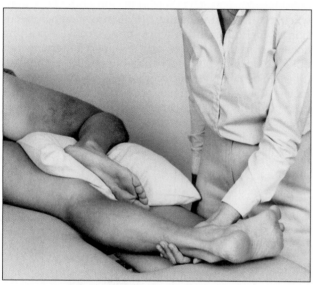

Figure 8-84 Start position: gastrocnemius.

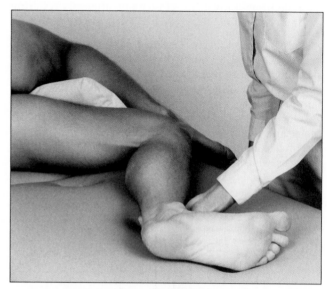

Figure 8-85 Start position: soleus.

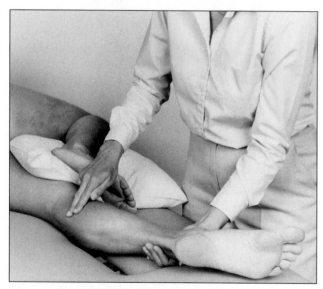

Figure 8-86 End position: gastrocnemius.

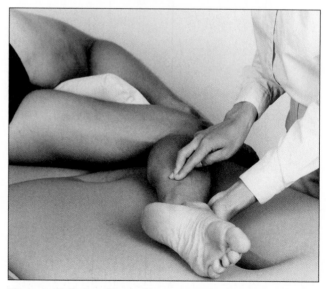

Figure 8-87 End position: soleus.

Foot Inversion

Against Gravity: Tibialis Posterior

Form 8-18

Accessory muscles: gastrocnemius, soleus, flexor digitorum longus, flexor hallucis longus, and tibialis anterior.

Start Position. The patient is in a side-lying position on the test side with the knee slightly flexed (Fig. 8-88). The foot projects over the end of the plinth. Because the tibialis anterior can invert the foot only from an everted position to the neutral position,[13] the foot and ankle are positioned in neutral.

Stabilization. The therapist stabilizes the lower leg proximal to the ankle.

Movement. The patient inverts the foot through full ROM with slight plantarflexion (Fig. 8-89). The patient is instructed to keep the toes relaxed or slightly extended.

Palpation. Between the tip of the medial malleolus and the navicular bone or proximal and posterior to the medial malleolus.

Substitute Movement. Toe flexion; tibialis anterior (ankle dorsiflexion).

Resistance Location. Applied on the medial border of the forefoot (Figs. 8-90 and 8-91).

Resistance Direction. Foot eversion.

Gravity Eliminated: Tibialis Posterior

Start Position. The patient is supine. The heel is off the plinth and the foot and ankle are in neutral (Fig. 8-92).

Stabilization. The therapist stabilizes the lower leg proximal to the ankle.

End Position. The patient inverts the foot through full ROM with slight plantarflexion (Fig. 8-93).

Substitute Movement. Toe flexion.

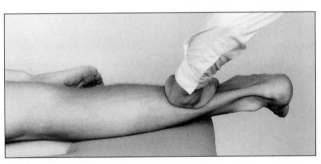
Figure 8-88 Start position: tibialis posterior.

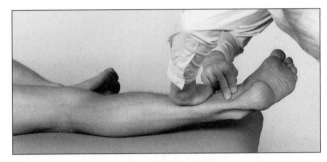
Figure 8-89 Screen position: tibialis posterior.

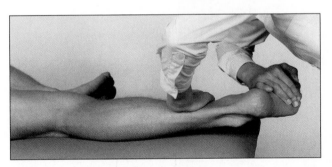
Figure 8-90 Resistance: tibialis posterior.

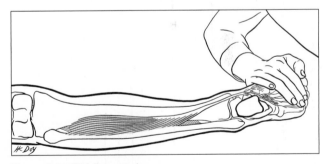
Figure 8-91 Tibialis posterior.

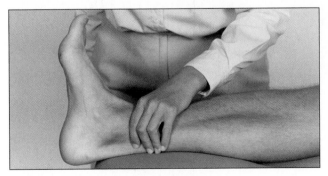
Figure 8-92 Start position: tibialis posterior.

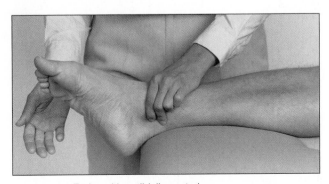
Figure 8-93 End position: tibialis posterior.

Foot Eversion

Against Gravity: Peroneus Longus and Peroneus Brevis

Accessory muscles: peroneus tertius and extensor digitorum longus.

Form 8-19 **Start Position.** The patient is in a side-lying position on the nontest side with the foot over the edge of the plinth (Fig. 8-94). The ankle is plantarflexed and the foot is inverted.

Stabilization. The therapist stabilizes the lower leg proximal to the ankle.

Movement. The patient everts the foot through full ROM while keeping the toes relaxed (Fig. 8-95).

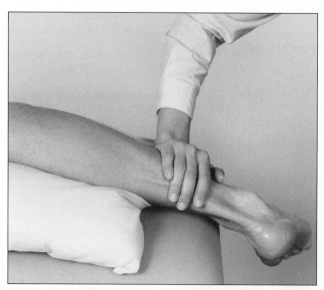

Figure 8-94 Start position: peroneus longus and brevis.

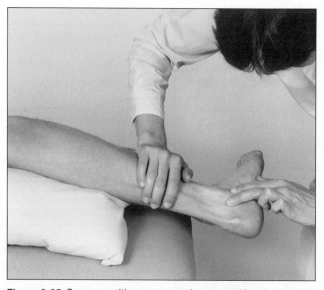

Figure 8-95 Screen position: peroneus longus and brevis.

Palpation. *Peroneus longus:* posterior to the lateral malleolus or distal to the head of the fibula. *Peroneus brevis:* proximal to the base of the fifth metatarsal on the lateral border of the foot.

Substitute Movement. Extensor digitorum longus and peroneus tertius.

Resistance Location. Applied on the lateral border of the foot and on the plantar surface of the first metatarsal (Figs. 8-96, 8-97, and 8-98).

Resistance Direction. Foot inversion and elevation of the first metatarsal.

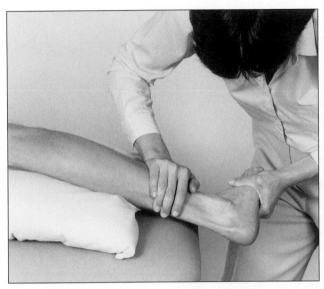

Figure 8-96 Resistance: peroneus longus and brevis.

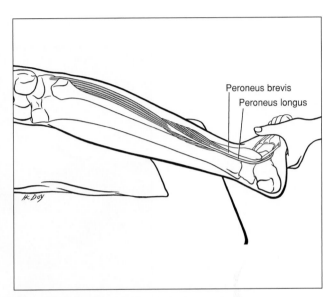

Figure 8-97 Peroneus longus and peroneus brevis.

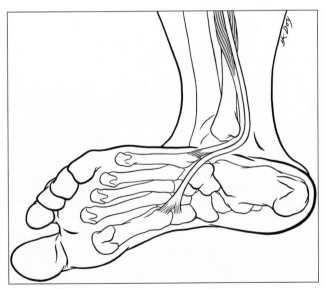

Figure 8-98 Insertions of peroneus longus and peroneus brevis.

Gravity Eliminated: Peroneus Longus and Peroneus Brevis

Start Position. The patient is supine with the heel over the edge of the plinth. The foot and ankle are in the inverted position (Fig. 8-99).

Stabilization. The therapist stabilizes the lower leg proximal to the ankle.

End Position. The patient everts the foot through full ROM (Fig. 8-100).

Substitute Movement. Peroneus tertius and extensor digitorum longus.

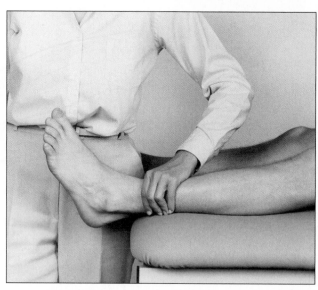

Figure 8-99 Start position: peroneus longus and brevis.

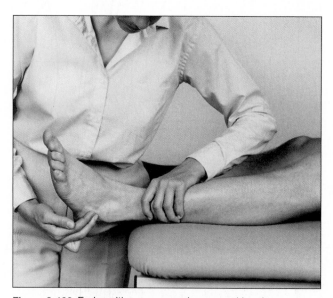

Figure 8-100 End position: peroneus longus and brevis.

TABLE 8-4	Grading for the Fingers and Toes
Numeral	**Description**
	The patient is able to actively move through:
5	The full available ROM against maximal resistance, gravity eliminated or against gravity
4	The full available ROM against moderate resistance, gravity eliminated or against gravity
3	The full available ROM, gravity eliminated or against gravity
2	Part of the available ROM, gravity eliminated or against gravity
1	None of the available ROM, but there is a palpable or observable flicker of a muscle contraction, gravity eliminated or against gravity
0	None of the available ROM, and there is no palpable or observable muscle contraction, gravity eliminated or against gravity

Toe Movements

Gravity is not considered to be a significant factor when testing the muscles of the toes. The muscles of the toes may be tested in either a gravity eliminated or an against gravity position for all grades. Table 8-4 gives a description of the grading for the toes.

Isolated movement of the toes is rarely required for activities of daily living (ADL) and it may not be possible or practical to perform isolated movements for specific muscle testing of the foot, although these tests are described below.

Metatarsophalangeal Flexion

Flexor Hallucis Brevis: Great Toe and Lumbricales: Lesser Four Toes

Form 8-20

Accessory muscles: flexor hallucis longus, flexor digitorum longus and brevis, abductor hallucis, abductor digiti minimi, and dorsal and plantar interossei.

Start Position. The patient is supine. The foot, ankle, and toes are in the anatomical position (Fig. 8-101).

Stabilization. The therapist stabilizes the metatarsals.

Movement. The patient flexes the MTP joint(s) while maintaining extension at the IP joint(s). The great toe is tested independently (Fig. 8-102) of the lateral four toes.

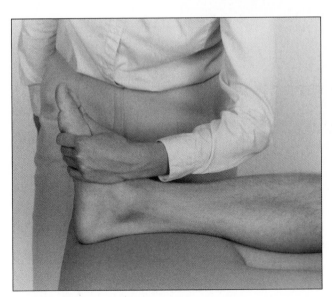

Figure 8-101 Start position: flexor hallucis brevis.

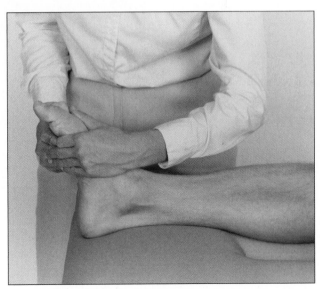

Figure 8-102 Screen position: flexor hallucis brevis.

Palpation. *Flexor hallucis brevis* is palpated on the medial border of the sole of the foot.

The *lumbricales* are not palpable.

Substitute Movement. Great toe: flexor hallucis longus. Lesser four toes: flexor digitorum longus and brevis, flexor digiti minimi, and plantar and dorsal interossei.

Resistance Location. Applied on the plantar surface of the proximal phalanges of the great toe (Figs. 8-103 and 8-104) and the lesser four toes (Fig. 8-105).

Resistance Direction. MTP joint extension.

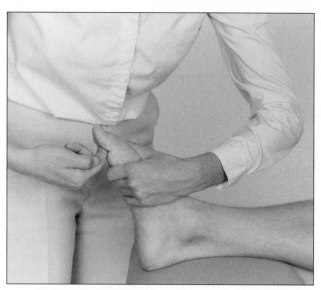

Figure 8-103 Resistance: flexor hallucis brevis.

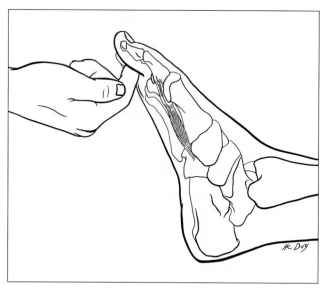

Figure 8-104 Flexor hallucis brevis.

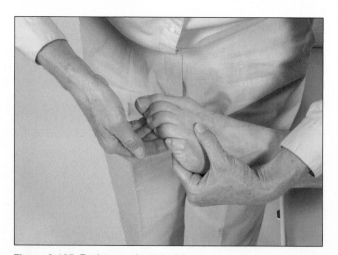

Figure 8-105 Resistance: lumbricales.

Interphalangeal Flexion

Flexor Hallucis Longus: Flexion of the IP Joint of the Great Toe; Flexor Digitorum Longus: Flexion of the DIP Joints of the Lateral Four Toes; and Flexor Digitorum Brevis: Flexion of the PIP Joints of the Lateral Four Toes

Form 8-21

Start Position. The patient is supine. The foot, ankle, and toes are in the anatomical position (Figs. 8-106 and 8-107).

Stabilization. The therapist stabilizes the MTP joints of each toe. If the gastrocnemius and soleus are paralyzed, the calcaneum should be stabilized to assist in fixing the origin of flexor digitorum brevis.

Movement. The great toe is tested independently of the lateral four toes. The patient flexes the IP joint of the great toe through full ROM (Fig. 8-108). The patient flexes the PIP and DIP joints of the lateral four toes through full ROM (Fig. 8-109).

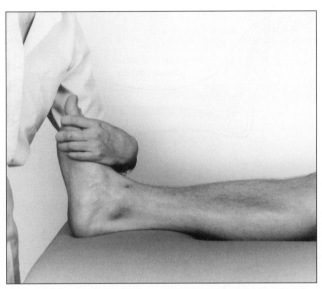

Figure 8-106 Start position: flexor hallucis longus.

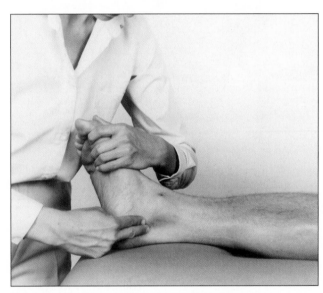

Figure 8-108 Screen position: flexor hallucis longus.

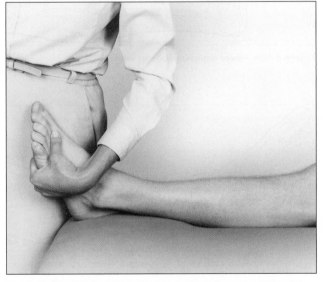

Figure 8-107 Start position: flexor digitorum longus and brevis.

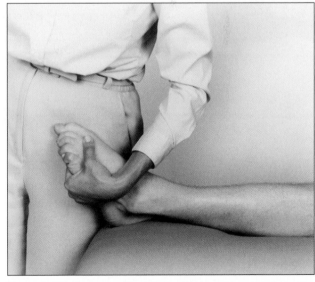

Figure 8-109 Screen position: flexor digitorum longus and brevis.

Palpation. *Flexor hallucis longus* may be palpated on the plantar surface of the proximal phalanx of the great toe or inferior to the medial malleolus. The *flexor digitorum brevis* is not palpable. *Flexor digitorum longus* may be palpated on some individuals on the plantar aspect of the proximal phalanges.

Resistance Location. Applied on the plantar surface of the distal phalanx of the great toe (Figs. 8-110 and 8-111) and the distal and middle phalanges of the lateral four toes (Figs. 8-112, 8-113, and 8-114).

Resistance Direction. Toe extension.

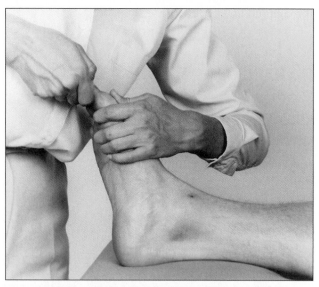

Figure 8-110 Resistance: flexor hallucis longus.

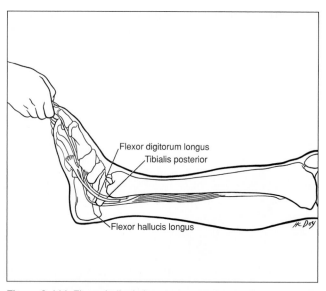

Flexor digitorum longus
Tibialis posterior

Flexor hallucis longus

Figure 8-111 Flexor hallucis longus.

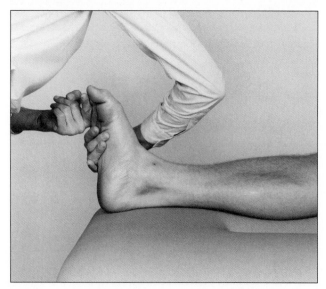

Figure 8-112 Resistance: flexor digitorum longus and brevis.

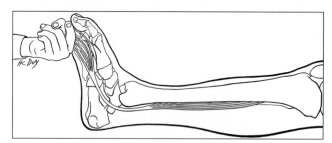

Figure 8-113 Flexor digitorum longus.

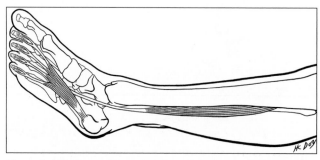

Figure 8-114 Flexor digitorum longus and flexor digitorum brevis.

Metatarsophalangeal Abduction of the Great Toe

Abductor Hallucis

Form 8-22

Start Position. The patient is supine. The ankle, foot, and toes are in the anatomical position (Fig. 8-115).

Stabilization. The therapist stabilizes the first metatarsal bone.

Movement. The patient abducts the great toe through full ROM (Fig. 8-116). The movement of abduction is accompanied by some flexion, as the abductor hallucis abducts and flexes the MTP joint of the great toe.

Palpation. Medial border of the foot superficial to the first metatarsal bone.

Resistance Location. Applied on the medial aspect of the proximal phalanx of the great toe (Figs. 8-117 and 8-118).

Resistance Direction. Great toe adduction.

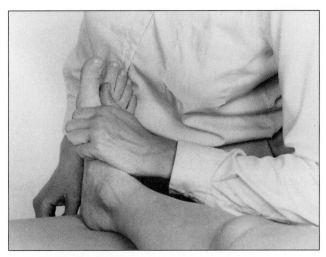

Figure 8-115 Start position: abductor hallucis.

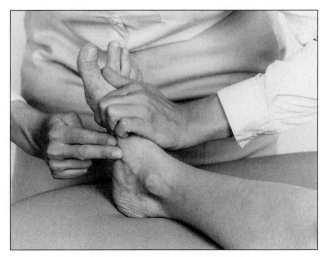

Figure 8-116 Screen position: abductor hallucis.

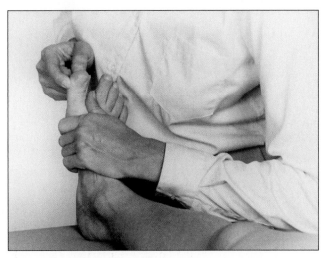

Figure 8-117 Resistance: abductor hallucis.

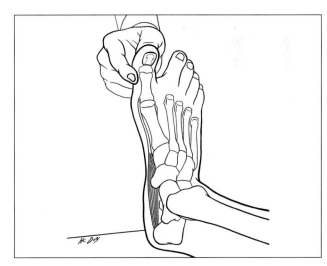

Figure 8-118 Abductor hallucis.

Metatarsophalangeal Abduction

Abductor Digiti Minimi and Dorsal Interossei

These two muscles are not isolated for grading. Function is determined through observation of abduction of the lateral three toes (Fig. 8-119). This movement is associated with flexion of the MTP joints. The therapist stabilizes the great toe.

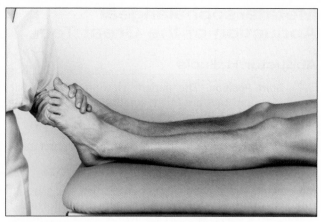

Figure 8-119 Observation of abductor digiti minimi and dorsal interossei.

Metatarsophalangeal and Interphalangeal Extension

Extensor Hallucis Longus: IP Extension of the Great Toe; Extensor Digitorum Brevis: MTP and IP Extension of the Middle Three Toes and MTP Extension of the Great Toe; and Extensor Digitorum Longus: MTP and IP Extension of the Lateral Four Toes

 Start Position. The patient is supine. The ankle is in the neutral position and the toes are flexed (Figs. 8-120 and 8-121).

Form 8-23

Stabilization. The therapist stabilizes the metatarsals.

Movement. The patient extends the great toe through full ROM (Fig. 8-122). The patient extends the lateral four toes through full ROM (Fig. 8-123). It may be difficult for the patient to extend the great toe and the lateral four toes separately; therefore, the toes may have to be tested as a group.

Palpation. *The extensor hallucis longus* is palpated on the dorsal aspect of the first MTP joint or on the anterior aspect of the ankle joint lateral to the tendon of tibialis anterior. *Extensor digitorum brevis* is palpated on the dorsolateral aspect of the foot anterior to the lateral malleolus. *Extensor digitorum longus* is palpated on the dorsal aspect of the metatarsal bones of the lateral four toes or on the anterior aspect of the ankle joint lateral to the tendon of extensor hallucis longus.

Note: The extensor digitorum brevis does not insert into the fifth toe; therefore, decreased extension strength of this toe indicates weakness of the extensor digitorum longus.[20] The portion of the extensor digitorum brevis that inserts into the base of the proximal phalanx of the great toe produces MTP joint extension of the great toe.

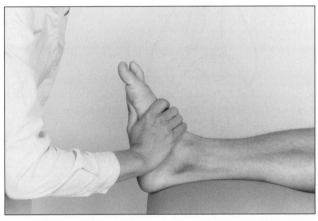

Figure 8-120 Start position: extensor hallucis longus and extensor hallucis brevis.

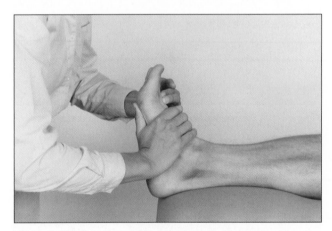

Figure 8-122 Screen position: extensor hallucis longus and extensor hallucis brevis.

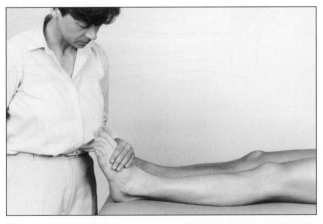

Figure 8-121 Start position: extensor digitorum longus and brevis.

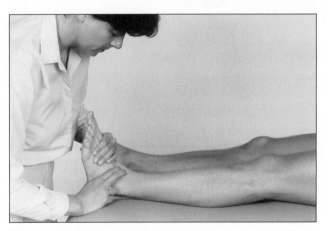

Figure 8-123 Screen position: extensor digitorum longus and brevis.

Resistance Location. *Extensor hallucis longus and extensor hallucis brevis* (Figs. 8-124 and 8-125): applied over the dorsal aspect of the distal phalanx of the great toe. *Extensor digitorum longus and brevis* (Figs. 8-126 and 8-127): applied over the dorsal surface of the lateral four toes.

Resistance Direction. Toe flexion.

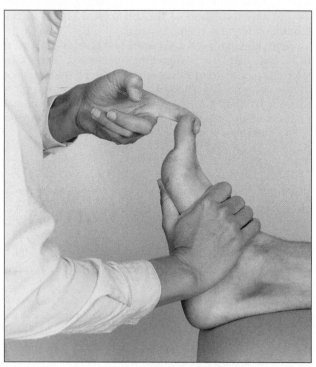

Figure 8-124 Resistance: extensor hallucis longus and brevis.

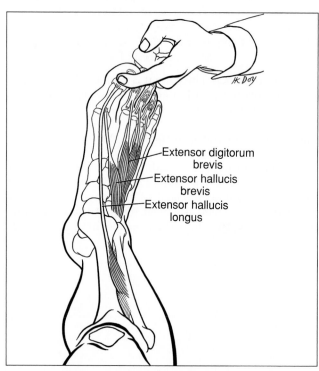

Figure 8-125 Extensor hallucis longus and brevis and extensor digitorum brevis.

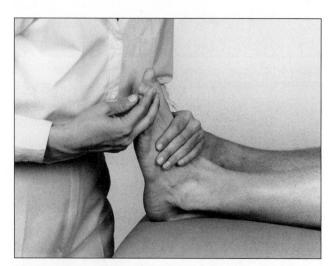

Figure 8-126 Resistance: extensor digitorum longus and brevis.

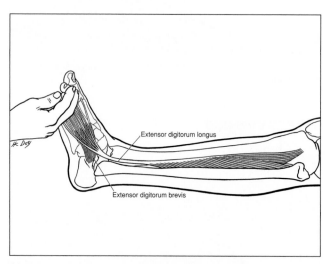

Figure 8-127 Extensor digitorum longus and extensor digitorum brevis.

FUNCTIONAL APPLICATION

Joint Function

The foot functions as a flexible base to accommodate rough terrain[13] and functions as a rigid lever during terminal stance of the walking pattern.[5] In transmitting forces between the ground and the leg, the foot absorbs shock.[13] With the foot planted, the ankle and foot elevate the body, and when off the ground, the foot is used to manipulate machinery.[13] When weight is taken through the foot, the MTP joints allow movement of the rigid foot over the toes.[5]

Functional Range of Motion (Table 8-5)

Ankle Dorsiflexion and Plantarflexion

The normal AROM of the ankle joint is 20° dorsiflexion and 50° plantarflexion. However, ankle dorsiflexion ROM measured in WB (e.g., on stairs, when rising from sitting, squatting, and kneeling) is greater than in NWB positions. The full range of ankle dorsiflexion is necessary to descend stairs (Fig. 8-128). Rising from sitting (Fig. 8-129) also requires significant ankle dorsiflexion ROM (i.e., an average of 28°[21]). Ankle dorsiflexion ROM is utilized by non-Western cultures accustomed to performing ADL such as kneeling and squatting.[25]

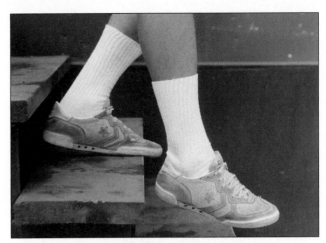

Figure 8-128 Full range of ankle dorsiflexion is required to descend stairs.

Full ankle plantarflexion may be required when climbing, jumping, or reaching high objects (Fig. 8-130). Less than the full range of ankle plantarflexion may be used to perform activities such as depressing the accelerator of a motor vehicle (Fig. 8-131) or the foot pedals of a piano, and wearing high-heeled shoes. Cross-legged sitting, a position essential in ADL used by Asian and Eastern cultures requires less than full ankle plantarflexion ROM of about 26°[25] to 29°.[26]

Livingston, Stevenson, and Olney[22] found that maximum ankle dorsiflexion ROM requirements to ascend and descend stairs ranged between averages of 14° and 27° to ascend and 21° and 36° to descend stairs. The

TABLE 8-5	Ankle and Great Toe ROM Required for Selected ADL		
Activity	**Ankle Dorsiflexion**	**Ankle Plantarflexion**	**Great Toe MTP Extension**
Rising from sitting*	28°		
Ascending stairs†	14–27°	23–30°	
Descending stairs†	21–36°	24–31°	
Walking	10°‡	20°‡	90°[23]
Running§	17°	32°	
Sitting cross-legged		26[25]–29°[26]	
Kneeling with ankles dorsiflexed	40°[25]		
Squatting with heels down	39°[25]		

*Average of young and elderly average values from original source.[21]

†Ankle dorsiflexion and plantarflexion ROM values for 15 subjects during ascent and descent of three stairs of different dimensions. Maximum ankle dorsiflexion and plantarflexion requirements varied depending on the stair dimensions and subject height.[22]

‡Data from the Rancho Los Amigos gait analysis forms as cited in the work of Levangie and Norkin.[5]

§There were no differences in average ankle ROM at fast-paced (faster than a 7.5-minute mile) and slow-paced (slower than an 8-minute mile) running.[24]

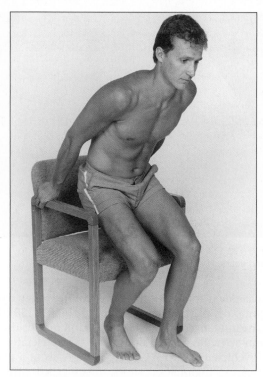

Figure 8-129 Ankle dorsiflexion is required to rise from sitting.

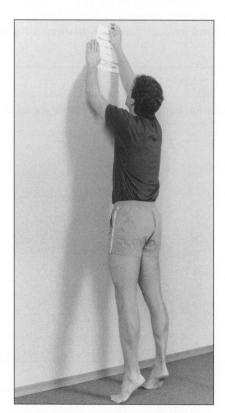

Figure 8-130 Toe extension, ankle plantarflexion, and contraction of the ankle plantarflexors.

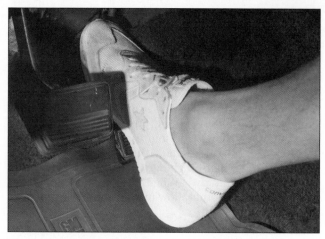

Figure 8-131 Ankle plantarflexion is used to depress the accelerator of a motor vehicle.

average maximum ankle plantarflexion ROM requirements ranged from 23° to 30° to ascend and 24° to 31° to descend stairs.[22]

Movements of the Foot

The AROM of the subtalar joint is 5° each for inversion and eversion without forefoot movement. The ranges of inversion and eversion may be augmented by forefoot movement of 35° and 15°, respectively. The subtalar, transverse tarsal joints, and joints of the forefoot must be fully mobile to allow the foot to accommodate to varying degrees of rough terrain (Fig. 8-132). With the foot across the opposite thigh, inversion is required to inspect the foot.

In standing, the MTP joints are in at least 25° extension due to the downward slope of the metatarsals.[2] Ranges approximating the full 90° of extension of the MTP joint of the great toe are required for many ADL.[23] Extension of the great toe and lesser four toes is essential for activities such as rising onto the toes to reach high objects (see Fig. 8-130) and squatting (Fig. 8-133). For

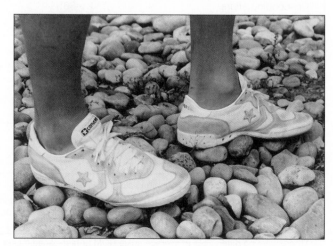

Figure 8-132 The mobile joints of the ankle and foot accommodate rough terrain.

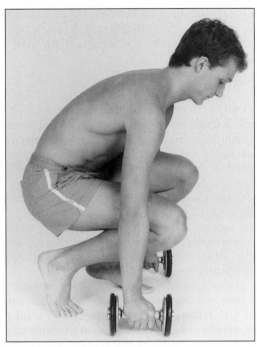

Figure 8-133 Extension of the toes is essential for squatting.

most ADL, only a few degrees of flexion are required at the great toe.[23] There appears to be no significant function that can be attributed to abduction and adduction at the MTP joints.[5]

Gait

Normal walking (see Appendix D) requires a maximum of 10° of ankle dorsiflexion at midstance to terminal stance as the tibia advances over the fixed foot and a maximum of 20° of plantarflexion at the end of preswing (from the Rancho Los Amigos gait analysis forms as cited in the work of Levangie and Norkin[5]). At the MTP joint of the great toe, almost 90° of extension is required at preswing.[23] Extension of the lesser four toes is also required.[23] Extension of the toes stretches the plantar aponeurosis, resulting in significant longitudinal arch support.[27]

Running requires a range of ankle joint motion from an average of 17° dorsiflexion at midstance to an average 32° maximum ankle plantarflexion at early swing.[24] Ankle ROM was the same when fast-paced running was compared to slow-paced running.[24]

Muscle Function

Ankle Plantarflexion

The triceps surae muscles, gastrocnemius and soleus, are the primary plantarflexors at the ankle joint. The gastrocnemius crosses the knee joint and is most effective as a plantarflexor when the knee is extended.[28] Gastrocnemius muscle activity and isometric ankle plantarflexion strength have been shown to decrease with increasing knee flexion, most significantly at knee flexion angles greater than 45°. Herman and Bragin[29] found the gastrocnemius contributes to plantarflexion when the ankle is in the plantarflexed position, when tension is developed rapidly, and when strong contraction is required.

Soleus muscle activity has been shown to be greatest at 90° knee flexion and less at full knee extension.[15] The soleus is mainly active in plantarflexing the ankle when the ankle is in a dorsiflexed position and when the contraction is minimal.[29] Tibialis posterior, flexor hallucis longus, flexor digitorum longus, and peroneus longus and brevis act as accessory plantarflexors at the ankle joint. The actions of the plantarflexors are illustrated in activities where the ankle is plantarflexed against resistance, for example, rising onto the toes (see Fig. 8-130), jumping, and depressing the gas pedal of a motor vehicle (see Fig. 8-131). The ankle plantarflexors also contract when movement is forced at the extreme of plantarflexion, such as when pulling on a sock. With the foot fixed on the ground, the plantarflexors control ankle dorsiflexion when descending stairs[30] (see Fig. 8-128).

Ankle Dorsiflexion

The dorsiflexors of the ankle include the tibialis anterior, extensor hallucis longus, extensor digitorum longus, and peroneus tertius. The function of the tibialis anterior is to initiate ankle dorsiflexion.[31] The tibialis anterior and extensor hallucis longus are strong dorsiflexors compared to the extensor digitorum longus and peroneus tertius.[32] The dorsiflexors contract and maintain the ankle in a dorsiflexed position in activities such as cutting toenails or tying shoelaces. These muscles also contract to control ankle plantarflexion when lowering the foot onto the ground, as illustrated when slowly tapping the foot on the floor and at loading response in the gait cycle (see Appendix D). When rising from the sitting to the standing position with the foot planted on the ground, the dorsiflexors contract to stabilize the tibia on the tarsus.[33]

Inversion and Eversion

The tibialis posterior, flexor hallucis longus, flexor digitorum longus, soleus, gastrocnemius, and tibialis anterior are responsible for inversion. The tibialis posterior is the principle invertor of the foot. The gastrocnemius and soleus muscles produce inversion of the calcaneus with plantarflexion of the ankle.[13] Opinions vary concerning the contribution made by tibialis anterior in inverting the foot. The line of action of tibialis anterior is along the subtalar joint axis[28] for inversion and eversion. For this reason, Soderberg[28] indicates there is no motion produced by the tibialis anterior around the subtalar joint axis. Smith, Weiss, and Lehmkuhl[13] state that tibialis anterior and the long toes flexor muscles may be weak invertors of the foot from a position of eversion to neutral position. O'Connell[31] concluded that the tibialis anterior only functions as an invertor when the medial border of the foot is elevated simultaneously. The action of the invertors is illustrated when the foot is positioned across the opposite thigh to inspect the foot for skin condition or when walking across rough terrain when the invertors assist in stabilizing the foot (see Fig. 8-132).

The peroneus longus and peroneus brevis, assisted by the extensor digitorum longus and peroneus tertius, perform eversion. The action of the evertors is illustrated when walking across rough ground (see Fig. 8-132).

Toe Flexion and Extension

The flexors of the great toe include the flexor hallucis longus, flexor hallucis brevis, and abductor hallucis brevis. The abductor hallucis brevis flexes the MTP joint and extends the IP joint of the great toe.[34] The flexor digitorum longus and flexor digitorum brevis flex the lesser four toes. The flexor digiti minimi and abductor digiti minimi also assist in flexion of the fifth toe. The toe flexors function so that the great toe presses firmly on the ground and the other four toes grip the ground to help maintain balance during unilateral stance[35] or when standing on the toes (see Fig. 8-130). The toe flexors contract eccentrically to control passive toe extension that occurs when crouching to pick up an object from the ground or walking.

The extensor apparatus of the foot is similar to the extensor apparatus of the hand. The extensors of the great toe include the extensor hallucis longus, extensor hallucis brevis, and abductor hallucis brevis. The extensor digitorum longus and extensor digitorum brevis extend the lesser four toes at the MTP joints. There is no extensor digitorum brevis to the fifth toe, but fibers from the abductor digiti minimi and flexor digiti minimi muscles make attachment to the dorsal digital expansion of the fifth toe[34] to assist with extension. The lumbricales and the interossei simultaneously flex the MTP joints and extend the IP joints of the lesser four toes. The toe extensors contract during walking and climbing stairs. The action of the toe extensors is illustrated when one extends the toes and maintains this position to cut the toenails.

Maintenance of the Arches

Unlike the hand, the intrinsic muscles of the foot do not perform specific functions but usually work as a group along with the extrinsic muscles to perform gross function. The intrinsic muscles function to stabilize the foot during propulsion.[36] Mann and Inman[36] explain that the main intrinsic muscles (abductor hallucis, flexor hallucis brevis, flexor digitorum brevis, and abductor digiti minimi) form the main muscle support of the arch by exerting a strong flexion force on the forefoot, to help stabilize the transverse tarsal joint. The intrinsic muscles contract to stabilize the foot when weight is taken through the forefoot in activities such as standing on the toes (see Fig. 8-130) or ascending and descending stairs or a ramp. The triceps surae, peroneus longus and brevis, and tibialis anterior and posterior contract with the intrinsic muscles to make the foot more rigid for activities such as running and climbing.[37]

Standing Posture

In standing, the line of gravity falls anterior to the ankle joint axis creating a dorsiflexion torque.[32] The dorsiflexion torque is opposed by the soleus muscle as it contracts to pull the tibia in a posterior direction.[32] Muscle activity is not required to support the arches of the foot when standing.[36]

Gait

The following description of muscle function during the gait cycle is based on the work of Norkin and Levangie,[32] and Inman, Ralston, and Todd.[38] The ankle dorsiflexors contract during the swing phase of the gait cycle to allow the foot to clear the ground. The tibialis anterior, extensor hallucis longus, and extensor digitorum longus contract concentrically to dorsiflex the ankle from preswing through midswing and then contract isometrically to hold the foot in this position. These same muscles contract eccentrically to control the lowering of the foot onto the floor from initial contact through loading response during the stance phase of the gait cycle.

The gastrocnemius and soleus muscles contract eccentrically from loading response to terminal stance to control ankle dorsiflexion produced by the forward movement of the tibia over the fixed foot as the body advances forward. In preswing the gastrocnemius, soleus, peroneus longus, peroneus brevis, and flexor hallucis longus contract concentrically and the heel is raised off the ground. Peroneus longus controls balance during normal gait, most notably at slower walking speeds.[39]

The intrinsic muscles of the foot contract during the stance phase of the gait cycle.[36] The contraction of the intrinsic muscles coincides with the period in the gait cycle when the foot requires maximal stability.

Reber and associates[40] describe the ankle muscle activity during running.

References

1. Kapandji AI. *The Physiology of the Joints. Vol. 2. The Lower Limb.* 6th ed. New York, NY: Churchill Livingstone Elsevier; 2011.
2. Soames RW. Skeletal system. Salmon S, ed. Muscle. In: *Gray's Anatomy.* 38th ed. New York: Churchill Livingstone; 1995.
3. Norkin CC, White DJ. *Measurement of Joint Motion: A Guide to Goniometry.* 4th ed. Philadelphia, PA: FA Davis; 2009.
4. Daniels L, Worthingham C. *Muscle Testing: Techniques of Manual Examination.* 5th ed. Philadelphia, PA: WB Saunders; 1986.
5. Levangie PK, Norkin CC. *Joint Structure & Function: A Comprehensive Analysis.* 3rd ed. Philadelphia, PA: FA Davis; 2001.
6. Woodburne RT. *Essentials of Human Anatomy.* 5th ed. London: Oxford University Press; 1973.
7. Magee DJ. *Orthopedic Physical Assessment.* 5th ed. St. Louis, MO: Saunders Elsevier; 2008.
8. American Academy of Orthopaedic Surgeons. *Joint Motion: Method of Measuring and Recording.* Chicago, IL: AAOS; 1965.
9. Berryman Reese N, Bandy WD. *Joint Range of Motion and Muscle Length Testing.* 2nd ed. St. Louis, MO: Saunders Elsevier; 2010.
10. Cyriax J. *Textbook of Orthopaedic Medicine. Vol. 1. Diagnosis of Soft Tissue Lesions.* 8th ed. London: Bailliere Tindall; 1982.
11. Taylor Major KF, Bojescul Captain JA, Howard RS, Mizel MS, McHale KA. Measurement of isolated subtalar range of motion: a cadaver study. *Foot Ankle Int.* 2001;22:426–432.

12. Costa ML, Logan K, Heylings D, Donell ST, Tucker K. The effects of achilles tendon lengthening on ankle dorsiflexion: a cadaver study. *Foot Ankle Int.* 2006;27(6):414–417.

13. Smith LK, Weiss EL, Lehmkuhl LD. *Brunnstrom's Clinical Kinesiology.* 5th ed. Philadelphia, PA: FA Davis; 1996.

14. Fiebert IM, Correia EP, Roach KE, Carte MB, Cespedes J, Hemstreet K. A comparison of EMG activity between the medial and lateral heads of the gastrocnemius muscle during isometric plantarflexion contractions at various knee angles. *Isokinet Exerc Sci.* 1996;6:71–77.

15. Signorile JE, Applegate B, Duque M, Cole N, Zink A. Selective recruitment of the triceps surae muscles with changes in knee angle. *J Strength Cond Res.* 2002;16(3):433–439.

16. Hébert-Losier K, Schneiders AG, Sullivan SJ, Newsham-West RJ, Garcia JA, Simoneau GG. Analysis of knee flexion angles during two clinical versions of the heel-raise test to assess soleus and gastrocnemius function. *J Orthop Sports Phys Ther.* 2011;41(7):505–513.

17. Lunsford BR, Perry J. The standing heel-rise test for ankle plantar flexion: criterion for normal. *Phys Ther.* 1995;75:694–698.

18. Jan MH, Chai HM, Lin YF, Lin JC, Tsai LY, Ou YC, Lin DH. Effects of age and sex on the results of an ankle plantar-flexor manual muscle test. *Phys Ther.* 2005;85(10):1078-1084.

19. Hébert-Losier K, Newsham-West RJ, Schneiders AG, Sullivan SJ. Raising the standards of the calf-raise test: a systematic review. *J Sci Med Sport.* 2009;12(6):594–602.

20. Janda V. *Muscle Function Testing.* London: Butterworth; 1983.

21. Ikeda ER, Schenkman ML, Riley PO, Hodge WA. Influence of age on dynamics of rising from a chair. *Phys Ther.* 1991;71:473–481.

22. Livingston LA, Stevenson JM, Olney SJ. Stairclimbing kinematics on stairs of differing dimensions. *Arch Phys Med Rehabil.* 1991;72:398–402.

23. Sammarco GJ, Hockenbury RT. Biomechanics of the foot and ankle. In: Nordin M, Frankel VH, eds. *Basic Biomechanics of the Musculoskeletal System.* 3rd ed. Philadelphia, PA: Lippincott Williams & Wilkins; 2001.

24. Pink M, Perry J, Houglum PA, Devine DJ. Lower extremity range of motion in the recreational sport runner. *Am J Sports Med.* 1994;22:541–549.

25. Hemmerich A, Brown H, Smith S, Marthandam SSK, Wyss UP. Hip, knee, and ankle kinematics of high range of motion activities of daily living. *J Orthop Res.* 2006;24:770–781.

26. Kapoor A, Mishra SK, Kewangan SK, Mody BS. Range of movements of lower limb joints in cross-legged sitting posture. *J Arthroplasty.* 2008;23:451–453.

27. Thordarson DB, Schmotzer H, Chon J, Peters J. Dynamic support of the human longitudinal arch. *Clin Orthop Relat Res.* 1995;316:165–172.

28. Soderberg GL. *Kinesiology: Application to Pathological Motion.* 2nd ed. Baltimore: Williams & Wilkins; 1997.

29. Herman R, Bragin SJ. Function of the gastrocnemius and soleus muscles. *Phys Ther.* 1967;47:105–113.

30. Andriacchi TP, Andersson GBJ, Fermier RW, Stern D, Galante JO. A study of lower-limb mechanics during stair-climbing. *J Bone Joint Surg [Am].* 1980;62:749–757.

31. O'Connell AL. Electromyographic study of certain leg muscles during movements of the free foot and during standing. *Am J Phys Med.* 1958;37:289–301.

32. Norkin CC, Levangie PK. *Joint Structure and Function: A Comprehensive Analysis.* 2nd ed. Philadelphia: FA Davis; 1992.

33. Houtz SJ, Walsh FP. Electromyographic analysis of the function of the muscles acting on the ankle during weight-bearing with special reference to the triceps surae. *J Bone Joint Surg [Am].* 1959;41:1469–1481.

34. Sarrafian SK, Topouzian LK. Anatomy and physiology of the extensor apparatus of the toes. *J Bone Joint Surg [Am].* 1969;51:669–679.

35. Cailliet R. *Foot and Ankle Pain.* Philadelphia, PA: FA Davis; 1968.

36. Mann R, Inman VT. Phasic activity of the intrinsic muscles of the foot. *J Bone Joint Surg [Am].* 1964;46:469–481.

37. Sammarco GJ. Biomechanics of the foot. In: Nordin M, Frankel VH, eds. *Basic Biomechanics of the Musculoskeletal System.* 2nd ed. Philadelphia, PA: Lea & Febiger; 1989.

38. Inman VT, Ralston HJ, Todd F. *Human Walking.* Baltimore, MD: Williams & Wilkins; 1981.

39. Louwerens JWK, van Linge B, de Klerk LWL, Mulder PGH, Snijders CJ. Peroneus longus and tibialis anterior muscle activity in the stance phase. *Acta Orthop Scand.* 1995;66:517–523.

40. Reber L, Perry J, Pink M. Muscular control of the ankle in running. *Am J Sports Med.* 1993;21:805–810.

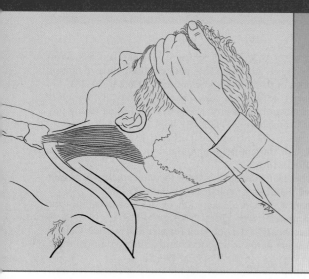

Chapter 9

Head, Neck, and Trunk

ARTICULATIONS AND MOVEMENTS: HEAD AND NECK

The articulations and joint axes of the temporomandibular joint (TMJ) and cervical spine are illustrated in Figs. 9-1, 9-2, and 9-3. The joint structure and movements of the TMJ and cervical spine are described below and summarized in Tables 9-1 and 9-2.

The Temporomandibular Joints

The TMJs, located on each side of the head just anterior to the ears, are individually described as condylar joints and together form a bicondylar articulation,[2] being linked via the mandible (lower jaw). The TMJs are evaluated together as a functional unit. The articular surfaces of the TMJ are incongruent mates, but an articular disc positioned between these surfaces promotes congruency

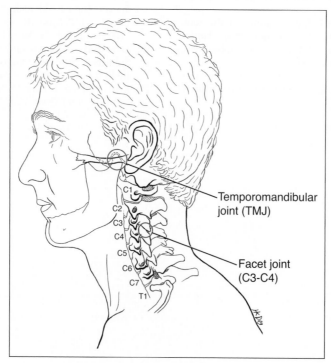

Temporomandibular joint (TMJ)

Facet joint (C3-C4)

Figure 9-1 TMJ and cervical spine articulations.

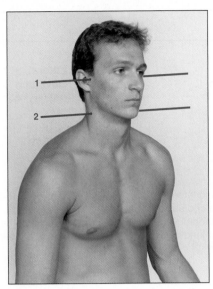

Figure 9-2 (1) TMJ axis: elevation–depression. (2) Cervical spine axis: flexion–extension.

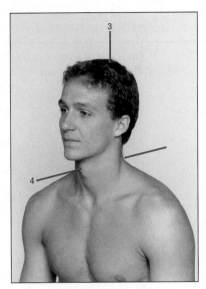

Figure 9-3 Cervical spine axes: (3) rotation; (4) lateral flexion.

and divides the TMJ into upper and lower compartments (Fig. 9-4C).

The upper compartment of each TMJ is formed superiorly by the concave mandibular fossa and the convex temporal articular eminence that lies anterior to the fossa. These bony surfaces together form the superior TMJ surface and articulate with the reciprocally shaped superior surface of the articular disc, which is anteroposteriorly concavoconvex. The inferior surface of the articular disc is concave and mated with the convex condyle of the mandible to form the lower compartment of the TMJ.

Simultaneous movement of the TMJs produces depression (to open the mouth), elevation (to close the mouth), protrusion, retraction, or lateral deviation of the mandible. Elevation and depression of the mandible occur in the sagittal plane with movement around a frontal axis (Fig. 9-2). On mouth opening, a two-part sequence of motion occurs within the lower compartment of each TMJ. First, the mandibular condyle rotates, and glides forward and downward on the articular disc. Second, because of the posterior attachment of the disc to the mandibular condyle, both structures move together anteriorly.[2] This motion results in the anterior gliding of the articular disc over the temporal joint surfaces within the upper compartment.[2] These motions are reversed with mouth closing.

When the lower jaw is protracted and retracted, the articular disc of each TMJ moves with the mandibular condyle[2] as the mandible moves in the transverse plane anteriorly and posteriorly, respectively. Movement within the upper compartment of each TMJ occurs between the articular disc and the temporal bone.[14]

Lateral deviation of the mandible includes rotation of the mandibular condyle in the mandibular fossa on the side toward which the deviation occurs and a gliding forward of the contralateral mandibular condyle over the mandibular fossa and temporal articular eminence.[2]

The Neck: Cervical Spine

There are seven vertebrae that make up the cervical spine (Fig. 9-1). The third through seventh vertebrae (C3–C7) have a similar structure, and C1 and C2 each have a different structure.

The first cervical vertebra, also referred to as C1 or the atlas, articulates with the occiput of the skull via the atlanto-occipital joints (Figs. 9-1 and 9-5A). These joints are formed superiorly by the convex condyles of the occiput articulating with the concave superior articular facets of C1, which lie in the transverse plane and face superiorly and medially. The orientation of the facets determines the motion at the atlanto-occipital articulations. The main movements being flexion and extension, there is slight lateral flexion,[14] and no rotation.[15]

There are three atlanto-axial articulations between the atlas (C1) and the axis (C2) (Figs. 9-1 and 9-5). A pivot is formed[2] between the odontoid process (dens) of C2 as it articulates anteriorly with the concave posterior surface of the anterior arch of C1, and posteriorly with the cartilaginous posterior surface of the transverse ligament. The transverse ligament retains the odontoid process in place. There are two facet joints, one on each side between C1 and C2, which lie posterior to the transverse ligament

	Opening of the Mouth (Depression of the Mandible)	**Closing of the Mouth (Occlusion)**	**Protrusion**	**Retrusion**	**Lateral Deviation**
TABLE 9-1 Joint Structure: Jaw Movements					
Articulation[1,2]	Temporomandibular (TM)	TM	TM	TM	TM
Plane	Sagittal	Sagittal	Horizontal	Horizontal	Horizontal
Axis	Frontal	Frontal			
Normal limiting factors[2,3]* **(see Fig. 9-4)**	Tension in the lateral/temporomandibular ligament and the retrodiscal tissue	Occlusion or contact of the teeth	Tension in the lateral/temporomandibular, sphenomandibular, and stylomandibular ligaments		Tension in the lateral/temporomandibular ligament
Normal AROM† (ruler)	35–50 cm[4]	Contact of teeth	3–7 mm[5]		10–15 mm[4]
Capsular pattern[4,6]	Limitation of mouth opening				

*There is a paucity of definitive research that identifies the normal limiting factors (NLF) of joint motion. The NLF and end feels listed here are based on knowledge of anatomy, clinical experience, and available references.

†AROM, active range of motion.

in the transverse plane. Each of the inferior facets of C1 articulates with a superior facet of C2. The orientation of the facets results in rotation being the primary motion at the atlanto-axial joints. Most of the rotation of the cervical spine occurs at the atlanto-axial joints.[15]

From C2 to C7, a vertebral segment consists of two vertebrae and the three articulations between these vertebrae. Anteriorly, the intervertebral disc is positioned between the adjacent vertebral bodies (Fig. 9-5B and C). Two facet joints are located posteriorly on each side of the vertebral segment. Each facet joint (Fig. 9-1) is formed by the inferior facet of the superior vertebra (oriented inferiorly and anteriorly) and the superior facet of the inferior vertebra (oriented superiorly and posteriorly). The surfaces of the facet joints lie at an angle of about 45°

to the transverse plane. The orientation of the facets from C2 through C7 permits cervical spine flexion, extension, lateral flexion, and rotation.

When assessing cervical spine range of motion (ROM), the combined motions of the segments between the occiput and C7 are assessed and measured, since segmental motion cannot be measured clinically. Cervical spine movements include neck flexion and extension, which occur in the sagittal plane about a frontal axis (Fig. 9-2); lateral flexion, which occurs in the frontal plane around a sagittal axis (Fig. 9-3); and rotation, which occurs in the transverse plane around a vertical axis (Fig. 9-3). About 40% of cervical flexion and 60% of cervical rotation occur at the occiput/C1/C2 complex of the cervical spine.[16]

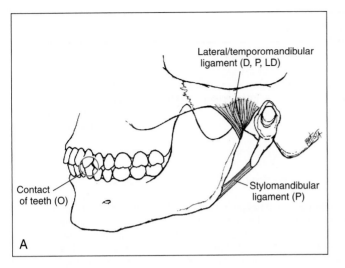

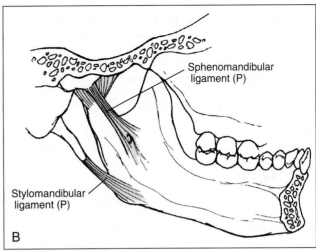

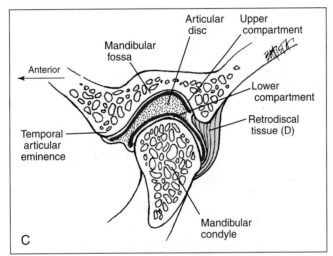

Figure 9-4 **Normal Limiting Factors: TMJ. (A)** Lateral view, **(B)** medial view (sagittal section), and **(C)** sagittal section showing noncontractile structures that normally limit motion. Motion limited by structures is identified in brackets, using the following abbreviations: *D,* depression of mandible; *O,* occlusion; *P,* protrusion; *LD,* lateral deviation.

TABLE 9-2 Joint Structure: Cervical Spine Movements

	Flexion	Extension	Lateral Flexion	Rotation
Articulation[1,2]	Atlanto-occipital Atlantoaxial Intervertebral	Atlanto-occipital Atlantoaxial Intervertebral	Atlanto-occipital Intervertebral (with rotation)	Atlanto-occipital Atlantoaxial Intervertebral (with lateral flexion)
Plane	Sagittal	Sagittal	Frontal	Transverse
Axis	Frontal	Frontal	Sagittal	Vertical
Normal limiting factors[7,8]★ (see Fig. 9-5)	Tension in the tectorial membrane, posterior atlantoaxial ligament, posterior longitudinal ligament, ligamentum nuchae, ligamentum flavum, posterior neck muscles, and posterior fibers of annulus; contact between anterior rim of foramen magnum of skull and dens (atlanto-occipital joint)	Tension in the anterior longitudinal ligament and anterior atlantoaxial neck muscles; anterior fibers of annulus; bony contact between the spinous processes	Tension in the alar ligament limits lateral flexion to the contralateral side; lateral fibers of annulus; uncinate processes	Tension in the alar ligament limits rotation to the ipsilateral side; tension in the annulus fibrosis
Normal AROM CROM[9]†	0–45°	0–65°	0–35°	0–60°
Tape Measure[10,11]‡	3 cm	20 cm	13 cm	11 cm
Inclinometer[12]	0–50°	0–60°	0–45°	0–80°
Universal Goniometer[13]	0–45°	0–45°	0–45°	

*There is a paucity of definitive research that identifies the normal limiting factors (NLF) of joint motion. The NLF and end feels listed here are based on knowledge of anatomy, clinical experience, and available references.

†AROM for 337 healthy subjects between 11 and 97 years of age. Values represent the means of the mean values (rounded to the nearest 5°) from each age group as derived from the original source.[9]

‡Values represent the mean (rounded to the nearest cm) of the mean values derived from both studies.[10,11]

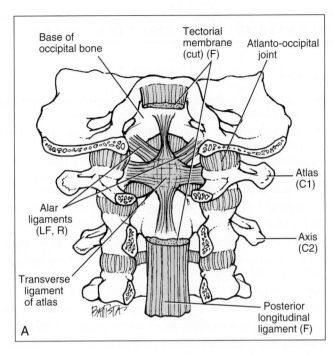

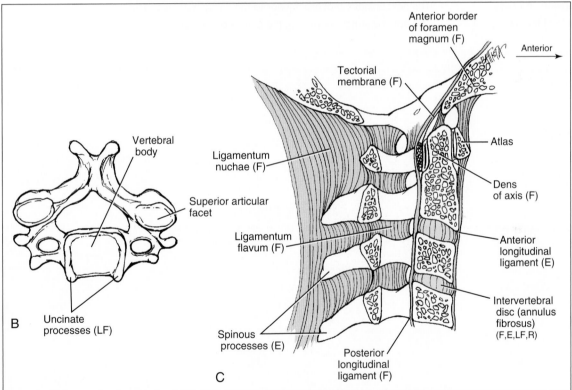

Figure 9-5 **Normal Limiting Factors. (A)** Posterior view (frontal section) of the occiput and upper cervical spine, **(B)** superior view of a cervical vertebra, and **(C)** sagittal section of the occiput and cervical spine (C1–4) showing noncontractile structures that normally limit motion. Motion limited by structures is identified in brackets, using the following abbreviations: *F,* flexion; *E,* extension; *LF,* lateral flexion; *R,* rotation. Muscles normally limiting motion are not illustrated.

SURFACE ANATOMY: HEAD AND NECK (Figs. 9-6 through 9-9)

Structure	Location
1. Suprasternal (jugular) notch	The rounded depression at the superior border of the sternum and between the medial ends of each clavicle.
2. Thyroid cartilage	The most prominent laryngeal cartilage located at the level of the fourth and fifth cervical vertebrae; subcutaneous projection (Adam's apple).
3. Hyoid bone	A submandibular U-shaped bone located above the thyroid cartilage at the level of the third cervical vertebra; the body is felt in the midline below the chin at the angle formed between the floor of the mouth and the front of the neck.
4. Angle of the mandible	The angle of the lower jaw located medially and distally to the earlobe.
5. Angle of the mouth	The lateral angle formed by the upper and lower lips.
6. Nasolabial fold	The fold of skin extending from the nose to the angle of the mouth.
7. Temporomandibular joint	The joint may be palpated anterior to the tragus of the external ear during opening and closing of the mouth.
8. Mastoid process	Bony prominence of the skull located behind the ear.
9. Acromion process	Lateral aspect of the spine of the scapula at the tip or point of the shoulder.
10. Spine of the scapula	The bony ridge running obliquely across the upper four fifths of the scapula.
11. C7 spinous process	Often the most prominent spinous process at the base of the neck.
12. T1 spinous process	The next spinous process inferior to the C7 spinous process.
13. Lobule of the ear	The soft lowermost portion of the auricle of the ear.

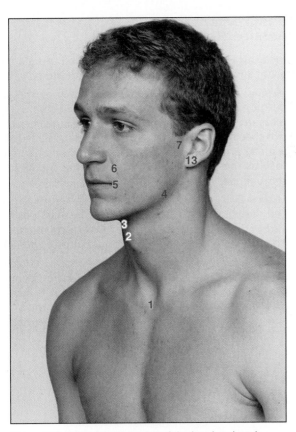

Figure 9-6 Anterolateral aspect of the head and neck.

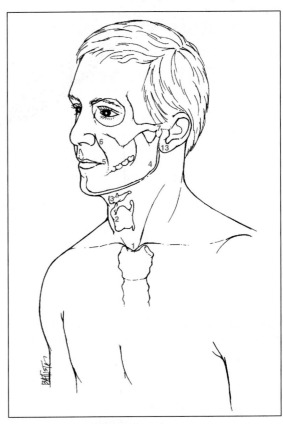

Figure 9-7 Surface anatomy, anterolateral aspect of the head and neck.

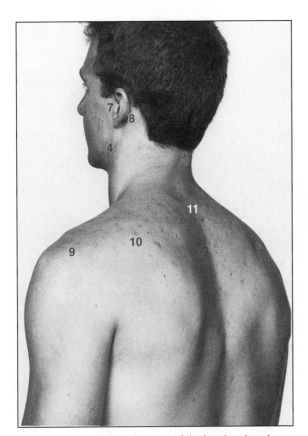

Figure 9-8 Posterolateral aspect of the head and neck.

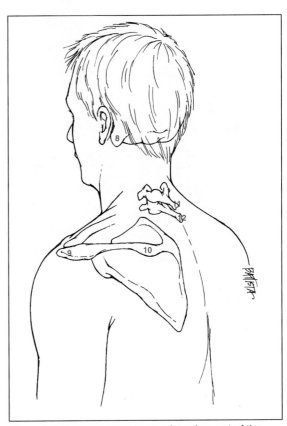

Figure 9-9 Bony anatomy, posterolateral aspect of the head and neck.

INSTRUMENTATION AND MEASUREMENT PROCEDURES: TMJ AND SPINE

Active ROM (AROM) measurements of the TMJs are made using a ruler or calipers. Instruments used to measure spinal AROM include the tape measure, standard inclinometer, the Cervical Range-of-Motion Instrument (CROM)[17] (Performance Attainment Associates, Roseville, MN), the Back Range-of-Motion Instrument (BROMII), and the universal goniometer. These instruments and the general principles for use of each instrument are described, with the exception of the universal goniometer and OB "Myrin" goniometer that are described in Chapter 1.

Tape Measure/Ruler/Calipers

A ruler or calipers are used to measure the AROM of the TMJs, and a tape measure is commonly used to measure AROM of the spine.

Measurement Procedure: Tape Measure/Ruler

A linear measurement of AROM is obtained using a tape measure and one of the following three methods:

Method 1 (Fig. 9-10): The patient moves to the end position for the motion being tested. Using a tape measure, the therapist measures the distance between two specified anatomical landmarks or a specified anatomical landmark and a stationary external surface, such as the plinth or floor to determine the ROM in centimeters.

Method 2 (Fig. 9-11): The distance between two specified vertebral levels is measured at the start position and at the end position for the ROM being measured. The difference between the two measures is the ROM in centimeters.

Method 3 (Fig. 9-12): The location of an anatomical landmark that moves with the test motion is marked on a stationary part of the body at the start and at the end of the ROM. The distance between the marks is the ROM for the movement.

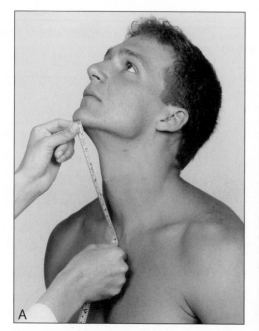
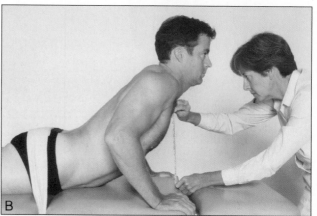

Figure 9-10 Tape measure method 1: the distance measured between **(A)** two anatomical landmarks, e.g., neck extension AROM, or **(B)** an anatomical landmark and an external surface, for example, the plinth for thoracolumbar extension AROM.

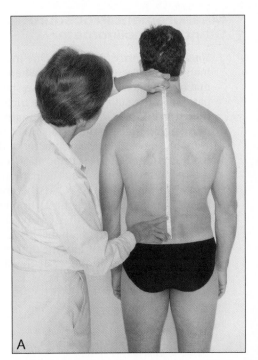
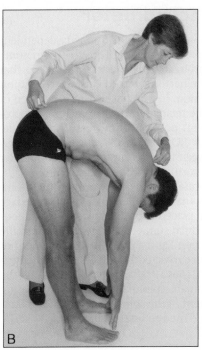

Figure 9-11 Tape measure method 2: e.g., thoracolumbar flexion AROM the difference between the distances measured between the two vertebral levels S2 and C7 at the **(A)** start position and **(B)** end position, is the AROM for thoracolumbar flexion.

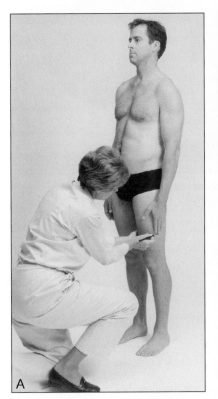
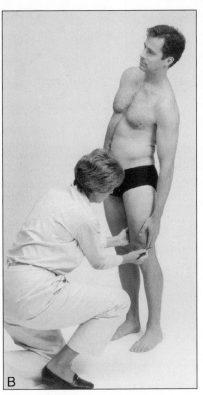
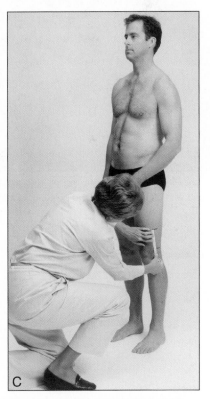

Figure 9-12 Tape measure method 3: e.g., trunk lateral flexion AROM – the location of the tip of the third finger is marked on the thigh at the **(A)** start position, **(B)** end position, and **(C)** the distance between the marks is the AROM for trunk lateral flexion.

Standard Inclinometer

The standard inclinometer contains a gravity-dependent needle and a 360° protractor scale (Fig. 9-13). On some inclinometers, the protractor scale can be rotated so that the gravity inclination needle is zeroed at the start position for the measured motion. In this case, the final position of the inclination needle relative to the protractor scale provides the ROM or joint position in degrees. If the needle cannot be zeroed, the ROM will be recorded as the difference in degrees between the readings on the inclinometer at the start and end positions for the assessed motion.

The therapist normally holds the standard inclinometer in place over an anatomical landmark(s). The surface of the inclinometer placed in contact with the patient may consist of a fixed flat surface, fixed feet, or adjustable feet. Adjustable feet (see Fig. 1-30) facilitate placement of the inclinometer over curved body surfaces. The American Medical Association (AMA)[12] has advocated using the inclinometer to evaluate spinal ROM when evaluating permanent impairment of the spine. One or two standard inclinometers may be used to assess ROM.

Measurement Procedure: Standard Inclinometer

Single Inclinometry (Fig. 9-13). One inclinometer is normally used to assess the AROM when either the proximal or distal joint body segment is stabilized. With the patient in the start position, the inclinometer is positioned in relation to a specified anatomical landmark, normally located on the distal end of the moving joint segment. If possible, the protractor of the inclinometer is adjusted to 0° in the start position, or the reading on the inclinometer is noted. The patient is instructed to move through the AROM. At the end of the movement, the therapist reads the inclinometer. If the inclinometer was zeroed in the start position, the reading is the ROM in degrees. If the inclinometer was not zeroed at the start position, the difference between the reading on the inclinometer at the start and the end positions is recorded as the ROM.

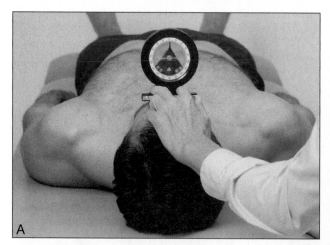 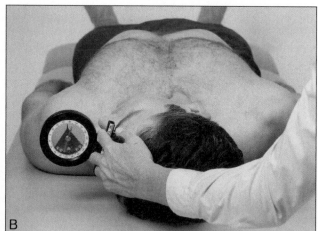

Figure 9-13 Single inclinometry. **(A)** Neck rotation AROM start position: supine with trunk stabilized, single inclinometer aligned on forehead with dial zeroed. **(B)** End position: reading on the inclinometer indicates neck rotation AROM.

Double Inclinometry (Fig. 9-14). When two standard inclinometers are used to assess AROM, the patient is in the start position with one inclinometer placed at a specified anatomical landmark at the inferior end of the spinal segments being measured. A second inclinometer is placed at a specified anatomical landmark at the superior end of the spinal segments being measured. The protractor of each inclinometer is either

i. Adjusted to 0° in the start position by a second therapist, or

ii. The readings on the inclinometers are noted at the start position.

The patient is instructed to move through the AROM.

At the end of the movement, the therapist reads each inclinometer.

If the inclinometers were zeroed in the start position, the difference between the two readings on the inclinometers at the end position is the AROM for the spinal movement being assessed.

If the inclinometers were not zeroed in the start position, the difference between the readings at the start and at the end positions on each inclinometer provides the ROM at each inclinometer location. The difference between the ROM at each inclinometer location is recorded as the ROM for the assessed movement.

When measuring ROM, the therapist ensures that sources of error (described in Chapter 1) do not occur or are minimized, so that ROM measurements will be reliable and the patient's progress can be meaningfully monitored. Note that Mayer and colleagues[18] studied the sources of error with inclinometric measurement of spinal ROM and found that "training and practice was the most significant factor (eliminating the largest source of error) improving overall test performance."[18(p. 1981)]

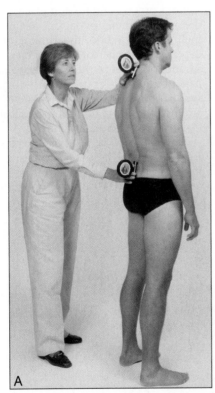
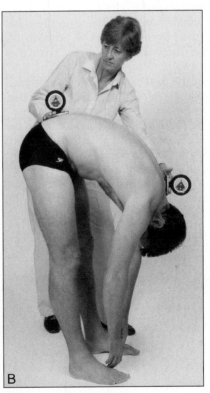

Figure 9-14 Double inclinometry. **(A)** Thoracolumbar spine flexion AROM start position with inclinometers placed over S2 and C7 and zeroed. **(B)** End position: the difference between the two inclinometer readings is the thoracolumbar flexion AROM.

Cervical Range-of-Motion Instrument (CROM)

The CROM[17] (Fig. 9-15) is designed to measure cervical spine motion. It consists of a headpiece (i.e., frame that holds three inclinometers) and a magnetic yoke. The inclinometers are located on the front and side of the CROM; each contains an inclination needle that is influenced by the force of gravity. The third inclinometer, situated in the transverse plane, contains a compass needle that reacts to earth's magnetic field for measurement of cervical spine rotation.

Measurement Procedure: CROM

The CROM is positioned on the patient's head with the bridge of the frame placed comfortably on the nose and the occipital strap snug (Fig. 9-15). The magnetic yoke is used when measuring cervical spine rotation ROM and serves to eliminate substitute trunk motion from the cervical spine rotation measurement. The magnetic yoke is positioned over the shoulders with the arrow on the yoke pointing north (indicated by observing the position of the red needle on the compass inclinometer with the yoke greater than 4 ft away).

With the patient in the start position for movements in either the sagittal plane (i.e., flexion/extension) or the frontal plane (i.e., lateral flexion), the gravity inclinometer situated in the same plane as that of the motion to be measured should read 0°. With the patient in the start position for movement in the transverse plane (i.e., rotation), both gravity inclinometers should read 0° by adjusting the patient's head position. The compass inclinometer is then rotated to read 0°.

The patient moves through the AROM to be measured. At the end of the test movement, the therapist reads the appropriate gravity or compass inclinometer and records the angular AROM measurement for the cervical spine movement being assessed.

Back Range-of-Motion Instrument (BROMII)

The Back Range-of-Motion Instrument (BROMII)[19] (Performance Attainment Associates, Roseville, MN) is a relatively new tool designed to measure AROM of the lumbar spine. It consists of two units for the measurement of back ROM. First, a frame that contains a protractor scale is positioned over S1 and held in place using Velcro straps. An L-shaped extension arm slides into the frame, and this device is used to measure lumbar flexion and extension ROM. Second, a frame that holds two inclinometers is positioned horizontally over the T12 spinous process and held in place by the therapist during the measurement of lateral flexion and rotation. One inclinometer lies in the frontal plane with a gravity-dependent needle for measurement of lateral flexion; a second, oriented in the transverse plane, contains a compass needle that reacts to Earth's magnetic field for measurement of rotation. A magnetic yoke is positioned around the pelvis to eliminate substitute pelvic motion from the rotation measurement.

The BROMII is relatively expensive, and from the research to date, it does not appear to be superior to other means of measuring AROM of the lumbar spine. For this reason, the BROMII is not used to demonstrate ROM assessment in this text.

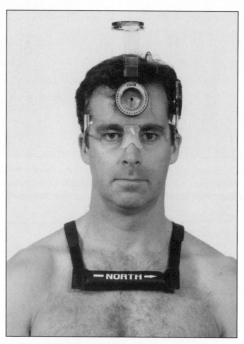

Figure 9-15 The Cervical Range-of-Motion Instrument (CROM).

ACTIVE RANGE OF MOTION ASSESSMENT AND MEASUREMENT: HEAD AND NECK

Practice Makes Perfect

To aid you in practicing the skills covered in this section, or for a handy review, use the practical testing forms found at http://thepoint.lww.com/Clarkson3e.

The use of the ruler and calipers to measure TMJ AROM are described and illustrated.

TMJ Movements

Start Position. The patient is sitting with the head, neck, and trunk in the anatomical position. The patient remains in this position throughout the test movements. It is important to maintain a standard position of the head and neck because the magnitude of mandibular opening is affected by head and neck position.[20,21] From the rest position (i.e., with the teeth not in contact), the patient performs elevation, depression, protrusion, or lateral deviation of the mandible.

Elevation of the Mandible

The patient elevates the lower jaw to a position where the teeth are in contact at full elevation (Fig. 9-16). The relative position of the mandibular teeth in relation to the maxillary teeth is observed.

Depression of the Mandible

Form 9-1

The patient is asked to open the mouth. On slow active opening of the mouth, the therapist observes for deviation of the mandible from the midline. In normal mouth opening, the mandible moves in a straight line. Deviation of the mandible to the left in the form of a C-type curve indicates hypomobility of the TMJ situated on the convex side of the C curve, or hypermobility of the joint on the concave side of the curve.[4] Deviation in the shape of an S-type curve may indicate a muscular imbalance or displacement of the condyle.[4]

Functional ROM normally required for daily activity is determined by placing two or three flexed proximal interphalangeal joints between the upper and lower central incisors[4] (Fig. 9-17). The fingers represent a distance of about 25 to 35 mm.[4]

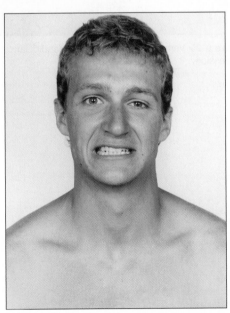

Figure 9-16 Occlusion of the teeth.

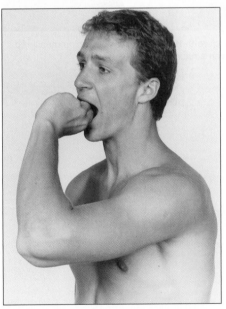

Figure 9-17 Functional ROM: opening of the mouth (depression of the mandible).

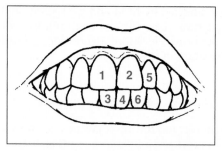

Figure 9-18 Teeth occluded. (1, 2) Maxillary central incisors. (3, 4) Mandibular central incisors. (5, 6) Lateral incisors.

Using a ruler and the edges of the upper and lower central incisors (Fig. 9-18) for reference, a measure of opening is obtained[22] for recording change (Fig. 9-19). Vernier calipers may also be used to measure the distance between the edges of the upper and lower central incisors to establish the range of mandibular depression (Fig. 9-20). Normal depression of the mandible (mouth opening) is 35 to 50 mm.[4]

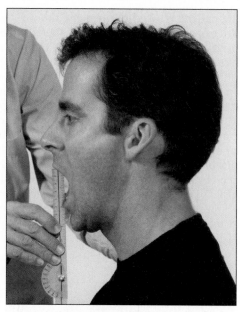

Figure 9-19 Mandibular depression measured with a ruler.

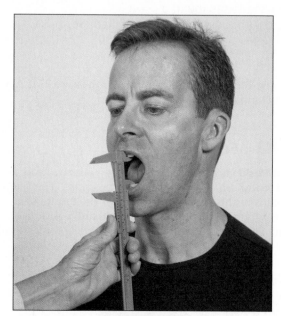

Figure 9-20 Vernier calipers measure mandibular depression.

Protrusion of the Mandible

Form 9-2

The patient protrudes the lower jaw (Fig. 9-21) to place the lower teeth beyond the upper teeth. A ruler measurement is obtained by measuring the distance between the upper and lower central incisors[22] (Fig. 9-21). From resting position, normal protrusion is 3 to 7 mm.[5]

Lateral Deviation of the Mandible

Form 9-3

The patient deviates the lower jaw to one side and then the other (Fig. 9-22). Lateral deviation of the mandible should be symmetrical. A measure is obtained for recording purposes by measuring the distance between two selected points that are level, one on the upper teeth and one on the lower teeth,[4] such as the space between the central incisors. The normal range of lateral deviation is 10 to 15 mm.[4]

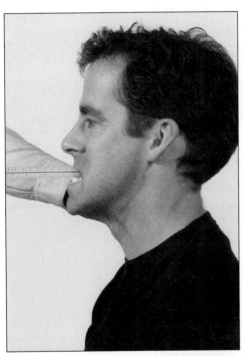

Figure 9-21 Ruler measurement of distance between the upper and lower central incisors, a measure of protrusion of the mandible.

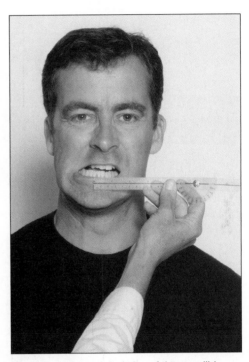

Figure 9-22 Lateral deviation of the mandible.

Neck Movements

Tests of head and neck movement are contraindicated in some instances. Contraindications include pathology that may result in spinal instability and pathology of the vertebral artery. In the absence of contraindications, cervical spine AROM may be assessed.

The measurement of cervical spine AROM is described and illustrated using the tape measure, inclinometer, CROM, and universal goniometer. When measuring cervical spine AROM, the start position (sitting) and the stabilization are the same for all neck movements regardless of the instrument used to measure the AROM, with one exception: the start position for active cervical spine rotation is supine when measured using an inclinometer.

Start Position. The patient is sitting in a chair with a back support. The feet are flat on the floor and the arms are relaxed at the sides. The head and neck are in the anatomical (neutral zero) position (Fig. 9-23).

Stabilization. The back of the chair provides support for the thoracic and lumbar spines. The patient is instructed to avoid substitute movement and the therapist can stabilize the trunk.

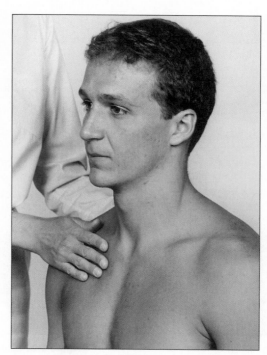

Figure 9-23 Start position for all movements of the neck with the exception of rotation when measured using the inclinometer.

Neck Flexion–Extension

End Positions. *Flexion:* The patient flexes the neck to the limit of the motion. *Extension:* The patient extends the neck to the limit of motion.

Substitute Movement. Mouth opening (for tape measurements), trunk flexion–extension.

Tape Measure Measurement

 Flexion. The distance is measured between the tip of the chin and the suprasternal notch. A measure is taken in the flexed position (Fig. 9-24). The linear measure reflects the neck flexion AROM (3 cm).

Forms 9-4, 9-5

Extension. The same reference points are used. A measure is taken in the extended position (Fig. 9-25). The linear measure reflects the range of neck extension AROM (20 cm).

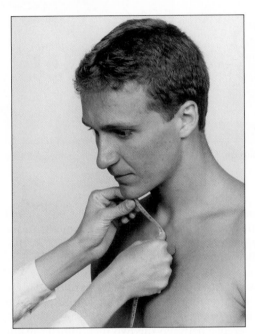

Figure 9-24 Neck flexion: limited AROM.

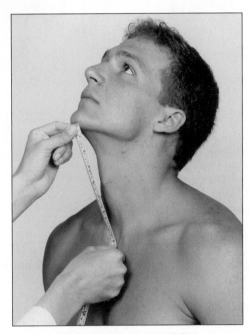

Figure 9-25 Neck extension: full AROM.

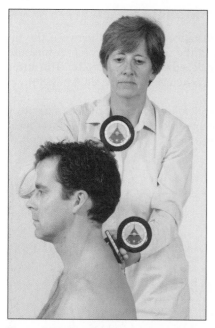

Figure 9-26 Start position: neck flexion and extension with inclinometers positioned on the vertex of the head and over the spine of T1.

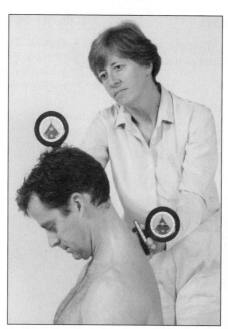

Figure 9-27 End position: neck flexion.

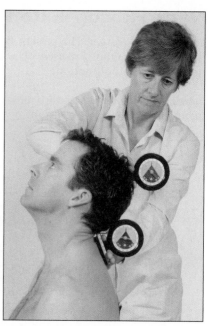

Figure 9-28 End position: neck extension.

Inclinometer Measurement

Forms 9-6, 9-7

Inclinometer Placement. *Superior:* On the vertex (i.e., top[23]) of the head. *Inferior:* On the spine of T1. In the start position (Fig. 9-26), the inclinometers are zeroed.

Alternate Inclinometer Placement

The inferior inclinometer is positioned over the spine of the scapula,[24] as shown in Fig. 9-29, if the position of the inclinometer over T1 hinders neck extension ROM or a large neck extension ROM displaces the inclinometer.

Flexion. At the limit of neck flexion (Fig. 9-27 or 9-30), the therapist records the angle measurements from both inclinometers. The neck flexion AROM (50°) is the difference between the two inclinometer readings.

Extension. At the limit of neck extension (Fig. 9-28 or 9-31), the therapist records the angle measurements from both inclinometers. The neck extension AROM (60°) is the difference between the two inclinometer readings.

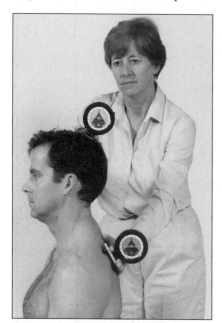

Figure 9-29 Alternate inclinometer placement, start position: neck flexion and extension with inclinometers positioned on the vertex of the head and over the spine of the scapula.

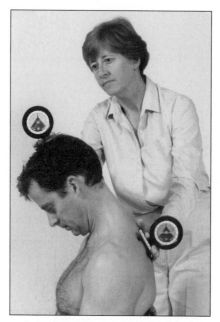

Figure 9-30 End position: neck flexion.

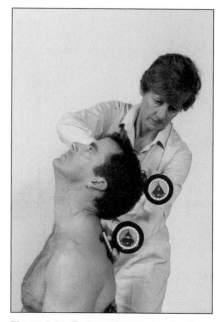

Figure 9-31 End position: neck extension.

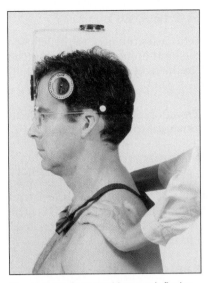

Figure 9-32 Start position: neck flexion and extension.

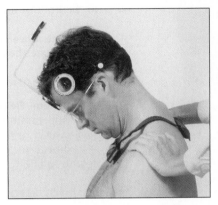

Figure 9-33 End position: neck flexion.

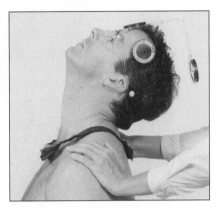

Figure 9-34 End position: neck extension.

CROM Measurement

 By positioning the patient's head, the inclinometer on the lateral aspect of the CROM is zeroed in the start position (Fig. 9-32).

Forms 9-8, 9-9

Flexion. The neck is flexed to the limit of motion and the reading on the lateral inclinometer is the neck flexion AROM (45°) (Fig. 9-33).

Extension. The neck is extended to the limit of motion and the reading on the lateral inclinometer is the neck extension AROM (65°) (Fig. 9-34).

Universal Goniometer Measurement

Goniometer Axis. Over the lobule of the ear (Fig. 9-35).

Stationary Arm. Perpendicular to the floor.

Movable Arm. Lies parallel to the base of the nares. In the start position (Fig. 9-35), the goniometer will indicate 90°. This is recorded as 0°.

Forms 9-10, 9-11

Flexion. The goniometer is realigned at the limit of neck flexion (Fig. 9-36). The number of degrees the movable arm lies away from the 90° position is recorded as the neck flexion AROM (45°).

Extension. The goniometer is realigned at the limit of neck extension (Fig. 9-37). The number of degrees the movable arm lies away from the 90° position is recorded as the neck extension AROM (45°).

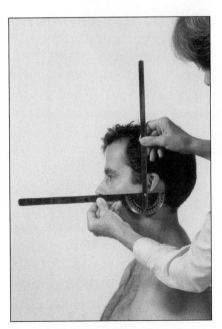

Figure 9-35 Start position: universal goniometer placement for neck flexion and extension.

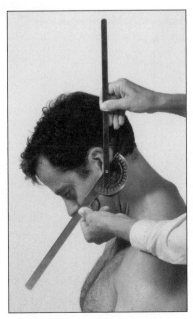

Figure 9-36 End position: neck flexion.

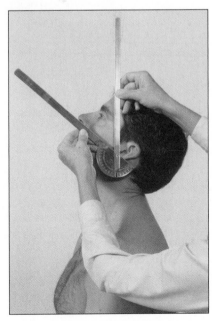

Figure 9-37 End position: neck extension.

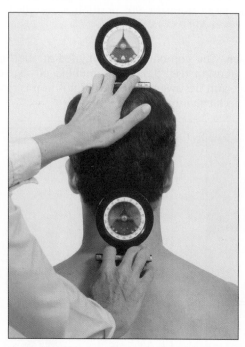

Figure 9-38 Neck lateral flexion.

Neck Lateral Flexion

End Positions. The patient flexes the neck to the left side (without rotation) to the limit of motion (Fig. 9-38). The patient flexes the neck to the right side (without rotation) to the limit of motion.

Substitute Movement. Elevation of the shoulder girdle to approximate the ear; ipsilateral trunk lateral flexion.

Tape Measure Measurement

Lateral Flexion. The distance is measured between the mastoid process of the skull and the lateral aspect of the acromion process (see Fig. 9-38). The linear measure reflects the range of neck lateral flexion AROM (13 cm) to the side measured.

Form 9-12

Inclinometer Measurement

Inclinometer Placement. *Superior:* On the vertex (i.e., top) of the head. *Inferior:* On the spine of T1. In the start position (Fig. 9-39), the inclinometers are zeroed.

Form 9-13

Lateral Flexion. At the limit of neck lateral flexion (Fig. 9-40), the therapist records the angle measurements from both inclinometers. The neck lateral flexion AROM (45°) is the difference between the two inclinometer readings.

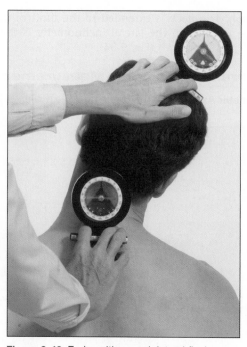

Figure 9-39 Start position: neck lateral flexion.

Figure 9-40 End position: neck lateral flexion.

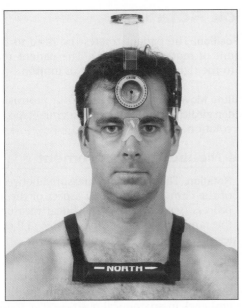

Figure 9-41 Start position: neck lateral flexion.

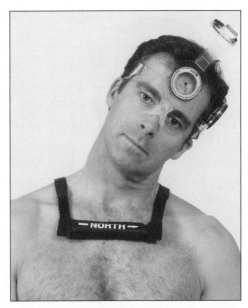

Figure 9-42 Neck lateral flexion.

CROM Measurement

Form 9-14

By positioning the patient's head, the inclinometer on the anterior aspect of the CROM is zeroed in the start position (Fig. 9-41).

Lateral Flexion. The neck is laterally flexed to the limit of motion, and the reading on the anterior inclinometer is the neck lateral flexion AROM (35°) to the side measured (Fig. 9-42).

Universal Goniometer Measurement

Form 9-15

Goniometer Axis. Over the C7 spinous process (Fig. 9-43).

Stationary Arm. Along the spine and perpendicular to the floor.

Movable Arm. Points toward the midpoint of the head. In the start position (Fig. 9-43), the goniometer will indicate 0°.

Lateral Flexion. The goniometer is realigned at the limit of neck lateral flexion (Fig. 9-44). The number of degrees the movable arm lies away from the 0° position is recorded as the neck lateral flexion AROM (45°) to the side measured.

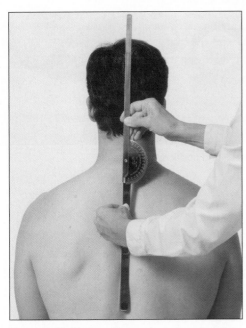

Figure 9-43 Start position: universal goniometer alignment neck lateral flexion.

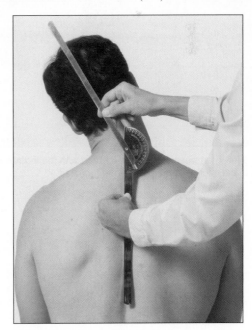

Figure 9-44 End position: neck lateral flexion.

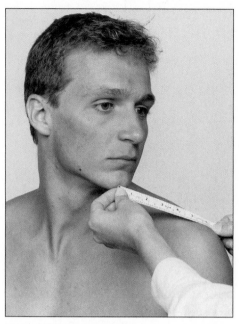

Figure 9-45 Neck rotation.

Neck Rotation

End Position. The patient rotates the head to the left to the limit of motion (Fig. 9-45). The patient rotates the head to the right side to the limit of motion.

Substitute Movement. Elevation and/or protrusion of the shoulder girdle to approximate the chin (tape measure); trunk rotation.

Tape Measure Measurement

Rotation. The distance is measured between the tip of the chin and the lateral aspect of the acromion process (see Fig. 9-45). The linear measure reflects the range of neck rotation AROM (11 cm) to the side measured.

Form 9-16

Inclinometer Measurement

Start Position. The patient is supine with the head and neck in anatomical position (Fig. 9-46).

Form 9-17

Inclinometer Placement. In the midline at the base of the forehead. In the start position, the inclinometer is zeroed.

Rotation. At the limit of neck rotation (Fig. 9-47), the therapist records the inclinometer reading as the neck rotation AROM (80°) to the side measured.

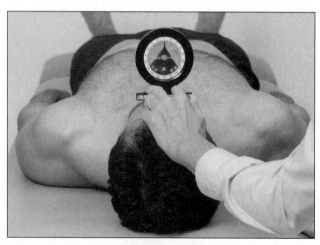

Figure 9-46 Start position for neck rotation with the inclinometer placed in the midline at the base of the forehead.

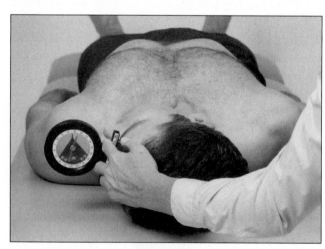

Figure 9-47 End position: neck rotation.

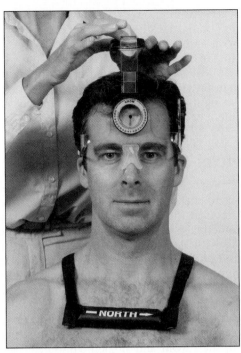

Figure 9-48 Start position: neck rotation.

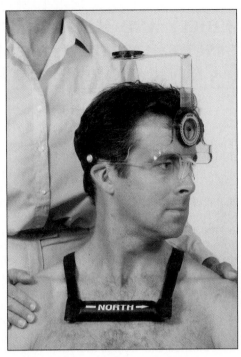

Figure 9-49 Neck rotation.

CROM Measurement

Form 9-18

The magnetic yoke is positioned over the shoulders with the arrow on the yoke pointing north. With the patient in the start position, both gravity inclinometers should read 0° (accomplished by adjusting the patient's head position). The compass inclinometer is then rotated to read 0° (Fig. 9-48).

Rotation. The neck is rotated to the limit of motion, and the reading on the compass inclinometer is the neck rotation AROM (60°) to the side measured (Fig. 9-49).

Universal Goniometer Measurement

Form 9-19

Goniometer Axis. Over the midpoint of the top of the head (Fig. 9-50).

Stationary Arm. Parallel to a line joining the two acromion processes.

Movable Arm. Aligned with the nose. In the start position (Fig. 9-50), the goniometer will indicate 90°. This is recorded as 0°.

Rotation. The goniometer is realigned at the limit of neck rotation (Fig. 9-51). The number of degrees the movable arm lies away from the 90° position is recorded as the neck rotation AROM.

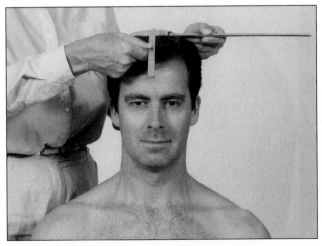

Figure 9-50 Start position: universal goniometer alignment neck rotation.

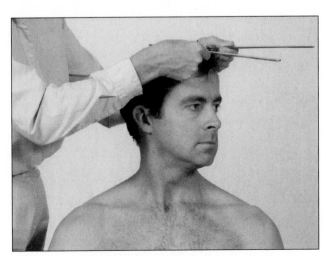

Figure 9-51 End position: neck rotation.

VALIDITY AND RELIABILITY: MEASUREMENT OF THE TMJ AND CERVICAL SPINE AROM

TMJ

The ruler and calipers are the tools used to measure TMJ AROM in this text.

Walker, Bohannon, and Cameron[25] evaluated the construct *validity* of using a ruler to measure AROM of the TMJs for mandibular depression, lateral deviation, and protrusion. The measurement of mouth opening was the only measure that demonstrated construct validity for identifying TMJ pathology. Therefore, the authors concluded that mouth opening measured by a ruler might be a possible method for documenting and monitoring the status of patients with TMJ disorders.

Evaluating the intra- and intertester *reliability* of the ruler for measuring mouth opening AROM, researchers[21,25–28] found the ruler to be reliable. Dijkstra and coworkers[26] pointed out that mandibular length might influence how much the mouth can be opened. Therefore, when comparing different subjects with the same linear mouth opening, one cannot conclude similar TMJ mobility. However, using a ruler to measure the distance between the central incisors in maximal mouth opening is a reliable and accurate measure of TMJ mobility when evaluating progress in the same subject over time.

Al-Ani and Gray[28] evaluated intra-instrument reliability of the ruler and an Alma bite gauge for measuring mouth opening. The Alma bite gauge is a set of calipers with recesses on the arms for ease of positioning against the edges of the central incisors. These researchers found the Alma bite gauge to have better reliability and ease of use when compared to the ruler.

For measurements of lateral deviation and protrusion of the TMJs using the ruler, Walker, Bohannon, and Cameron[25] found acceptable intratester reliability and good-to-excellent intertester reliability, but Dworkin and colleagues[27] found less-than-desirable intertester reliability. Dworkin and colleagues[27] also found that examiners trained in the standardized procedure for the measurement of TMJ AROM demonstrated better intertester reliability than untrained examiners, supporting the importance of using standardized procedures for reliable clinical measurement of TMJ AROM.

Cervical Spine

Reviews[29–31] of *validity and reliability* studies of tools and tests used to measure cervical spine ROM convey the present status of the research on this topic. This type of review, undertaken to select an appropriate measurement tool to assess ROM, is difficult due to the lack of optimized study designs, poor reporting in studies, lack of studies of some measurement methods, and studies having been conducted on a limited number of patient populations.[31]

Reviews by Williams, and associates[31] and de Koning and colleagues[30] concluded that although more research is needed, the CROM and single inclinometer were the most valid and reliable instruments for use in assessing cervical spine ROM. Jordon,[29] in an earlier review of the literature on the reliability of tools used to measure cervical spine ROM in clinical settings, could give "no strong recommendation for any tool" but found the CROM to be the most reliable tool. He also noted the CROM shows promise but may not be the most practical tool in the clinical setting due to cost, portability, and specificity for use in measuring only cervical spine ROM. Jordan[29] suggested the tape measure might be the preferred clinical option as it is inexpensive, portable, and clinically acceptable, but he found the tape measure needs more support in the literature. Williams, and associates[31] found visual estimation to be the least reliable and concurrently valid method, and along with de Koning and colleagues[30] recommended visual estimation not be used to measure cervical spine ROM.

MUSCLE STRENGTH ASSESSMENT: MUSCLES OF THE FACE (TABLE 9-3)

Practice Makes Perfect

To aid you in practicing the skills covered in this section, or for a handy review, use the practical testing forms found at http://thepoint.lww.com/Clarkson3e.

The muscles of the face and eyes (Figs. 9-52 through 9-55) are innervated by the cranial nerves (CN). The motor functions of CN III, IV, V, VI, VII, and XII are tested as a component part of a neurological examination. The objectives of testing are to determine the presence or absence of dysfunction and the functional implications of weakness or paralysis to the patient. The muscles are tested in groups according to their CN supply and common function.

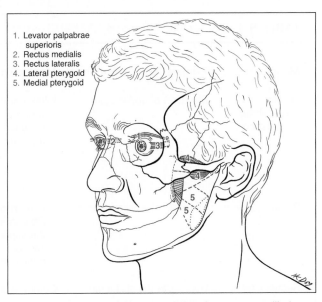

1. Levator palpabrae superioris
2. Rectus medialis
3. Rectus lateralis
4. Lateral pterygoid
5. Medial pterygoid

Figure 9-53 Muscles of the eye region and temporomandibular region.

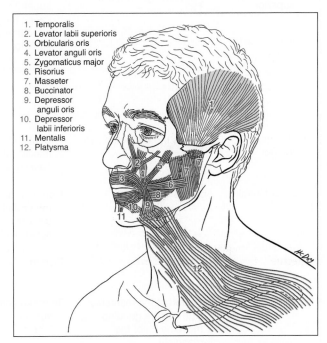

1. Temporalis
2. Levator labii superioris
3. Orbicularis oris
4. Levator anguli oris
5. Zygomaticus major
6. Risorius
7. Masseter
8. Buccinator
9. Depressor anguli oris
10. Depressor labii inferioris
11. Mentalis
12. Platysma

Figure 9-54 Muscles of the mouth, temporomandibular region, and platysma.

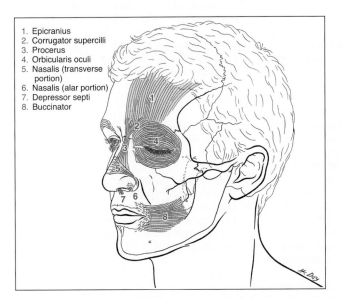

1. Epicranius
2. Corrugator supercilli
3. Procerus
4. Orbicularis oculi
5. Nasalis (transverse portion)
6. Nasalis (alar portion)
7. Depressor septi
8. Buccinator

Figure 9-52 Deep muscles of the eye, nose, and cheek.

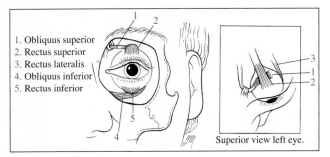

1. Obliquus superior
2. Rectus superior
3. Rectus lateralis
4. Obliquus inferior
5. Rectus inferior

Superior view left eye.

Figure 9-55 Muscles controlling eye movements.

TABLE 9-3   Muscle Actions, Attachments, and Nerve Supply: The Face and Eyes[2]

Muscle	Primary Muscle Action	Muscle Origin	Muscle Insertion	Cranial Nerve
Levator palpebrae superioris	Elevation of upper eyelid	Inferior surface of the small wing of the sphenoid, superior and anterior to the optic canal	Skin of the upper eyelid; anterior surface of the superior tarsus; the superior conjunctival fornix; tubercle on the zygomatic bone; superior aspect of the orbital septum	III
Rectus superior	Elevates the abducted eye	Common annular tendon (fibrous ring surrounding the superior, medial and inferior margins of the optic canal)	The sclera superiorly, posterior to the margin of the cornea	III
Rectus inferior	Depresses the abducted eye	Common annular tendon	The sclera inferiorly, posterior to the margin of the cornea	III
Obliquus superior	Depresses the adducted eye	Body of the sphenoid superomedial to the optic canal; the tendinous attachment of the rectus superior	The tendon passes through the trochlea (a fibrocartilaginous loop attached to the fossa of the frontal bone) and then passes posteriorly, laterally and downward to insert into the sclera posterior to the equator on the superolateral aspect of the eyeball	IV
Obliquus inferior	Elevates the adducted eye	Orbital surface of the maxilla lateral to the nasolacrimal groove	Lateral part of the sclera, posterior to the equator of the eyeball	III
Rectus lateralis	Abducts the eye	Common annular tendon; the orbital surface of the greater wing of the sphenoid bone	The sclera laterally, posterior to the margin of the cornea	VI
Rectus medialis	Adducts the eye	Common annular tendon	The sclera medially, posterior to the margin of the cornea	III
Temporalis	Elevation of the mandible; side-to-side grinding movements of the mandible	Temporal fossa; deep surface of the temporal fascia	The coronoid process of the mandible; anterior border of the ramus of the mandible nearly as far as the last molar	V
Masseter	Elevation of the mandible; small effect in side-to-side movements, protraction, and retraction of the mandible	a. Superficial layer: maxillary process of the zygomatic bone; anterior two thirds of the zygomatic arch b. Middle layer: medial aspect of the anterior two thirds of the zygomatic arch; lower border of the posterior third of the mandibular ramus c. Deep layer: deep surface of the zygomatic arch	a. Superficial layer: angle and inferior half of the lateral surface of the mandibular ramus b. Middle layer: central part of the mandibular ramus c. Deep layer: upper part of the ramus of the mandible; the coronoid process of the mandible	V

TABLE 9-3 *Continued*

Muscle	Primary Muscle Action	Muscle Origin	Muscle Insertion	Cranial Nerve
Medial pterygoid	Elevation of the mandible; protrusion of the mandible (with the lateral pterygoid); side-to-side movements of the jaw	Medial aspect of the lateral pterygoid plate; pyramidal process of the palatine bone; tuberosity of the maxilla	Posteroinferior part of the medial surfaces of the ramus and angle of the mandible	V
Lateral pterygoid	Protrusion of the mandible (with the medial pterygoid); opening of the mouth; control of the posterior movement of the articular disc of the temporomandibular joint and condyle of the mandible during mouth closing; side-to-side movements of the mandible	a. Upper head: inferior part and lateral surface of the great wing of the sphenoid bone b. Lower head: the lateral surface of the lateral pterygoid plate	Depression on the anterior aspect of the neck of the mandible; articular capsule and disc of the temporomandibular articulation	V

Suprahyoid muscles (diagastric, stylohyoid, mylohyoid, and geniohyoid)

Muscle	Primary Muscle Action	Muscle Origin	Muscle Insertion	Cranial Nerve
Digastric	Depression of the mandible; elevation of the hyoid bone (swallowing, chewing)	Posterior belly: mastoid process of the temporal bone Anterior belly: digastric fossa on the base of the mandible near the midline	The course of the muscle changes direction as it passes through a fibrous loop attached to the hyoid bone	V, VII
Stylohyoid	Elevation and retraction of the hyoid bone (swallowing)	Posterior aspect of the styloid process of the temporal bone	The body of the hyoid bone at its junction with the greater cornu	VII
Mylohyoid	Elevation of the floor of the mouth (swallowing); elevation of the hyoid bone; depression of the mandible	The entire mylohyoid line of the mandible	Body of the hyoid bone; median fibrous raphe from the symphysis menti of the mandible to the hyoid bone	V
Geniohyoid	Elevation and protraction of the hyoid bone; depression of the mandible	Inferior mental spine on the posterior aspect of the symphysis menti	Anterior aspect of the body of the hyoid bone	XII
Epicranius occipitof- rontalis	Elevation of the eyebrows and skin over the root of the nose, resulting in transverse wrinkling of the forehead	Frontal part: epicranial aponeurosis anterior to the coronal suture	Fibers are continuous with procerus, corrugator supercilii and orbicularis oculi; the skin of the eyebrows and the root of the nose	VII

(continued)

TABLE 9-3 Continued

Muscle	Primary Muscle Action	Muscle Origin	Muscle Insertion	Cranial Nerve
Corrugator supercilii	Draws the eyebrows together, resulting in vertical wrinkles on the supranasal strip of the forehead	Medial end of the superciliary arch	The skin above the supraorbital margin	VII
Procerus	Draws the medial angle of the eyebrow inferiorly to wrinkle the skin transversely over the bridge of nose	Fascia covering the inferior portion of the nasal bone; superior portion of the lateral nasal cartilage	Skin over the inferior aspect of the forehead between the eyebrows	VII
Orbicularis oculi	a. Orbital part: closes the eyelids tightly drawing the skin of forehead, temple and cheek medially towards the nose b. Palpebral part: closes the eyelids gently	a. Orbital part: nasal part of the frontal bone; frontal process of the maxilla; medial palpebral ligament b. Palpebral part: the medial palpebral ligament and bone immediately above and below the ligament c. Lacrimal part: the lacrimal fascia; the upper part of the crest and adjacent part of the lacrimal bone	The fibers sweep around the circumference of the orbit; skin and subcutaneous tissues of the eyebrow; tarsi of the eyelids; the lateral palpebral raphe	VII
Nasalis				
1. Alar portion	Widens the nasal opening	Maxilla superior to the lateral incisor tooth	Alar cartilage of the nose	VII
2. Transverse-portion	Narrows the nasal opening	Maxilla lateral to the nasal notch	By an aponeurosis that merges on the bridge of the nose with the muscle of the contralateral side; the aponeurosis of the procerus muscle	VII
Depressor septi	Widens the nasal opening	Maxilla superior to the central incisor tooth	The nasal septum	VII
Orbicularis oris	Closure of the lips; protrusion of the lips	The modiolus at the lateral angle of the mouth; several strata of muscle fibers of other facial muscles that insert into the lips, principally buccinator	The majority of fibers, into the deep surface of the skin and mucous membrane	VII
Buccinator	Compression of the cheeks against the teeth	The alveolar processes of the mandible and maxilla, opposite the three molar teeth; the anterior border of the pterygomandibular raphe	The skin and mucosa of the lips blending with orbicularis oris; the modiolus	VII

TABLE 9-3   *Continued*

Muscle	Primary Muscle Action	Muscle Origin	Muscle Insertion	Cranial Nerve
Levator anguli oris	Elevation of the angle of the mouth; produces the nasolabial furrow	Canine fossa of the maxilla just inferior to the infraorbital foramen	The modiolus at the lateral angle of the mouth blends with orbicularis oris, depressor anguli oris; the dermal floor of the lower part of the nasolabial furrow	VII
Risorius	Retraction of the angle of the mouth	The parotid fascia over the masseter; parotid fascia; zygomatic arch; fascia enclosing pars modiolaris of platysma; fascia over mastoid process	The modiolus at the lateral angle of the mouth	VII
Zygomaticus major	Draws the angle of the mouth superiorly and laterally	Zygomatic bone anterior to the zygomaticotemporal suture	The modiolus at the lateral angle of the mouth blending with levator anguli oris, and orbicularis oris	VII
Platysma	Depression of the corner of the mouth and lower lip; depression of the jaw; tenses skin over the neck	The fascia covering the superior portion of the pectoralis major and deltoid muscles	Inferior border of the mandible; the skin and subcutaneous tissues of the inferior aspect of the face and corner of the mouth into the modiolus; blends with the contralateral platysma medially; lateral half of the lower lip	VII
Depressor anguli oris	Depression of the angle of the mouth	Oblique line of the mandible	The modiolus at the lateral angle of the mouth	VII
Depressor labii inferioris	Depression and lateral movement of the lower lip	Oblique line of the mandible, between the mental foramen and the symphysis menti	Skin of the lower lip blending with the contralateral depressor labii inferioris and orbicularis oris	VII
Levator labii superioris	Elevation and eversion of the upper lip	Inferior margin of the orbital opening immediately superior to the infraorbital foramen, from the maxilla and zygomatic bones	The muscular substance of the lateral half of the upper lip	VII
Zygomaticus minor	Elevation of the upper lip	Lateral aspect of the zygomatic bone immediately posterior to the zygomaticomaxillary suture	The muscular substance of the lateral aspect of the upper lip	VII
Levator labii superioris alaeque-nasi	Elevation of the upper lip; dilation of the nostril	Superior aspect of the frontal process of the maxilla	Ala of the nose; skin and muscular substance on the lateral aspect of the upper lip	VII

(continued)

TABLE 9-3 Continued

Muscle	Primary Muscle Action	Muscle Origin	Muscle Insertion	Cranial Nerve
Mentalis	Elevation and protrusion of the lower lip	Incisive fossa of the mandible	Skin of the chin	VII
Genioglossus	Tongue protrusion; depression of the middle region of the tongue	Upper genial tubercle on the inner surface of the symphysis of the mandible	Under surface of the tongue from the root to the apex of the tongue; via an aponeurosis to the superior aspect of the anterior surface of the hyoid bone	XII

Conventional grading is not applied to the results of testing as it is not always practical or possible to palpate the muscle, apply resistance, or position the patient. The results of the tests can be descriptive or recorded according to a defined set of parameters as follows[8]:

- 5   N (normal)   For completion of the test movement with ease and control
- 3   F (fair)   For performance of test movement with difficulty
- 1   T (trace)   No motion, minimal muscle contraction
- 0   0 (zero)   When no contraction can be elicited
- Observation of asymmetrical movement is documented.

A description of the test for the infrahyoid muscles is included with the facial muscles due to the functional significance of these muscles in mastication and swallowing. Swallowing is a complex process that involves the participation of the muscles of the jaw, tongue, lips, soft palate, pharynx, larynx, and suprahyoid and infrahyoid muscle groups. Weakness or paralysis in any of these muscles can affect the ability of the patient to move food from the tongue to the pharynx and esophagus. Head control is also necessary for swallowing. When testing the facial, submandibular, and neck muscles, the therapist should routinely ask the patient if any difficulty is experienced in swallowing, or observe the patient as liquid or a bolus of food is swallowed.

Oculomotor, Trochlear, and Abducens Nerves (CN III, IV, and VI)

Motor Function. Motor functions are opening of the eyelid (levator palpebrae superioris) (Fig. 9-53) and control of eye movements (the six extraocular muscles) (Figs. 9-53 and 9-55).

Component Movements Tested. Component movements are elevation of the upper eyelids and elevation, abduction, depression, and adduction of the eyeballs.

Elevation of the Upper Eyelid

Levator Palpebrae Superioris

Form
9-20

Test. The patient elevates or raises the upper eyelid (Fig. 9-56). The clinical term used to describe the inability to perform this movement is ptosis.

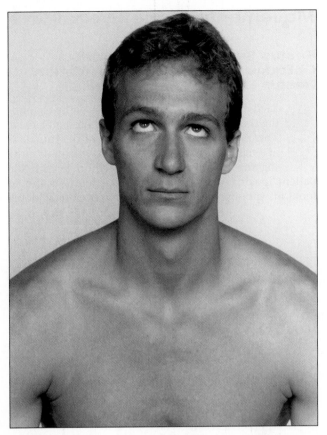

Figure 9-56 Elevation of the upper eyelid.

Movements of the Eyeball

Rectus Superior, Rectus Inferior, Obliquus Superior, Obliquus Inferior, Rectus Lateralis, Rectus Medialis

Forms
9-21 to
9-26

Each extraocular muscle can be tested by examining the muscle in its position of greatest efficiency. This position is when the action of the muscle is at a right angle to the axis around which it is moving the eyeball.[32] The start position is with the patient looking straight ahead. The patient is asked to look in various directions. The presence of diplopia (double vision) should be determined in conjunction with individual muscle tests.[32–34] *All test movements described pertain to the right eye of the patient* (Figs. 9-57 through 9-62). Simultaneous observation of specific movements of both eyes combines muscle tests and may be preferred. The muscle combinations are:

1. Right rectus superior and left obliquus inferior (see Fig. 9-57)
2. Right rectus inferior and left obliquus superior (see Fig. 9-58)
3. Right obliquus superior and left rectus inferior (see Fig. 9-59)

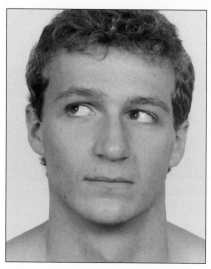

Figure 9-57 Rectus superior is tested by asking the patient to look upward and outward. Observe for limitation in elevation.

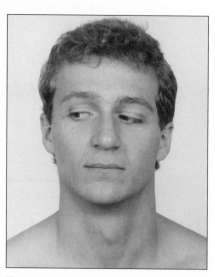

Figure 9-58 Rectus inferior is tested by asking the patient to look down and out. Observe for limitation in depression.

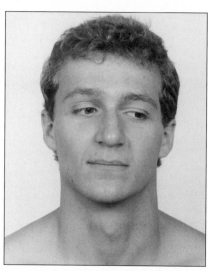

Figure 9-59 Obliquus superior is tested by asking the patient to look downward and inward. Observe for limitation in depression.

4. Right obliquus inferior and left rectus superior (see Fig. 9-60)
5. Right rectus lateralis and left rectus medialis (see Fig. 9-61)

6. Right rectus medialis and left rectus lateralis (see Fig. 9-62)

Observe whether the movement is normal (i.e., smooth through the full ROM) or abnormal.[8]

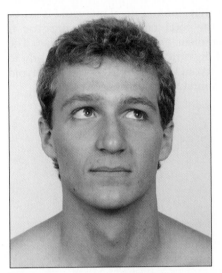

Figure 9-60 Obliquus inferior is tested by asking the patient to look upward and inward. Observe for limitation in elevation.

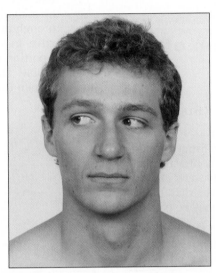

Figure 9-61 Rectus lateralis is tested by asking the patient to look outward (abduction). Observe the limitation in abduction.

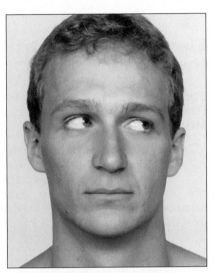

Figure 9-62 Rectus medialis is tested by asking the patient to look inward (adduction). Observe for limitation in adduction.

Trigeminal Nerve (CN V)

Motor Function. Motor function is mastication.

Component Movements Tested. Component movements are elevation, depression, protrusion, and retrusion of the mandible.

Elevation and Retrusion of the Mandible

Temporalis, Masseter, Medial Pterygoid, Lateral Pterygoid (Superior Head)

Form 9-27

Test. The patient closes the jaw and firmly clenches the teeth (Fig. 9-63). The force of contraction and muscle bulk of temporalis and masseter may be determined by palpation. Temporalis may be palpated over the temporal bone. Masseter may be palpated over the angle of the mandible.

Depression of the Mandible

Lateral Pterygoid, Suprahyoids (Mylohyoid, Digastric, Stylohyoid, Geniohyoid)

Form 9-28

Test. The patient opens the mouth by depressing the mandible (Fig. 9-64). Lateral pterygoid is active throughout the total range and the digastric is active in complete or forceful depression.[35] The anterior portion of digastric can be palpated inferiorly to the mandible. The hyoid bone is fixed by the infrahyoid muscles when the suprahyoid muscles contract.[36]

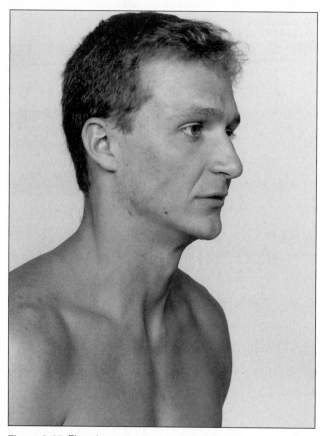

Figure 9-63 Elevation and retrusion of the mandible.

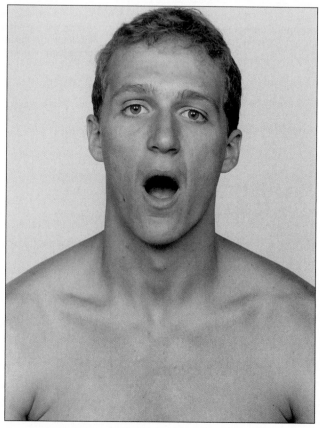

Figure 9-64 Depression of the mandible.

Protrusion of the Mandible

Medial and Lateral Pterygoids

 Test. With the mouth partially open, the patient protrudes the mandible (Fig. 9-65).

Form
9-29

Lateral Deviation of the Mandible

Temporalis, Medial and Lateral Pterygoids, Masseter

 Test. With the mouth slightly open, the patient deviates the lower jaw to one side and then the other (Fig. 9-66).

Form
9-30

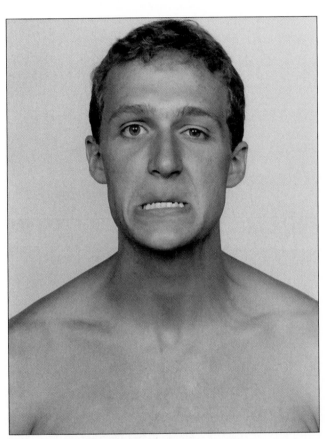

Figure 9-65 Protrusion of the mandible.

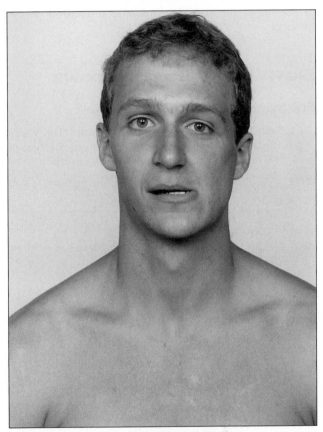

Figure 9-66 Contraction of the left temporalis and right medial and lateral pterygoids produces left lateral deviation of the mandible.

Facial Nerve (CN VII)

Motor Function. Motor functions are facial expression and control of the musculature of the eyebrows, eyelids, nose, and mouth.

Component Movements Tested. Component movements are (1) eyebrows: elevation, adduction, and depression; (2) eyelids: closure; (3) nose: dilation and constriction of the nasal opening; and (4) mouth: closure and protrusion of the lips; compression of the cheeks; elevation, retraction, and depression of the angle of the mouth; elevation of the upper lip; and elevation and protrusion of the lower lip.

Elevation of the Eyebrows

Epicranius (Occipitofrontalis)

Form 9-31

Test. The patient elevates the eyebrows (Fig. 9-67). The action forms transverse wrinkles of the skin of the forehead and the expression of surprise.

Adduction of the Eyebrows

Corrugator Supercili

Form 9-32

Test. The patient pulls the medial aspect of the eyebrows together (Fig. 9-68). This action forms vertical wrinkles between the eyebrows and the expression of frowning.

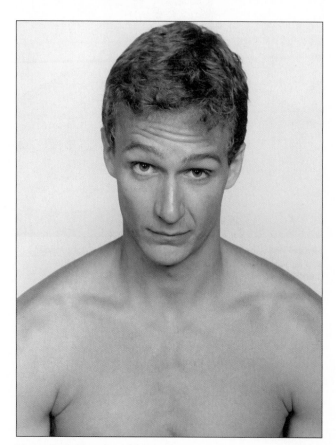

Figure 9-67 Elevation of the eyebrows.

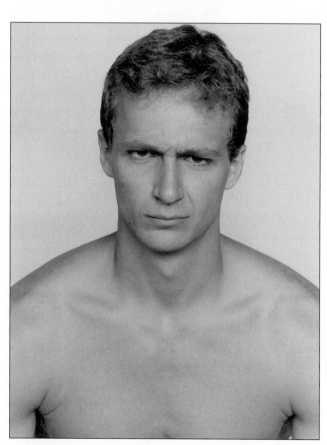

Figure 9-68 Adduction and depression of the eyebrows.

Depression of the Medial Angle of the Eyebrow

Procerus

Form 9-33

Test. The patient draws the medial angle of the eyebrows down and elevates the skin of the nose (Fig. 9-69). This action produces transverse wrinkles over the bridge of the nose. The patient may be asked to wrinkle the skin over the bridge of the nose as in the expression of distaste.

Closure of the Eyelids

Orbicularis Oculi

Form 9-34

Test. The patient closes the eyelids tightly (Fig. 9-70). This action pulls the skin of the forehead, temple, and cheek medially toward the nose.

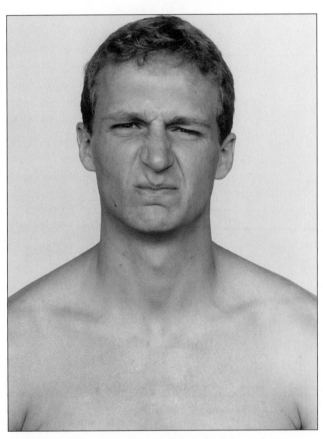

Figure 9-69 Depression of the medial angle of the eyebrow.

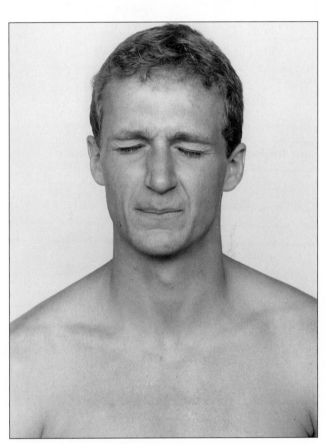

Figure 9-70 Closure of the eyelids.

Dilation of the Nasal Aperture

Nasalis (Alar Portion) Depressor Septi

 Test. The patient dilates or widens the nostrils (Fig. 9-71). To accomplish the movement, the patient may be asked to take a deep breath.

Form
9-35

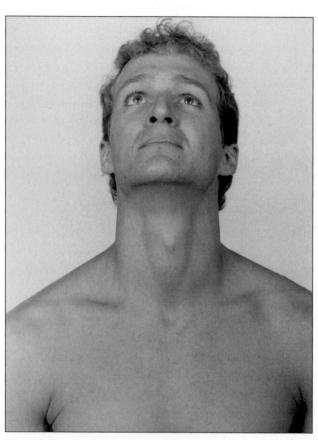

Figure 9-71 Dilation of the nasal aperture.

Constriction of the Nasal Aperture

Nasalis (Transverse Portion)

 Test. The patient compresses the nostrils together (Fig. 9-72).

Form
9-36

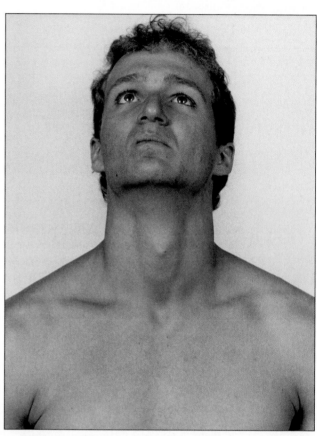

Figure 9-72 Constriction of the nasal aperture.

Closure and Protrusion of the Lips

Orbicularis Oris

 Test. The patient closes and protrudes the lips (Fig. 9-73). The patient may be asked to simulate whistling by pursing the lips.

Form 9-37

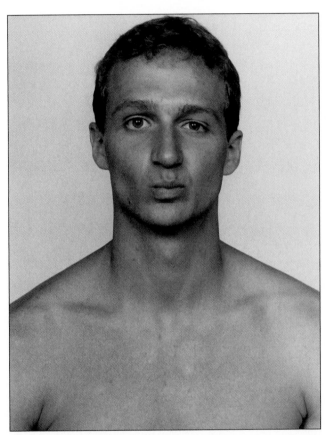

Figure 9-73 Closure and protrusion of the lips.

Compression of the Cheeks

Buccinator

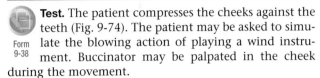 **Test.** The patient compresses the cheeks against the teeth (Fig. 9-74). The patient may be asked to simulate the blowing action of playing a wind instrument. Buccinator may be palpated in the cheek during the movement.

Form 9-38

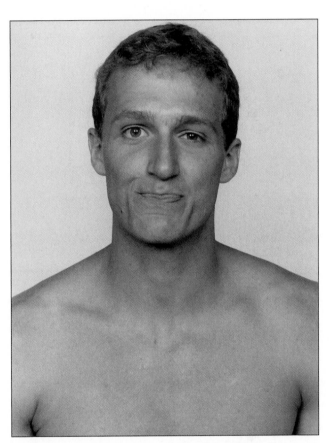

Figure 9-74 Compression of the cheeks against the teeth.

Elevation of the Angle of the Mouth

Levator Anguli Oris

Test. The patient raises the angle or corner of the mouth (Fig. 9-75). This action deepens the nasolabial fold.

Form 9-39

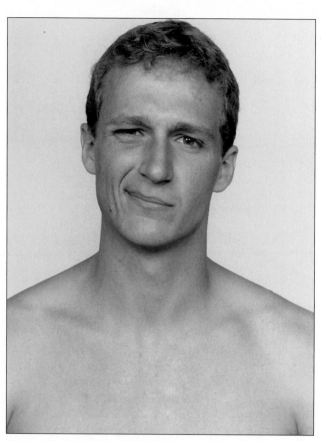

Figure 9-75 Elevation of the angle of the mouth.

Elevation and Retraction of the Angle of the Mouth

Zygomaticus Major

Test. The patient draws the angle of the mouth upward and laterally (Fig. 9-76). This action forms the facial expression of smiling. The muscle can be palpated above and lateral to the angle of the mouth.

Form 9-40

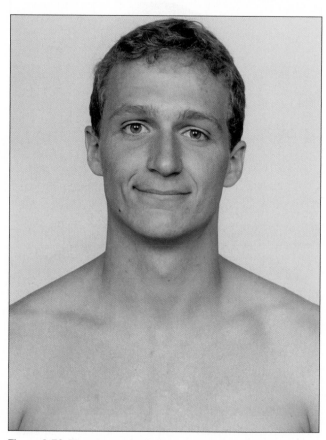

Figure 9-76 Elevation and retraction of the angle of the mouth.

Retraction of the Angle of the Mouth

Risorius

 Test. The patient retracts or draws the angle of the mouth in a posterior direction (Fig. 9-77). This action forms the facial expression of a grimace.

Form 9-41

Depression of the Angle of the Mouth and Lower Lip

Platysma, Depressor Anguli Oris, Depressor Labii Inferioris

 Test. The patient depresses the lower lip and angles of the mouth by drawing down the corners of the mouth and tensing the skin between the chin and the clavicle (Fig. 9-78). The patient may be asked to simulate the movement of easing the pressure of a tight shirt collar.

Form 9-42

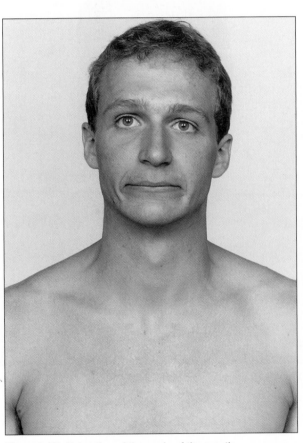

Figure 9-77 Retraction of the angle of the mouth.

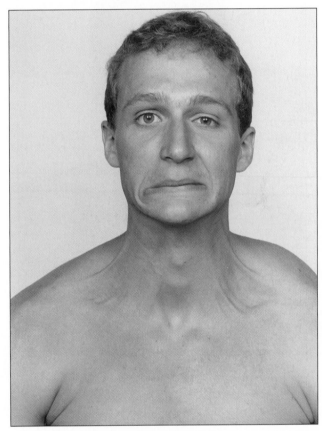

Figure 9-78 Depression of the angle of the mouth.

Elevation of the Upper Lip

Levator Labii Superioris, Zygomaticus Minor

Form 9-43

Test. The patient elevates and protrudes (everts) the upper lip (Fig. 9-79) as in showing the incisors or upper gums.

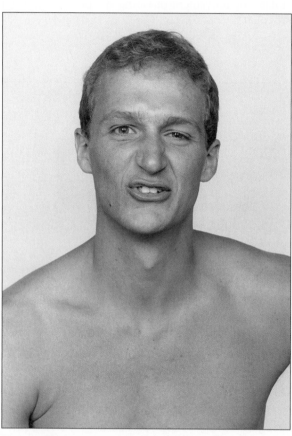

Figure 9-79 Elevation of the upper lip.

Elevation and Protrusion of the Lower Lip

Mentalis

Form 9-44

Test. The patient elevates the skin of the chin and protrudes the lower lip (Fig. 9-80). This action forms the facial expression of pouting.

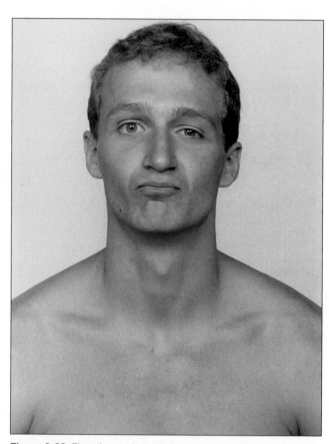

Figure 9-80 Elevation and protrusion of the lower lip.

Hypoglossal Nerve (CN XII)

Motor Function. The muscles supplied by the hypoglossal nerve act to produce tongue movements for the functions of mastication, taste, deglutition, speech, and oral hygiene.

Component Movements Tested. Tongue protrusion is the only movement tested.

Protrusion of the Tongue

Genioglossus

Form 9-45

Test. The mouth is open and the tongue is resting on the floor of the mouth. A wooden tongue depressor is placed on the midline of the chin to obtain a reference line for the midline of the

tongue.[33] The patient is asked to protrude the tongue so that the tip of the tongue touches the tongue depressor (Fig. 9-81). Note any deviation to the side of the lesion by observing the line formed by the lingual septum line and the edge of the tongue blade. During tongue movement, the geniohyoid muscle pulls the hyoid bone in an antero-superior direction. The movement of the hyoid bone may be palpated. The tongue is inspected for atrophy on the side of the lesion.

Note: Should there be risk of infection or contact with body fluids, the therapist must use universal precautions and be gloved, masked, and gowned as required.

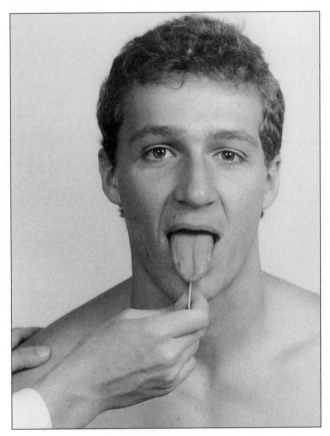

Figure 9-81 Protrusion of the tongue.

Depression of the Hyoid Bone

Infrahyoid (Strap) Muscles: Sternohyoid, Thyrohyoid, Omohyoid

Form 9-46

The primary function of the infrahyoid muscles is to depress the hyoid bone during swallowing and speaking.

Component Movements Tested. Depression of the hyoid bone (infrahyoid muscles) with depression of the tongue (hyoglossus muscle).

Test. The patient is asked to depress the root of the tongue as in swallowing (Figs. 9-82 and 9-83). The therapist may palpate the contraction of the infrahyoid muscles inferiorly to the hyoid bone.

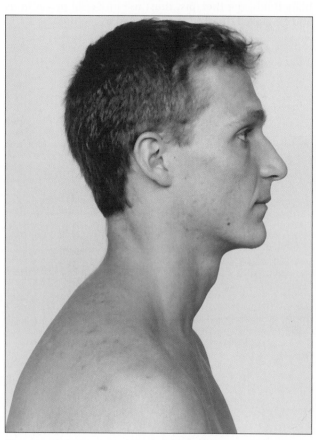

Figure 9-82 Relaxed position of the hyoid bone.

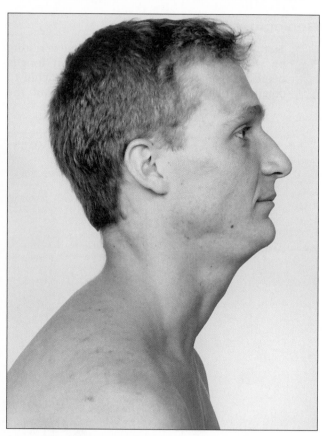

Figure 9-83 Depression of the hyoid bone.

MUSCLE STRENGTH ASSESSMENT: MUSCLES OF THE HEAD AND NECK (TABLE 9-4)

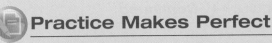

Practice Makes Perfect

To aid you in practicing the skills covered in this section, or for a handy review, use the practical testing forms found at http://thepoint.lww.com/Clarkson3e.

TABLE 9-4 Muscle Actions, Attachments, and Nerve Supply: The Head and Neck[2]

Muscle	Primary Muscle Action	Muscle Origin	Muscle Insertion	Peripheral (Cranial) Nerve	Nerve Root
Infrahyoid muscles (sternohyoid, sternothyroid, and thyrohyoid)					
Sternohyoid	Depression of the hyoid bone	Posterior aspect of the medial end of the clavicle; posterior sternoclavicular ligament; superior and posterior aspect of the manubrium	Inferior aspect of the body of the hyoid bone	Ansa cervicalis	C123
Sternothyroid	Depression of the larynx	Posterior aspect of the manubrium below the origin of the sternohyoid and from the edge of the first costal cartilage	Oblique line on the lamina of the thyroid cartilage	Ansa cervicalis	C123
Thyrohyoid	Depression of the hyoid bone; elevation of the larynx	Oblique line on the lamina of the thyroid cartilage	Inferior border of the greater cornu and the adjacent part of the body of the hyoid bone	(Hypoglossal CN XII)	C1
Omohyoid	Depression of the hyoid bone	Superior border of the scapula near the scapular notch; superior transverse scapular ligament	A band of deep cervical fascia holds the intermediate portion of the muscle down towards the clavicle and first rib and the course of the muscle changes direction at this point; lower border of the body of the hyoid bone	Ansa cervicalis	C123
Sternomastoid	Neck extension; neck flexion; contralateral neck rotation; ipsilateral neck side flexion	a. Sternal head: superior aspect of the manubrium b. Clavicular head: superior surface of the medial third of the clavicle	Lateral aspect of the mastoid process; lateral half of the superior nuchal line	(CN XI)	C234

(continued)

TABLE 9-4   *Continued*

Muscle	Primary Muscle Action	Muscle Origin	Muscle Insertion	Peripheral (Cranial) Nerve	Nerve Root
Longus colli	Neck flexion; contralateral neck rotation (inferior oblique fibers); neck side flexion (oblique fibers)	a. Inferior oblique part: anterior aspect of the bodies T1 to T3 b. Superior oblique part: the anterior tubercles of the transverse processes of C3 to C5 c. Vertical part: anterior aspect of the bodies of T1 to T3 and C5 to C7	a. Inferior oblique part: the anterior tubercles of the transverse processes of C5 and C6 b. Superior oblique part: anterolateral surface of the tubercle on the anterior arch of the atlas c. Vertical part: anterior aspects of the bodies of C2 to C4		C23456
Longus capitis	Flexes the head	Anterior tubercles of the transverse processes of C3 to C6	Inferior surface of the basilar aspect of the occipital bone		C123
Rectus capitis anterior	Flexes the head	Anterior aspect of the lateral mass of the atlas; root of the transverse process of the atlas	Inferior surface of the basilar aspect of the occipital bone anterior to the occipital condyle		C12
Rectus capitis lateralis	Ipsilateral lateral flexion of the head	Superior aspect of the transverse process of the atlas	Inferior aspect of the jugular process of the occipital bone		C12
Scalenus anterior	Neck flexion and ipsilateral neck lateral flexion Contralateral neck rotation	Anterior tubercles of the transverse processes of C3 to C6	Scalene tubercle on the inner border of the first rib and the ridge on the upper surface of the rib anterior to the groove for the subclavian artery		C456
Scalenus medius	Ipsilateral neck lateral flexion	Transverse process of the axis; anterior aspect of the posterior tubercles of the transverse processes of C3 to C7	Superior aspect of the first rib between the tubercle of the rib and the groove for the subclavian artery		C3–8
Scalenus posterior	Ipsilateral neck lateral flexion	Posterior tubercles of the transverse processes of C4 to C6	Lateral surface of the second rib		C678
Upper fibers of trapezius	Head and neck extension	Medial third of the superior nuchal line of the occipital bone; external occipital protuberance; ligamentum nuchae	Posterior border of the lateral one third of the clavicle	(CN XI)	
Splenius capitis	Neck extension; ipsilateral neck rotation	Inferior half of the ligamentum nuchae; the spinous processes of C7 and T1 to T4 and the corresponding supraspinous ligaments	Mastoid process of the temporal bone; the occipital bone inferior to the lateral third of the superior nuchal line	Middle cervical spinal nerves	

TABLE 9-4 *Continued*

Muscle	Primary Muscle Action	Muscle Origin	Muscle Insertion	Peripheral (Cranial) Nerve	Nerve Root
Splenius cervicis	Neck extension; ipsilateral neck rotation	The spinous processes of T3 to T6	Posterior tubercles of the transverse processes of the upper three cervical vertebrae	Lower cervical spinal nerves	
Rectus capitis posterior major	Head extension and ipsilateral head rotation	Spinous process of the axis	Lateral part of the inferior nuchal line and area of bone just inferior to the line	First cervical spinal nerve	
Rectus capitis posterior minor	Head extension	Tubercle on the posterior arch of the atlas	Medial part of the inferior nuchal line and the area of bone between the line and foramen magnum	First cervical spinal nerve	
Obliquus capitis inferior	Ipsilateral head rotation	Lateral aspect of the spine and adjacent superior aspect of the lamina of the axis	Inferior and posterior aspect of the transverse process of the atlas	First cervical spinal nerve	
Obliquus capitis superior	Head extension and ipsilateral head lateral flexion	Superior surface of the transverse process of the atlas	Occipital bone between the superior and inferior nuchal lines lateral to the semispinalis capitis	First cervical spinal nerve	

Note: **See Table 9-6** for other neck extensor muscles.

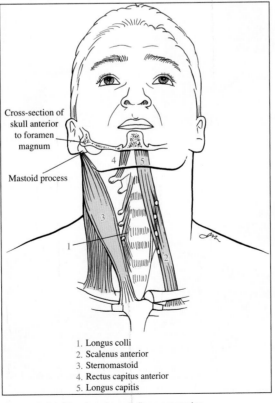

1. Longus colli
2. Scalenus anterior
3. Sternomastoid
4. Rectus capitus anterior
5. Longus capitis

Cross-section of skull anterior to foramen magnum

Mastoid process

Figure 9-84 Head and neck flexor muscles.

Note: Manual muscle testing of the head and neck is contraindicated in some instances. Contraindications include pathology that may result in spinal instability and pathology of the vertebral artery. In the absence of contraindications to resisted head and neck movements, resistance is applied with care not to apply too much resistance for the muscles being tested.

Head and Neck Flexion

Rectus Capitis Anterior, Longus Capitis, Longus Colli, Scalenus Anterior, Sternomastoid

Form 9-47

Accessory muscles: Scalenus medius, scalenus posterior, suprahyoids, infrahyoids, and rectus capitis lateralis.

The head and neck flexors (Fig. 9-84) are tested in the against gravity position. The anterior head and neck flexors are tested as a group; followed by isolation of the sternomastoid muscles.

Start Position. The patient is supine (Fig. 9-85). The arms are over the head resting on the plinth. The elbows are flexed.

Stabilization. The trunk is stabilized by the plinth. The anterior abdominal muscles must be strong enough to provide anterior fixation of the thorax on the pelvis.[36] In a patient with weak abdominals, stabilization is provided by downward pressure of the therapist's hand on the thorax (Fig. 9-86).

Movement. The patient flexes the head and neck through partial (grade 2) or full range (grade 3) (Fig. 9-87). The patient is instructed to keep the chin depressed (i.e., tucked in toward the manubrium sternum) as the neck is flexed.

Palpation. *Longus capitis, longus colli, and rectus capitis anterior* are too deep to palpate. The *sternomastoid* muscle may be palpated proximal to the clavicle or sternum. The muscle is more easily palpated in the isolated test involving rotation. The *scalenus anterior* may be palpated above the clavicle and behind the sternomastoid.

Resistance Location. Applied on the forehead (Fig. 9-88).

Resistance Direction. Head and neck extension.

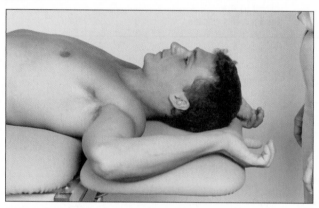

Figure 9-85 Start position for head and neck flexion.

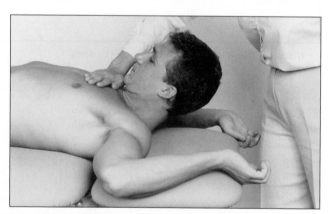

Figure 9-86 Screen position: head and neck flexion with stabilization.

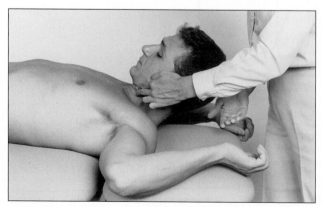

Figure 9-87 Screen position: head and neck flexion.

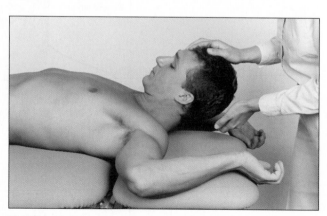

Figure 9-88 Resistance: head and neck flexors.

Head and Neck Flexion, Rotation and Lateral Flexion

Sternomastoid

Start Position. The patient is supine (Fig. 9-89). The arms are over the head resting on the plinth. The elbows are flexed.

Form 9-48

Stabilization. The trunk is stabilized by the plinth. With abdominal muscle weakness, stabilization of the thorax is required.[37]

Movement. The patient laterally flexes on the test side and rotates the neck to the opposite side (Fig. 9-90). Each side is tested. The patient laterally flexes through partial (grade 2) or full range (grade 3).

Palpation. Each sternomastoid muscle can be palpated at any point along the oblique ridge of the muscle from the mastoid process to the sternum or clavicle.

Resistance Location. The therapist's fingers are used to apply resistance on the temporal region of the head (Figs. 9-91 and 9-92).

Resistance Direction. Oblique posterior direction and ipsilateral rotation.

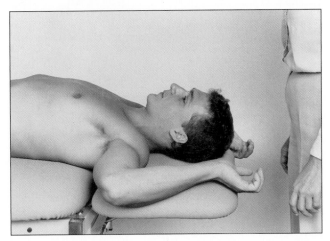

Figure 9-89 Start position: sternomastoid.

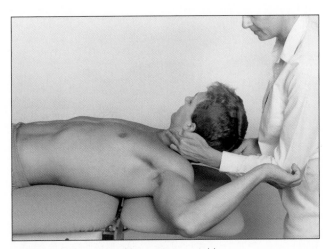

Figure 9-90 Screen position: sternomastoid.

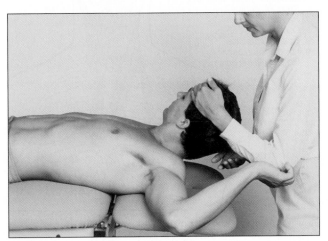

Figure 9-91 Resistance: sternomastoid.

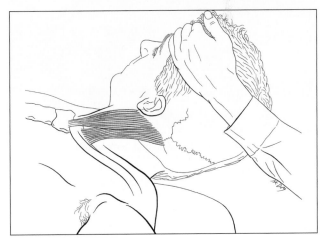

Figure 9-92 Sternomastoid.

Head and Neck Extension

The head and neck extensors are tested as a group in the against gravity position. The muscles include semispinalis capitis, rectus capitis posterior (major and minor), obliquus capitis (inferior and superior), splenius capitis, semispinalis cervicis, longissimus capitis and cervicis, splenius cervicis, spinalis capitis and cervicis, and iliocostalis cervicis.

Form 9-49

The strength of upper trapezius is tested as an elevator of the scapula.

Start Position. The patient is prone (Fig. 9-93). The arms are over the head resting on the side of the plinth. The elbows are flexed.

Stabilization. The patient grasps the end of the plinth for stabilization. The therapist may stabilize the upper thoracic region to prevent trunk extension.

Movement. The patient extends and rotates the head and neck (Fig. 9-94).

Palpation. The extensor muscles (Fig. 9-96) are palpated as a group paravertebrally.

Resistance Location. Applied on the head just proximal to the occiput (Fig. 9-95).

Resistance Direction. Head and neck flexion and rotation.

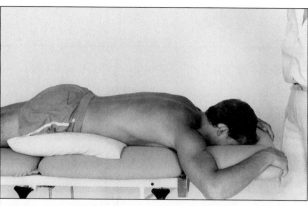

Figure 9-93 Start position: head and neck extensors.

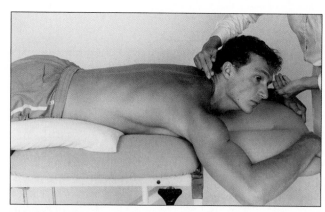

Figure 9-94 Screen position: right head and neck extensors.

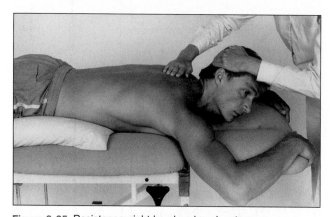

Figure 9-95 Resistance: right head and neck extensors.

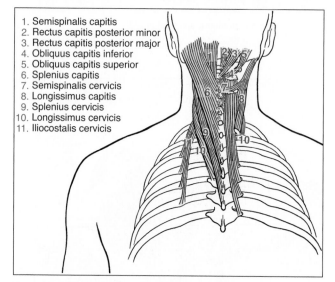

1. Semispinalis capitis
2. Rectus capitis posterior minor
3. Rectus capitis posterior major
4. Obliquus capitis inferior
5. Obliquus capitis superior
6. Splenius capitis
7. Semispinalis cervicis
8. Longissimus capitis
9. Splenius cervicis
10. Longissimus cervicis
11. Iliocostalis cervicis

Figure 9-96 Head and neck extensors.

ARTICULATIONS AND MOVEMENTS: TRUNK

The Trunk: Thoracic and Lumbar Spines

The articulations and joint axes of the trunk are illustrated in Figs. 9-97, 9-98, and 9-99. The joint structure and movements of the trunk are described below and summarized in Table 9-5.

There are 12 vertebrae in the thoracic spine and 5 in the lumbar spine (Fig. 9-97). Vertebral segments are referred to when describing the articulations of the spine. A vertebral segment consists of two vertebrae and the three articulations between them (Fig. 9-100). Anteriorly, intervertebral discs are positioned between the adjacent vertebral bodies. However, it is the orientation of the facet joints, located posteriorly on each side of the vertebral segment that determines the predominant motions that occur between the vertebral segments. Each facet joint is formed by the inferior facet of the superior vertebra articulating with the superior facet of the inferior vertebra.

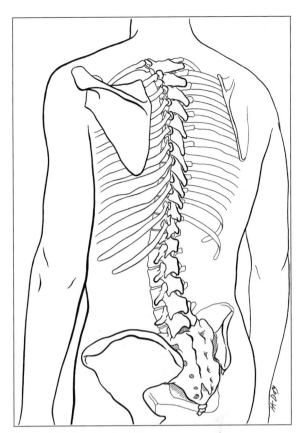

Figure 9-97 Trunk articulations.

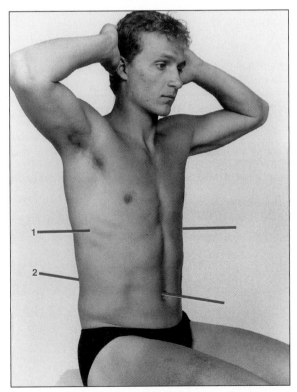

Figure 9-98 Trunk axes: (1) flexion–extension; (2) lateral flexion.

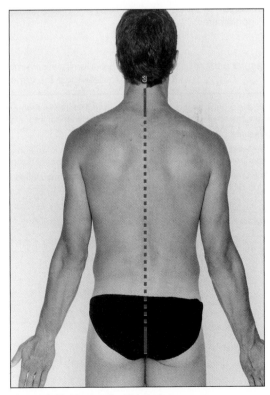

Figure 9-99 Trunk axis: (3) rotation.

TABLE 9-5 Joint Structure: Trunk Movements

	Flexion	Extension	Lateral Flexion	Rotation
Articulation[38]	Lumbar spine, thoracic spine (mainly T6–12)	Lumbar spine, thoracic spine (mainly T6–12)	Lumbar spine, thoracic spine	Thoracic spine, lumbosacral articulation
Plane	Sagittal	Sagittal	Frontal	Horizontal
Axis	Frontal	Frontal	Sagittal	Vertical
Normal limiting factors[8,9,39]* **(see Fig. 9-100)**	Tension in the posterior longitudinal, supraspinous, interspinous and intertransverse ligaments, the ligamentum flavum, facet joint capsules and spinal extensor muscles; compression of the intervertebral discs anteriorly and tension in the posterior fibers of the annulus; apposition of articular facets thoracic spine; rib cage	Tension in the anterior longitudinal ligament, abdominal muscles, facet joint capsules and the anterior fibers of the annulus; contact between adjacent spinous processes; apposition of articular facets thoracic spine	Contact between the iliac crest and thorax; tension in the contralateral trunk side flexors, intertransverse and iliolumbar ligaments and facet joint capsules; tension in the contralateral fibers of the annulus; apposition of articular facets lumbar spine	Tension in the costovertebral, supraspinous, interspinous, intertransverse, and iliolumbar ligaments and facet joint capsules lumbar spine and annulus fibrosus of the intervertebral discs; tension in the ipsilateral external and contralateral internal abdominal oblique muscles; apposition of articular facets lumbar spine
Normal AROM Tape measure	10 cm[5]† 6 cm[40]§		22 cm[41]‡	
Inclinometer[12] Universal goniometer[3]	0–60+° L spine	0–25° L spine	0–25° L spine 0–35°	0–30° T spine
Capsular pattern	It is difficult to perform passive movements of the trunk due to its size and weight. It is difficult to determine the capsular pattern for the trunk[6].			

*There is a paucity of definitive research that identifies the normal limiting factors (NLF) of joint motion. The NLF and end feels listed here are based on knowledge of anatomy, clinical experience, and available references.

†Measured between C7 and S1.

‡Measured between level of middle finger on thigh in anatomical position and at end of lateral flexion ROM. Value represents the mean of mean values from the original source[41] for right and left lateral flexion ROM of 39 healthy subjects.

§Measured between level of PSIS and 15 cm proximal. Value represents the rounded mean of mean values from the original source[40] for L spine flexion ROM of 104 children 13 to 18 years of age.

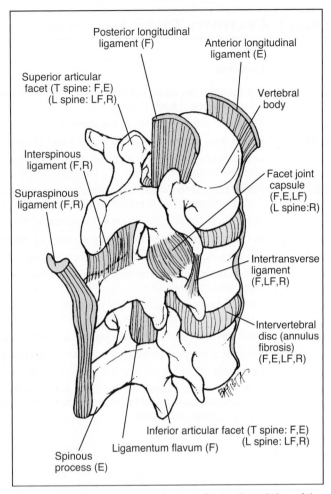

Superior articular
facet (T spine: F,E)
(L spine: LF,R)

Posterior longitudinal
ligament (F)

Anterior longitudinal
ligament (E)

Vertebral
body

Interspinous
ligament (F,R)

Facet joint
capsule
(F,E,LF)
(L spine:R)

Supraspinous
ligament (F,R)

Intertransverse
ligament
(F,LF,R)

Intervertebral
disc (annulus
fibrosis)
(F,E,LF,R)

Inferior articular facet (T spine: F,E)
(L spine: LF,R)

Ligamentum flavum (F)

Spinous
process (E)

Figure 9-100 Normal Limiting Factors. Posterolateral view of the vertebral column to illustrate noncontractile structures that normally limit motion in the thoracic and lumbar spines. Motion limited by structures is identified in brackets, using the following abbreviations: *F,* flexion; *E,* extension; *LF,* lateral flexion; *R,* rotation. Muscles normally limiting motion are not illustrated.

Although all segments of the thoracic and lumbar spines contribute to flexion, extension, lateral flexion, and rotation of the trunk, the regional contribution to these motions varies. The surfaces of the facets in the thoracic spine lie in the frontal plane, favoring the motions of lateral flexion and rotation. The facet joint surfaces of the lumbar spine are oriented in the sagittal plane, favoring flexion and extension.

When assessing thoracic and lumbar spine ROM, the combined motions of the segments are assessed and measured since segmental motion cannot be measured clinically. Thoracic and lumbar spine movements include flexion and extension, which occur in the sagittal plane around a frontal axis (Fig. 9-98); lateral flexion, which occurs in the frontal plane around a sagittal axis (Fig. 9-98); and rotation, which occurs in the transverse plane around a vertical axis (Fig. 9-99).

SURFACE ANATOMY: TRUNK (Figs. 9-101 through 9-104)

Structure	Location
1. Suprasternal (jugular) notch	The rounded depression at the superior border of the sternum, between the medial ends of each clavicle.
2. Xiphoid process	The lower end of the body of the sternum.
3. Anterior superior iliac spine (ASIS)	Round bony prominence at the anterior end of the iliac crest.
4. Iliac crest	Upper border of the ilium; a convex bony ridge, the top of which is level with the space between the spines of L4 and L5.
5. Posterior superior iliac spine (PSIS)	Round bony prominence at the posterior end of the iliac crest, felt subcutaneously at the dimples on the proximal aspect of the buttocks.
6. S2 spinous process	At the midpoint of a line drawn between each PSIS.
7. Inferior angle of the scapula	At the inferior aspect of the vertebral border of the scapula.
8. Spine of the scapula	The bony ridge running obliquely across the upper four fifths of the scapula.
9. T7 spinous process	Midline of the body at the level of the inferior angle of the scapula with the body in the anatomical position.
10. T3 spinous process	With the body in the anatomical position, it is at the midpoint of a line drawn between the roots of the spines of each scapula.
11. C7 spinous process	Often the most prominent spinous process at the base of the neck.
12. T1 spinous process	The next spinous process inferior to the C7 spinous process.
13. Acromion process	Lateral aspect of the spine of the scapula at the tip or point of the shoulder.
14. Greater trochanter	With the tip of the thumb on the lateral aspect of the iliac crest, the tip of the third digit placed distally on the lateral aspect of the thigh locates the upper border of the greater trochanter.

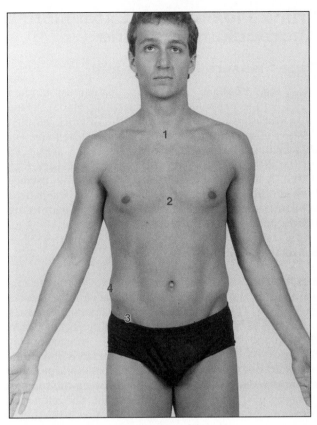

Figure 9-101 Anterior aspect of the trunk.

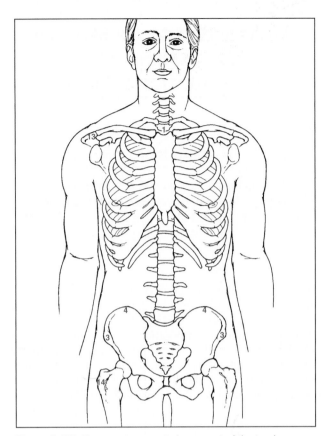

Figure 9-102 Bony anatomy, anterior aspect of the trunk.

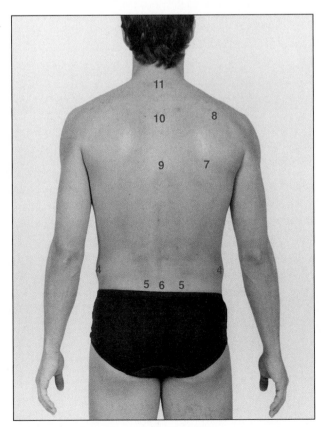

Figure 9-103 Posterior aspect of the trunk.

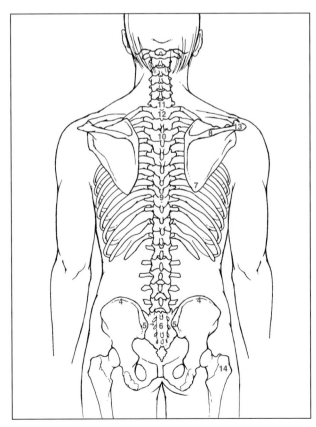

Figure 9-104 Bony anatomy, posterior aspect of the trunk.

ACTIVE RANGE OF MOTION ASSESSMENT AND MEASUREMENT: TRUNK

Practice Makes Perfect

To aid you in practicing the skills covered in this section, or for a handy review, use the practical testing forms found at http://thepoint.lww.com/Clarkson3e.

The tape measure, universal goniometer, and standard inclinometer are the tools used to objectively measure spinal AROM as presented in this text. Description of the general principles of application for the tape measure, standard inclinometer, and BROMII can be found in the section "Instrumentation and Measurement Procedures: TMJ and Spine" at the beginning of this chapter. The measurement of spinal AROM is described and illustrated.

Trunk Flexion and Extension: Thoracolumbar Spine

Tape Measure Measurement

Forms 9-50, 9-51

Start Positions. *Flexion:* The patient is standing with feet shoulder width apart (Fig. 9-105). A tape measure is used to measure the distance between the spinous processes of C7 and S2. *Extension:* For thoracolumbar extension, the patient's hands are placed on the iliac crests and into the small of the back (Fig. 9-106). A tape measure is used to measure the distance between the spinous processes of C7 and S2. The patient is instructed to keep the knees straight when performing the test movements.

Substitute Movement. None.

End Positions. *Flexion:* The patient flexes the trunk forward to the limit of motion for thoracolumbar flexion (Fig. 9-107). The distance between the spinous processes of C7 and S2 is measured again. The difference between the start and end position measures is the thoracolumbar flexion ROM. *Extension:* The patient extends the trunk backward to the limit of motion for thoracolumbar extension (Fig. 9-108). The distance between the spinous processes of C7 and S2 is measured again. The difference between the start and end position measures is the thoracolumbar extension ROM.

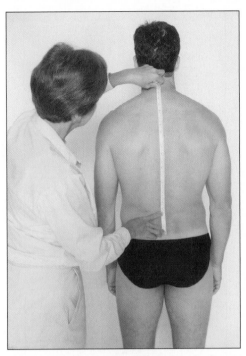

Figure 9-105 Start position: thoracolumbar spinal flexion. The distance is measured between the spinous processes of C7 and S2.

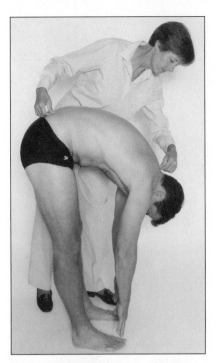

Figure 9-107 End position: thoracolumbar spinal flexion.

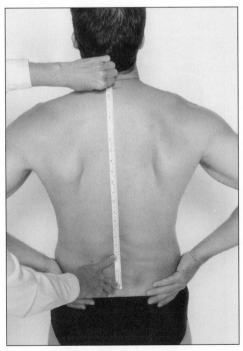

Figure 9-106 Start position for thoracolumbar extension.

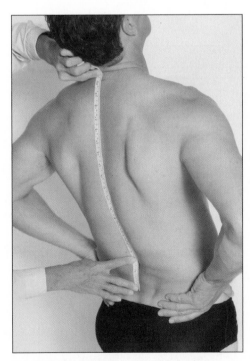

Figure 9-108 End position: thoracolumbar extension.

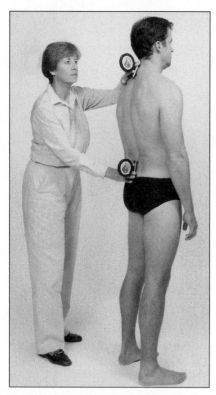

Figure 9-109 Start position: thoracolumbar flexion with inclinometer placement over the spines of C7 and S2.

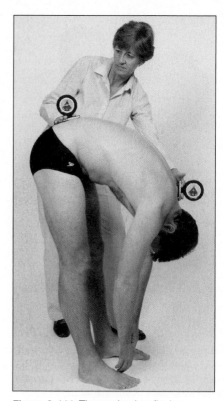

Figure 9-111 Thoracolumbar flexion.

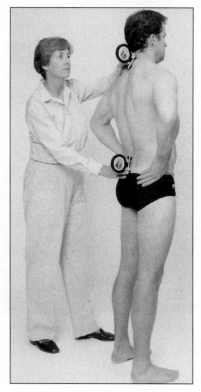

Figure 9-110 Start position: thoracolumbar extension.

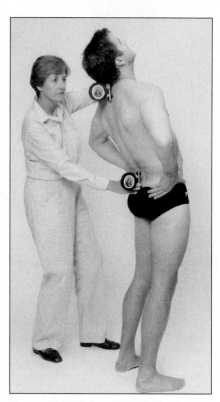

Figure 9-112 End position: thoracolumbar spine extension.

Trunk Flexion and Extension: Thoracolumbar Spine

Inclinometer Measurement

 Start Positions. The patient is standing with feet shoulder width apart (Fig. 9-109). For thoracolumbar extension, the patient's hands are placed on the iliac crests and into the small of the back (Fig. 9-110). The inclinometers are positioned and zeroed in each start position. The patient is instructed to keep the knees straight when performing the test movements.

Forms 9-52, 9-53

Substitute Movement. None.

Inclinometer Placement. *Superior:* On the spine of C7. *Inferior:* On the spine of S2.

End Positions. The patient flexes the trunk forward to the limit of motion for thoracolumbar flexion (Fig. 9-111).

The patient extends the trunk backward to the limit of motion for thoracolumbar extension (Fig. 9-112). At the end position for each movement, the therapist records the angle measurements from both inclinometers.

The AROM for the movement measured is the difference between the inclinometer readings.

Trunk Extension: Thoracolumbar Spine

Tape Measure Measurement (Prone Press-Up)

Start Position. The patient is prone (Fig. 9-113). The hands are positioned on the plinth at shoulder level.

Form 9-54

Stabilization. A strap is placed over the pelvis.

Substitute Movement. Lifting the pelvis from the plinth.

End Position. The patient extends the elbows to raise the trunk and extends the thoracolumbar spine (Fig. 9-114). A tape measure is used to measure the perpendicular distance between the suprasternal notch and the plinth at the limit of motion. This method is unsuitable for patients who have upper extremity muscle weakness or who find the prone position uncomfortable. In these cases, spinal extension is assessed in standing using a tape measure.

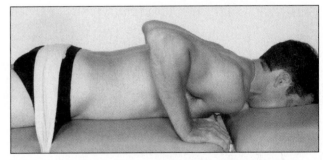

Figure 9-113 Start position: thoracolumbar spinal extension.

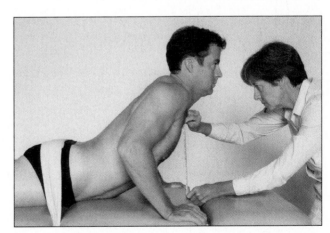

Figure 9-114 End position: thoracolumbar spinal extension.

Trunk Flexion and Extension: Lumbar Spine

Tape Measure Measurement

Start Positions. *Flexion*[40]: The patient is standing with feet shoulder width apart. A tape measure is used to measure a distance and mark a point 15 cm above the midpoint of the line connecting the PSISs (i.e., the spinous process of S2) with the patient in the start position (Fig. 9-115). *Extension:* For lumbar extension, the patient's hands are placed on the iliac crests and into the small of the back (Fig. 9-116). The patient is instructed to keep the knees straight when performing the test movements.

Forms 9-55, 9-56

End Positions. *Flexion:* The patient flexes the trunk forward to the limit of lumbar flexion motion (Fig. 9-117). A second measure is taken to measure the distance between the PSIS and the 15-cm skin mark at the limit of lumbar flexion ROM. The difference between the start and end measures is the lumbar spinal flexion ROM. This method of measurement is referred to as the modified-modified Schöber method. *Extension:* The patient extends the trunk backward to the limit of motion for lumbar extension (Fig. 9-118). A second measure is taken to measure the distance between the PSIS and the 15-cm skin mark at the limit of lumbar extension ROM. The difference between the start and end measures is the lumbar spinal extension ROM.

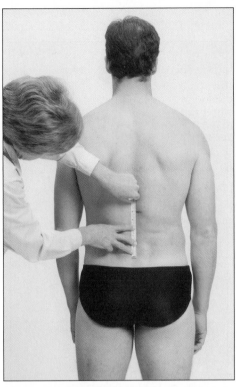

Figure 9-115 Start position: lumbar flexion, modified-modified Schöber method. The distance measured is between the spine of S2 and a point 15 cm above S2.

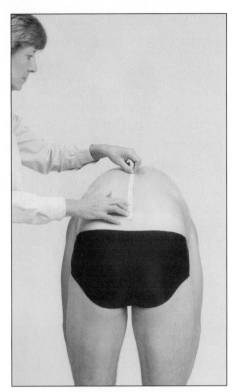

Figure 9-117 End position: lumbar flexion, modified-modified Schöber method.

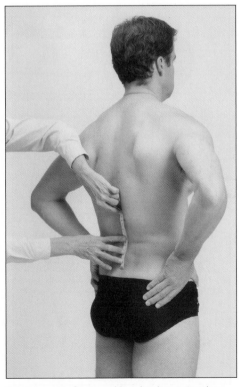

Figure 9-116 Start position: lumbar extension.

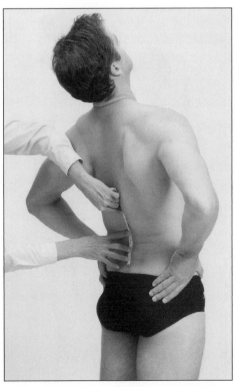

Figure 9-118 End position: lumbar extension.

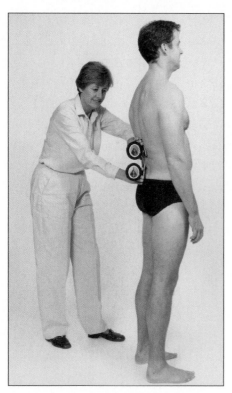

Figure 9-119 Start position: lumbar flexion with inclinometer placement over the spine of S2 and over a mark 15 cm above the spine of S2.

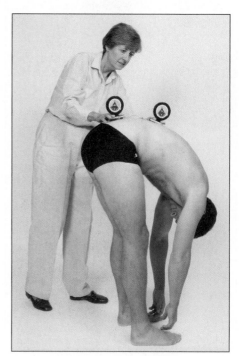

Figure 9-121 Lumbar spine flexion.

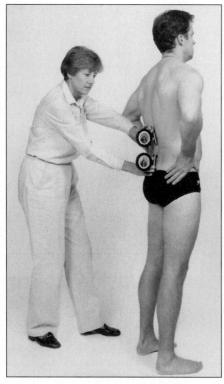

Figure 9-120 Start position: lumbar spine extension.

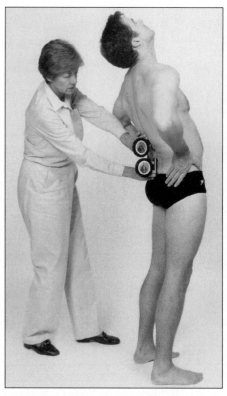

Figure 9-122 Lumbar spine extension.

Trunk Flexion and Extension: Lumbar Spine

Inclinometer Measurement

 Start Positions. *Flexion:* For lumbar flexion, the patient is standing with feet shoulder width apart (Fig. 9-119). *Extension:* For lumbar extension, the patient's hands are placed on the iliac crests and into the small of the back (Fig. 9-120).

Forms 9-57, 9-58

The inclinometers are positioned and zeroed in each start position. The patient is instructed to keep the knees straight when performing the test movements.

Inclinometer Placement. *Superior:* On a mark 15 cm above the spinous process of S2. *Inferior:* On the spine of S2.

End Positions. *Flexion*: The patient flexes the trunk forward to the limit of motion for lumbar flexion (Fig. 9-121). *Extension*: The patient extends the trunk backward to the limit of motion for lumbar extension (Fig. 9-122). At the end position for each movement, the therapist records the angle measurements from both inclinometers.

The AROM for lumbar spine flexion or extension is the difference between the inclinometer readings in the end position for the movement being measured.

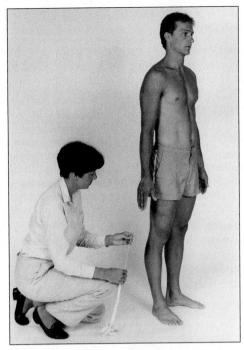

Figure 9-123 Start position: trunk lateral flexion.

Trunk Lateral Flexion

Tape Measure Measurement

 Start Position. The patient is standing with the feet shoulder width apart (Fig. 9-123). The patient is instructed to keep both feet flat on the floor when performing the test movements.

Form 9-59

Stabilization. None.

Substitute Movement. Trunk flexion, trunk extension, ipsilateral hip and knee flexion, raising the contralateral or ipsilateral foot from the floor.

End Position. The patient laterally flexes the trunk to the limit of motion (Fig. 9-124). A tape measure is used to measure the distance between the tip of the third digit and the floor.

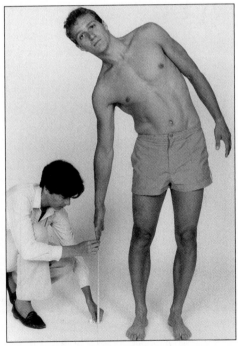

Figure 9-124 End position: trunk lateral flexion.

Alternate Tape Measure Measurement[41]

Start Position. The patient is standing with the feet shoulder width apart. A mark is placed on the thigh at the level of the tip of the middle finger (Fig. 9-125). The patient is instructed to keep both feet flat on the floor when performing the test movements.

Form 9-60

Stabilization. None.

End Position. The patient laterally flexes the trunk to the limit of motion. A second mark is placed on the thigh at the level of the tip of the middle finger (Fig. 9-126).

Measurement. A tape measure is used to measure the distance between the marks placed on the thigh at the level of the tip of the middle finger at the start position and at the end position (Fig. 9-127). The distance measured represents the lateral flexion ROM.

Inclinometer Measurement

Start Position. The patient stands with feet shoulder width apart. The inclinometers are positioned and zeroed (Fig. 9-128). The patient is instructed to keep both feet flat on the floor when performing the test movements.

Form 9-61

Inclinometer Placement. *Superior:* On the spine of T1. *Inferior:* On the spine of S2.

End Position. The patient laterally flexes the trunk to the limit of motion (Fig. 9-129). At the end position, the therapist records the angle measurements from both inclinometers. The AROM for lateral flexion is the difference between the inclinometer readings.

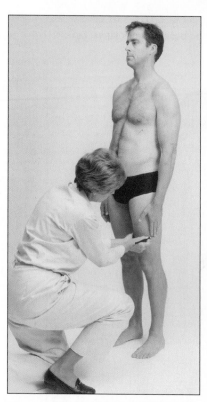

Figure 9-125 Start position: trunk lateral flexion.

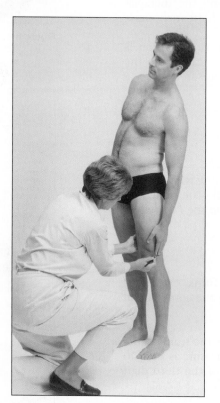

Figure 9-126 End position: trunk lateral flexion.

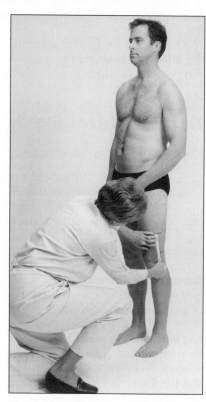

Figure 9-127 Measurement: trunk lateral flexion.

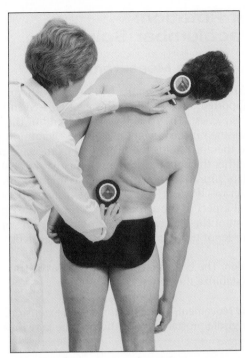

Figure 9-128 Inclinometer placement (spines of T1 and S2) for trunk lateral flexion.

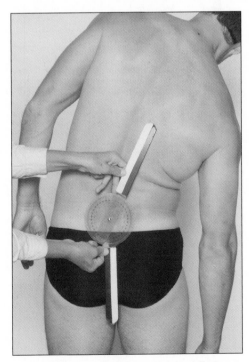

Figure 9-129 End position: trunk lateral flexion.

Universal Goniometer Measurement

Form 9-62

Start Position. Standing (Fig. 9-130).

Goniometer Axis. In the midline at the level of the PSIS (i.e., over the S2 spinous process).

Stationary Arm. Perpendicular to the floor.

Movable Arm. Points toward the spine of C7.

Lateral Flexion. The goniometer is realigned at the limit of trunk lateral flexion (Fig. 9-131). The number of degrees the movable arm lies away from the 0° position is recorded as the thoracolumbar lateral flexion ROM to the side measured.

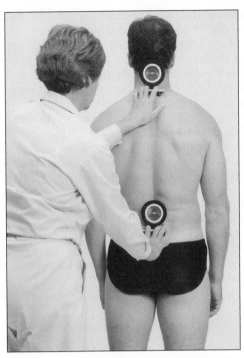

Spine of C7

Figure 9-130 Start position: universal goniometer placement trunk lateral flexion.

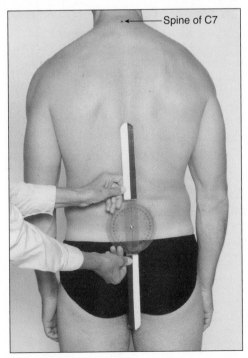

Figure 9-131 End position: trunk lateral flexion.

Trunk Rotation: Thoracolumbar Spine

Tape Measure Measurement

Start Position. The patient is sitting with the feet supported on a stool and the arms crossed in front of the chest. The patient holds the end of the tape measure on the lateral aspect of the acromion process. The therapist holds the other end of the tape measure on either the uppermost point of the iliac crest at the midaxillary line (not shown) or on the upper border of the greater trochanter (Fig. 9-132). The distance between the lateral aspect of the acromion process and the uppermost point of the iliac crest at the midaxillary line or the upper border of the greater trochanter is measured.

Form 9-63

Stabilization. The body weight on the pelvis; the therapist can also stabilize the pelvis.

Substitute Movement. Trunk flexion, trunk extension, and shoulder girdle protraction (on the side the tape measure is held).

End Position. The patient rotates the trunk to the limit of motion (Fig. 9-133). The distance between the lateral aspect of the acromion process and either the uppermost point of the iliac crest at the midaxillary line or the upper border of the greater trochanter is measured at the limit of rotation. The difference between the start position and end position measures is the thoracolumbar rotation ROM. The surface landmarks used in the assessment should be documented.

Frost and colleagues[42] described the use of the tape measure to measure trunk rotation (using the posterior clavicular prominence and the greater trochanter as landmarks) and noted that the accurate definition and palpation of the landmarks used in the assessment are critical for reliable assessment.

Clarkson recommends using the lateral aspect of the acromion process and the uppermost point of the iliac crest as the preferred surface landmarks, as these are easily palpated.

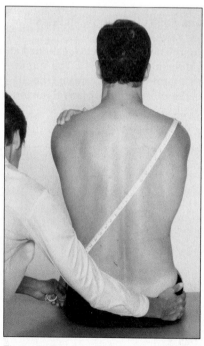

Figure 9-132 Start position: trunk rotation.

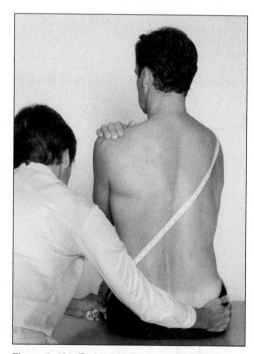

Figure 9-133 End position: trunk rotation.

Trunk Rotation: Thoracic Spine

Inclinometer Measurement

Start Position. The patient is standing with the arms crossed in front of the chest. The patient leans forward with the head and trunk parallel to the floor or as close to this position as possible. The inclinometers are positioned and zeroed (Fig. 9-134).

Form 9-64

Inclinometer Placement. *Superior:* On the spine of T1. *Inferior:* On the spine of T12.

End Positions. The patient rotates the trunk to the limit of motion (Fig. 9-135). At the end position, the therapist records the angle measurements from both inclinometers. The AROM for thoracic spine rotation is the difference between the inclinometer readings.

Substitute Movement. Trunk flexion and trunk extension. The range of trunk rotation when measured in the forward lean or stooped posture is less than when measured in sitting.[43] This may be caused by the contraction of the back muscles required to sustain the stooped posture that splint the spine and restrict trunk rotation.[43]

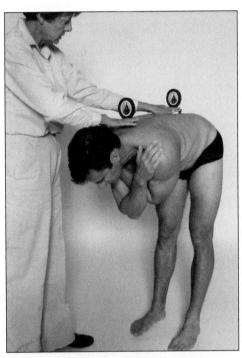

Figure 9-134 Start position: thoracic spine rotation with inclinometers placed over the spines of T1 and T12.

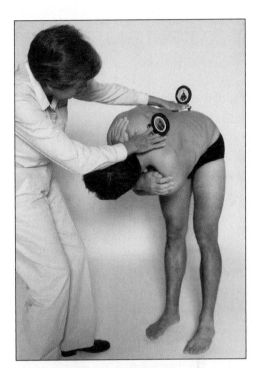

Figure 9-135 End position: thoracic spine rotation.

Chest Expansion

Tape Measure Measurement

Start Position. The patient is sitting. The patient makes a full expiration (Fig. 9-136).

Form
9-65   **End Position.** The patient makes a full inspiration (Fig. 9-137).

Measurement. A tape measure is used to measure the circumference of the chest at the level of the xiphisternal joint. Measures are taken at full expiration and at full inspiration. The difference between the two measures is the chest expansion. The chest expansion may also be measured at the levels of the nipple line and anterior axillary fold. The chest expansion measured at the latter points is slightly less than that at the xiphisternal joint. It is recommended[44] that two measurement sites, specifically the xiphoid and axilla, and a consistent patient position be used to provide a thorough evaluation of pulmonary status. A wide range of normal values exists for normal chest expansion and, beginning in the late 30s, chest expansion gradually decreases with increasing age.[45] Decreased chest expansion may indicate costovertebral joint involvement in certain pathological conditions[46] or may occur with chronic obstructive pulmonary disease (e.g., emphysema).

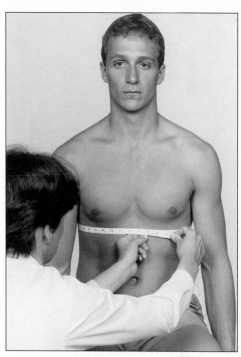

Figure 9-136 Start position: full expiration measured at the level of the xiphisternal joint.

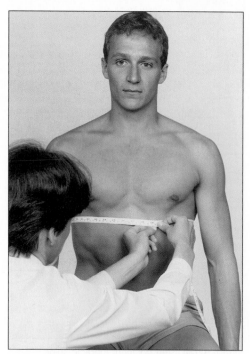

Figure 9-137 End position: full inspiration measured at the level of the xiphisternal joint.

Validity and Reliability: Measurement of the Thoracic and Lumbar Spine AROM

Littlewood and May[47] reviewed studies of the *validity* of low-tech clinical procedures, that is, clinically common, simple to use, and noninvasive methods, compared to x-ray (gold standard) measures of lumbar spine ROM in patients with nonspecific low-back pain. Only four studies were found that matched the criteria for inclusion for qualitative review. Littlewood and May[47] found limited evidence of validity of the modified-modified Schöber method for lumbar spine flexion ROM, and the double inclinometry method for measuring total lumbar flexion/extension, and lumbar extension ROM. There was also conflicting evidence of the validity of the double inclinometry method for lumbar flexion ROM. Therefore, Littlewood and May[47] were not able to make "convincing conclusions." These researchers indicate[47] that there is a need for high-quality meaningful research and reporting of the validity (using radiographic comparison) of low-tech clinical methods used to measure lumbar spine ROM in patient populations.

The *reliability* of tests of the low back assessment of ROM, strength, and endurance was reviewed by Essendrop, Maul, Läubli et al.[48] This research team searched databases for studies published from 1980 until 1999 from the Danish, German, and English language and literature. Only six studies that pertained to the reliability of tests of the low back assessment of ROM met the predetermined quality criteria and qualified for review. The most reliable methods of measuring mobility of the low back, when groups but not single individuals are compared, appeared to be the tape measure for trunk flexion, the tape measure and Cybex EDI 320 goniometric measurements for trunk lateral flexion, and no reliable measurement methods were found for trunk extension or rotation. Essendrop, Maul, Läubli et al.[48] could not make a recommendation for consensus, and indicate a need for more quality research and reporting of reliability studies of measures of low back function.

MUSCLE LENGTH ASSESSMENT AND MEASUREMENT: TRUNK

 Practice Makes Perfect

To aid you in practicing the skills covered in this section, or for a handy review, use the practical testing form found at http://thepoint.lww.com/Clarkson3e.

Trunk Extensors and Hamstrings (Toe-Touch Test)

Form 9-66

The trunk extensors are the erector spinae (iliocostalis thoracis and lumborum, longissimus thoracis, spinalis thoracis, semispinalis thoracis, and multifidus); the hip extensor and knee flexor muscles are the hamstrings (semitendinosus, semimembranosus, and biceps femoris). The toe-touch test provides a composite measure of hip, spine, and shoulder girdle ROM.

Start Position. The patient is standing (Fig. 9-138).

Substitute Movement. Knee flexion.

Stabilization. None.

End Position. The patient flexes the trunk and hips and reaches toward the toes to the limit of motion (Fig. 9-139).

Measurement. A tape measure is used to measure the distance between the floor and the most distant point reached by both hands. Normal ROM is present if the patient can touch the toes. If the patient can reach beyond floor level, the test can be carried out with the patient standing on a step or platform to measure reach distance beyond the supporting surface.

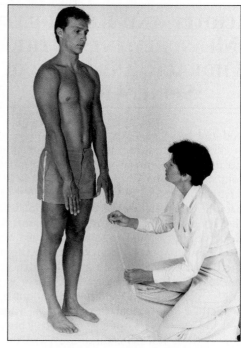

Figure 9-138 Start position: toe-touch test.

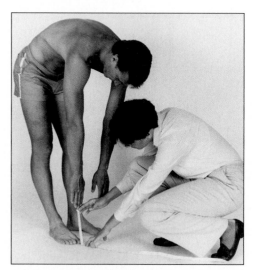

Figure 9-139 End position: trunk extensor and hamstring muscle length.

MUSCLE STRENGTH ASSESSMENT: MUSCLES OF THE TRUNK (TABLE 9-6)

 Practice Makes Perfect

To aid you in practicing the skills covered in this section, or for a handy review, use the practical testing forms found at http://thepoint.lww.com/Clarkson3e.

TABLE 9-6 Muscle Actions, Attachments, and Nerve Supply: The Trunk, Head, and Neck[2]

Muscle	Primary Muscle Action	Muscle Origin	Muscle Insertion	Peripheral Nerve	Nerve Root
Rectus abdominis	Trunk flexion	Crest and superior ramus of the pubis; ligaments covering the anterior surface of the symphysis pubis	Fifth, sixth, and seventh costal cartilages	Lower six or seven thoracic spinal nerves	T5–12
External abdominal oblique	Trunk rotation; trunk flexion	Eight digitations from the external and inferior surfaces of the lower eight ribs	Anterior half of the outer lip of the iliac crest; by an aponeurosis to merge with a similar aponeurosis from the opposite side into the linea alba from the xiphoid process to the symphysis pubis; as the inguinal ligament into the anterior superior iliac spine and the pubic tubercle	Lower six thoracic spinal nerves	T6–12
Internal abdominal oblique	Trunk rotation; trunk flexion	Lateral two thirds of the inguinal ligament; anterior two thirds of the iliac crest; the thoracolumbar fascia	Inferior borders of the lower three or four ribs; pubic crest and medial aspect of the pecten pubis; by an aponeurosis that splits around the rectus abdominus and inserts into the linea alba and the cartilages of ribs seven, eight, and nine	Lower six thoracic and first lumbar spinal nerves	T6–12, L1
Transversus abdominus	Compresses the abdominal contents	Lateral third of the inguinal ligament; anterior two thirds of the inner lip of the iliac crest; the thoracolumbar fascia between the iliac crest and rib twelve; the internal aspects of the costal cartilages of the lower six ribs	By an aponeurosis into the crest and pecten of the pubis and linea alba	Lower six thoracic and first lumbar spinal nerves	T6–12, L1
Quadratus lumborum	Elevation of the pelvis; trunk side flexion	The iliolumbar ligament and the adjacent posterior aspect of the iliac crest	Medial half of the inferior border of the 12th rib; by four small tendons into the tips of the transverse processes of the upper four lumbar vertebrae	Twelfth thoracic and upper three or four lumbar spinal nerves	T12, L1–4

(continued)

TABLE 9-6 *Continued*

Muscle	Primary Muscle Action	Muscle Origin	Muscle Insertion	Peripheral Nerve	Nerve Root
Erector spinae	The erector spinae lies along the sides of the vertebral column. The muscle is composed of three major columns of muscle mass (from lateral to medial: iliocostalis, longissimus and spinalis) all having a common origin:				C1–8 T1–12 L1–5
		The posterior aspects of the sacrum and iliac crest; the sacrotuberous and dorsal sacroiliac ligaments; the L1 to L5 and T11 and T12 spinous processes, and corresponding supraspinous ligament			
	The three columns have origins of attachment in addition to the common origin. The three columns become identifiable at different levels of the lumbar region. Each column is composed of three smaller parts that span from six to ten segments of the vertebral column.				
a. Iliocostalis 1. Iliocostalis lumborum	Trunk extension; trunk side flexion		Inferior borders of the angles of ribs five to twelve	Lower cervical, thoracic and upper lumbar spinal nerves	
2. Iliocostalis thoracis	Trunk extension; trunk side flexion	The superior borders of the angles of ribs six to twelve	Superior borders of the angles of ribs one to six; posterior aspect of the C7 transverse process		
3. Iliocostalis cervicis	Neck extension; neck side flexion	The angles of ribs three to six	Posterior tubercles of the transverse processes of C4 to C6		
b. Longissimus 1. Longissimus thoracis	Trunk extension	The posterior aspects of the transverse processes and accessory process of L1 to L5; the middle layer of the thoracolumbar fascia	The tips of the transverse processes of T1 to T12; between the tubercles and angles of the lower nine to ten ribs	Lower cervical, thoracic and lumbar spinal nerves	
2. Longissimus cervicis	Neck extension	Transverse processes of T1 to T5	Posterior tubercles of the transverse processes of C2 to C6		
3. Longissimus capitis	Head and neck extension Head and neck rotation (ipsilateral)	Transverse processes of T1 to T5; articular processes of C3 to C7	Mastoid process		
c. Spinalis 1. Spinalis thoracis	Trunk extension	Spinous processes of L1, L2, T11, and T12	Spinous processes of T1 to T4 or T8	Lower cervical and thoracic spinal nerves	

TABLE 9-6 *Continued*

Muscle	Primary Muscle Action	Muscle Origin	Muscle Insertion	Peripheral Nerve	Nerve Root
2. Spinalis cervicis	Neck extension	Inferior aspect of the ligamentum nuchae, spinous processes of C7, T1, and T2	The spinous processes of C1 to C3		
3. Spinalis capitis	Head extension	Tips of the transverse processes of C7 and T1 to T7; articular processes of C5 to C7	Region between the superior and inferior nuchal lines of the occiput		
Transverso-spinalis a. Semispinalis 1. Semispinalis thoracis	Trunk extension; contralateral trunk rotation	Transverse processes of T6 to T10	Spinous processes of C6, C7 and T1 to T4	Cervical and thoracic spinal nerves	
2. Semispinalis cervicis	Neck extension; contralateral neck rotation	Transverse processes of T1 to T6	Spinous processes of C2 to C5		
3. Semispinalis capitis	Head extension; contralateral rotation of head	Tips of the transverse processes of C7 and T1 to T7; articular processes of C4 to C6	Medial aspect of the region between the superior and inferior nuchal lines of the occipital bone		
b. Multifidus	Trunk extension; trunk side flexion; trunk rotation (control of posture)	Posterior aspect of the sacrum; aponeurosis of erector spinae; posterior superior iliac spine; dorsal sacroiliac ligament; transverse processes of C4 through L5	Into the spinous processes of from one to four of the vertebrae above	Dorsal rami of the spinal nerves	
Rotatores	Trunk rotation (control of posture)	Superior and posterior aspect of the transverse processes of the vertebrae in the cervical, thoracic and lumbar regions	Inferior and lateral aspect of the lamina of the vertebra above in the cervical, thoracic and lumbar regions	Dorsal rami of the spinal nerves	
Interspinales	Trunk extension (control of posture)	Short muscular fasciculi between the spines of contiguous vertebrae lateral to the interspinous ligament bilaterally in the cervical, thoracic and lumbar regions		Dorsal rami of the spinal nerves	
Intertransversarii	Trunk side flexion (control of posture)	Short muscles between the transverse processes of contiguous vertebrae in the cervical, thoracic and lumbar regions		Dorsal and ventral rami of the spinal nerves	

Trunk Flexion

The strength of the neck and hip flexors should be tested before testing the strength of the abdominal muscles.[36] If the neck flexors are weak, the head will have to be supported during the testing.

A half curl-up is performed to assess abdominal muscle strength. The movement begins from a supine position with the feet unsupported. The patient initially tilts the pelvis posteriorly to flex the lumbar spine, flexes the cervical spine, and then flexes the thoracic spine to lift the head and scapulae off the plinth.

Using the curl-up movement with the feet unsupported is more effective in activating the rectus abdominus muscle than performing the full sit-up from the supine position with the feet supported.[49] The first phase of the curl-up, start position to 45°, is primarily performed by the rectus abdominis, whereas the second phase, from 45° to the sitting position, is primarily performed by the iliacus muscle.[50] Therefore, a half curl-up is used to test abdominal muscle strength.

Rectus Abdominis

 Accessory muscles: iliopsoas, rectus femoris, internal abdominal oblique, and external abdominal oblique.

Form 9-67 The rectus abdominis muscle (Fig. 9-145) is tested in the against gravity position for all grades.

Start Position. The patient is supine.

Stabilization. Flexion of the cervical spine serves to fix the thorax and when combined with a posterior pelvic tilt provides the optimal posture for decreasing the lumbar lordosis, reducing the stress on the low back, and activating the abdominal muscles[51] in performing the curl-up. If the patient is unable to perform a posterior pelvic tilt and maintain the lumbar spine in a flexed position when being tested for abdominal muscle strength, the test is discontinued.

To prevent contraction of the iliopsoas muscle and greater hyperextension of the lumbar spine, the therapist should not stabilize the feet.[52]

Movement. The patient initially tilts the pelvis posteriorly to flex the lumbar spine, flexes the cervical spine lifting the head off the plinth, and then flexes the thoracic spine to perform a curl-up. The movement is performed slowly.

Substitute Movement. Hip flexors (lumbar lordosis).[36]

Palpation. Lateral to the midline on the anterior abdominal wall midway between the sternum and the pubis.

Grading

- Grade 0: No movement, and no palpable contraction is evident.
- Grade 1: No movement is possible but a flicker of a muscle contraction may be palpated. When testing for grade 1, the patient may also be asked to cough while the therapist observes and palpates for the presence of muscle contraction (Fig. 9-140).
- Grade 2 (Fig. 9-141): With the arms held outstretched in front of the trunk, the patient lifts the head and cervical spine off the plinth. The scapulae remain on the plinth.
- Grade 3 (Fig. 9-142): With the arms held outstretched in front of the trunk, the patient lifts the inferior angles of the scapulae clear of the plinth.

Resistance. Resistance is not applied manually by the therapist but is provided through positioning of the arms. The resistance of the head, trunk, and upper limbs increases as the upper limbs are moved toward the head. Accordingly, the arms are positioned across the chest (Fig. 9-143) or at above shoulder level with the hands beside the ears (Fig. 9-144) throughout the movement, for grades of 4 and 5, respectively. *Note:* For grade 5 testing, the hands are positioned beside the ears, rather than behind the head, to prevent stress being placed on the cervical spine inadvertently during testing.

Grading

- Grade 4 (Fig. 9-143): With the arms positioned across the chest, the patient lifts the inferior angles of the scapulae clear of the plinth.
- Grade 5 (Fig. 9-144): With the hands positioned beside the ears, the patient lifts the inferior angles of the scapulae clear of the plinth.

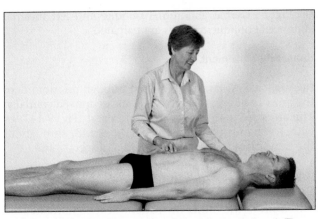

Figure 9-140 Test position: rectus abdominis, grade 0 or 1. The therapist asks the patient to cough while palpating for muscle contraction.

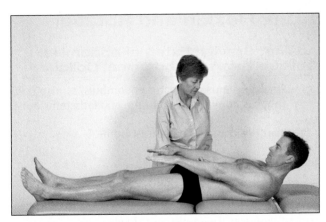

Figure 9-141 Test position: rectus abdominis, grade 2.

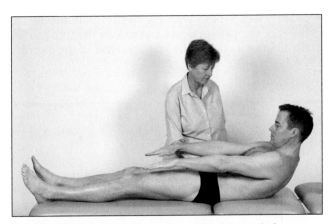

Figure 9-142 Screen position: rectus abdominis, grade 3.

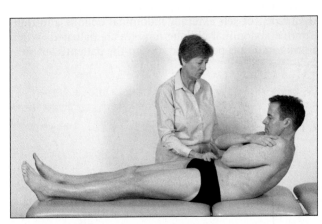

Figure 9-143 Test position: rectus abdominis, grade 4.

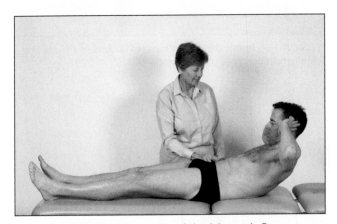

Figure 9-144 Test position: rectus abdominis, grade 5.

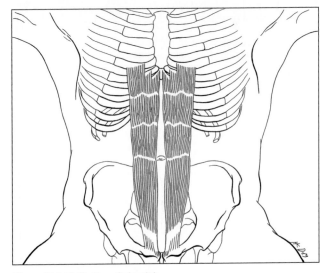

Figure 9-145 Rectus abdominis.

Trunk Flexion and Rotation

Against Gravity: External Abdominal Oblique, Internal Abdominal Oblique

Accessory muscles: rectus abdominus, semispinalis thoracis, multifidus, rotatores, and latissimus dorsi.

Form 9-68 **Start Position.** The patient is supine.

Stabilization. None.

Movement. The patient flexes and rotates the trunk to perform a half curl-up with rotation (Fig. 9-146). The patient performs the movement slowly.

Palpation. *External abdominal oblique:* at the lower edge of the rib cage. *Internal abdominal oblique:* medial to and above the anterior superior iliac spine.

When trunk rotation is performed toward the patient's right side, the left external abdominal oblique and right internal abdominal oblique muscles are palpated. When trunk rotation is performed toward the patient's left side, the right external abdominal oblique and left internal abdominal oblique muscles are palpated.

Substitute Movement. None.

Resistance. Resistance is provided through positioning of the arms[37] and increases as the arms are moved cranially. The arms are positioned across the chest (Fig. 9-147) or with the hands beside the ears (Fig. 9-148) throughout the movement, for grades of 4 and 5, respectively.

Grading

- Grade 3 (Fig. 9-146): With the arms held outstretched in front of the trunk, the patient flexes and rotates the trunk to lift the inferior angles of the scapulae clear of the plinth.
- Grade 4 (Fig. 9-147): With the arms positioned across the chest, the patient flexes and rotates the trunk to lift the inferior angles of the scapulae clear of the plinth.
- Grade 5 (Fig. 9-148): With the hands positioned beside the ears, the patient flexes and rotates the trunk to lift the inferior angles of the scapulae clear of the plinth.

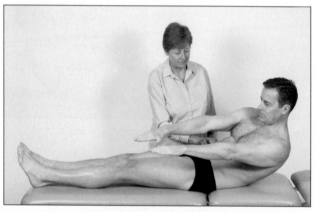

Figure 9-146 Screen position: right external abdominal oblique and left internal abdominal oblique, grade 3.

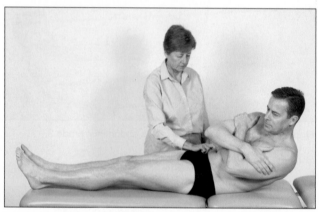

Figure 9-147 Test position: right external abdominal oblique and left internal abdominal oblique, grade 4.

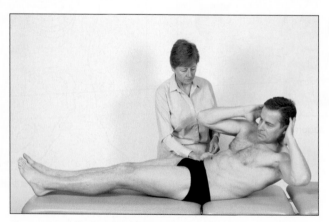

Figure 9-148 Test position: right external abdominal oblique and left internal abdominal oblique, grade 5.

Gravity Eliminated: External Abdominal Oblique, Internal Abdominal Oblique

Start Position. The patient is sitting with the hands off the plinth and the feet supported (Fig. 9-149).

Stabilization. The pelvis is stabilized by the patient's body weight.

End Position. The patient rotates the thorax with slight flexion (Figs. 9-150 and 9-151).

Substitute Movement. None.

Deviation of the umbilicus[36]: With marked weakness of the abdominal muscles deviation of the umbilicus can occur during testing. The umbilicus will be pulled toward the stronger muscle(s) and away from the weaker muscle(s). The umbilicus may also be pulled by and deviated toward a muscle that is shortened and being stretched. Palpation of the muscles can be used to confirm the presence of deviation of the umbilicus due to muscle imbalance.

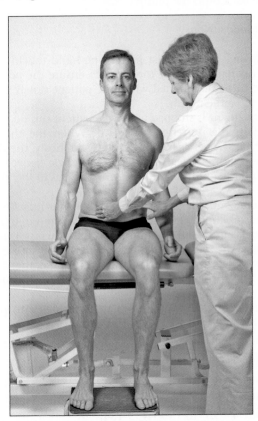

Figure 9-149 Start position: external abdominal oblique, internal abdominal oblique.

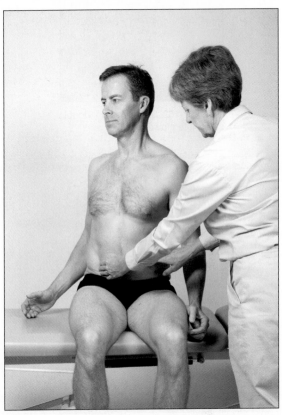

Figure 9-150 End position: left external abdominal oblique, right internal abdominal oblique, grade 2.

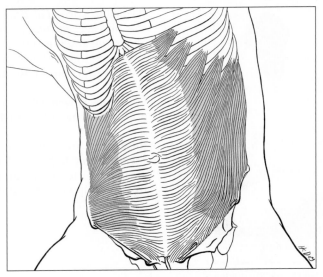

Figure 9-151 Left external abdominal oblique, right internal abdominal oblique.

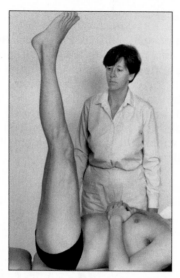

Figure 9-152 Start position: double straight leg lowering.

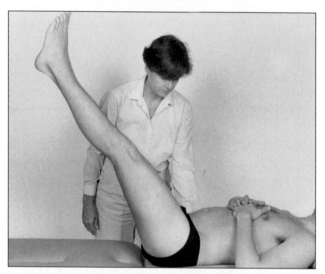

Figure 9-153 Test position: hip flexion 60°, grade 3+.

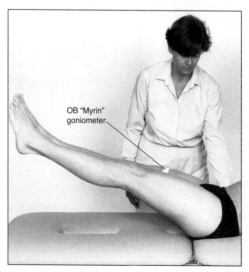

OB "Myrin" goniometer

Figure 9-154 Test position: hip flexion 20°, grade 4−.

Double Straight Leg Lowering[53]

External Abdominal Oblique, Internal Abdominal Oblique, Rectus Abdominis

Start Position. The patient is lying supine. The therapist raises the legs to a position of 90° hip flexion (Fig. 9-152). The patient posteriorly tilts the pelvis to flex the lumbar spine and flatten the small of the back onto the plinth.

Form 9-69

Stabilization. None.

Movement. The therapist places one hand touching the posterolateral aspect of the ilium to ensure the posterior pelvic tilt is maintained while the patient slowly lowers the legs to the plinth.

Movement is stopped when the patient can no longer maintain the posterior pelvic tilt. When the therapist feels that the pelvis begins to rotate anteriorly, the therapist supports the legs and notes the angle between the legs and the plinth before lowering the legs to the plinth.

Measurement. The OB "Myrin" goniometer may be used to measure the angle of hip flexion at the limit of motion. This measurement procedure allows the therapist to easily assess the angle of hip flexion without assistance. The strap is placed around the distal thigh and the dial is placed on the lateral aspect of the thigh (Fig. 9-154).

Grading.[36] Angles of hip flexion are translated into grades as follows:

- Grade 3: 90° to 75°
- Grade 3+: 74° to 60° (Fig. 9-153)
- Grade 4−: 59° to 45°
- Grade 4: 44° to 30°
- Grade 4+: 29° to 15° (Fig. 9-154)
- Grade 5: 14° to 0°.

Palpation. *External abdominal oblique:* at the lower edge of the rib cage. *Internal abdominal* oblique: medial to and above the anterior superior iliac spine. *Rectus abdominus:* lateral to the midline on the anterior abdominal wall midway between the sternum and the pubis.

Substitute Movement. Increased lumbar lordosis due to anterior tilting of the pelvis.

Resistance. Resistance is not applied manually by the therapist but is provided through the increased torque created by the lower extremities as the limbs are moved from 90° hip flexion to the surface of the plinth.

Trunk Extension

Erector Spinae: Iliocostalis Thoracis and Lumborum, Longissimus Thoracis, Spinalis Thoracis, Semispinalis Thoracis, and Multifidus

Accessory muscles: interspinales, quadratus lumborum, and latissimus dorsi.

Form 9-70

The strength of the neck and hip extensors should be tested before testing the strength of the trunk extensor muscles.[37] If the neck extensors are weak, the head will have to be supported during testing. If the hip extensors are weak or paralyzed, the pelvis cannot be adequately fixed in an extended position on the thigh as the patient attempts trunk extension and the patient will be unable to extend the trunk.[36]

The trunk extensors are tested as a group in the against gravity position.

Start Position. The patient is prone-lying with the feet over the end of the plinth and a pillow under the abdomen (Fig. 9-155).

Stabilization. A strap is placed over the pelvis to isolate the lumbar extensor muscles[54] and the therapist stabilizes the legs proximal to the ankles.

Substitute Movement. None.

Palpation. The trunk extensor muscles (Fig. 9-160) are palpated as a group paravertebral to the lumbar or thoracic spines.

Grading

- Grade 0: No movement, and no palpable contraction is evident.
- Grade 1: No movement is possible but a flicker of a muscle contraction can be palpated or observed as the patient attempts to lift the head.
- Grade 2: With the arms at the sides, the patient lifts the head and upper portion of the sternum off the plinth (Fig. 9-156).
- Grade 3: With the hands held behind the low back, the patient extends the trunk through partial ROM (Fig. 9-157).

Resistance. Resistance is not applied manually by the therapist. Resistance is provided through positioning of the arms and increases as the upper limbs are positioned toward the head. The hands are positioned behind the low back (Fig. 9-158) or behind the head (Fig. 9-159) to test for grades 4 and 5, respectively.[37]

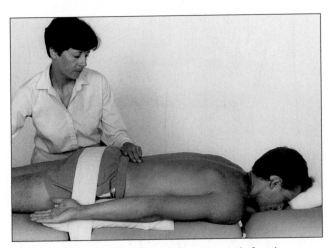

Figure 9-155 Test position: trunk extensors, grade 0 or 1.

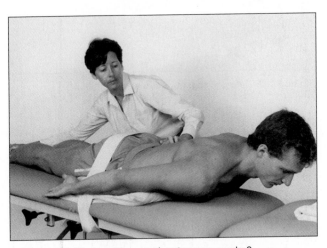

Figure 9-156 Test position: trunk extensors, grade 2.

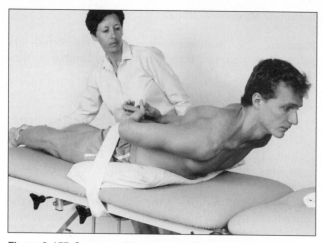

Figure 9-157 Screen position: trunk extensors, grade 3.

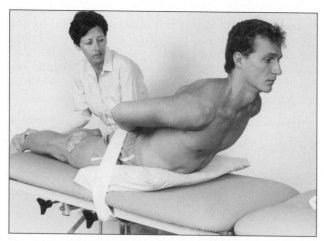

Figure 9-158 Test position: trunk extensors, grade 4.

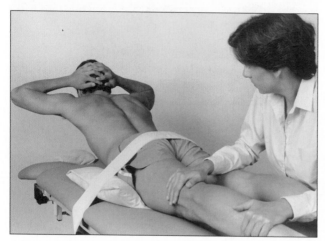

Figure 9-159 Test position: trunk extensors, grade 5.

Grading

- Grade 4: With the hands held behind the back, the patient extends the trunk through the full ROM, that is, lifts the head and upper portion of the sternum, so that the xiphoid process is off the plinth (Fig. 9-158).
- Grade 5: With the hands held behind the head, the patient extends the trunk through the full ROM and lifts the head and the sternum, so that the xiphoid process is off the plinth (Fig. 9-159).

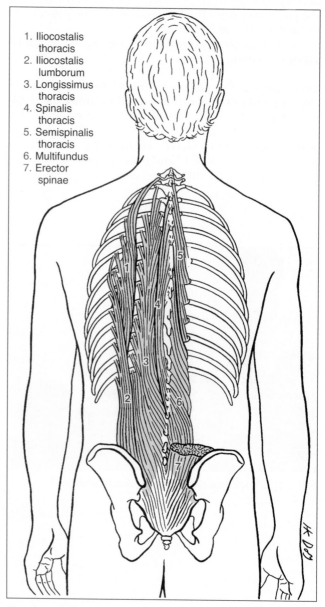

1. Iliocostalis thoracis
2. Iliocostalis lumborum
3. Longissimus thoracis
4. Spinalis thoracis
5. Semispinalis thoracis
6. Multifundus
7. Erector spinae

Figure 9-160 Trunk extensors.

Pelvic Elevation

Gravity Eliminated: Quadratus Lumborum

Form
9-71

Accessory muscles: latissimus dorsi, contralateral hip abductors, internal abdominal oblique, external abdominal oblique, and erector spinae.
The quadratus lumborum muscle is tested in the gravity eliminated position.

Start Position. The patient lies supine or prone (Fig. 9-161) with the feet off the end of the plinth, the hip in abduction, and slight extension.

Stabilization. The weight of the trunk; the patient holds the edges of the plinth.

Palpation. Above the crest of the ilium, lateral to the paravertebral extensor muscle mass, although quadratus lumborum is difficult to palpate.

Substitute Movement. Lateral fibers of the external abdominal oblique and internal abdominal oblique, latissimus dorsi, and erector spinae.

Grading

- Grade 0: No movement, and no palpable contraction is evident.
- Grade 1: No movement but a flicker of a muscle contraction may be palpated (see note under palpation above) as the patient attempts to elevate the iliac crest toward the ribs.
- Grade 2: The patient elevates the iliac crest toward the ribs through the full ROM (Fig. 9-162).

Resisted Gravity Eliminated: Quadratus Lumborum

Start Position. The patient lies supine or prone (Fig. 9-161) with the feet off the end of the plinth, with the hip in abduction and slight extension.

Stabilization. The weight of the trunk; the patient holds the edges of the plinth.

Movement. The patient elevates the iliac crest toward the ribs through the full ROM.

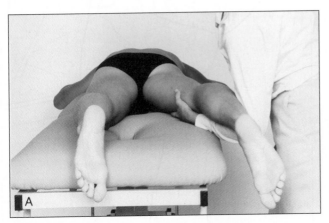
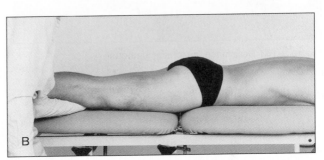

Figure 9-161 Start position: quadratus lumborum.

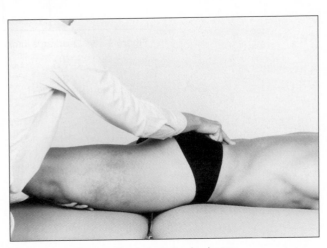

Figure 9-162 End position: quadratus lumborum.

Resistance Location. Anterior aspect of the distal end of the femur (Fig. 9-163). Alternatively, resistance can be applied on the posterolateral aspect of the iliac crest if hip pathology is present (Fig. 9-164).

Resistance Direction. A traction force equal to the weight of the leg is applied to the femur when performing a screen test and additional resistance is applied for grades 4 and 5.

Grading

- Grade 3: The patient elevates the iliac crest toward the ribs through the full ROM against resistance equal to the weight of the lower extremity (Fig. 9-163).

- Grade 4: The patient elevates the iliac crest toward the ribs through the full ROM against resistance equal to the weight of the lower extremity and moderate resistance.

- Grade 5: The patient elevates the iliac crest toward the ribs through the full ROM against resistance equal to the weight of the lower extremity and maximal resistance.

Alternatively, quadratus lumborum may be tested against gravity in standing. The therapist must ensure the contralateral hip abductors do not contract to depress the ipsilateral pelvis and elevate the iliac crest on the test side for quadratus lumborum.[37]

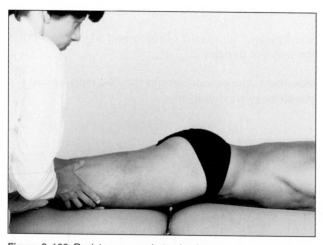

Figure 9-163 Resistance: quadratus lumborum.

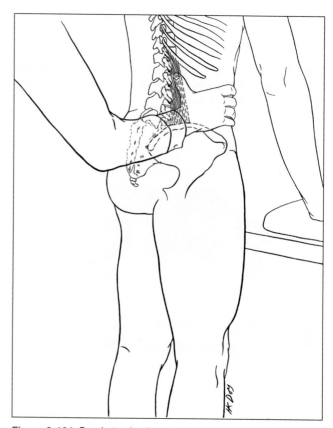

Figure 9-164 Quadratus lumborum.

FUNCTIONAL APPLICATION: NECK AND TRUNK

Joint Function: Neck and Trunk

The trunk complex articulations include the vertebral column, sacrum and coccyx, ribs, costal cartilages, and sternum. The vertebral column and its system of linkages have particular significance in functional application of ROM and strength. The stability function of the spine includes resisting compressive forces; supporting the major portion of the body weight; supporting the head, arms, and trunk against the force of gravity; shock absorption; protection of the spinal cord; and providing a stable structure for movement of the extremities.[7,55]

The articulations at the intervertebral body and facet joints of the vertebral column permit movement in flexion, extension, lateral flexion, and rotation to allow neck and back mobility. The functional range of the lower region of the spine is increased by the tilt of the pelvis. The total motion of the spine is the result of the collective movements of the articulations of the various segments of the vertebral column[7,14,56] with functional ranges varying between individuals.[56] Restriction of motion at any level may result in increased motion at another level.[56] Mobility in all planes is the greatest at the cervical spine segment. The thoracic spine has limited mobility in all planes due to the limitations imposed by the thorax.[1,7,14] Through movements of the thoracic wall, intrathoracic volume is increased or decreased for inspiration and expiration. The lumbar spine is most mobile in the sagittal plane. Functional ROM is described for the cervical and the thoracic and lumbar spines.

Functional Range of Motion

Cervical Spine

The movement components of the cervical spine allow movement for functioning of the sense organs within the head[57] and expression of nonverbal communication, including affirmative (nodding) or negative responses. Maintenance of ROM in flexion, extension, lateral flexion, and rotation is of particular importance to the individual for interacting with the environment through the sense of vision. The significance of the interdependence between vision and neck movements is demonstrated in many self-care, leisure, and occupational tasks.

During ADL, neck flexion and extension are the most frequently performed neck movements, occurring twice as often as lateral flexion and rotation.[58] Full ROM in all planes is not required for most self-care activities (Table 9-7) (Figs. 9-165 and 9-166). The majority of neck ROM performed during normal daily activities is less than 15° (i.e., median ROM of 13° for flexion, extension, and rotation; and 10° for lateral flexion).[58]

Ranges approximating full values may be required for such activities as driving (in a left-hand drive car: neck rotation occasionally reaching 36° left and 43° right rotation[60] (Fig. 9-167), painting a ceiling, placing an object on a high shelf (Fig. 9-168), gazing at the stars (extension), and many specific leisure and occupational tasks linking vision and neck movements. When eye mobility is restricted, greater cervical spine ROM may be required[62] or head posture may be affected[63] to accommodate for the restricted field of gaze.

Neck extension is required when drinking (Fig. 9-169). The shape of the body of the glass and the diameter of the rim are factors that determine the amount of neck extension required to drink from a glass.[64] "Pot-bellied" and narrow-rimmed glasses require more neck

Activity	Flexion ROM Max	Extension ROM Max	Rotation ROM Max	Lateral Flexion ROM Max
TABLE 9-7 Cervical Spine ROM Required for Selected ADL[59,60*,61*]				
Cervical Spine ROM				
Shampooing hair[59]	46°	—	—	—
Washing face[59]	16°	—	—	—
Eating[59]	—	8°	—	—
Driving[60*] (left hand drive car)	—	—	36° left 43° right	—
Lumbar Spine ROM				
Putting on a sock in sitting[61*]	48°	—	3°	4°

*Mean values from original source[60,61] rounded to the nearest degree.

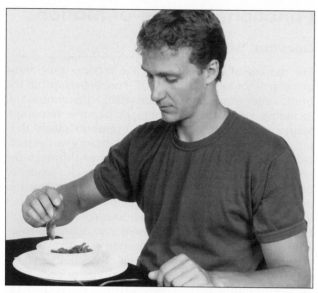

Figure 9-165 Eating: an activity requiring less than full neck flexion ROM.

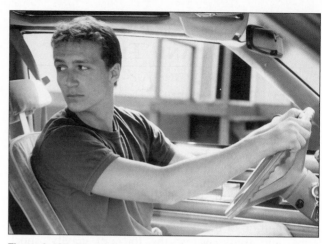

Figure 9-167 An activity requiring full neck rotation ROM.

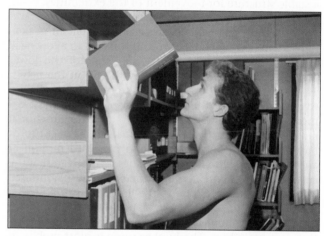

Figure 9-168 An activity requiring full neck extension ROM.

extension.[64] For example, nearly full neck extension (i.e., a mean of 40°) is required to drink from a narrow champagne flute compared to 0° for a saucer-shaped champagne glass.[64]

Thoracic and Lumbar Spines

Trunk rotation extends the reach of the hands beyond the contralateral side of the body, permits the individual to face different directions without foot movement (Fig. 9-170), and assists one to roll over while in the recumbent position. Rotation of the trunk is achieved through

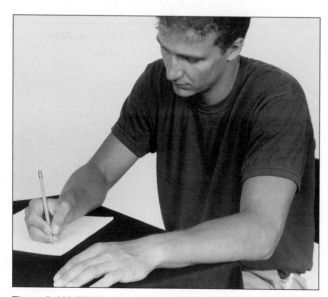

Figure 9-166 Writing at a desk: an activity requiring less than full neck flexion ROM.

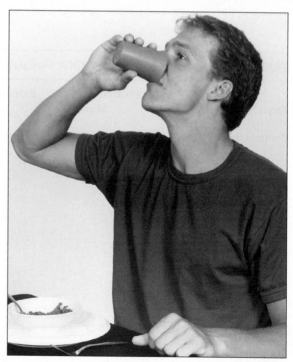

Figure 9-169 Drinking: an activity requiring neck extension.

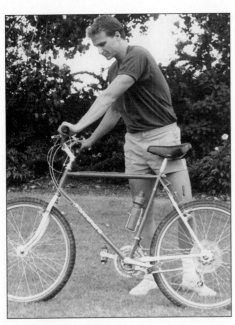

Figure 9-170 Trunk rotation.

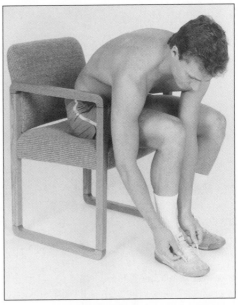

Figure 9-172 Tying a shoelace with the foot flat on the floor requires thoracic and lumbar flexion and neck extension.

the movement components of the thoracic and lumbar spine and is coupled with slight lateral flexion.[35,55,56] Rotation is a movement that is most free in the upper spinal segments and progressively diminishes in the lower segments.[35]

The major contribution of the mobility in the lumbar spine to daily functioning is through flexion and extension movements. When combined with the thoracic and

cervical segments, the individual can reach the more distal parts of the lower extremities and objects in the environment (Figs. 9-168, 9-171, 9-172 and 9-173). The final degrees of functional range are achieved through the interaction of the pelvis and hip.[7,14]

When forward flexing to touch the toes (see Figs. 9-138 and 9-139) a coordinated pattern of movement occurs between the lumbar spine and pelvis, called

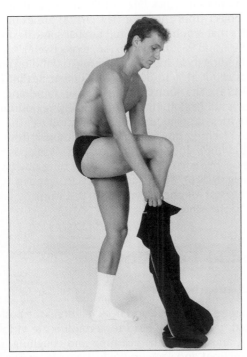

Figure 9-171 Donning a pair of trousers requires flexion of the thoracic and lumbar spines.

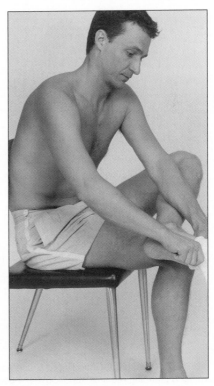

Figure 9-173 Lumbar flexion.

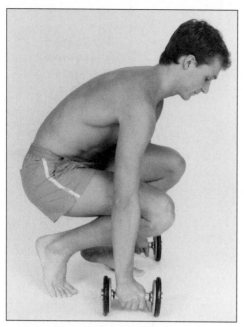

Figure 9-174 Squatting to pick up an object from the floor requires almost full lumbar flexion (i.e., about 95% of full flexion).[68]

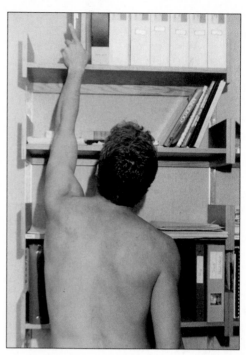

Figure 9-176 Reaching objects overhead requires trunk lateral flexion.

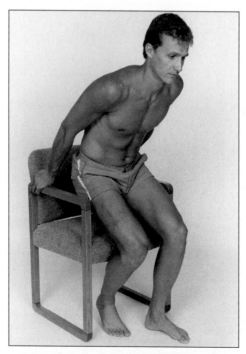

Figure 9-175 Moving from standing to sitting and returning to standing requires about 56% to 66% of full lumbar flexion ROM.[68]

"lumbar-pelvic rhythm,"[65] providing smooth movement and a large excursion of movement for the lower extremity and trunk. The lumbar spine and hip (i.e., as the pelvis moves on the femur) contribute an average of about 40° lumbar spine flexion and 70° hip flexion, respectively, to complete this forward bending motion.[66] Lumbar and pelvic motions are nearly simultaneous with varying degrees of contribution from the lumbar spine and pelvis throughout range.[66,67] Changing the speed of motion, lifting various size loads, and past history of low back pain may influence the lumbar-pelvic rhythm.[66,67]

Normal ROM for lumbar spine flexion is about 60°.[68] Sitting to put on a sock (Fig. 9-173) and squatting to pick up an object from the floor (Fig. 9-174) are examples of activities that require almost full lumbar spine flexion (i.e., about 90% and 95% of full flexion, respectively).[68] Moving from standing to sitting and returning to standing position requires about 56% to 66% of full lumbar flexion ROM[68] (Fig. 9-175). The joints in the lumbar spine and L5/S1 approach full flexion in the slouched sitting position.[69]

Activities that require lateral flexion of the spine include reaching down to pick up an object from a low surface at one's side, moving from a side-lying position to sitting on the edge of a bed, and reaching objects overhead (Fig. 9-176). To mount a bicycle, one leg is lifted over the seat of the bicycle and the trunk is laterally flexed to the same side.

Muscle Function

Head and Neck

The muscles of the head and neck maintain the posture of the head, position the head to accommodate vision and feeding, and assist with breathing and coughing. Group muscle actions and some individual muscle actions of the head and neck are described relative to function.

Head and Neck Flexors. The longus colli, longus capitis, sternocleidomastoid, and scalenus anterior, medius, and posterior contracting bilaterally flex the head and neck. The sternocleidomastoids contracting bilaterally flex the cervical spine relative to the thoracic spine and flex the head when the prevertebral muscles contract to flatten the cervical spine and keep it rigid.[1] The scaleni muscles contracting bilaterally also flex the cervical spine on the thoracic spine when the prevertebral muscles hold the cervical spine rigid.[1] Chewing, swallowing, and speaking are the main functions of the infrahyoid and suprahyoid muscles as these muscles act on the hyoid bone, mandible, and thyroid cartilage.[55] These muscles also flex the cervical spine when the masseter and temporalis muscles contract to keep the mandible closed.[1] The rectus capitis anterior and lateralis muscles contracting bilaterally, flex the head on the cervical spine.[1]

The head and neck flexors contract when flexion occurs against a resistance, such as the weight of the head. The flexors flex the head and neck and hold the head in this flexed position when the head is lifted off the supporting surface in the supine position, as illustrated in getting out of bed (Fig. 9-177). The flexors control neck extension when the head is lowered back onto the supporting surface when lying down supine. In upright postures, the head and neck flexors contract when flexion is full and forced such as, when one looks down to manipulate buttons at the top of a shirt and when doing up the clasp of a necklace at the back of the neck.

When eating, bilateral contraction of the sternocleidomastoid pulls the head forward and assists the longus colli to flex the cervical spine.[2] Electromyographic study has demonstrated sufficient bilateral activity in the longus colli and sternocleidomastoid muscles on anterior protrusion of the head to maintain the head in this position[70] (Fig. 9-178).

Head and Neck Extensors. The extensor muscles of the head and neck include the semispinalis capitis and cervicis, splenius capitis and cervicis, rectus capitis posterior major and minor, obliquus capitis inferior and superior, and the erector spinae (i.e., iliocostalis cervicis, longissimus

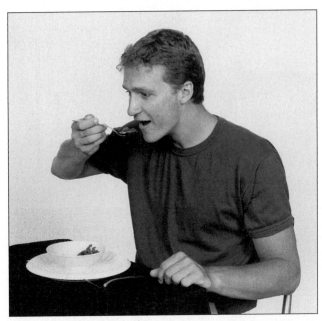

Figure 9-178 Sternocleidomastoid and longus colli function to anteriorly protrude the head.

capitis and cervicis, and spinalis capitis and cervicis muscles). The levator scapulae, sternocleidomastoid, and upper fibers of trapezius also act to extend the head and neck. The sternocleidomastoid contracting bilaterally acts as an extensor of the head and flexes the cervical spine on the thoracic spine when the cervical spine is flexible and not flattened and held rigid by the prevertebral muscles.[1] Unilateral contraction of sternocleidomastoid produces neck extension with lateral flexion to the same side and rotation to the opposite side.[1] The obliquus capitis inferior and superior and rectus capitis posterior major and minor, contracting bilaterally, extend the head and upper cervical spine.[1] Bilateral contraction of the head and neck extensor muscles produces neck extension eliminating the actions of lateral flexion and rotation that occur when these muscles contract unilaterally.

The head and neck extensors contract when extension is forced at the end of the ROM or occurs against a resistance. Activities carried out overhead require contraction of the extensors at the end of the ROM, such as, when reaching for a book on a high shelf (Fig. 9-179). Other activities that require contraction at the end of the ROM include drinking from a glass (Fig. 9-180) and looking down the bowling lane as the bowling ball is released from the hand. The neck extensors contract and work against resistance to lift the head off the supporting surface when lying prone and control neck flexion when the head is lowered to the surface again. The extensors contract in activities where the head is inclined forward, such as writing (Fig. 9-166) and reading.[55] Activity in the neck extensors ceases when the neck becomes fully flexed and the tension in the ligamentum nuchae maintains the position of the head.[55]

Head and Neck Lateral Flexors. Unilateral contraction of the head and neck extensors, and many of the head and

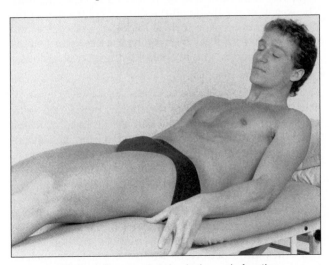

Figure 9-177 Neck flexor and abdominal muscle function.

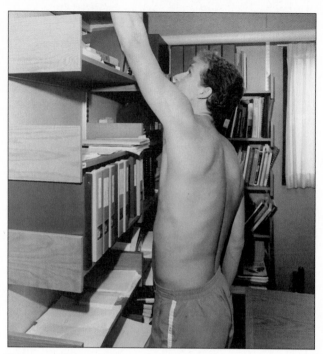

Figure 9-179 Neck extensor muscle function.

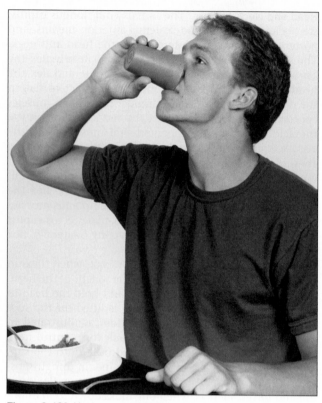

Figure 9-180 Neck extensors contract at full neck extension, when drinking from a glass.

neck flexors, laterally flex the head and neck to the same side. Functionally, these muscles contract to laterally flex the cervical spine and position and control the tilt of the head so that one can correctly see objects that are not in level. The lateral flexors can contract to position the head and assist in realigning the body in the upright posture from either a recumbent or inverted posture. The lateral flexors contract to hold the head in position when one moves from a side-lying position to a sitting position to get out of bed.

Head and Neck Rotators. The rectus capitis major and minor, obliquus capitis superior and inferior, sterno-cleidomastoid, scalenus anterior, medius and posterior, upper fibers of trapezius, semispinalis cervicis, splenius capitis and cervicis, multifidus, rotatores, and the erector spinae (i.e., iliocostalis cervicis and longissimus capitis and cervicis) muscles rotate the head and neck when contraction occurs unilaterally. The main function of the rotators is to rotate the head and neck to look from side to side as one would do to shoulder check when driving (Fig. 9-167) or track the ball during a tennis match. In rolling from supine to side-lying or prone-lying positions, the movement of the trunk may be initiated by rotating the head and neck in the direction of the move. The rotators contract when indicating a negative response to a question. When performing activities, such as combing the hair that require placement of the hand at the back of the head, the cervical spine and head may be rotated.

Breathing.[55] Some of the muscles of the neck assist with breathing. Scalenus anterior, medius, and posterior are primary muscles of inspiration and elevate the first and second ribs when the cervical spine is fixed.

Sternocleidomastoid, suprahyoid, and infrahyoid muscles act as accessory muscles of inspiration, being recruited on forceful breathing, for example, when exercising. Coughing requires contraction from the primary, accessory, and stabilizing muscles of respiration.

Posture. The position of the line of gravity anterior to the atlanto-occipital joint of the neck produces a flexion moment that tends to cause the head to fall forward. Forward flexion of the head in sitting and standing is prevented by the contraction of the head and neck extensors. The weight of the head and the force of contraction of the neck extensors increase cervical lordosis.[71] The contraction of longus colli stabilizes and counteracts the forces tending to increase lordosis, thus maintaining the cervical lordosis.[71]

Trunk

The trunk muscles stabilize the thorax, pelvis, and spine for movements of the head and extremities, maintain posture, and assist with breathing, coughing, and straining. The abdominals also support and protect the abdominal viscera, contribute to a normal walking pattern, and contract to protect the spine in lifting activities.

Trunk Flexion. The psoas major muscle and the abdominal and erector spinae muscle groups are responsible for trunk flexion. The abdominal muscles contract when trunk flexion is performed against a resistance such as body weight. The abdominal muscles are therefore the prime movers when one rises from the supine position to get out of bed (see Fig. 9-177). In the supine position, the rectus abdominis is the most active abdominal muscle when the head is raised,[72] contracting to stabilize the thorax. The abdominal muscles contract isometrically and function to stabilize the thorax and pelvis when performing pushing, pulling, or lifting activities.[59]

Flexion of the trunk in standing position occurs as one picks up an object from the floor or ties a shoelace. Trunk flexion is initiated by contraction of the abdominals and the vertebral portion of the psoas major muscle.[56] Once the trunk is inclined forward gravity takes over to flex the trunk. Flexion of the trunk is then controlled through contraction of the erector spinae muscle until a "critical position" is reached when the erector spinae muscle relaxes and further flexion occurs through hip flexion.[73] The posterior layer of the thoracolumbar fascia,[74] elastic forces generated in the extensor musculature as a result of the passive stretch on the muscles,[75] and the posterior intervertebral ligaments support the trunk in the fully flexed position when the erector spinae is relaxed. Wolf and coworkers[76] identify the critical position to be at greater than 70° of trunk flexion, most often between 80° and 90°. If further trunk flexion is required at the end of the movement, the abdominal muscles must contract to force the movement.[77]

Trunk Extension. The erector spinae muscle contracts to initiate trunk extension in the standing position and once started, gravity pulls the trunk into further extension and the movement is controlled by the contraction of the abdominal muscles.[56] The erector spinae contracts again, if required, to force extension at the end of the ROM.[56] When trunk extension is performed against resistance, the erector spinae muscle contracts to perform the entire movement. This occurs when the trunk is extended from a forward lean position in sitting, and in the prone position when the trunk is extended to reach for a light switch located at the head of the bed.

When lifting objects off the floor from a forward flexed position, the pattern of muscle activity is the reverse of that required to flex forward in standing. There is no contraction of the erector spinae muscles at the beginning of the lift, the thoracolumbar fascia, elastic forces generated in the extensor musculature, and the posterior intervertebral ligaments take the load and the movement to extend occurs initially at the hip joints, as the pelvis rotates posteriorly. As the movement continues the erector spinae muscle contracts close to the critical position and the contraction continues until the erect position is reached.[73] Great forces are placed on the trunk when lifting in the forward flexed position; therefore, this position should be discouraged and the lift performed with the back straight and the knees flexed[78] with the object being lifted positioned as close to the body as possible. When heavy weights are lifted and large forces are placed on the spine, the abdominal (primarily the transversus abdominus[79]), diaphragm, and intercostal muscles contract to increase the intra-abdominal and intrathoracic pressures so that the thorax and abdomen become semirigid cylinders.[80] This results in some of the force

from the weight being transmitted through the arms to the thorax and abdomen and then to the pelvis, taking some of the load off the spine.[80] This also results in additional trunk stabilization and an extensor moment is applied to the lumbar spine[79] through activation of the transversus abdominus and subsequent increased tension in the thoracolumbar fascia.

Trunk Lateral Flexion. The erector spinae, intertransversarii, and posterolateral fibers of the external abdominal oblique, quadratus lumborum, and iliopsoas muscles contribute to lateral flexion of the trunk. Lateral flexion is not used often in activities unless to pick an object up from a low table at one's side or when moving from a side-lying position to sitting on the edge of a bed or sitting to a side-lying position. The lateral flexors contract on the ipsilateral side to initiate movement and contract on the contralateral side to modify the movement in the upright position.[56]

Trunk Rotation. The trunk rotator muscles include the erector spinae, multifidus, rotatores, and internal and external abdominal oblique muscles. The internal and external abdominal obliques are the prime rotators of the trunk.[81] The extensor muscles function to counteract the flexion torque created by the oblique abdominal muscles during trunk rotation.[81] The muscles contract to rotate the trunk to change position while recumbent and when one turns to look in a posterior direction, or reaches with the hand(s) in directions lateral or posterior to the trunk.

Posture. Electromyographic studies report slight activity in the erector spinae muscle[73] and slight contraction in the internal abdominal oblique muscle[72] in standing. The erector spinae contracts during unsupported upright sitting but is relaxed when sitting in the "slumped" position with the spine in full flexion.[73]

Breathing. The erector spinae is active during inspiration when ventilatory demand is increased.[82] With an increased inspiratory effort, forces are transmitted to the spine through the costovertebral and costotransverse articulations encouraging flexion of the spine. Spinal flexion will cause a deflationary effect on the rib cage. This deflationary effect is counteracted by the erector spinae contracting to stiffen and extend the vertebral column.

The abdominal muscles are inactive during expiration at rest. When ventilatory demands increase, the abdominal muscles (rectus abdominus, external abdominal oblique, internal abdominal oblique, and transversus abdominus) contract to pull the rib cage down and increase the intra-abdominal pressure, thus pushing the abdominal contents and diaphragm upward into the thoracic cavity, decreasing the lung volume to expel air.[83]

Gait.[7] As the pelvis rotates forward on the side of the advancing leg, the trunk rotates forward on the opposite side to keep the body facing forward during the gait cycle. The erector spinae muscles contract on the contralateral side to the supporting leg to prevent the trunk falling forward due to the hip flexion moment created on the stance leg. The erector spinae muscles contract at initial contact and preswing. The abdominal muscles do not normally contract when walking on the level.[84]

References

1. Kapandji AI. *The Physiology of the Joints. Vol 3. The Spinal Column, Pelvic Girdle and Head.* 6th ed. London: Churchill Livingstone Elsevier; 2008.
2. Soames RW, ed. Skeletal system. Salmon S, ed. Muscle. In: *Gray's Anatomy.* 38th ed. New York: Churchill Livingstone; 1995.
3. Berryman Reese N, Bandy WD. *Joint Range of Motion and Muscle Length Testing.* 2nd ed. St. Louis, MO: Saunders Elsevier; 2010.
4. Magee DJ. *Orthopedic Physical Assessment.* 4th ed. Philadelphia, PA: Saunders; 2002.
5. American Academy of Orthopaedic Surgeons. *Joint Motion: Method of Measuring and Recording.* Chicago, IL: AAOS; 1965.
6. Cyriax J. *Textbook of Orthopaedic Medicine. Vol 1. Diagnosis of Soft Tissue Lesions.* 8th ed. London: Bailliere Tindall; 1982.
7. Levangie PK, Norkin CC. *Joint Structure and Function: A Comprehensive Analysis.* 3rd ed. Philadelphia, PA: FA Davis; 2001.
8. Daniels L, Worthingham C. *Muscle Testing: Techniques of Manual Examination.* 5th ed. Philadelphia, PA: WB Saunders; 1986.
9. Youdas JW, Garrett TR, Suman VJ, Bogard CL, Hallman HO, Carey JR. Normal range of motion of the cervical spine: an initial goniometric study. *Phys Ther.* 1992;72:770–780.
10. Balogun JA, Abereoje OK, Olaogun MO, Obajuluwa VA. Inter- and intratester reliability of measuring neck motions with tape measure and Myrin gravity-reference goniometer. *J Orthop Sports Phys Ther.* 1989;10:248–253.
11. Hsieh C-Y, Yeung BW. Active neck motion measurements with a tape measure. *J Orthop Sports Phys Ther.* 1986;8:88–92.
12. American Medical Association. *Guides to the Evaluation of Permanent Impairment.* 5th ed. Chicago, IL: AMA Press; 2001.
13. American Medical Association. *Guides to the Evaluation of Permanent Impairment.* 2nd ed. Chicago, IL: AMA Press; 1984.
14. Soderberg GL. *Kinesiology: Application to Pathological Motion.* 2nd ed. Baltimore, MD: Williams & Wilkins; 1997.
15. Iglarsh ZA, Snyder-Mackler L. Temporomandibular joint and the cervical spine. In: Richardson JK, Iglarsh ZA. *Clinical Orthopaedic Physical Therapy.* Philadelphia, PA: WB Saunders; 1994.
16. Moskovich R. Biomechanics of the cervical spine. In: Nordin M, Frankel VH. *Basic Biomechanics of the Musculoskeletal System.* 3rd ed. Philadelphia, PA: Lippincott Williams & Wilkins; 2001.
17. Performance Attainment Associates. *CROM Procedure Manual: Procedure for Measuring Neck Motion with the CROM.* St. Paul, MN: University of Minnesota; 1988 (copyright University of Minnesota).
18. Mayer TG, Kindraske G, Beals SB, Gatchel RJ. Spinal range of motion: accuracy and sources of error with inclinometric measurement. *Spine.* 1997;22:1976–1984.
19. Performance Attainment Associates, 958 Lydia Drive, Roseville, MN: 55113.
20. Calder I, Picard J, Chapman M, O'Sullivan C, Crockard HA. Mouth opening: a new angle. *Anesthesiology.* 2003;99:799–801.
21. Higbie EJ, Seidel-Cobb D, Taylor LF, Cummings GS. Effect of head position on vertical mandibular opening. *J Orthop Sports Phys Ther.* 1999;29:127–130.

22. Thurnwald PA. The effect of age and gender on normal temporomandibular joint movement. *Physiotherapy Theory Practice.* 1991;7:209–221.
23. Venes D, ed. *Taber's Cyclopedic Medical Dictionary.* 19th ed. Philadelphia, PA: FA Davis; 2001.
24. American Medical Association. *Guides to the Evaluation of Permanent Impairment.* 3rd ed (Revised). Chicago, IL: AMA Press; 1990.
25. Walker N, Bohannon RW, Cameron D. Discriminant validity of temporomandibular joint range of motion measurements obtained with a ruler. *J Orthop Sports Phys Ther.* 2000;30:484–492.
26. Dijkstra PU, De Bont LGM, Stegenga B, Boering G. Temporomandibular joint mobility assessment: a comparison between four methods. *J Oral Rehab.* 1995;22:439–444.
27. Dworkin SF, LeResche L, DeRouen T, VonKorff M. Assessing clinical signs of temporomandibular disorders: reliability of clinical examiners. *J Prosthet Dent.* 1990;63:574–579.
28. Al-Ani MZ, Gray RJ. Evaluation of three devices used for measuring mouth opening. *Dent Update.* 2004;31(6):346–348, 350.
29. Jordan K. Assessment of published reliability studies for cervical range-of-motion measurement tools. *J Manip Physiol Ther.* 2000;23:180–195.
30. de Koning CHP, van den Heuvel SP, Staal JB, Smits-Engelsman BCM, Hendriks EJM. Clinimetric evaluation of active range of motion measures in patients with non-specific neck pain: a systematic review. *Eur Spine J.* 2008;17:905-921.
31. Williams MA, McCarthy CJ, Chorti A, Cooke MW, Gates S. Literature Review. A systematic review of reliability and validity studies of methods for measuring active and passive cervical range of motion. *J Manipulative Physiol Ther.* 2010;33(2):138.
32. Moore KL. *Clinically Oriented Anatomy.* Baltimore, MD: Williams & Wilkins; 1980.
33. Gilroy J, Holliday PL. *Basic Neurology.* New York, NY: MacMillan, 1982.
34. Mancall EL. *Alpers and Mancall's Essentials of the Neurologic Examination.* 2nd ed. Philadelphia, PA: FA Davis; 1981.
35. MacConaill MA, Basmajian JV. *Muscles and Movements: A Basis for Human Kinesiology.* Huntington, NY: RE Krieger; 1977.
36. Kendall FP, McCreary EK, Provance PG. *Muscles Testing and Function.* 4th ed. Baltimore, MD: Williams & Wilkins; 1993.
37. Kendall FP, McCreary EK. *Muscles Testing and Function.* 3rd ed. Baltimore, MD: Williams & Wilkins; 1983.
38. White AA, Panjabi MM. *Clinical Biomechanics of the Spine.* Philadelphia, PA: JB Lippincott; 1978.
39. Neumann DA. *Kinesiology of the Musculoskeletal System: Foundations for Rehabilitation.* 2nd ed. St. Louis, MO: Mosby Elsevier; 2010.
40. van Adrichem JAM, van der Korst JK. Assessment of the flexibility of the lumbar spine. *Scand J Rheumatol.* 1973;2:87–91.
41. Mellin GP. Accuracy of measuring lateral flexion of the spine with a tape. *Clin Biomechanics.* 1986;1:85–89.
42. Frost M, Stuckey S, Smalley LA, Dorman G. Reliability of measuring trunk motions in centimeters. *Phys Ther.* 1982;62:1431–1437.
43. Pearcy MJ. Twisting mobility of the human back in flexed postures. *Spine.* 1993;18:114–119.
44. Harris J, Johansen J, Pedersen S, LaPier TK. Site of measurement and subject position affect chest expansion measurements. *Cardiopulmonary Phys Ther.* 1997;8:12–17.
45. Moll JMH, Wright V. An objective clinical study of chest expansion. *Ann Rheum Dis.* 1972;31:1–8.
46. Neustadt DH. Ankylosing spondylitis. *Postgrad Med.* 1977;61:124–135.

47. Littlewood C, May S. Measurement of range of movement in the lumbar spine – what methods are valid? A systematic review. *Physiotherapy.* 2007;93:201–211.

48. Essendrop M, Maul I, Läubli T, Riihimäki H, Schibye B. Measures of low back function: a review of reproducibility studies. *Phys Ther in Sport.* 2003;4:137-151. Reprinted from *Clinical Biomech.* 2002;17:235–249.

49. Beim GM, Giraldo JL, Pincivero DM, Borror MJ, Fu FH. Abdominal strengthening exercises: a comparative EMG study. *Sport Rehabil.* 1997;6:11–20.

50. Flint MM. An electromyographic comparison of the function of the iliacus and the rectus abdominis muscles. *J Am Phys Ther Assoc.* 1965;45:248–253.

51. Shirado O, Toshikazu I, Kaneda K, Strax TE. Electromyographic analysis of four techniques for isometric trunk muscle exercises. *Arch Phys Med Rehabil.* 1995;76:225–229.

52. Norris CM. Abdominal muscle training in sport. *Br J Sports Med.* 1993;27:19–27.

53. Gilleard WL, Brown JMM. An electromyographic validation of an abdominal muscle test. *Arch Phys Med Rehabil.* 1994;75:1002–1007.

54. Graves JE, Webb DC, Pollock ML, Matkozich J, Leggett SH, Carpenter DM, Foster DN, Cirulli J. Pelvic stabilization during resistance training: its effect on the development of lumbar extension strength. *Arch Phys Med Rehabil.* 1994;75: 210–215.

55. Smith LK, Weiss EL, Lemkuhl LD. *Brunnstrom's Clinical Kinesiology.* 5th ed. Philadelphia, PA: FA Davis; 1996.

56. Lindh M. Biomechanics of the lumbar spine. In: Nordin M, Frankel VH. *Basic Biomechanics of the Musculoskeletal System.* 2nd ed. Philadelphia, PA: Lea & Febiger; 1989.

57. Cailliet R. *Neck and Arm Pain.* 3rd ed. Philadelphia, PA: FA Davis; 1991.

58. Sterling AC, Cobian DG, Anderson PA, Heiderscheit C. Annual frequency and magnitude of neck motion in healthy individuals. *Spine.* 2008;33(17):1882–1888.

59. Henmi S, Yonenobu K, Masatomi T, Oda K. A biomechanical study of daily living using neck and upper limbs with an optical three-dimensional motion analysis system. *Mod Rheumatol.* 2006;16:289–293.

60. Shugg JAJ, Jackson CD, Dickey JP. Cervical spine rotation and range of motion: pilot measurements during driving. *Traffic Inj Prev.* 2011;12:82–87.

61. Shum GLK, Crosbie J, Lee RYW. Symptomatic and asymptomatic movement coordination of the lumbar spine and hip during an everyday activity. *Spine.* 2005;30(23):E697–E702.

62. Hutton JT, Shapiro I, Christians B. Functional significance of restricted gaze. *Arch Phys Med Rehabil.* 1982;63:617–619.

63. Muñoz M. Congenital absence of the inferior rectus muscle. *Am J Ophthalmol.* 1992;121:327–329.

64. Pemberton PL, Calder I, O'Sullivan C, Crockard HA. The champagne angle. *Anaesthesia.* 2002;57:402–403.

65. Cailliet R. *Low Back Pain Syndrome.* 5th ed. Philadelphia, PA: FA Davis; 1995.

66. Esola M, McClure PW, Fitzgerald GK, Siegler S. Analysis of lumbar spine and hip motion during forward bending in subjects with and without a history of low back pain. *Spine.* 1996;21(1):71–78.

67. Granata KP, Sanford AH. Lumbar-pelvic coordination is influenced by lifting task parameters. *Spine.* 2000;25(11): 1412–1418.

68. Hsieh CJ, Pringle RK. Range of motion of the lumbar spine required for four activities of daily living. *J Manipulative Physiol Therap.* 1994;17:353–358.

69. Dunk NM, Kedgley AE, Jenkyn TR, Callaghan JP. Evidence of a pelvis-driven flexion pattern: are the joints of the lower lumbar spine fully flexed in seated postures? *Clin Biomech.* 2009;24:164–168.

70. Vitti M, Fujiwara M, Basmajian JV, Iida M. The integrated roles of longus colli and sternomastoid muscles: an electromyographic study. *Anat Rec.* 1973;177:471–484.

71. Mayoux-Benhamou MA, Revel M, Vallee C, Roudier R, Barbet JP, Bargy F. Longus colli has a postural function on cervical curvature. *Surg Radiol Anat.* 1994;16:367–371.

72. Carman DJ, Blanton PL, Biggs NL. Electromyographic study of the anterolateral abdominal musculature utilizing indwelling electrodes. *Am J Phys Med.* 1972;51:113–129.

73. Floyd WF, Silver PHS. The function of the erectores spinae muscles in certain movements and postures in man. *J Physiol.* 1955;129:184–203.

74. Bogduk N, Macintosh JE. The applied anatomy of the thoracolumbar fascia. *Spine.* 1984;9:164–170.

75. McGill SM, Kippers V. Transfer of loads between lumbar tissues during the flexion-relaxation phenomenon. *Spine.* 1994;19:2190–2196.

76. Wolf SL, Basmajian JV, Russe TC, Kutner M. Normative data on low back mobility and activity levels. *Am J Phys Med.* 1979;58:217–229.

77. Basmajian JV, DeLuca CJ. *Muscles Alive: Their Functions Revealed by Electromyography.* 5th ed. Baltimore, MD: Williams & Wilkins; 1985.

78. Davis PR, Troup JDG, Burnard JH. Movements of the thoracic and lumbar spine when lifting: a chrono-cyclophotographic study. *J Anat (Lond).* 1965;99:13–26.

79. Cresswell AG, Thorstensson A. Changes in intra-abdominal pressure, trunk muscle activation and force during isokinetic lifting and lowering. *Eur J Appl Physiol.* 1994;68: 315–321.

80. Morris JM, Lucas DB, Bresler B. Role of the trunk in stability of the spine. *J Bone Joint Surg [Am].* 1961;43:327–351.

81. Macintosh JE, Pearcy MJ, Bogduk N. The axial torque of the lumbar back muscles: torsion strength of the back muscles. *Aust NZJ Surg.* 1993;63:205–212.

82. Cala SJ, Edyvean J, Engel LA. Chest wall and trunk muscle activity during inspiratory loading. *Appl Physiol.* 1992;73: 2373–2381.

83. Epstein SK. An overview of respiratory muscle function. *Clin Chest Med.* 1994;15:619–639.

84. Sheffield FJ. Electromyographic study of the abdominal muscles in walking and other movements. *Am J Phys Med.* 1962;41:142–147.

SECTION III
Appendices

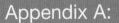

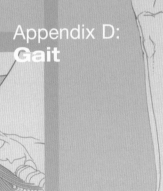

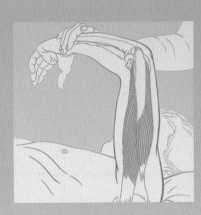

Appendix A

Sample Numerical Recording Form: Range of Motion Assessment and Measurement

Range of Motion Assessment and Measurement

Patient's Name _____

Diagnosis _____

Therapist Name _____

    Signature _____

Date of Birth/Age _____

Date of Onset _____

AROM ☐   PROM ☐

Recording:

1. The Neutral Zero Method defined by the American Academy of Orthopaedic Surgeons[1] is used for measurement and recording.

2. Average ranges defined by the American Academy of Orthopaedic Surgeons,[1] are provided in parentheses.

3. The columns designated with asterisks (*) are used for indicating limitation of range of motion and referencing for summarization.

4. Space is left at the end of each section to record hypermobile ranges and comments regarding positioning of the patient or body part, measuring instrument, edema, pain, and/or end feel.

Left Side					Right Side			
	*		*	Therapist Initials	*		*	
				Date of Measurement				
				Head, Neck, and Trunk				
				Mandible: Depression				
				Protrusion				
				Lateral deviation				
				Neck: Flexion (0–45°)				
				Extension (0–45°)				
				Lateral flexion (0–45°)				
				Rotation (0–60°)				
				Trunk: Flexion (0–80°, 10 cm)				
				Extension (0–20–30°)				
				Lateral flexion (0–35°)				
				Rotation (0–45°)				
				Hypermobility: Comments:				

Patient's Name _____

	*		*	Therapist Initials	*		*	
				Date of Measurement				
				Scapula				
				Elevation				
				Depression				
				Abduction				
				Adduction				
				Shoulder Complex				
				Elevation through Flexion (0–180°)				
				Elevation through Abduction (0–180°)				
				Shoulder (Glenohumeral) Joint				
				Flexion (0–120°)[2]				
				Abduction (0–90° to 120°)[2]				
				Extension (0–60°)				
				Horizontal abduction (0–45°)				
				Horizontal adduction (0–135°)				
				Internal rotation (0–70°)				
				External rotation (0–90°)				
				Hypermobility: Comments:				
				Elbow and Forearm				
				Flexion (0–150°)				
				Supination (0–80°)				
				Pronation (0–80°)				
				Hypermobility: Comments:				

Left Side / **Right Side**

Patient's Name _____

Left Side				Therapist Initials	Right Side			
	*		*	Date of Measurement	*		*	
				Wrist				
				Flexion (0–80°)				
				Extension (0–70°)				
				Ulnar deviation (0–30°)				
				Radial deviation (0–20°)				
				Hypermobility:				
				Comments:				
				Thumb				
				CM flexion (0–15°)				
				CM extension (0–20°)				
				Abduction (0–70°)				
				MCP flexion (0–50°)				
				IP flexion (0–80°)				
				Opposition				
				Hypermobility:				
				Comments:				
				Fingers				
				MCP digit 2 flexion (0–90°)				
				extension (0–45°)				
				abduction				
				adduction				
				MCP digit 3 flexion (0–90°)				
				extension (0–45°)				
				abduction (radial)				
				adduction (ulnar)				
				MCP digit 4 flexion (0–90°)				
				extension (0–45°)				
				abduction				
				adduction				

Patient's Name _____

Left Side					Right Side			
	*		*	**Therapist Initials**	*		*	
				Date of Measurement				
				MCP digit 5 flexion (0–90°)				
				extension (0–45°)				
				abduction				
				adduction				
				PIP digit 2 flexion (0–100°)				
				3 flexion (0–100°)				
				4 flexion (0–100°)				
				5 flexion (0–100°)				
				DIP digit 2 flexion (0–90°)				
				3 flexion (0–90°)				
				4 flexion (0–90°)				
				5 flexion (0–90°)				
				Composite finger abduction/thumb extension— Distance between:				
				Thumb–digit 2				
				Digit 2–digit 3				
				Digit 3–digit 4				
				Digit 4–digit 5				
				Composite flexion—Distance between:				
				Finger pulp-distal palmar crease				
				Finger pulp-proximal palmar crease				
				Hypermobility: Comments:				

Patient's Name _____

Left Side				Therapist Initials	Right Side			
	*		*	Therapist Initials	*		*	
				Date of Measurement				
				Hip				
				Flexion (0–120°)				
				Extension (0–30°)				
				Abduction (0–45°)				
				Adduction (0–30°)				
				Internal rotation (0–45°)				
				External rotation (0–45°)				
				Hypermobility:				
				Comments:				
				Knee				
				Flexion (0–135°)				
				Tibial rotation				
				Patellar mobility—Distal glide				
				Patellar mobility—Medial-lateral glide				
				Hypermobility:				
				Comments:				
				Ankle				
				Dorsiflexion (0–20°)				
				Plantarflexion (0–50°)				
				Inversion (0–35°)				
				Eversion (0–15°)				
				Hypermobility:				
				Comments:				

Patient's Name _____

	*		*	Therapist Initials	*		*	
				Date of Measurement				
				Toes				
				MTP great toe flexion (0–45°)				
				extension (0–70°)				
				abduction				
				MTP digit 2 flexion (0–40°)				
				extension (0–40°)				
				MTP digit 3 flexion (0–40°)				
				extension (0–40°)				
				MTP digit 4 flexion (0–40°)				
				extension (0–40°)				
				MTP digit 5 flexion (0–40°)				
				extension (0–40°)				
				IP great toe flexion (0–90°)				
				PIP digit 2 flexion (0–35°)				
				PIP digit 3 flexion (0–35°)				
				PIP digit 4 flexion (0–35°)				
				PIP digit 5 flexion (0–35°)				
				Hypermobility: Comments:				

Left Side / Right Side

Summary of Limitation:

Additional Comments:

[1]American Academy of Orthopaedic Surgeons: *Joint Motion: Method of Measuring and Recording*. Chicago: AAOS; 1965.
[2]Levangie PK, Norkin CC. *Joint Structure and Function: A Comprehensive Analysis*. 3rd ed. Philadelphia: FA Davis; 2001.

Appendix B

Sample Recording Form:
Manual Muscle Strength Assessment

Manual Muscle Strength Assessment

Patient's Name _____ Date of Birth/Age _____ ID _____

Diagnosis _____ Date of Onset _____

Therapist Name _____

     Signature _____

Manual Muscle Testing (MMT) Method Used

Date of Assessment: _____ MMT method used: _____

Date of Assessment: _____ MMT method used: _____

Date of Assessment: _____ MMT method used: _____

Date of Assessment: _____ MMT method used: _____

Key: MMT Method Used.

C   Conventional "through range" grading

I   "Isometric" grading: **b** break test or **m** make test
     (eg: **Ib** indicates "Isometric" break test)

Left Side						Right Side		
			Therapist Initials					
			Date of Assessment					
			Motion	**Muscle**	**Nerve supply**			
			Eye					
			Eyelid elevation	Levator palpebrae superioris	CN III			
			Eyelid closure	Obicularis oculi	CN VII			
			Eyeball elevation	Rectus superior / Obliquus inferior	CN III / CN III			
			Eyeball depression	Rectus inferior / Obliquus superior	CN III / CN IV			
			Eyeball abduction	Rectus lateralis	CN VI			
			Eyeball adduction	Rectus medialis	CN III			
			Eyebrows					
			Elevation	Epicranius	CN VII			
			Adduction	Corrugator supercilli	CN VII			
			Depression	Procerus	CN VII			
			Mandible					
			Elevation	Temporalis/masseter/medial pterygoid	CN V			
			Depression	Lateral pterygoid/suprahyoid	CN V			
			Protrusion	Pterygoids	CN V			

Remarks:

Patient's Name/ID _____

Left Side						Right Side		
			Therapist Initials					
			Date of Assessment					
			Motion	Muscle	Nerve supply			
			Nasal Aperture					
			Dilation	Nasalis/depressor septi	CN VII			
			Constriction	Nasalis	CN VII			
			Lips/Mouth					
			Lip closure	Obicularis oris	CN VII			
			Cheek compression	Buccinator	CN VII			
			Elevation of angle	Levator anguli oris	CN VII			
			Retraction of angle	Zygomaticus major/risorius	CN VII			
			Depression of angle	Platysma/depressor anguli oris/ depressor labii inferioris	CN VII			
			Upper lip elevation	Levator labii superioris/zygomaticus minor	CN VII			
			Lower lip elevation	Mentalis	CN VII			
			Tongue					
			Protrusion	Genioglossus	CN XII			
			Neck					
			Hyoid bone depression	Infrahyoid group	Cervical			
			Flexion	Flexor group	Cervical			
				Sternomastoid	Cervical			
			Extension	Extensor group	Cervical			
			Scapula					
			Abduction Lateral rotation	Serratus anterior	Long Thoracic			
			Elevation	Upper trapezius Levator scapulae	Accessory, CN XI Dorsal Scapular			
			Adduction	Middle trapezius	Accessory, CN XI			
			Adduction Medial rotation	Rhomboids	Dorsal Scapular			
			Depression	Lower trapezius	Accessory, CN XI			

Remarks:

Patient's Name/ID _____

Left Side						Right Side		
			Therapist Initials					
			Therapist Initials					
			Date of Assessment					
			Motion	**Muscle**	**Nerve supply**			
			Shoulder					
			Flexion	Anterior deltoid	Axillary			
			Flexion–Adduction	Coracobrachialis	Musculocutaneous			
			Extension	Latissimus dorsi Teres major	Thoracodorsal Subscapular			
			Abduction	Middle deltoid Supraspinatus	Axillary Suprascapular			
			Adduction	Pectoralis major Teres major Latissimus dorsi	Pectoral Subscapular Thoracodorsal			
			Horizontal adduction	Pectoralis major	Pectoral			
			Horizontal abduction	Posterior deltoid	Axillary			
			Internal rotation	Subscapularis	Subscapular			
			External rotation	Infraspinatus Teres minor	Suprascapular Axillary			
			Elbow/Forearm					
			Flexion	Biceps	Musculocutaneous			
				Brachioradialis Brachialis	Radial Musculocutaneous/radial			
			Extension	Triceps	Radial			
			Supination	Supinator	Radial			
			Pronation	Pronator teres Pronator quadratus	Median			
			Wrist					
			Flexion	Flexor carpi radialis	Median			
				Flexor carpi ulnaris	Ulnar			
			Extension	Extensor carpi radialis longus Extensor carpi radialis brevis	Radial Radial			
				Extensor carpi ulnaris	Radial			

Remarks:

Patient's Name/ID _____

Left Side						Right Side		
			Therapist Initials					
			Date of Assessment					
			Motion	Muscle	Nerve supply			
			Fingers					
			MCP extension	Extensor digitorum Extensor indicis proprius Extensor digiti minimi	Radial Radial Radial			
			MCP abduction	Dorsal interossei	Ulnar			
				Abductor digiti minimi	Ulnar			
			MCP adduction	Palmar interossei	Ulnar			
			MCP flexion-IP extension	Lumbricales 1 and 2 Lumbricales 3 and 4	Median Ulnar			
			5th MCP flexion	Flexor digiti minimi	Ulnar			
			PIP flexion digit 2	Flexor digitorum superficialis	Median			
			digit 3					
			digit 4					
			DIP flexion digit 2	Flexor digitorum profundus	Median			
			digit 3		Median			
			digit 4		Ulnar			
			digit 5		Ulnar			
			Thumb					
			IP flexion	Flexor pollicis longus	Median			
			MCP flexion	Flexor pollicis brevis	Ulnar			
			IP extension	Extensor pollicis longus	Radial			
			MCP extension	Extensor pollicis brevis	Radial			
			Radial abduction	Abductor pollicis longus	Radial			
			Palmar abduction	Abductor pollicis brevis	Median			
			Adduction	Adductor pollicis	Ulnar			
			Opposition	Opponens pollicis	Median			
				Opponens digiti minimi	Ulnar			
			Trunk					
			Flexion	Rectus abdominis	Thoracic			
			Rotation	External oblique Internal oblique	Thoracic Thoracic			
			Extension	Extensor group	Thoracic			
			Pelvic elevation	Quadratus lumborum	Lumbar			

Remarks:

Patient's Name/ID _____

Left Side						Right Side		
			Therapist Initials					
			Date of Assessment					
			Motion	**Muscle**	**Nerve supply**			
			Hip					
			Flexion	Psoas major Iliacus	Lumbar Femoral			
				Sartorius	Femoral			
			Extension	Gluteus maximus Biceps femoris Semitendinosus Semimembranosus	Gluteal Sciatic Sciatic Sciatic			
			Abduction	Gluteus medius Gluteus minimus	Gluteal Gluteal			
				Tensor fascia latae	Gluteal			
			Adduction	Adductor group	Obturator			
			Internal rotation	Gluteus medius Gluteus minimus Tensor fascia latae	Gluteal Gluteal Gluteal			
			External rotation	External rotator group	Sacral/lumbar			
			Knee					
			Flexion	Biceps femoris	Sciatic			
				Semitendinosus Semimembranosus	Sciatic Sciatic			
			Extension	Quadriceps	Femoral			
			Ankle					
			Dorsiflexion	Tibialis anterior	Peroneal			
			Plantarflexion	Gastrocnemius	Tibial			
				Soleus	Tibial			
			Inversion	Tibialis posterior	Tibial			
			Eversion	Peroneus longus Peroneus brevis	Peroneal Peroneal			
			Toes					
			MTP flexion	Flexor hallucis brevis	Tibial			
				Lumbricales	Tibial			
			IP flexion	Flexor hallucis longus	Tibial			
				Flexor digitorum longus Flexor digitorum brevis	Tibial			
			MTP abduction	Abductor hallucis	Tibial			
				Abductor digiti minimi	Tibial			
				Dorsal interossei	Tibial			
			Extension	Extensor hallucis longus	Peroneal			
				Extensor digitorum brevis Extensor digitorum longus				

Remarks:

Appendix C

Summary of Patient Positioning for the Assessment and Measurement of Joint Motion, Muscle Length, and Muscle Strength

This summary chart is a resource the therapist may use to facilitate an organized and efficient assessment of joint range of motion (ROM), muscle length, and muscle strength to avoid unnecessary patient position changes and fatigue.

The assessment and measurement of joint motion, that is, joint ROM and muscle length, and the manual assessment of muscle strength presented in this book, first shows the *preferred start position* for these assessment techniques based on the position that offers the best

stabilization. In some instances, *alternate start positions* are documented if commonly used in clinical practice. The following chart summarizes the *preferred (P)* and *alternate (A)* start positions used by the therapist when assessing and measuring joint motion and manually testing muscle strength. For assessment of muscle strength greater than grade 2, the patient is positioned *against gravity (AG)* for the test motion, and for strength less than or equal to grade 2, the patient is in a *gravity eliminated (GE)* position, unless stated otherwise.

Joint Motion	Sitting	Supine	Prone	Sidely	Standing	Muscle Strength	Sitting	Supine	Prone	Sidely	Standing
Shoulder Complex						**Shoulder Complex**					
Scapular movements	P			P		Serratus anterior	P(GE)/A(AG)	P(AG)			
Elevation through flexion	A	P				Upper trapezius, levator scapulae	P(AG)		P(GE)		
Glenohumeral joint flexion		P				Middle trapezius	P(GE)		P(AG)		
Extension	A		P			Rhomboids	P(GE)		P/A(AG)		
Elevation through abduction	A	P				Lower trapezius			P(GE)/P(AG)		
Glenohumeral joint abduction		P				Anterior deltoid	P(AG)			P(GE)	
Adduction	A	P				Coracobrachialis		P(AG)		P(GE)	
Horizontal adduction/abduction	P		P			Latissimus dorsi, teres major			P(AG)	P(GE)	
Internal rotation	A		P			Middle deltoid, supraspinatus	P(AG)	P(GE)			
External rotation	A	P				Pectoralis major	P(GE)	P(AG)			
Pectoralis major length		P				Posterior deltoid	P(GE)		P(AG)		
Pectoralis minor length		P				Subscapularis	P(GE)/A(GE)		P(AG)		
						Infraspinatus, teres minor	P(GE)		P(AG)		
Elbow and Forearm						**Elbow and Forearm**					
Flexion/extension	A	P				Biceps	P(GE)	P(AG)			
Supination/pronation	P					Brachioradialis/brachialis	P(GE)	P(AG)			
Biceps brachii length	P	P				Triceps	P(GE)	P(AG)	A(AG)	A(GE)	
Triceps length	P	A				Supinator	P(AG)	P(GE)			
						Pronator teres, pronator quadratus	P(AG)	P(GE)			
Wrist and Hand						**Wrist and Hand**					
All wrist movements	P					All muscles	P				
All finger and thumb movements	P										
Long finger flexors length	A	P									
Long finger extensors length	P										
Lumbricales length	P										
Hip						**Hip**					
Flexion	P	P				Iliopsoas	P(AG)	A(AG)		P(GE)	

Joint Motion	Sitting	Supine	Prone	Sidely	Standing	Muscle Strength	Sitting	Supine	Prone	Sidely	Standing
Extension			P			Sartorius	P/A(AG) P(AssistedAG)*					
Abduction/adduction		P				Gluteus maximus, hamstrings		A(AG)	A(AG)	P(GE)	P(AG)	
Internal/external rotation	P	A	A			Gluteus medius, gluteus minimus			A	P(AG)		
Hip flexors length		P				Tensor fascia latae		P(GE)		P(AG)		
Hamstrings length (SLR)		P				Adductors		P(GE)		P(AG)		
Tensor fascia latae length			A	P		Internal rotators	P(AG)	P(GE)				
Adductors length		P				External rotators	P(AG)	P(GE)				
Knee						**Knee**						
Flexion/extension		P	P			Hamstrings			P(AG)	P(GE)		
Patellar glides		P				Quadriceps	P(AG)			P(GE)		
Tibial rotation	P											
Rectus femoris length		A	P									
Hamstrings length	A	P										
Ankle and Foot						**Ankle and Foot**						
Dorsiflexion	A	P			A	Tibialis anterior	P(AG)			P(GE)		
Plantarflexion	A	P				Gastrocnemius			P(AG) NWB	P(GE)	P(AG)WB	
Supination/pronation: Inversion/eversion components	P					Soleus			P(AG) NWB	P(GE)	P(AG)WB	
Subtalar joint inversion/eversion		P	A			Tibialis posterior		P(GE)		P(AG)		
All toes movements		P				Peroneus longus, peroneus brevis		P(GE)		P(AG)		
Gastrocnemius length		A			P	All foot muscles		P				
Soleus length					P							
Spine						**Trunk**						
Flexion					P	Rectus abdominis		P				
Extension			P		A	External oblique, internal oblique	P(GE)	P(AG)				
Rotation	P					Extensor muscle group			P			

Joint Motion	Sitting	Supine	Prone	Sidely	Standing	Muscle Strength	Sitting	Supine	Prone	Sidely	Standing
Lateral flexion					P	Quadratus lumborum			P(ResistedGE)[†] P(GE)		
Trunk extensors, hamstrings (toe-touch test)					P						
Neck						**Neck**					
All neck movements	P					Infrahyoid muscle group	P				
						Flexor group		P			
						Sternomastoid		P			
						Extensor group			P		
TMJ						**Mandible and Face**					
All TMJ movements	P					All muscles of mandible and face	P				

*P(GE) is equivalent to P(AssistedAG): when the patient is positioned AG to test strength less than or equal to grade 2, the therapist offers assistance equal to the weight of the limb to resemble the gravity eliminated situation.

†P(AG) is equivalent to P(ResistedGE): when the patient is positioned GE to test strength greater than grade 2, the therapist offers resistance equal to the weight of the limb to resemble the against gravity situation.

Appendix D

Gait

The gait cycle consists of a series of motions that occur between consecutive initial contacts of one leg.[1] The gait cycle is divided into two phases: the stance phase, when the foot is in contact with the ground and the body advances over the weight-bearing limb, and the swing phase, when the limb is unweighted and advanced forward in preparation for the next stance phase. Each phase is further subdivided into a total of eight instants[1] or freeze frames. Five instants occur in the stance phase and three occur in the swing phase of the gait cycle. The description of the normal gait pattern is provided so that the implications of the findings on assessment of joint range of motion and manual muscle strength can be understood in relation to gait. The average positions and the motions of the joints during the gait cycle that are reported in this appendix were adapted from the Rancho Los Amigos gait analysis forms as cited in Levangie and Norkin.[2] The right leg is used to illustrate the joint positions and motions of the lower limb throughout the gait cycle.

Stance Phase

The lower limb is advanced in front of the body during the swing phase and the stance phase begins at initial contact (Fig. D-1) when the heel makes the first contact between the foot and the ground. At initial contact the pelvis is rotated forward and the trunk is rotated backward on the stance side. The rotation of the pelvis counteracts the trunk rotation to prevent excessive trunk motion. On the opposite side the upper extremity is flexed at the shoulder. As the body advances over the supporting limb through the stance phase, the pelvis rotates backward and the trunk rotates forward on the swing side. As the weight-bearing leg extends at the hip, the upper limb on the opposite side extends. The average joint positions and the motions of the right lower limb in the sagittal plane are described and illustrated.

Motion from *A* to *B* (Figs. D-1 and D-2): *hip:* extension (from 30 to 25° flexion); *knee:* flexion (from 0 to 15° flexion); *ankle:* plantarflexion (from 0 to 15° plantarflexion); *MTP joints of toes:* 0°.

Motion from *B* to *C* (Figs. D-2 and D-3): *hip:* extension (from 25 to 0° flexion); *knee:* extension (from 15 to 5° flexion); *ankle:* dorsiflexion (from 15° plantarflexion to 5 to 10° dorsiflexion); *MTP joints of toes:* remain at 0°.

Motion from *C* to *D* (Figs. D-3 and D-4): *hip:* extension (from 0° flexion to 10 to 20° extension); *knee:* extension (from 5° flexion to 0°); *ankle:* dorsiflexion (from 5 to 10° dorsiflexion to 0° dorsiflexion); *MTP joints of toes:* extension (from 0 to 20° extension).

Motion from *D* to *E* (Figs. D-4 and D-5): *hip:* flexion (from 10 to 20° extension to 0°); *knee:* flexion (from 0 to 30° flexion); *ankle:* plantarflexion (from 0 to 20° plantarflexion); *MTP joints of toes:* extension (from 30° extension to 50 to 60° extension).

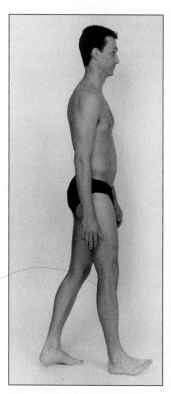

Figure D-1 Initial contact (*A*).

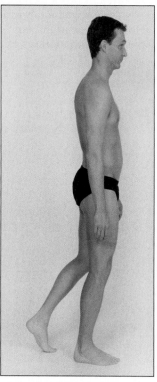

Figure D-2 Loading response (*B*).

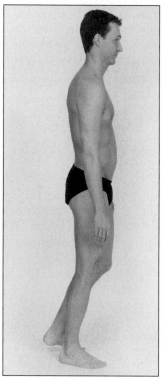

Figure D-3 Midstance (*C*).

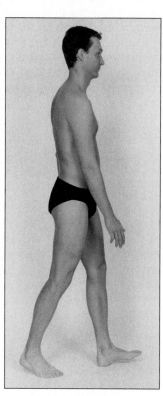

Figure D-4 Terminal stance (*D*).

Swing Phase

The swing phase begins after preswing when the foot leaves the ground and is advanced forward in the line of progression in preparation for initial contact. The positions and motions of the right lower limb are described and illustrated.

Motion from *E* to *F* (Figs. D-5 and D-6): *hip:* flexion (from 0 to 20° flexion); *knee:* flexion (from 30° flexion to 60° flexion); *ankle:* dorsiflexion (from 20° plantarflexion to 10° plantarflexion).

Motion from *F* to *G* (Figs. D-6 and D-7): *hip:* flexion (from 20° flexion to 30° flexion); *knee:* extension (from 60° flexion to 30° flexion); *ankle:* dorsiflexion (from 10° plantarflexion to 0°).

Motion from *G* to *H* (Figs. D-7 and D-8): *hip:* remains flexed at 30°; *knee:* extension (from 30° flexion to 0°); *ankle:* remains at 0°.

Motion from *H* to *A* (Figs. D-8 and D-1): *hip:* remains flexed at 30°; *knee:* remains extended at 0°; *ankle:* remains at 0°.

References

1. Koerner I. *Observation of Human Gait.* Edmonton, Alberta: Health Sciences Media Services and Development, University of Alberta; 1986.
2. Levangie PK, Norkin CC. *Joint Structure & Function: A Comprehensive Analysis.* 3rd ed. Philadelphia: FA Davis; 2001.

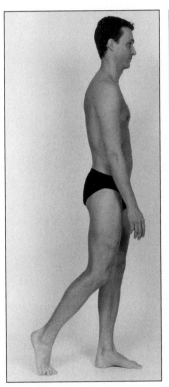

Figure D-5 Preswing (*E*).

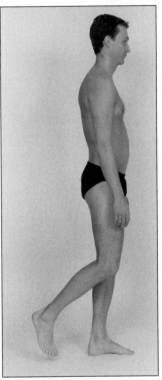

Figure D-6 Initial Swing (*F*).

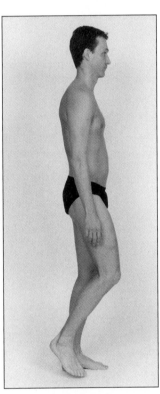

Figure D-7 Midswing (*G*).

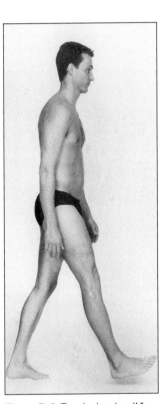

Figure D-8 Terminal swing (*H*).

Index